# Radioguided Surgery

# Radioguided Surgery

## A Comprehensive Team Approach

Edited by

Giuliano Mariani, MD
*Regional Center of Nuclear Medicine, University of Pisa Medical School,*
*Pisa, Italy*

Armando E. Giuliano, MD
*Chief of Science and Medicine, John Wayne Cancer Institute,*
*Saint John's Health Center, Santa Monica, California, USA*

H. William Strauss, MD
*Nuclear Medicine Service, Department of Radiology, Memorial Sloan-Kettering*
*Cancer Center, New York, New York, USA*

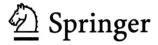 Springer

Giuliano Mariani, MD
Regional Center of Nuclear
    Medicine
University of Pisa Medical School
Pisa, Italy

Armando E. Giuliano, MD
Chief of Science and Medicine
John Wayne Cancer Institute
Saint John's Health Center
Santa Monica, CA
USA

H. William Strauss, MD
Nuclear Medicine Service
Department of Radiology
Memorial Sloan-Kettering
    Cancer Center
New York, NY
USA

Library of Congress Control Number: 2006925262

ISBN: 978-0-387-33684-8 (hardcover)          e-ISBN: 978-0-387-38327-9
ISBN: 978-1-4419-1618-1 (softcover)

Printed on acid-free paper

9 8 7 6 5 4 3 2 1

springer.com

# Preface

The fields of nuclear medicine, surgery, and general oncology have changed dramatically in the past two decades. Surgical oncologists are being asked to resect smaller and often radiographically occult tumors. The accurate staging of many malignancies is now performed with identification and resection of sentinel lymph nodes, almost always with the aid of nuclear medicine. *Radioguided Surgery: A Comprehensive Team Approach* presents an interdisciplinary approach to performing radioguided surgical resection. Experienced surgeons, nuclear medicine physicians, physicists and radiopharmacists describe how to effectively apply these techniques.

The book is divided into three sections. The first discusses the chemistry and physics of radiopharmaceuticals, intraoperative probes, site-directed biopsy, radiation safety, and training requirements. This section will be extremely helpful to any group wishing to initiate or improve their own radioguided surgical approach to malignancies.

Part two describes sentinel lymph node surgery, the field that has benefited extensively by and revitalized the comprehensive team approach. Tumor cells express a large number of growth factors, including many members of the vascular endothelial growth factor (VEGF) family. Expression of VEGFs by a neoplasm is associated with the growth of lymphatics in the region of tumors. In addition to entering these new lymphatic vessels, tumor cells can enter existing host lymphatics by secreting metalloproteinases and collagenases to dissolve the basement membrane, allowing the tumor cells to enter the lumen. Once in the lumen, the tumor cells are carried to the regional lymph nodes. The sentinel node is the first lymph node along this path. Sentinel lymph node (SLN) biopsy and lymphatic mapping were initially developed in patients with penile cancer, and further refined in patients with melanoma, under the assumption that examining the first regional lymph node that drains the lesion would predict the status of the remainder of the nodes in that region. If no tumor cells are seen in the sentinel node, the morbidity associated with an extensive lymph node dissection could be avoided. This hypothesis was confirmed in multiple clinical trials in patients with breast cancer, melanoma as well as penile and vulvar cancer. As a result, sentinel node evaluation has become an integral component of treatment planning in patients with these tumors. In this book, leading world experts present both the state-of-the art and the latest advances in radioguided SLN biopsy in a variety of solid tumors, discussing in general the anatomy and physiology of lymph nodes and lymph node staging, and then SLN biopsy for specific malignancies. The histopathology of sentinel nodes and histopathologic examination intraoperatively and postoperatively is discussed. In addition, the technique and role of molecular assessment of sentinel nodes in the basic science laboratory is described.

The third section describes a particularly vexing problem for the clinical surgeon—the detection and removal of lesions which were not detected by traditional imaging. In this section the origins of radioguided surgery from radio-immunoimaging is described. The localization and resection of occult lesions in the breast, parathyroid, lung, and other organ systems are described.

The authors hope that this text will serve both as a reference for those who encounter the occasional patient with these problems and as a guide for those immersed in the field. Clinical judgments and opinions of experts in each chapter should be of great aid to the management of patients with malignancy.

Finally, the authors wish to acknowledge their colleagues and associates who contributed to the many chapters and revisions that occurred prior to publication. We wish to thank our editorial assistants at Springer Science+Business Media, LLC; our Developmental Editor Margaret Burns; our individual assistants around the globe, especially Vicky E. Norton and Gwen Berry from Santa Monica; and finally, of course, our families who lovingly bear the burden we place on them by additional work and time away from home.

*Giuliano Mariani, MD*
*Armando E. Giuliano, MD*
*H. William Strauss, MD*

# Contents

# Contributors

*Stefan Adams, MD*
Department of Nuclear Medicine, PET Center, Zentralklinik Bad Berka, Bad Berka, Germany

*Farin Amersi, MD*
Department of Molecular Oncology, John Wayne Cancer Institute, Santa Monica, CA, USA

*Preya Ananthakrishnan, MD*
Department of Breast and Endocrine Surgery, John Wayne Cancer Institute, Saint John's Health Center, Santa Monica, CA, USA

*Fausto Badellino, MD*
Former Chief, Division of Surgical Oncology, National Institute for Cancer Research (IST), Genoa, Italy

*Richard P. Baum, MD*
Department of Nuclear Medicine, PET Center, Zentralklinik Bad Berka, Bad Berka, Germany

*Emilio Bombardieri, MD*
Division of Nuclear Medicine, National Cancer Institute, Milan, Italy

*Giuseppe Boni, MD*
Regional Center of Nuclear Medicine, University of Pisa Medical School, Pisa, Italy

*Elisa Borsò, MD*
Regional Center of Nuclear Medicine, University of Pisa Medical School, Pisa, Italy

*Roberto Bruschini, MD*
Division of Head and Neck Surgery, European Institute of Oncology, Milan, Italy

*Luca Calabrese, MD*
Division of Head and Neck Surgery, European Institute of Oncology, Milan, Italy

*Carlo Chiesa, PhD*
Department of Nuclear Medicine, National Cancer Institute, Milan, Italy

*Fausto Chiesa, MD*
Division of Head and Neck Surgery, European Institute of Oncology, Milan, Italy

*Marco Chinol, PhD*
Division of Nuclear Medicine, European Institute of Oncology, Milan, Italy

*Charles E. Cox, MD*
Departments of Surgery and Interdisciplinary Oncology, H. Lee Moffitt Cancer Center and Research Institute, University of South Florida, Tampa, FL, USA

*John M. Cox, MD*
Comprehensive Breast Program, H. Lee Moffitt Cancer Center and Research Institute, University of South Florida, Tampa, FL, USA

*Concetta De Cicco, MD*
Division of Nuclear Medicine, European Institute of Oncology, Milan, Italy

*Rudy A. Dierckx, MD*
Division of Nuclear Medicine, University Hospital, Ghent, Belgium; Department of Nuclear Medicine and Molecular Imaging, University Hospital, Groningen, The Netherlands

*Paola A. Erba, MD*
Regional Center of Nuclear Medicine, University of Pisa Medical School, Pisa, Italy

*Richard Essner, MD*
Roy E. Coats Research Laboratories, John Wayne Cancer Institute, Santa Monica, CA, USA

*Einat Even-Sapir, MD*
Nuclear Medicine Institute, Tel-Aviv Sourasky Medical Centre, and the Sackler Faculty of Medicine, Tel-Aviv University, Tel Aviv, Israel

*Rosanna Fontanelli, MD*
Division of Gynecologic Oncology, National Cancer Institute, Milan, Italy

*Giovanna Gatti, MD*
Division of Senology, European Institute of Oncology, Milan, Italy

*Jeffrey E. Gershenwald, MD*
Department of Surgical Oncology, University of Texas M.D. Anderson Cancer Center, Houston, TX, USA

*Armando E. Giuliano, MD*
Chief of Science and Medicine, John Wayne Cancer Institute, Saint John's Health Center, Santa Monica, CA, USA

*Edwin C. Glass, MD*
Department of Nuclear Medicine, John Wayne Cancer Institute, Santa Monica, CA; V.A. Greater Los Angeles Healthcare System, Los Angeles, CA, USA

*Fiorella Guadagni, MD*
Department of Laboratory Medicine and Advanced Biotechnologies, S. Raffaele IRCCS, Rome, Italy

*Rolf Harzmann, MD*
Department of Urology, Klinikum Augsburg, Augsburg, Germany

*Danielle M. Hasson, BS*
Department of Surgery, H. Lee Moffitt Cancer Center and Research Institute, University of South Florida, Tampa, FL, USA

*Dave S.B. Hoon, MSc, PhD*
Department of Molecular Oncology, John Wayne Cancer Institute, Santa Monica, CA, USA

*Simon Horenblas, MD*
Department of Urology, Netherlands Cancer Institute-Antoni van Leeuwenhoek Hospital, Amsterdam, The Netherlands

*Gyozo A. Janoki, PharmD, PhD*
Fodor Jozsef National Center of Public Health, Budapest, Hungary

*Samira Khera, MD*
Comprehensive Breast Program, H. Lee Moffitt Cancer Center and Research Institute, University of South Florida, Tampa, FL, USA

*Yuko Kitagawa, MD, PhD, FACS*
Department of Surgery, Keio University School of Medicine, Tokyo, Japan

*Masaki Kitajima, MD, PhD, FACS*
Department of Surgery, Keio University School of Medicine, Tokyo, Japan

*Bin K. Kroon, MD*
Department of Urology, Netherlands Cancer Institute-Antoni van Leeuwenhoek Hospital, Amsterdam, The Netherlands

*Marco Lucchi, MD*
Department of Cardiothoracic, Division of Thoracic Surgery, University of Pisa Medical School, Pisa, Italy

*Alberto Luini, MD*
Division of Senology, European Institute of Oncology, Milan, Italy

*Marco Maccauro, MD*
Division of Nuclear Medicine, National Cancer Institute, Milan, Italy

*Eugenio Maiorano, MD, MS*
Department of Pathological Anatomy, University of Bari, Bari, Italy

*Gianpiero Manca, MD*
Regional Center of Nuclear Medicine, University of Pisa Medical School, Pisa, Italy

*Giuliano Mariani, MD*
Regional Center of Nuclear Medicine, University of Pisa Medical School, Pisa, Italy

*Mario Mariani, PhD*
Department of Nuclear Engineering, Politecnico di Milano, Milan, Italy

*Giovanni Mazzarol, MD*
Department of Pathology and Laboratory Medicine, European Institute of Oncology, Milan, Italy

*Franca M.A. Melfi, MD*
Department of Cardiothoracic, Division of Thoracic Surgery, University of Pisa Medical School, Pisa, Italy

*Luciano Moresco, MD*
Surgical Oncology, Department of Oncology, Biology, and Genetics, University of Genoa Medical School, and National Institute for Research on Cancer, Genoa, Italy

*Alfredo Mussi, MD*
Department of Cardiothoracic, Division of Thoracic Surgery, University of Pisa Medical School, Pisa, Italy

*Santo V. Nicosia, MD*
Departments of Pathology and Interdisciplinary Oncology, University of South
Florida College of Medicine, Tampa, FL, USA

*Omgo E. Nieweg, MD*
Department of Surgery, Netherlands Cancer Institute-Antoni van Leeuwenhoek
Hospital, Amsterdam, The Netherlands

*James Norman, MD*
Norman Endocrine Surgery Clinic, Tampa, FL, USA

*Esteban Obenaus, PhD*
National Atomic Energy Commission, Ezeiza, Buenos Aires, Argentina

*Michael J. O'Doherty, MD*
Department of Nuclear Medicine, Guy's and St. Thomas' NHS Foundation Trust,
London, UK

*Giovanni Paganelli, MD*
Division of Nuclear Medicine, European Institute of Oncology, Milan, Italy

*Ilaria Pastina, MD*
Division of Medical Oncology, University Hospital, Pisa, Italy

*Maria Rosa Pelizzo, MD*
Department of Surgery, University of Padua, Padua, Italy

*Marzio Perri, MD*
Regional Center of Nuclear Medicine, University of Pisa Medical School, Pisa, Italy

*Francesco Raspagliesi, MD*
Division of Gynecologic Oncology, National Cancer Institute, Milan, Italy

*Sergio Ricci, MD*
Division of Medical Oncology, University Hospital, Pisa, Italy

*Lary A. Robinson, MD*
Division of Thoracic and Cardiovascular Surgery, H. Lee Moffitt Cancer Center
and Research Institute, Tampa, FL, USA

*Mario Roselli, MD*
Department of Internal Medicine, Clinical Oncology, University of Rome Tor
Vergata, Rome, Italy

*Domenico Rubello, MD*
Nuclear Medicine Service, PET Center, S. Maria della Misericordia Hospital, Istituto Oncologico Veneto (IOV), Rovigo, Italy.

*Sukamal Saha, MD, FACS, FRCS*
Department of Surgery and Anatomy, College of Human Medicine and Depart-
ment of Surgery, Michigan State University; McLaren Regional Medical Center,
Flint, MI, USA

*Massimo Salvatori, MD*
Nuclear Medicine Service, Policlinico Gemelli, Catholic University of the Sacred
Heart, Rome, Italy

*Sergio Sandrucci, MD*
Surgical Oncology Unit, University of Turin Medical School, Turin, Italy

*Schlomo Schneebaum, MD*
Radioguided Surgery Unit, Department of Surgery A, Tel-Aviv Sourasky Medical
Centre, and the Sackler Faculty of Medicine, Tel-Aviv University, Tel Aviv, Israel

*Francesco Scopinaro, MD*
Nuclear Medicine Unit, Department of Radiological Sciences, Second Medical School, University of Rome La Sapienza, Rome, Italy

*Alberto Signore, MD*
Department of Nuclear Medicine, University of Rome La Sapienza, Rome, Italy

*Alessandro Soluri, PhD*
Institute of Biomedical Engineering, Italian National Research Council, Rome, Italy

*David Soutar, MD*
Department of Radiology, Canniesburn Hospital, Glasgow, Scotland, UK

*H. William Strauss, MD*
Nuclear Medicine Service, Department of Radiology, Memorial Sloan-Kettering Cancer Center, New York, NY, USA

*John F. Thompson, MD*
Sydney Melanoma Unit, Sydney Cancer Centre, Royal Prince Alfred Hospital, Camperdown; Discipline of Surgery, University of Sydney, Sydney, Australia

*Francesca Toscano, PhD*
Department of Nuclear Engineering, Politecnico di Milano, Milan, Italy

*Roger F. Uren, MD*
Sydney Melanoma Unit, Sydney Cancer Centre, Royal Prince Alfred Hospital, Camperdown; Nuclear Medicine and Diagnostic Ultrasound, RPAH Medical Centre and Discipline of Medicine, University of Sydney, Sydney, Australia

*Renato A. Valdés Olmos, MD*
Department of Nuclear Medicine, Netherlands Cancer Institute-Antoni van Leeuwenhoek Hospital, Amsterdam, The Netherlands

*Christophe Van de Wiele, MD*
Division of Nuclear Medicine, University Hospital, Ghent, Belgium

*Giuseppe Viale, MD, FRCPath*
Department of Pathology and Laboratory Medicine, European Institute of Oncology, Milan and University of Milan, Milan, Italy

*Harry Vogt, MD*
Department of Nuclear Medicine, Klinikum Augsburg, Augsburg, Germany

*Wendy A. Waddington, PhD*
Institute of Nuclear Medicine, Middlesex Hospital, University College London Hospitals, London, UK

*Friedhelm Wawroschek, MD*
Department of Urology and Pediatric Urology, Hospital Oldenburg, Oldenburg, Germany

*Dorothea Weckermann, MD*
Department of Urology, Klinikum Augsburg, Augsburg, Germany

*Jochen Werner, MD*
Department of Otolaryngology, University of Marburg, Marburg, Germany

*Laura B. White, BS*
Comprehensive Breast Program, H. Lee Moffitt Cancer Center and Research Institute, University of South Florida, Tampa, FL, USA

*Eric D. Whitman, MD, FACS*
Melanoma Center, Mountainside Hospital, Montclair, NJ, USA

*Caren E.G. Wilkie, MD*
Comprehensive Breast Program, H. Lee Moffitt Cancer Center and Research Institute, University of South Florida, Tampa, FL, USA

*Alexander Winter, MD*
Department of Urology and Pediatric Urology, Hospital Oldenburg, Oldenburg, Germany

# Part I
## Chemistry and Physics

# 1
# Radiopharmaceuticals for Radioguided Surgery

Esteban Obenaus, Paola A. Erba, Marco Chinol, Christophe Van de Wiele, Gyozo A. Janoki, Rudy A. Dierckx, Francesco Scopinaro, and Alberto Signore

## Sentinel Lymph Node Localization

The most common radioguided surgery procedure is sentinel lymph node localization with radiolabeled colloids. Cabanas described the sentinel node methodology in patients with penile cancer in his groundbreaking 1977 publication (1). In that study, sentinel lymph node localization was accomplished with lymphangiography, using iodinated contrast material. Lymphangiography requires cannulation of lymphatic channels for the direct injection of an oily iodinated contrast agent. Lymph nodes are visualized on the radiographs as the contrast material passes from the injection site through the node. In contrast to the radiographic technique, when using radiocolloids no skin incision is required to study lymphatic drainage from a specific site. As a result, the radionuclide technique has replaced the x-ray technique.

The radionuclide method relies on the physiologic function of lymphatics in the skin and in most organs to transport the radiocolloid (2). The lymphatic vessels serve 2 major purposes in most tissues: first, the vessels transport extracellular fluid leaking from the capillary back to the central circulation; and second, the fenestrated lymph vessels pick up and transport small particulates (most likely intended for bacteria) to local lymph nodes, where the particles are phagocytized (3). The radionuclide technique exploits the latter property. Following intradermal, subcutaneous, or deep injections of radiolabeled colloids, the radiotracer localizes in lymph nodes draining the site of injection. This technique works well, although there are differences in the incidence of visualization of secondary and tertiary nodes, depending on the size of the colloidal particle.

In the mid-1950s, radionuclides (principally [198]Au colloidal gold) were used to evaluate lymphatic drainage of the breast (4). This tracer had the major disadvantage of emitting beta particles, which caused a high radiation burden at the injection site. The development of colloids labeled with technetium-99m reduced the radiation burden at the site of injection and set the stage for radioguided surgery to identify sentinel lymph nodes.

In addition to the radionuclide methodology, magnetic resonance agents and optical dyes have been advocated for identification of sentinel nodes (5). The magnetic resonance approach, however, requires imaging before and about 24 hours after administration of intravenous contrast material (6). The blue dye optical approach is widely employed in the operating room, but is limited by the transient localization of the dye in the nodes. The concept of histologic interrogation of a sentinel lymph node to identify the spread of tumor, coupled with the commercial availability of sensitive and handheld intraoperative gamma-detecting probes, has led to the wide acceptance of the radioguided technique by surgeons and oncologists (7).

## Physiology and Anatomy

About 3 liters of lymph is produced daily. The average speed of lymphatic circulation varies in different regions of the body: for example, it is 1.5 cm/min in the head and neck regions, and 10.2 cm/min in the limbs. The speed of lymph circulation can be accelerated by ten- to thirtyfold when the muscles draining into the local lymphatic basin are working. Every 2 to 3 minutes, lymph vessels contract to propel lymph in the interstitial tissue to the lymph nodes (see Figure 1-1). The structure of the lymphatic capillaries and their connections with the surrounding tissues are represented in Figure 1-2. When lymph arrives at a lymph node, the fluid traverses a gauntlet consisting of exposed lymphocytes, plasma cells, and macrophages. Particulate materials in the lymph, such as radiocolloids, are phagocytosed by macrophages. Depending on the particle size and the particular path through the lymph node, some of the colloidal material (especially the smaller particles) proceeds through the efferent lymph vessel to the next node.

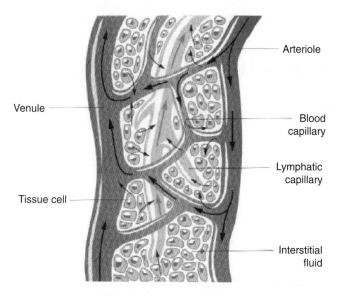

FIGURE 1-1. Lymphatic circulation and its environment.

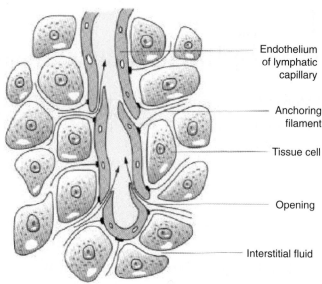

FIGURE 1-2. The structure of the lymphatic capillary system.

## Sentinel Lymph Node Detection

Colloidal particles are introduced into the lymphatic circulation at or adjacent to the tumor site (8). Large colloids (between 200 to 1000 nm) are most useful to pinpoint the sentinel lymph node (see Figure 1-3, see Color Plate). Radiopharmaceuticals considered for detecting sentinel nodes should have the following characteristics:

- Labeled with technetium-99m
- A narrow range of particle size (to avoid high dispersion)
- Fast transport across the lymphatic chain and high retention in the node

- In vivo stability of the label
- Registered for human use

The characteristics of the colloidal agents—such as the particle size, pH, and the use of stabilizers—will influence the rate of tracer migration into the nodes, discomfort at the injection site, and the number of second- and third-tier lymph nodes visualized. Moreover, when the size is less than 4 to 5 nm, the particles are quickly cleared from the injection site through the blood capillaries. If the particles are less than 30 nm, they migrate rapidly and only a small proportion remains in the first lymph node, generating undesired visualization of additional nodes. On the other hand, particles between 30 to

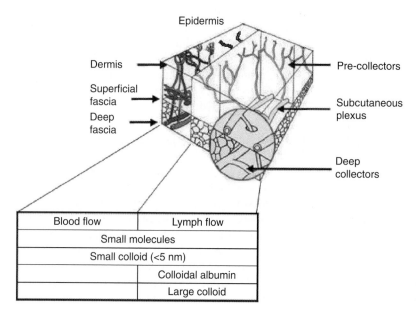

| Blood flow | Lymph flow |
|---|---|
| Small molecules | |
| Small colloid (<5 nm) | |
| | Colloidal albumin |
| | Large colloid |

FIGURE 1-3. The effect of particle size on the colloid clearance pathway. Blood is represented in red and blue, and the lymphatic vessels in yellow. (See Color Plate.)

2000 nm reduce the number of lymph nodes detected—only 1 or 2 nodes are visualized (9–14)—but increase the residual activity at the injection site (15). For a colloid size between 20 to 1000 nm, an average 1.3 nodes are observed, compared to an average 1.7 lymph nodes shown with particle sizes of less than 80 nm (16). A disadvantage of larger particles, however, is that they fail to enter the lymphatic system in some patients, resulting in delayed or nonvisualization of lymph nodes (10,11,16). In our opinion, the colloidal particle size should be at least 80 nm, and ideally around 200 nm (17).

Numerous radiocolloids have been clinically evaluated to detect the sentinel lymph node intraoperatively. Technetium-99m-antimony colloid, nanocolloid, and colloidal sulphur are the most widely used agents (the radiopharmaceutical varies in different countries, depending on drug approval). Technetium-99m-nanocolloid is the predominant agent in Europe, while technetium-99m-antimony colloid is used in Canada and Australia (16,17), and technetium-99m-colloidal sulphur in the United States. In addition, other radiopharmaceuticals such as technetium-99m-stannous phytate, denatured technetium-99m-collagen colloid, or technetium-99m-stannous fluoride could be used. Technetium-99m-Dextran 70, a sucrose polymer of high molecule weight, is another option for sentinel lymph node detection; although not a true colloid, it behaves in a similar fashion following interstitial injection.

Generally, the labeling procedure consists of the adsorption of technetium-99m on the particle's surface at nonspecific sites. Colloid quantity, hence the available adsorption surface, must be used in excess. In other cases, the labeling procedure is carried out like a co-precipitation process; for example, in the labeling of colloidal sulphur, technetium heptasulfide ($Tc_2S_7$) is formed, eliminating the likelihood of separation of the tracer technetium-99m from the colloid.

## Technetium-99m-Albumin Colloid

Technetium-99m-albumin colloids are obtained by controlled protein coagulation. Depending on the process, the colloid can be produced in different particle sizes. Several commercial kits have been developed, which differ according to the final particle sizes. These kits are ready for labeling with technetium-99m, and basically contain human albumin particles and stannous chloride. The kit most frequently used in Europe has the following characteristics: 95% of the particles are less than 80 nm in size, around 4% are between 80 to 100 nm in size, and 1% are larger than 100 nm. Different particle sizes could be obtained by changing some parameters in the production process. For example, it is possible to make a useful preparation of technetium-99m-labeled human serum albumin colloid ($^{99m}$Tc-HSAC) in the laboratory from a mixture of human serum albumin (HSA) and $SnCl_2 \cdot 2H_2O$ as a reducing agent. Briefly, a 20% HSA solution is added to 0.1M HCl containing the necessary $SnCl_2 \cdot 2H_2O$. The pH is adjusted to 7.4, and the solution is then placed into a water bath at 96°C with constant stirring. After 3 minutes, it is removed from the bath and cooled at 4°C for 20 minutes (18). Adding a tensoactive agent is recommended in colloid preparation to avoid particle aggregation. At this point, it is possible to label the colloid with technetium-99m, or to make a lyophilized kit. To label the lyophilized preparation, it is redissolved with 1 mL of saline and labeled by the addition of fresh $^{99m}$TcO$_4^-$. It is important to optimize the time of agitation, method and intensity, temperature, protein concentration, and tensoactive addition, as these parameters influence considerably the final characteristics of the radiopharmaceutical.

## Technetium-99m-Antimony Trisulphide Colloid

Technetium-99m-antimony trisulphide colloid (ATC), like albumin colloid, is a preformed particulate agent that can be labeled with $^{99m}$Tc by chemical reaction on its surfaces. Its range of particle size is smaller than that of albumin colloid, usually between 3 to 30 nm. The formulation of a cold ATC kit does not contain a reducing agent, but requires the addition of potassium antimonyl tartrate, a dispersant in aqueous solution, hydrogen sulphide, potassium sulphide, and tartaric acid (19). Radiolabeling is carried out by adding first $^{99m}$TcO$_4^-$ and then hydrochloric acid to the ATC kit. Afterward, it is heated at 100°C for 30 minutes, cooled at room temperature, and finally neutralized using an antimony buffer. The radiolabeling yield for technetium-99m colloidal antimony preparations is greater than 95%. Some studies report $^{111}$In-labeling of this kit, attaining radiochemical purity higher than 95%. The product shows useful properties for prolonged lymphoscintigraphic studies (20). This kit could also be labeled with Rhenium-188, by introducing some modifications in the labeling procedure.

## Technetium-99m Colloidal Sulphur

Radiolabeling is performed using thiosulfate as the sulphur source, and depending on the condition and preparation method, a wide distribution of particle size from 100 to 5000 nm is obtained. A final filtration is necessary to remove colloidal particles of larger size (21); however, some authors claim unfiltered sulphur colloid to be superior (22,23). The formulation of technetium-99m-colloidal sulphur is commonly reported as $^{99m}$Tc$_2$S$_7$, but the exact stoichiometry of technetium bound

TABLE 1-1. Summary of the radiopharmaceuticals available for lymphoscintigraphic uses and their average particle size.

| Radiocolloid | Range of size (nm) |
| --- | --- |
| $^{99m}$Tc-albumin colloid I | <80 |
| $^{99m}$Tc-albumin colloid II | 200–3000 |
| $^{99m}$Tc-antimony trisulphide colloid | 3–30 |
| $^{99m}$Tc-colloidal sulphur | 100–1000 |
| $^{188}$Re-colloidal sulphur | 3–500 |
| $^{198}$Au-colloid | 5–30 |
| $^{99m}$Tc-stannous phytate | 200–1000 |
| $^{99m}$Tc-dextran 70 (no colloid) | 2–3 |

to sulphur is unknown. It has been speculated that S-Tc-S bonds may be involved (24).

Table 1-1 shows a summary of the radiopharmaceuticals available for lymphoscintigraphic uses and their average particle size.

# Biodistribution and Quality Control

Radiocolloid behavior is often evaluated during preclinical biological studies in animals. These studies in larger animals are important in the screening of a new colloidal preparation and are included in the documentation submitted to the regulatory agencies for commercial approval of the product. Figure 1-4 shows an experiment carried out in a beagle dog injected subcutaneously with 1 mL of $^{99m}$Tc-HSAC (15 MBq/0.1 mL). Static images were recorded at 30 minutes, and at 1, 3, 6, and 22 hours postinjection. The images on the left are the native ones, while those on the right show the injection site shielded using a lead plate to detect a possible secondary lymph node. The images reveal that particle sizes of 100 to 600 nm enter the lymph circulation and show adequate lymph node retention. Radiocolloids of this size range could be used to detect sentinel nodes during surgery, even 24 hours postinjection. Their high retention and

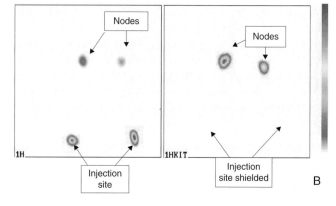

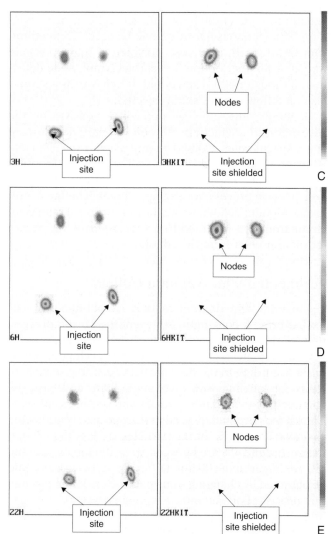

FIGURE 1-4. Static images showing the distribution of 15 MBq of $^{99m}$Tc-Senti Scint subdermally injected into a beagle's abdominal perimammary region in both sides. The left column shows the native images, the right column (name extension KIT) shows images taken with the injection site shielded. Note that in the shielded images, even after 22 hours postinjection, only the first nodes were detected.

activity remaining in the sentinel lymph node may allow for easy and fast surgical location.

Kits to prepare radiocolloids usually show high stability. For example, lyophilized human albumin kits are stable for 1 year on the shelf; following addition of the radionuclide, the material remains stable for more than 24 hours. With albumin colloids, the particles tend to increase in size due to particle agglomerations after formulation, so the agent should be used promptly after preparation. An alternative approach adds a tensoactive agent to minimize agglomeration.

# Non-Sentinel Lymph Node Radioguided Surgery

A major goal of radioguided surgery is not only lesion localization, but also assuring the complete removal of the lesion. Lesions may be identified by several factors, including increased perfusion, increased receptor expression, increased substrate utilization, and expression of novel epitopes on the surface of the lesion. These characteristics are usually present to some degree throughout the lesion. Radiolabeling one of these characteristics allows the lesion to be identified with the probe at surgery. Following extirpation of the lesion, any residual radiation found on re-evaluation of the surgical bed with the radiation detector suggests residual lesion. A host of radiopharmaceuticals measuring a wide variety of cellular processes are available to identify these lesions.

## The Basic Principles of Radiopharmaceutical Localization

Radionuclide imaging can depict specific biochemical processes at the cellular and subcellular level. The imaging technique uses pico- or micromolar mass amounts of radiopharmaceutical and sensitive radiation detection equipment to delineate the biological process of interest. The radiolabeled agents emit gamma rays (in the case of single photon agents) or annihilation radiation (in the case of positron emission, a pair of 511 keV gamma rays are emitted simultaneously when the positively charged positron interacts with a negatively charged electron in tissue, with the conversion of mass to energy). Single photon detectors can be either imaging devices, gamma cameras, which acquire two-dimensional images of the object in the field of view, or probes, which detect radiation but do not provide an image. With an imaging device, multiple images can be recorded around the object of interest, which can be reconstructed as cross-sectional slices (single photon emission tomography, or SPECT). Most single photon gamma cameras use a sodium iodide crystal of 0.95 to 2.54 cm thickness as the radiation sensor. Sodium-iodide scintillators of this thickness are most suitable for radionuclides with gamma-ray energies between 80 and 300 keV. The main radionuclides that are used in current nuclear medicine procedures are iodine ($^{123}$I, $t_{1/2} = 12.8$ hours; $^{131}$I, $t_{1/2} = 8.2$ days; and $^{125}$I, $t_{1/2} = 60$ days), gallium ($^{67}$Ga, $t_{1/2} = 78.3$ hours), thallium ($^{201}$Tl, $t_{1/2} = 73$ hours), indium ($^{111}$In, $t_{1/2} = 67.9$ hours), and technetium ($^{99m}$Tc, $t_{1/2} = 6$ hours).

Radiopharmaceuticals labeled with technetium-99m are used in more than 85% of studies in a general nuclear medicine department. The basic principle of technetium-99m-labeling involves reduction of the atom from the +7 oxidation state (as found in pertechnetate) to a lower oxidation state that binds to a chelating molecule of interest. In the past 30 years, advances in organometallic chemistry and enhanced understanding of the unique chemistry of technetium have led to the development of technetium-99m-labeling for peptides, proteins, and a variety of lipophilic and hydrophilic molecules (25,26).

Positron-emitting radionuclides can also be incorporated in molecules of biologic interest. The 511 keV gamma rays, emitted 180° apart, are detected simultaneously for imaging purposes. The gamma ray pairs define the location of the radionuclide along a line between the 2 detectors. Tomographic images are generated by reconstructing the data after correction for scatter and accidental coincident events. Isotopes of carbon ($^{11}$C, $t_{1/2} = 20.38$ min), oxygen ($^{15}$O, $t_{1/2} = 2.03$ min), nitrogen ($^{13}$N, $t_{1/2} = 9.96$ min), and fluorine ($^{18}$F, $t_{1/2} = 109.72$ min) can be readily produced in medical cyclotrons; other positron-emitting nuclides can be made in high-energy cyclotrons or linear accelerators. From a biochemical perspective, positron emission tomographic (PET) molecular probes are often preferred, because incorporation of atoms of carbon-11, nitrogen-13, and oxygen-15 into molecules renders compounds biochemically indistinguishable from their natural counterparts. In other cases, fluorine-18 can be used to substitute for hydroxyl groups, or to replace native fluorine-19 atoms in molecules of interest, to trace biochemical or pharmacologic processes in a predictable manner (27). One advantage of labeling substances with positron emitters for radioguided surgery is the ability to use the beta particle for detection. This eliminates the requirement for a bulky collimator and makes the device easier to use in surgery.

## Requirements of Radiopharmaceuticals

In addition to localizing sentinel lymph nodes, tissues with altered substrate utilization (most often with $^{18}$F-fluorodeoxyglucose), local hypoxia (using $^{18}$F-labeled misonidazole), or increased cell proliferation ($^{11}$C-thymidine) can also be identified with radioguided surgery. This is particularly helpful if radioguided surgery is performed after radionuclide imaging. The imaging procedure provides a region of tracer localization for investigation in the operating room.

## Mechanisms of Tissue Retention of Radiopharmaceuticals

Many different radiopharmaceutical agents are available for use in the operating room. The selection of a particular agent is driven by clinical needs, such as localizing sentinel lymph nodes for biopsy, localizing tumor tissue for biopsy, or determining if the known lesion has been completey removed. The following is a brief list of mechanisms of tracer localization which, in addition to phagocytosis of colloidal materials, may be useful for radioguided surgery:

*Dilution or compartmental localization:* If the agent is not metabolized, the tracer will enter the compartment and equilibrate in proportion to the local volume. This approach is helpful in measuring the local concentration of some drugs or the blood volume or protein space of a lesion or tissue. The dilution principle is often used for quantitative evaluation of red blood cell volume ($^{51}$Cr-RBCs), plasma volume ($^{125}$I-HSA), and total blood volume (28). It is important that the radiopharmaceutical remains only in the blood volume to be measured (nondiffusible intravascular tracer). The use of technetium-99m-red blood cells to measure cardiac ejection fraction or extravasation in gastrointestinal bleeding studies are other applications of this principle (29).

*Mechanical trapping (capillary blockade):* The regional distribution of perfusion to an organ or tissue may be determined by trapping radiolabeled particles (microembolization) in the capillary bed of an organ following intrarterial injection. Pulmonary circulation represents a special case, in that blood perfusion is assessed by injecting the microembolizing agents (technetium-99m-human albumin macroaggregates) in a peripheral vein rather than intrarterially. After reaching the right heart chambers via systemic venous circulation, the radiolabeled particles microembolize the first arteriolo-capillary bed they encounter, thus depicting the predominant distribution of blood flow in the lungs, one supplied by the pulmonary rather than by the bronchial arteries. Intra-arterial injection of particles is also used for treating hepatoma, where yttrium-90-labeled glass spheres are injected into the vessel(s) supplying the tumor, allowing the local delivery of radiation to the tumor, with minimal radiation of normal tissue.

*Ion exchange (chemiabsorption):* Chemiabsorption is the typical way technetium-99m-labeled phosphonates accumulate in the hydroxyapatite crystal matrix of bone and in the amorphous calcium phosphate (30) seen in tissue necrosis.

*Chemotaxis:* Radiolabeled cells follow a chemical concentration gradient to localize in a site of disease (e.g. technetium-99m-HMPAO- or $^{111}$I-Oxine-leukocytes in infectious foci (31), or indium-111-platelets in thrombus formation and heat-damaged technetium-99m-red blood cells in the spleen).

*Membrane transport:* Membrane transport may be a simple diffusion process from a higher to a lower concentration, if the concentration of each side is at chemical equilibrium. Diffusion is often followed by intracellular metabolism (binding or degradation to polar metabolites or charged complexes) that prevents subsequent washout of the tracer by back-diffusion. A number of lipophilic, cationic technetium-99m-radiopharmaceuticals enter cells by passive diffusion and subsequently bind to cytosolic components (technetium-99m-tetrofosmin) or mitochondria (technetium-99m-sestamibi) (32), allowing the agents to achieve a high intracellular concentration. The efflux of tetrofosmin and sestamibi is mediated by p-Glycoprotein, a 170-Kd plasma membrane lipoprotein encoded by the human-MDR gene (33,34), which actively transports these substances out of the cell. Increased capillary and plasma membrane permeability may augment the transport of macromolecules across leakier tumor blood vessels. Facilitated diffusion mediated by transport proteins is responsible for $^{18}$F-2-fluoro-2-deoxy-d-glucose (FDG) uptake in normal and neoplastic cells (GLUT 1–5) (35). In active transport, the translocation of a solute molecule through a cell membrane against its concentration gradient requires the expenditure of energy (ATP hydrolysis, electrochemical gradient of $Na^+$ or $H^+$) across the membrane. Active transport is the mechanism through which iodide symporter accumulates iodine and certain other anions (technetium-99m-pertechnetate) into the thyroid cells (36). In addition, active transport is involved in thallous ion ($^{201}$Tl) and $^{82}$Ru accumulation: acting as analogues of $K^+$ ions, they accumulate in cells due to the $Na^+/K^+$ ATPase pump within cell membranes (37).

*Enzyme-mediated intracellular trapping:* Some radiotracers are characterized by trapping in tissue, the result of a specific interaction of the molecular probe with an enzyme. This interaction normally produces a chemical transformation of the original probe, catalyzed by the enzyme that is being targeted. The product of the enzyme-mediated transformation (e.g. phosphorylated substrate) is impermeable to cell membranes and is therefore retained in tissue in proportion to the rate of reaction of the enzyme-mediated process. The process has been called metabolic trapping. The best example of a molecular imaging probe going through this pathway is FDG. Another class of radiopharmaceuticals employing this approach is the methyl-substituted fatty acids, such as beta-methyl heptadecanoic acid. In this case, after the fatty acid is transported into the cell by facilitated diffusion, the molecule cannot be metabolized because the methyl group in the beta position does not allow beta-oxidation.

*Receptor-mediated probes:* Receptor-mediated probes (or receptor ligand) compete with physiologic ligands for the target. Because the number of target sites is limited (typically in the nanomolar concentration), binding specificity is highly dependent on the activity of the radiopharmaceutical. When probe-specific activity decreases (the mass of cold or unlabeled component increases per unit amount of radioisotope), receptor site occupancy may reach saturation, reducing image contrast. On the other hand, this important property of receptor sites can be exploited, using molecular imaging probes to determine receptor occupancy by drugs. Therefore, imaging probes using receptors as targets should typically have high specific activity, to preclude mass effects during the in-vivo determination. The binding affinity of these probes for their target should typically be in the nanomolar range.

Examples of receptor-specific radiopharmaceuticals are somatostatin analogues (octreotide and lanreotide) (38). These agents can help localize receptor-expressing tissues in the operating room. They are most helpful when patients have altered anatomy, such as after multiple surgical procedures. Under that circumstance, computed tomography, ultrasound, and magnetic resonance imaging are of limited value compared to "hot spot" detection with a radiolabeled agent.

*Non-receptor-mediated binding (antibodies):* Radiolabeled antibodies or antibody-derived large peptides (engineered mini-bodies) recognize specific epitopes on the surface of tumor cells (39). In developing radiolabeled antibodies, the most important requirement is to identify an antigen or an epitope specific to a particular type or class of cancer or tissue. Most tumor cells synthesize many proteins or glycoproteins that are antigenic in nature. These antigens may be intracellular, expressed on the cell surface, or shed or secreted from the cell into extracellular fluid or circulation. While tumor-associated antigens, such as carcinoembryonic antigen (CEA), tumor-associated glycoprotein (TAG)-72, prostate-specific antigen (PSA), and prostate-specific membrane antigen (PSMA), may be expressed in a small amount in normal cells, typically cancer cells produce them in much larger amounts. A number of radiolabeled antibodies and their fragments specific to tumor-associated antigens have been developed for tumor localization (immunoscintigraphy) and treatment (radioimmunotherapy).

*Apoptosis:* Cells undergoing programmed cell death (apoptosis) redistribute phosphatidylserine (PS) from the inner leaflet of the plasma membrane lipid bilayer to the outer leaflet (40). Externalization of PS is a general feature of apoptosis, occurring before membrane bleb formation and DNA degradation. Annexin V binds selectively to membrane-bound PS and has been labeled with fluorescent or biotinylated materials to identify cells undergoing apoptosis in vitro. It also has been radioiodinated and coupled with a wide variety of linker molecules, such as diamide dimercaptide ($N_2S_2$) or hydrazine nicotinamide for complexation with technetium-99m, for imaging of apoptosis in vivo. For imaging of apoptosis with PET, the molecule has been labeled with $^{18}$F (N-succimidyl-4–$^{18}$F-fluorobenzoate) (41).

## Concluding Remarks

In this chapter we have reviewed the main concepts concerning localization of radiopharmaceuticals in vivo and how this process relates to radioguided surgery. For the most common procedure of radioguided surgery, sentinel lymph node localization, there is consensus on using technetium-99m-labeled colloids with well-defined properties in terms of particle size. The tracers are injected either interstitially, intradermally, subcutaneously, peritumorally, or intratumorally, depending on the tissue and on the experience of the specific laboratory. The injection site is related to the rapidity of radiocolloid uptake in the lymphatics. Particle size also determines how efficiently the radiocolloid is retained in the sentinel lymph node (or, conversely, how fast additional nodes along the same lymphatic channels are visualized). The trapping of radiocolloids in the nodes is due to the physiologic function of macrophages in lymph nodes, and does not correlate with the possible presence of tumor deposits in the nodes.

The amounts of radioactivity commonly employed for sentinel lymph node localization (approximately 20 MBq, or 500 µCi) are minute when compared to the doses employed for most diagnostic nuclear medicine procedures. The ensuing radiation dosimetry to both patients and dedicated staff (nuclear medicine personnel, surgical team, pathology) is minimal and in general negligible, as reviewed in chapter 5. Highly sensitive intraoperative gamma-detecting probes (as those described in chapter 2) make it possible to efficiently detect the sentinel lymph nodes up to 18 to 24 hours postinjection with high target/background ratios, despite the short physical half-life of technetium-99m (6 hours only). Applications of the radioguided sentinel lymph node procedure in various types of cancer are reviewed in Chapters 9 to 17.

Nonsentinel lymph node applications of radioguided surgery can roughly be distinguished by 2 main categories: those based on radiopharmaceuticals that do not have any tumor-seeking property (such as nonspecific particulate agents that do not appreciably move from the site of interstitial, intralesional injection); and those based on different tumor-seeking radiopharmaceuticals that accumulate preferentially at tumor sites after systemic administration.

By adopting the interstitial, intralesional route of administration (a procedure most commonly defined as "radioguided occult lesion localization," or ROLL), the former instance can be somewhat assimilated to the procedures of sentinel lymph node localization (in terms of, e.g. small amounts of radioactivity injected and high target/background ratios), the only difference being in the size of the radiolabeled particles. In fact, technetium-99m-human albumin macroaggregates employed to this purpose are so large (up to 50 μm in diameter) that they cannot enter the lymphatic vessels as radiocolloids do, and are therefore retained indefinitely at the site of interstitial injection, thus providing an extremely efficient and selective signal for radioguided resection of the tumor lesion. Applications of the ROLL procedure are reviewed in Chapters 22 and 25.

Radioguided surgery based on systemic administration of tumor-seeking agents implies administration of radioactivity amounts in the order of a full diagnostic dose, and intraoperative detection is more or less heavily affected by a relatively high radioactivity concentration in normal tissues surrounding the tumor. Moreover, the period of radioactivity retention in the tumor of the radiopharmaceuticals (which can be labeled with single-photon emitting radionuclides or with positron-emitting radionuclides) is highly variable, which in turn affects the target/background ratios at different times postinjection. There are some immediate consequences of such conditions, at variance with the ROLL procedures: (1) intraoperative detecting probes must be narrowly collimated in such a way to exclude as much as possible count rates originated by surrounding nontarget tissues; (2) the optimal time window for radioguided surgery must be identified specifically for each procedure, to ensure the highest possible target/background ratio; (3) intraoperative probes designed specifically to detect positron emission or the high-energy gamma emission originated from positron-electron annihilation must be employed when using PET tracers (such equipment is reviewed in chapter 3); (4) intraoperative definition of the target volume can sometimes be facilitated by the availability of small dedicated imaging probes (as reviewed in chapter 4); and (5) radiation dosimetry to patients and personnel is usually higher than that from sentinel lymph node or ROLL procedures. Chapters 21, 23, 24, 26 and 27 review current clinical experience in the field of radioguided surgery following systemic administration of tumor-seeking radiopharmaceuticals.

# References

1. Cabanas RM. An approach for the treatment of penile carcinoma. *Cancer*. 1977;39:456–466.
2. Schneebaum S, Even-Sapir E, Cohen M, et al. Clinical applications of gamma-detection probes—radioguided surgery. *Eur J Nucl Med*. 1999;26:S26–S35.
3. Szuba A, Strauss W, Sirsikar SP, Rockson SG. Quantitative radionuclide lymphoscintigraphy predicts outcome of manual lymphatic therapy in breast cancer-related lymph-edema of the upper extremity. *Nucl Med Commun*. 2002;23:1171–1175.
4. Leborgne FE, Leborgne R, Schaffner E, Leborgne FE Jr. Study of the lymphatics of the mammary gland with radioactive gold 198. *Torax*. 1955;4:233–244.
5. Cheng LY, Chen XD, Zhang YX, Feng XD. Clinical significance of sentinel lymph node detection by combining the dye-directed and radioguided methods in gastric cancer. *Zhonghua Wai Ke Za Zhi*. 2005;43:569–572.
6. Harisinghani MG, Barentsz J, Hahn PF, Deserno WM, Tabatabaei S, van de Kaa CH, et al. Noninvasive detection of clinically occult lymph-node metastases in prostate cancer. *N Engl J Med*. 2003;348:2491–2499.
7. Liang WC, Sickle-Santanello BJ, Nims TA. Is a completion axillary dissection indicated for micrometastases in the sentinel lymph node? *Am J Surg*. 2001;182:365–368.
8. Perkins AC, Frier M. Nuclear medicine techniques in the evaluation of pharmaceutical formulations. *Pharm World Sci*. 1996;18:97–104.
9. Trifirò G, Viale G, Gentilini O, Travaini LL, Paganelli G. Sentinel node detection in pre-operative axillary staging. *Eur J Nucl Med Mol Imaging*. 2004;31:S46–S55.
10. Leidenius MH, Leppanen EA, Krogerus LA, Smitten KA. The impact of radiopharmaceutical particle size on the visualization and identification of sentinel nodes in breast cancer. *Nucl Med Commun*. 2004;25:233–238.
11. Wilhelm AJ, Mijnhout GS, Franssen EJ. Radiopharmaceuticals in sentinel lymph-node detection—an overview. *Eur J Nucl Med*. 1999;26:S36-S42.
12. Paganelli G, De Cicco C, Cremonesi M, et al. Optimized sentinel node scintigraphy in breast cancer. *Q J Nucl Med*. 1998;42:49–53.
13. De Cicco C, Cremonesi M, Luini A, et al. Lymphoscintigraphy and radioguided biopsy of the sentinel axillary node in breast cancer. *J Nucl Med*. 1998;39:2080–2084.
14. Noguchi M. Sentinel lymph node biopsy and breast cancer. *Br J Surg*. 2002;89:21–34.
15. Mariani G, Moresco L, Viale G, et al. Radioguided sentinel lymph node biopsy in breast cancer surgery. *J Nucl Med*. 2001;42:1198–1215.
16. Chinol M, Paganelli G. Current status of commercial colloidal preparations for sentinel lymph node detection. *Eur J Nucl Med*. 1999;26:560.
17. Nieweg OE, Jansen L, Valdes Olmos RA, et al. Lymphatic mapping and sentinel lymph node biopsy in breast cancer. *Eur J Nucl Med*. 1999;26:S11–S16.
18. Edreira MM, Colombo LL, Perez JH, Sajaroff EO, de Castiglia SG. In vivo evaluation of 3 different $^{99m}$Tc-labeled radiopharmaceuticals for sentinel lymph node identification. *Nucl Med Commun*. 2001;22:499–504.
19. Tsopelas C. Understanding the radiolabeling mechanism of $^{99m}$Tc-antimony sulphide colloid. *Appl Radiat Isot*. 2003;59:321–328.
20. Tsopelas C, Cooper R. Radiolabeling and biodistribution of $^{111}$In-antimony trisulphide colloid. *Hell J Nucl Med*. 2005;8:109–112.
21. Goldfarb LR, Alazraki NP, Eshima D, Eshima LA, Herda SC, Halkar RK. Lymphoscintigraphic identification of sentinel lymph nodes: clinical evaluation of 0.22-micron

filtration of Tc-99m sulfur colloid. *Radiology*. 1998;208: 505–509.

22. Klimberg VS, Rubio IT, Henry R, Cowan C, Colvert M, Korourian S. Subareolar versus peritumoral injection for location of the sentinel lymph node. *Ann Surg*. 1999;229: 860–864; discussion 864–865.

23. Tafra L, Chua AN, Ng PC, Aycock D, Swanson M, Lannin D. Filtered versus unfiltered technetium sulfur colloid in lymphatic mapping: a significant variable in a pig model. *Ann Surg Oncol*. 1999;6:83–87.

24. Billinghurst M. Radiolabeled particulates in routine use. Part 1: colloids and suspension. In: Arshady R, ed. *Radiolabeled and Magnetic Particulates in Medicine and Biology*. Vol 3. London: Citus Books; 2001:1965.

25. Banerjee S, Pillai MR, Ramamoorthy N. Evolution of Tc-99m in diagnostic radiopharmaceuticals. *Semin Nucl Med*. 2001;31:260–277.

26. Arano Y. Recent advances in [99m]Tc radiopharmaceuticals. *Ann Nucl Med*. 2002;16:79–93.

27. Saha GB, MacIntyre WJ, Go RT. Cyclotrons and positron emission tomography radiopharmaceuticals for clinical imaging. *Semin Nucl Med*. 1992;22:150–161.

28. International Committee for Standardization in Haematology. Recommended methods for measurement of red-cell and plasma volume. *J Nucl Med*. 1980;21:793–800.

29. Callahan RJ, Rabito CA. Radiolabeling of erythrocytes with technetium-99m: role of band-3 protein in the transport of pertechnetate across the cell membrane. *J Nucl Med*. 1990;31:2004–2010.

30. Volkert WA, Edwards B, Simon J, et al. In vivo skeletal localization properties of [99m]Tc complexes of large phosphonate ligands. *Int J Rad Appl Instrum B*. 1986;13:31–37.

31. Barrow SA, Graham W, Jyawook S, et al. Localization of indium-111-immunoglobulin G, technetium-99m-immunoglobulin G, and indium-111-labeled white blood cells at sites of acute bacterial infection in rabbits. *J Nucl Med*. 1993;34:1975–1979.

32. Fukumoto M. Single-photon agents for tumor imaging: [201]Tl, [99m]Tc-MIBI, and [99m]Tc-tetrofosmin. *Ann Nucl Med*. 2004;18:79–95.

33. Piwnica-Worms D, Chiu ML, Budding M, et al. Functional imaging of multidrug resistant P-Glycoprotein with an organotechetium complex. *Cancer Res*. 1993;53:977–984.

34. Hendrikse NH, Franssen EJ, van der Graaf WT, et al. [99m]Tc-sestamibi is a substrate for P-glycoprotein and the multidrug resistance-associated protein. *Br J Cancer*. 1998;77:353–358.

35. Mueckler M. Facilitative glucose transporters. *Eur J Biochem*. 1994;219:713–725.

36. DH, Kloos RT, Mazzaferri EL, Jhian SM. Sodium iodide symporter in health and disease. *Thyroid*. 2001;11:415–425.

37. Sessler MJ, Geck P, Maul FD, Hor G, Munz DL. New aspects of cellular thallium uptake: Tl$^+$-Na$^+$-2Cl$^-$-cotransport is the central mechanism of ion uptake. *Nuklearmedizin*. 1986;25:24–27.

38. Yuksel M, Eziddin S, Ladwein E, Haas S, Biersack HJ. [111]In-pentetreotide and [123]I-MIBG for detection and resection of lymph node metastases of a carcinoid not visualized by CT, MRI, or FDG-PET. *Ann Nucl Med*. 2005;19:611–615.

39. Kenanova V, Wu AM. Tailoring antibodies for radionuclide delivery. *Expert Opin Drug Deliv*. 2006;3:53–70.

40. Blankenberg FG, Katsikis PD, Tait JF, et al. In vivo detection and imaging of phosphatidylserine expression during programmed cell death. *Proc Natl Acad Sci USA*. 1998;95: 6349–6354.

41. Toretsky J, Levenson A, Weinberg IN, Tait JF, Uren A, Mease RC. Preparation of F-18 labeled annexin V: a potential PET radiopharmaceutical for imaging cell death. *Nucl Med Biol*. 2004;31:747–752

# 2
# Physical Performance Parameters of Intraoperative Probes

Carlo Chiesa, Francesca Toscano, Mario Mariani, and Emilio Bombardieri

In 1951, the neurosurgeon William Sweet described the value of intraoperative gamma probes to demarcate brain tumors in the operating room (1). Since then the increase of applications, especially sentinel lymph node biopsy, has prompted a number of commercial manufacturers to offer intraoperative probes for radioguided surgery (2). Their basic physical principle relies on a radiation detector (usually a scintillator or semiconductor detector) and associated electronics to provide a visual and auditory signal related to the amount of radiation detected (3). Many investigators have compared the performance of these instruments (4–9), and some have suggested using a figure of merit (10–12). This chapter summarizes the most important characteristics of non-imaging intraoperative gamma probes. The performance of the most widely used models is discussed in detail, to assist in the selection of one that best fits a specific application. In order to make such a comparison *rigorously* objective, a set of well defined experimental conditions was developed, and this goal constitutes the core of the Italian protocol for quality control of intraoperative probes. In this regard, the current protocol for quality control adopted by the National Electrical Manufacturers Association (NEMA) does not define a standard energy window for assessing the most important probe parameter, sensitivity.

## The Structure of a Gamma Probe

A schematic diagram of the structure of an intraoperative gamma probe is shown in Figure 2-1. A gamma sensitive detector is positioned inside a collimator, keeping a distance between the detector face and the collimator border on the photon entrance side. The collimation goal is to reduce the contribution of radiation coming from the sides of the detector (noise), which makes it difficult to precisely localize the uptake region (signal) in front of the detector. Collimation is extremely important in radioimmunoguided surgery, where a large amount of radioactivity (~400 MBq) is administered as the labeled antibody. The tracer circulates for days, and it diffuses into the tissues. Uptake in the target site(s) may be only slightly greater than background in the non-antigen-expressing tissues. Specific identification of the lesion's margins with the probe requires therefore excellent collimation. On the other hand, sentinel lymph node studies use a limited amount of locally administered radiocolloid (20 MBq), which migrates from the injection site to the node via lymphatic flow and is trapped in the node with an extremely high concentration compared to the surrounding tissues.

Two detector materials—scintillators or semiconductors—are used in probes. In general, the higher density and $Z_{eff}$ of scintillators offers a greater likelihood of a photon having a photopeak interaction in the detector (photopeak efficiency). Since the photoelectric interaction probability is roughly proportional to the fourth to fifth power of $Z_{eff}$, even a small difference in $Z_{eff}$ between two materials (see Table 2-1) can have a major effect on their sensitivity (S), i.e., the ratio between count rate and activity of a source at a fixed distance.

Geometry also has a key role in gamma photon detection (geometrical efficiency), and crystal dimensions (diameter and thickness) and design properties (the crystal's depth inside the collimator) determine a probe's physical properties. Scintillators are preferred, because current crystal manufacturing techniques can produce reliable crystals of any dimension at a reasonable price. The primary drawback of scintillator probes is the instability of energy calibration, i.e., the peak position within the energy window, due to changes in temperature and humidity (13). Such factors also affect the response of the photomultiplier tubes, and for this reason, energy calibration of the peak is left to the user. The calibration is usually done manually, using a known source; only one manufacturer peaks the probe automatically (C-Trak® Automatic).

TABLE 2-1. Effective atomic number of crystal detector of probes.

| Scintillators | Z effective | Semiconductors | Z effective |
|---|---|---|---|
| NaI(Tl) | 53 | Cadmium telluride | 42 |
| CsI (Tl) | 54 | Cadmium zinc telluride | 47 |

*Source:* Data from Zanzonico P. et al. (3).

Semiconductors, on the other hand, produce a signal based on the number of electrons conducted as the photon traverses the depletion layer, making the amplitude, i.e., the peak position, independent of the applied voltage, and thus resulting in better stability.

The energy discrimination window influences probe performance by defining the fraction of detected events that are displayed on the readout. The selection of this parameter is left to the user (Figure 2-2). Energy discrimination allows the rejection of diffused (scattered) gamma rays that enter the detector after single or multiple Compton events (14). These events start from the source site (the injection site in sentinel nodes, or circulating activity in radioimmunoguided surgery), but follow a random deflection path to the detector, being degraded in energy at each collision with an electron in the biological medium. These photons must be rejected, since they do not carry any information about the original position of the source and instead constitute a sort of disturbing "noise" for its localization. Luckily, they do not keep the primary photon energy (i.e., 140 keV for $^{99m}$Tc), and therefore rejection is performed on the basis of their degraded energy. Thus, photons whose energy is within

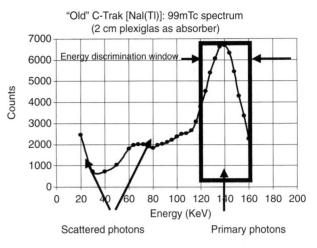

FIGURE 2-2. The energy discrimination window method.

a window around the photopeak of the "primary photons" are accepted, and those with energy falling below the lower level are rejected as "scattered" photons.

# A Short Description of Probes

The following provides descriptions of the commercial models studied.

## Scintillation Probes

The "old" C-Trak®, the first model produced by Care Wise (US) in 1998, has a NaI(Tl) crystal. The energy threshold and width are adjustable, as is applied high voltage. Two additional collimators are available. A different probe is available for $^{111}$In medium-energy photon detection.

C-Trak® Automatic, also produced by Care Wise (US), is a CsI(Tl) probe. Omniprobe is the standard angled probe. Two collimators for low energy ($^{99m}$Tc) are available: wide and narrow. Only the wide collimator was tested. One heavier collimator is designed to shield the higher energy photons of $^{111}$In. The "laparoscopic" probe is 46.6 cm long. A source holder is delivered, together with a 200 KBq $^{57}$Co "coin-shaped" point source for daily operational checks and, in case of failure, automatic calibration. Calibration is performed using software control of step-by-step high voltage variation to define the point of count rate maximization.

Europrobe, a CsI(Tl) probe produced by Eurorad (France), is equipped with one optional additional external collimator. A small display allows spectrum visualization.

Gammasonics™ (Institute for Medical Research Pty Ltd) is an Australian 6 mm CsI(Tl) crystal probe. For a rough daily check, the front panel contains a built-in 33 KBq $^{241}$Am point source (half-life 432 years).

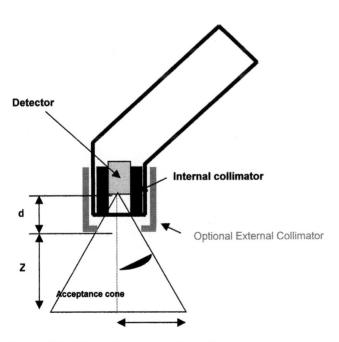

FIGURE 2-1. Schematic cross-section of a gamma intraoperative probe.

Pol.Hi.Tech, an Italian company, offers the Scinti-Probe MR100, which can be connected to different types of probes: fixed collimator probes 11-C and 15–3; variable collimator probes 15 LVR, 18 LVR, and 22 LVR; and laparoscopic probe 11-L. Number in the name indicates the external probe diameter (in mm). An interesting design feature of the LVR probes is the 4-step variation of the relative crystal collimator position (parameter "d" in Figure 2-1). This allows the investigation of the important influence of d on sensitivity. Position 0 indicates the minimum d, while position 3 is maximum d. The largest diameter available is conceived and collimated for detection of the [131]I 364 keV photons.

Gammafinder, produced by World of Medicine (Germany), is a CsI(Tl) wireless probe. This is the simplest probe available, contained in one handheld unit. However, its simplicity limits the possible controls by the user: spectrum and energy thresholds are not accessible, nor the counter time setting.

## Semiconductor Probes

Neoprobe Corporation (US) produces a set of probes based on cadmium zinc telluride (CdZnTe) crystals, which can be connected to the same power-analysis unit. The 14 mm rectilinear probe may be equipped with an optional additional external collimator. Neoprobe BlueTip line uses a universal pre-sterilized, single-use handle with 3 reusable probe tip configurations: 19 mm, not internally collimated; 12 mm, internally collimated; and 12 mm, not internally collimated.

Navigator was produced by United States Surgical Corporation (USSC) at the time of the tests. No external collimator is available.

## Methods

Probes designed for the operating room are used quite differently from the other nuclear medicine machines. Probes are switched on and off daily, while photomultiplier tubes in imaging devices are designed to have continuous high voltage. Probes are made to function well over a range of temperatures, from ambient room temperature to body temperature, while imaging devices are designed to work in a temperature- and humidity-controlled environment. Handheld probes are moved rapidly and are used in various positions, while imaging devices allow for only slow movements and relatively fixed orientations. Probes may be in contact with biological fluids such as blood or serum when the seam at the end of the sterile plastic sheath is not waterproof; in contrast, imaging devices are not designed to get wet.

The tough environment raises the probability of probe failure (15). To assure the operator that the system is functioning, the unit should be tested with a small radioactive source before use. These issues created the need for quality control procedures (16). Two protocols were developed: the Italian protocol, and the NEMA protocol.

## The Italian Protocol

An Italian law, derived from European Community Directive 97/43 EURATOM, states that nuclear medicine devices must undergo quality control procedures. The first quality control protocol was developed in March 2001 by the Italian Association of Medical Physics (AIFM, President L. Conte—C. Chiesa reference physicist), the Italian Association of Nuclear Medicine (AIMN, President E. Bombardieri), the Italian Study Group for Radioguided Surgery and ImmunoScintigraphy (GISCRIS, President A. Mussa), and the National Task Group for Breast Cancer (FONCAM President U. Veronesi) (17).

The first goal of the Italian protocol is developing reproducible tests. The main tests performed require measurements with the probe in contact with a sealed [57]Co or [99m]Tc point source (Figure 2-3) to assure reproducibility. Tests in scatter medium are limited to sensitivity, spatial and angular resolution, and employ 4 1-cm-thick polymethylmethacrylate (PMMA) plates (Figure 2-4).

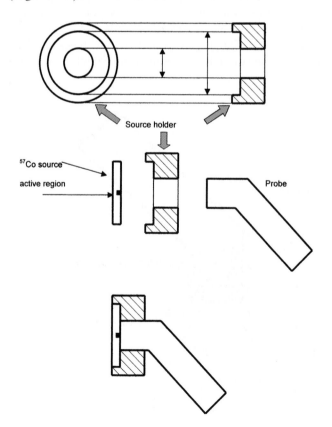

FIGURE 2-3. Experimental setup for the measurements of sensitivity, energy resolution, short-term sensitivity, and stability. (Italian Protocol, modified by permission from GISCRIS.)

**A Experimental setup**

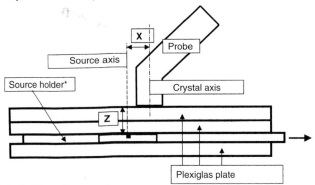

**B Definition of parameters**

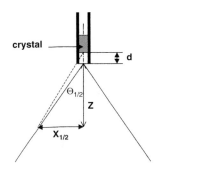

FIGURE 2-4. Spatial and angular resolution test showing: (A) experimental setup, and (B) the definition of parameters. (Italian Protocol, reprinted with permission.)

The second aim is to measure probe performance under standardized experimental conditions to allow meaningful comparison between different commercial models. The width of the energy window plays a critical role in this regard: the larger the energy window, the

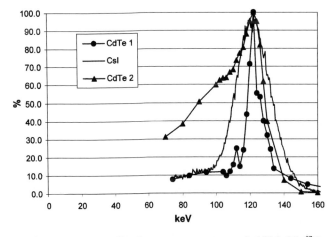

FIGURE 2-5. Normalized energy spectra of 122 keV $^{57}$Co photons. Energy resolution is the percentage full width at half maximum, divided by the peak energy. Semiconductors (Navigator, Eurorad CdTe) usually have sharper—but often asymmetrical—peaks than scintillators. (Italian Protocol, reprinted with permission.)

higher the sensitivity and the lower the angular resolution, because more scattered photons are accepted. Because energy spectra are quite different between crystals of different types, the window width should be properly chosen in order to compare probe sensitivities (see Figure 2-5).

The width of the photoelectric peak of semiconductor detectors is usually much narrower than that for a scintillator, so a comparison using identical window widths would penalize scintillator performance. The most homogeneous experimental conditions are obtained using the "standard window," defined in the Italian protocol as an energy window centered on the photopeak with a width twice the peak full width at half maximum (FWHM). In this way, the same portion of the energy spectrum is accepted for any probe, regardless of its width. For asymmetric peaks, the standard window width is twice the upper half width at half maximum (UHWHM).

Spatial resolution ($R_S$) is measured according to the experimental setup shown in Figure 2-4, at 4 depths of 10, 20, 30, and 40 mm in tissue-equivalent scatter medium (PMMA). The small difference (2%) between the linear attenuation coefficient in PMMA and in water with $^{57}$Co photons becomes a difference of 8% at a depth of 40 mm; nevertheless, PMMA is more practical in respect to water as scatter medium. $R_S$ is defined as twice the distance $X_{1/2}$ at which counts drop to one-half of the maximum.

$R_S$ worsens at increasing depth, since a probe accepts photons coming from an ideal cone—known as the acceptance cone—whose vertex is the crystal and whose limits are given by the collimator border. An ideally depth-independent resolution parameter is the angular resolution ($R_A$), which is defined as twice the half opening of the acceptance cone:

$$R_A = 2\Theta_{1/2} = 2 \text{ arc tg}(X_{1/2}/Z)$$

As shown in Figure 2-4B, the formula makes the approximation considering the distance (Z) between the probe tip and the source, rather than the true distance (Z + d) between the cone vertex and the source. Increasing Z diminishes this approximation, so determining angular resolution at 40 mm is best. Moreover, a dependence of angular resolution upon the distance could be explained by the variation of the scatter contribution.

If one adopts a different experimental setup, as in the NEMA protocol, choosing a circular geometry (with a probe tip at the center and source moved on an arc of a circle), higher $R_A$ will be obtained.

## The NEMA Protocol

The current NEMA protocol is NU-3 2004 (18) (purchasable at www.nema.org). It is comprehensive,

TABLE 2-2. Summary of the tests required by the Italian protocol and the National Electrical Manufacturers Association protocol.

| Test | Performance | Quality control monthly | Per use |
|---|---|---|---|
| Sensitivity (air) | IT and NEMA | | IT and NEMA |
| Sensitivity (scatter medium) | IT and NEMA | | |
| Sensitivity through side shielding in air | IT and NEMA | | |
| Sensitivity to scatter | NEMA | | |
| Spatial resolution (scatter medium) | IT and NEMA | | |
| Volume sensitivity to distributed activity | NEMA | | |
| Short-term sensitivity stability | IT and NEMA | IT | |
| Count rate capability | IT (air) | | |
| Angular resolution (scatter medium) | NEMA (medium) | | |
| Energy resolution | IT and NEMA | IT | |
| Side and back shielding | IT (side) NEMA (both) | | |
| Visual inspection | IT and NEMA | | IT and NEMA |
| Power source | IT and NEMA | | IT and NEMA |
| Timer and counter | IT | | |
| Background (wide window) | IT | IT | |
| Background (usual window) | IT | | IT |
| Energy calibration (peak position) | IT | IT | |

Legend:
IT—Italian protocol
NEMA—National Electrical Manufacturers Association protocol
*Source:* Data from references (17,18).

consisting of a larger number of performance tests than the Italian protocol, such as acceptance and reference tests after major maintenance. Quality control tests, such as those to be performed on a regular basis, are limited to sensitivity in air, visual inspection, and a battery test (the Italian protocol requires a monthly set of measurements that include energy resolution, sensitivity in air, short-term sensitivity stability, and background with a wide window). The NEMA protocol is, in general, more accurate, but it is also more demanding and more difficult to reproduce. For example, the scatter influence is carefully investigated: sensitivity at source-probe tip distances of 0, 10, 30, and 50 mm have to be measured both in air, with the source distant from scatter objects, and in water. Two additional tests are introduced: sensitivity to scatter, and volume sensitivity to distributed activity. For this reason, more refined materials are required, like a $20 \times 20 \times 15$ cm water bath for the scatter test, and a system for probe-source distance or angle ("a travelling stage with screw controlled position" is suggested). A disadvantage of the NEMA protocol is that the energy window width used during tests is not fixed, making it difficult to compare the results of different probes.

Table 2-2 summarizes the list of tests required by the two standards. The importance of a simple test on any day of use (the Italian protocol) or "per use" (the NEMA protocol) is remarked in both documents.

# Physical Comparison Between Commercial Models

The following section reports on the results of a systematic comparison between several commercial models (12). All the tests were performed in the year 2000, according to the Italian protocol then under development. In most of the histogram plots in the chapter, data are divided in two sections: scintillators' data (upper part) and semiconductors' data (lower part). In each plot section, data are listed in alphabetic order of the producer company.

## Energy Resolution

According to the Italian protocol, the first parameter to be determined is the energy resolution, i.e., the full width at half maximum (FWHM) of the photoelectric peak of $^{57}$Co divided by 122 keV photon energy. Figure 2-6 shows the measured energy resolution. Since it is not possible to measure the energy spectrum for each commercial model, energy resolution could not always be determined. Neoprobe shows the best resolution, which allows for an excellent scatter discrimination. The other semiconductors also show good UHWHM, but this cannot be exploited to reject scattered photons, since their peak is strongly asymmetrical and deformed at low energies.

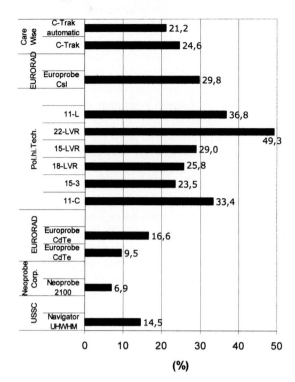

FIGURE 2-6. Measured probe energy resolution. (Data from Chiesa C. et al. [12].)

the highest values seen with the scintillators (Pol. Hi.Tech 15 LVR 0, 22 LVR 0). For scintillators, there is only a negligible increase in sensitivity passing from the standard energy window width to that suggested by the company.

These data indicate that sensitivity is quite different between different models, but this fact is seldom considered one of the most important criteria for selection of an instrument.

In Pol.Hi.Tech probes, sensitivity is reduced by increasing the crystal-probe tip distance (d) (Figure 2-4B), keeping the source in contact with the probe tip (Z = 0). This is an almost pure example of the inverse square distance law.

Adding the external optional collimator reduces the sensitivity of the Neoprobe (from 25.6 to 3.7 cps/KBq), while the reduction in sensitivity is much less with the C-Trak® Automatic (from 31.6 to 29.1 cps/KBq with the wide collimator, to 14.6 cps/KBq with the narrow collimator). This effect is dependent upon the probe and collimator design, and will be investigated in the next section.

## Sensitivity at Contact of a $^{57}$Co Source

All the tests were performed with the same $^{57}$Co source, whose activity was around 50 KBq at the beginning of the study. The source was so weak that dead time count loss was negligible. In Figure 2-7, the highest value of the Neoprobe BlueTip 19 mm is due to the absence of an internal or external collimator, and to its large diameter.

The Neoprobe 14 mm has a sensitivity of 25.6 cps/KBq, obtained with the Italian protocol standard window (108 keV, 124 keV), an excellent value for a semiconductor. However, this value is almost half of the value of 45 cps/KBq obtained with the default window (98 keV, 600 keV), which is automatically set when the device is switched on. This window is quite large and is misleading, because it accepts a large contribution of scatter from high-energy $^{57}$Co photons emitted at 692 keV (with a low probability of 0.15%). Navigator has a rather limited sensitivity of 3.6 cps/KBq, with a standard window (110 keV, ∞), which becomes 6.9 cps/KBq if an 80 keV threshold is adopted; the relationship of sensitivity to the energy window width is illustrated in Figure 2-8. Care Wise's C-Trak® Automatic is at 31.6 cps/KBq with a (96 keV, 148 keV) standard window, i.e., around

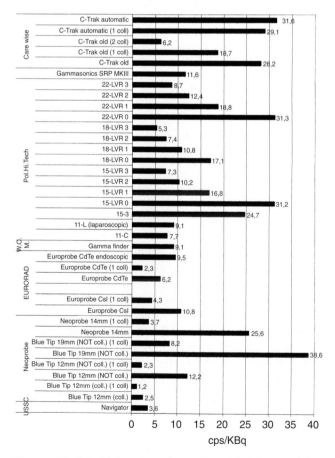

FIGURE 2-7. Sensitivity with a "standard window" defined in the Italian protocol (i.e., width twice the energy resolution) at contact of a $^{57}$Co point source. (Data from Chiesa C. et al. [12].)

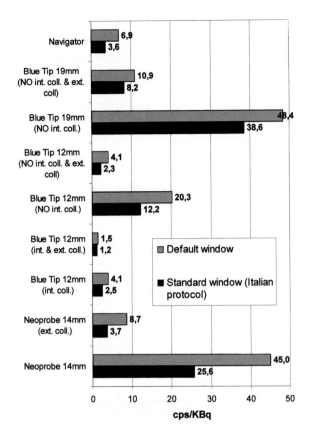

FIGURE 2-8. Probe sensitivity increases by broadening the energy window, but more scattered photons are accepted. (Data from Chiesa C. et al. [12].)

## Relative Sensitivity as a Function of Depth

Since lymph nodes are embedded in tissue, it is important to evaluate the sensitivity of the probe as a function of the depth (Z) of the radiation source in tissue (simulated by PMMA in Figure 2-4A). Table 2-3 reports values of percentage sensitivity studied with $^{99m}$Tc, with respect to the value at contact.

Relative sensitivity decreases dramatically with the depth of the lesion, due to a combination of effects from the inverse square distance law and from tissue attenuation. But even this physical property varies among models. Some probes maintain their sensitivity better than others when the source is deeper in tissues. Ignoring the thicker probes (Neoprobe BlueTip 19 mm and Pol. Hi.Tech. 22), which are very dedicated instruments, Neoprobe relative sensitivity falls at 16% at 1 cm, C-Trak® Automatic at 21.6%, Navigator at 26.5%. To understand these differences, the variable collimator probe Pol. Hi.Tech 15 LVR will be considered (Figure 2-9).

If the collimator is fully retracted (position 0), the crystal probe tip distance is at its minimum and absolute sensitivity at contact is at its maximum, but the relative sensitivity loss with depth is also the highest. If the collimator is fully extracted (position 3), the crystal probe tip distance is at its maximum and absolute sensitivity at

contact is at its minimum, but the relative sensitivity loss with depth is reduced: the curve for position 3 is less steep than its analogue for position 0. The critical role played by the crystal position inside the internal collimator is clear (parameter d in Figures 2-1 and 2-4). As the source goes deeper and deeper, we encounter the inverse square distance law, which must be properly thought of as $1/(d + Z)^2$. In the clinical interval of Z from 0 to 4 cm, this mathematical function is steeper if d is smaller, i.e. starting very close to the crystal. Probes with crystal very exposed to the entrance hole show the maximum possible sensitivity for that crystal material and shape, but lose sensitivity more rapidly if the source goes deeper. Neoprobe 14 mm is an extreme example of this. On the other hand, probes designed with a crystal well embedded inside the internal collimator lose less sensitivity with depth, although their sensitivity at contact is something less than the maximum possible for that crystal material and shape. This behavior can be clearly seen when we add an external collimator, which adds thickness in front of the probe.

## Absolute Sensitivity in Operative Conditions

To compare the sensitivity of probes in probable operative settings, Figure 2-10 reports the calculated absolute sensitivity curves as a function of depth. Values are obtained starting at contact with $^{57}$Co (Figure 2-7), measured with default windows (wider than the standard window required by the Italian protocol), multiplied by the relative factor of Table 2-3, obtained by $^{99m}$Tc. The discrepancy in photon energy (122 keV vs 140 keV) is of minor effect on the conclusions. Under these conditions (i.e. with a rather wide energy window), the semiconductor Neoprobe 14 mm definitely has a sensitivity higher than other semiconductors, and one close to the values of scintillators.

## Spatial and Angular Resolution

Spatial resolution at 4 cm depth in PMMA is reported in Figure 2-11. Angular resolution $R_A$ is indirectly computed by means of the approximated formula

$$R_A = 2 \text{ arc tg}(X_{1/2}/Z)$$

In Figure 2-12, the less approximated angular resolutions at 4 cm depth in PMMA are reported.

In all models, the addition of an external collimator improves the resolution (but reduces the sensitivity). Neoprobe 14 mm is among the probes with lower spatial resolution and a correspondingly wider acceptance cone (apart from the BlueTip 19 mm, which is not internally collimated). All the Pol.Hi.Tech LVR probes have higher values of $R_S$ and $R_A$ (low spatial and angular resolution) with the collimator retracted in position 0, with respect

TABLE 2-3. Relative sensitivity (%) to 0 mm as a function of depth in polymethylmethacrylate with $^{99m}$Tc.

| | Probe | Sensitivity relative to 0 mm (%) | | | |
|---|---|---|---|---|---|
| | | 10 mm | 20 mm | 30 mm | 40 mm |
| Care-Wise | C-Trak® Automatic | 21.6 | 8.2 | 4.1 | 2.3 |
| | C-Trak® Automatic, 1 collimator | 22.1 | 8.9 | 4.4 | 2.4 |
| | C-Trak® old | 23.2 | 8.6 | 4.4 | 2.5 |
| | C-Trak® old, 1 collimator | 28.5 | 11.5 | 5.9 | 3.4 |
| | C-Trak® old, 2 collimators | 37.7 | 17.9 | 10.2 | 6.3 |
| | Gammasonics SRP MKIII | | | | |
| Pol.Hi.Tech. | 11C | 23.8 | 10.2 | 5.3 | 3.2 |
| | 11L | 34.0 | 14.1 | 7.3 | 4.1 |
| | 15–3 | 33.8 | 13.8 | 6.8 | 4.1 |
| | 15 LVR 0 | 27.4 | 10.8 | 5.8 | 3.3 |
| | 15 LVR 1 | 30.1 | 12.3 | 6.6 | 3.7 |
| | 15 LVR 2 | 33.2 | 14.7 | 8.3 | 5.1 |
| | 15 LVR 3 | 37.8 | 17.0 | 9.7 | 5.9 |
| | 18LVR 0 | 30.8 | 14.3 | 7.5 | 4.4 |
| | 18LVR 1 | 31.4 | 17.2 | 8.2 | 5.2 |
| | 18LVR 2 | 34.2 | 17.0 | 9.4 | 5.8 |
| | 18LVR 3 | 36.9 | 18.8 | 10.9 | 6.6 |
| | 22 LVR 0 | 49.4 | 20.5 | 10.6 | 6.5 |
| | 22 LVR 1 | 42.6 | 21.8 | 10.0 | 6.5 |
| | 22 LVR 2 | 43.0 | 21.1 | 10.8 | 7.2 |
| | 22 LVR 3 | 41.6 | 21.9 | 11.8 | 8.7 |
| World of Medicine | Gammafinder | 16.6 | 6.1 | 2.8 | 1.6 |
| Eurorad | Europrobe CdTe | 38.7 | 14.8 | 6.8 | 3.9 |
| | Europrobe CdTe, 1 collimator | 29.8 | 12.4 | 6.2 | 3.5 |
| | Europrobe CdTe endoscopic | 12.8 | 3.8 | 1.9 | 1.0 |
| | Europrobe CsI | 31.2 | 13.9 | 7.5 | 4.6 |
| | Europrobe CsI, 1 collimator | 38.2 | 18.7 | 11.0 | 6.5 |
| Neoprobe | Neoprobe 2100 14 mm | 16.0 | 5.4 | 2.6 | 1.2 |
| | Neoprobe 2100 14 mm, 1 collimator | 29.9 | 13.6 | 7.0 | 4.0 |
| | BlueTip 12 mm (with internal collimator) | 30.6 | 13.3 | 7.1 | 4.1 |
| | BlueTip 12 mm (with internal collimator) 1 external collimator | 36.9 | 17.5 | 9.7 | 5.9 |
| | BlueTip 12 mm (no internal collimator) | 26.5 | 9.8 | 5.0 | 2.8 |
| | BlueTip 12 mm (no internal collimator) 1 external collimator | 30.4 | 13.1 | 6.9 | 4.0 |
| | BlueTip 19 mm (no internal collimator) | 44.2 | 19.3 | 10.1 | 16.1 |
| | BlueTip 19 mm (no internal collimator) 1 external collimator | 45.1 | 22.7 | 12.9 | 7.7 |
| USSC | Navigator | 26.5 | 10.9 | 5.7 | 3.2 |

*Source:* Adapted from Chiesa C. et al. (12) with permission from Springer.

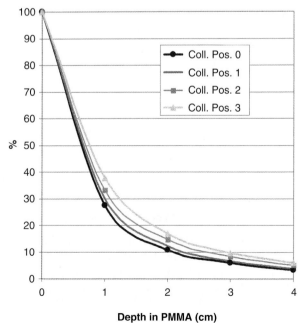

FIGURE 2-9. Relative sensitivity of a probe as a function of depth (using the Pol.Hi.Tech 15 LVR). (Data from Chiesa C. et al. [12].)

to other collimator positions. The fully extracted collimator, on the other hand, gives the best spatial and angular resolution. These observations confirm the importance of the distance (d) between the crystal and the probe face. A small d value implies maximum possible sensitivity at contact, but marked sensitivity loss with depth and low spatial and angular resolution (broad acceptance cone). A higher d value makes the acceptance cone narrower and reduces the changes in sensitivity with depth, but also lessens sensitivity at contact. Such a tradeoff between sensitivity and resolution is intrinsic in the geometry of intraoperative probes.

## Lateral Shielding

Figure 2-13 reports the probes' lateral penetration probability. The effectiveness of lateral shielding was measured with a $^{57}$Co point source positioned at contact in front of and at the side of the probe. The lowest shielding efficacy was found in the Neoprobe BlueTip, as a consequence of the absence of an internal collimator.

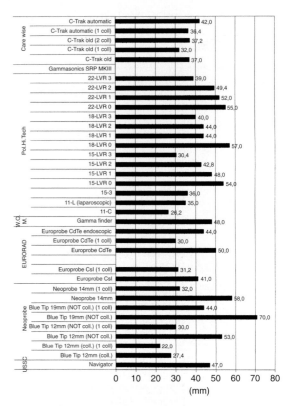

FIGURE 2-11. Probe spatial resolution measured with a $^{99m}$Tc point source at 4 cm depth in polymethylmethacrylate. (Data from Chiesa C. et al. [12].)

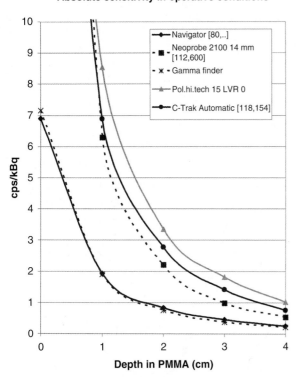

FIGURE 2-10. Comparison of probe absolute sensitivity in scatter medium. For a further comparison in operative conditions, semiconductor probes are evaluated with default windows (wider than the standard window required by the Italian protocol). (Data from Chiesa C. et al. [12].)

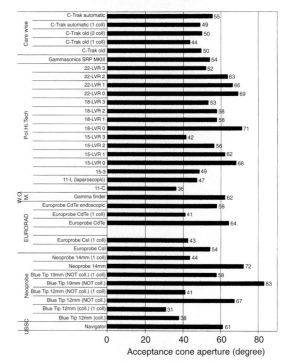

FIGURE 2-12. Probe angular resolution deduced from spatial resolution at 4 cm depth in polymethylmethacrylate. (Data from Chiesa C. et al. [12].)

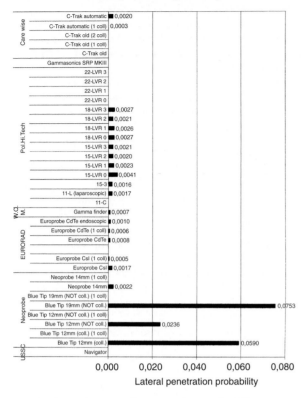

FIGURE 2-13. Probe lateral penetration probability measured with $^{57}$Co 122 keV photons. (Data from Chiesa C. et al. [12].)

indicator, the quality of service, and cost (19). The considerations here, however, have been limited to physical parameters that can be put together in a "figure of merit." Two different approaches to calculate the figure of merit have been published, the first by Britten (10) and the second by our group (12). In the method by Britten, the figure of merit is the ability of distinguishing the lymph node from the injection site; only 5 probes were compared, and the method is rather complicated and demanding. We proposed a figure of merit (G) that can easily be deduced from the 2 most important physical parameters of a probe: its sensitivity (S) and its angular resolution ($R_A$). To overcome the problem of the tradeoff between the two, G is defined as the ratio between S and the fraction of solid angle $\Delta\Omega/2\pi$ subtended by $\theta$ (the solid angle is the three-dimensional portion of space delimited by a cone). In practice, our figure of merit is a sort of sensitivity independent of the three-dimensional aperture of the acceptance cone. We evaluated 17 commercial models, and the results are shown in Figure 2-15. Although a figure of merit is a useful parameter, a general consensus about the weighting factors to calculate it have not been discussed.

## Count Rate Capability

The system's ability to handle high count rate is rarely clinically relevant, since most systems are operating far below their saturation level. This is usually true in radio-immunoguided surgery, or monitoring of leakage of a chemotherapic agent during operative treatment of limb cancer. On the contrary, high count rates are typical of the performance tests, where the choice of high activity test source aims to shorten the test duration. For this reason, it is important to know the limit at which the linearity between activity and count rate is preserved. Clearly, dead time problems affect scintillators more than semiconductors, as in other fundamental physics detectors (Figure 2-14). A rule of thumb puts a limit rate for scintillators around 5 to 10,000 counts per second, and 10 to 30,000 counts per second (cps) for semiconductors. In sentinel lymph node biopsy, typical rates are around 10 to 100 cps.

## The Best Probe

Several factors should be considered when choosing a medical instrument: physical performance, display and analysis software, ergonomics, the quality of the sound

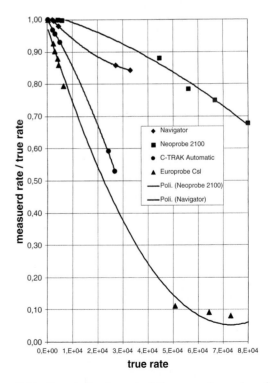

FIGURE 2-14. Count rate characteristic curves for probes. (Data from Chiesa C. et al. [12].)

**Figure of merit G = S/(ΔΩ/2π)**

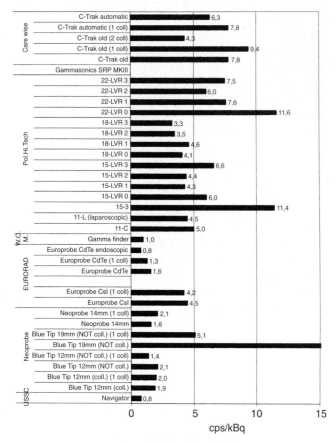

FIGURE 2-15. Comparison of probes according to the proposed figure of merit. G = S/(ΔΩ/2π) evaluated at 4 cm depth in polymethylmethacrylate. (Data from Chiesa C. et al. [12].)

## References

1. Sweet WH. The uses of nuclear disintegration in the diagnosis and treatment of brain tumor. *N Engl J Med.* 1951; 245:875–887.
2. Hoffman EJ, Tornai MP, Janacek M, Patt BE, Iwanczy JS. Intraoperative probes and imaging probes. *Eur J Nucl Med.* 1999;26:913–935.
3. Zanzonico P, Heller S. The intraoperative gamma probe: basic principles and choices available. *Semin Nucl Med.* 2000;30:33–48.
4. Barber HB, Barret HH, Hickernell TS, et al. Comparison of NaI(Tl), CdTe, and HgI2 surgical probes: physical characterization. *Med Phys.* 1991;18:373–381.
5. Kwo DP, Barber HB, Barrett HH, Hickernell TS, Woolfenden JM. Comparison of NaI(Tl), CdTe, and HgI2 surgical probes: effects of scatter compensation on probe performance. *Med Phys.* 1991;18:382–389.
6. Tiourina T, Arends B, Huysmans D, Rutten H, Lemaire B, Muller S. Evaluation of surgical gamma probes for radioguided sentinel node localization. *Eur J Nucl Med.* 1998;25:1224–1231.
7. van Lingen A, Bosma AM, Pijpers R. Evaluation of surgical gamma probes. *Eur J Nucl Med.* 1999;26:183–184.
8. Kopp J, Wengenmair H, Vogt H, Heidenreich P. Intraoperative gamma probes: performances of commercially available systems—a comparison. *Eur J Nucl Med.* 1999; 26(suppl):S59.
9. Brands PJM, Arends AJ, Tiourina TB, Rutten HJT, Huysmans D. Physical aspects of surgical gamma probe selection and practical use in radioguided sentinel node localization. *Eur J Nucl Med.* 1999;26(suppl): S59.
10. Britten AJ. How to choose a probe. *Eur J Nucl Med.* 1999; 26:76–83.
11. van Lingen A, Bosma AM, Pijpers R, Hoekstra OS, Teule GJ. The need for a figure-of-merit for the comparison of surgical gamma probe performances. *Eur J Nucl Med.* 1999;26(suppl):S61.
12. Chiesa C, Toscano F, Mariani M, Bombardieri E. Intraoperative gamma probes: systematic inter-comparison of 14 commercial devices under identical experimental conditions—introduction of a simple physical figure of merit. *Eur J Nucl Med.* 2001;28(suppl):1110.
13. van Lingen A, Bosma AM, Pijpers R, Hoekstra OS, Teule GJJ. On the detection of drift in gamma probe sensitivity. *Eur J Nucl Med.* 1999;26(suppl);S61.
14. Muller SH. Scatter suppression in sentinel node detection. *Eur J Nucl Med.* 1999;26(suppl);S60.
15. Chiesa C, Toscano F, Maffioli L, Bombardieri E. Intraoperative probes: constancy of performances. *Eur J Nucl Med.* 2000;27:989.
16. Evans WD, Bodey RK, Clarke D, Mansel RE. A laboratory assessment of gamma radiation probes for the localization of sentinel lymph nodes at operation. *Eur J Nucl Med.* 1999;26(suppl):S59.
17. *Sonde intraoperatorie per chirurgia radioguidata—protocollo per il controllo di qualita.* Italian Association of Medical Physics (AIFM), Italian Association of Nuclear Medicine (AIMN), Italian Group for Radioguided Surgery and ImmunoScintigraphy (GISCRIS), and National Operative Breast Cancer Force (FONCAM), eds. March 6, 2001. Available in Italian at: http://www.aifm.it; keyword "intraoperatorie".
18. National Electrical Manufacturers Association (NEMA). *Performance Measurements and Quality Control Guidelines for Non-Imaging Intraoperative Gamma Probes.* NEMA Standard Publication NU3-2004. Purchasable at www.NEMA.org.
19. Mariani G, Vaiano A, Nibale O, Rubello S. Is the "ideal" γ-probe for intraoperative radioguided surgery conceivable? *J Nucl Med.* 2005;46:388–390.

# 3
# Positron-Sensitive Probes

Schlomo Schneebaum, Richard Essner, and Einat Even-Sapir

Radioguided surgery is a surgical technique that uses specific tissue characteristics (e.g., receptor or epitope expression, increased metabolism, or protein synthesis) to mark tissue with a radionuclide before surgery. The surgeon then uses a radiation-sensitive probe to define the tissue margins at the time of surgery.

Although most intraoperative probes use single photon radionuclides, such as $^{99m}$Tc, $^{111}$In, or an isotope of iodine, there is increasing interest in defining lesion borders based on tissue metabolism, membrane, or protein synthesis. $^{18}$F-fluorodeoxyglucose (FDG) (1) is a positron-emitting analog of glucose, which is useful to define the increase in glycolysis often associated with tumors. The FDG molecule is transported into cells by facilitative glucose transporters and is phosphorylated to FDG-6 phosphate (2), which is retained in the tissue. Since tumor cells often have higher metabolic rates than normal tissue, they can be identified by their localized increase in counts from the FDG-6 phosphate trapped in the cancer cells. Although positron emission tomography (PET) with FDG is widely used for cancer patients, the limited resolution of this imaging technique does not allow for reliable detection of lesions that are less than 5 mm in diameter or those adjacent to sites of normal tissue with high physiological uptake of FDG (e.g., heart, kidney, or bladder) (3).

The information provided by positron emission tomography-computed tomography (PET-CT) delineates the extent of disease, often modifying the surgical procedure (4,5). At times, lesions found on FDG-PET imaging are not visually obvious at the operating table; this is particularly true for lesions in the abdomen, for example, where a lymph node clearly visible on the image may be visually indistinguishable from the others. Therefore, surgeons have tried to perform PET-radioguided surgery.

Radioguided surgery was originally developed to: 1) detect tumors suspected to be in the abdomen due to elevated tumor markers in the blood, e.g., carcinoembryonic antigen (CEA); 2) identify tumors that were missed by other imaging modalities and localize them during the operation; 3) assess the completeness of resection (margins). Radioguided surgery added therefore another tool to the inspection and palpation used during abdominal surgery.

## Positron Emission Tomographic Probes

### The Gamma-Detecting Probe

The idea of using a handheld probe for the intraoperative localization of diseased tissue was first discussed by Sweet in 1951 (6). Since then, there have been numerous reports, as summarized in Chapter 21. The first reported use of the probe for radioguided surgery was in 1981 (7), when it was employed to intraoperatively localize lesions in bone and soft tissues. This was extended to the localization of accessory spleens in 3 patients with persistent idiopathic thrombocytopenic purpura following splenectomy, and to a patient with a CEA-producing tumor (8).

There are several different probe designs, including gas-filled detectors, plastic scintillators and optical fibers (to conduct the light to an external photomultiplier tube), and semiconductor detectors. One semiconductor detector uses cadmium telluride as the radiation detector, together with a preamplifier, in a collimated handheld unit. Its small size enables adapting the probe size according to its use in radioimmunoguided surgery or sentinel lymph node mapping. The surgeon can identify the presence of a concentration of radioactivity by watching a digital numerical display and/or listening to an auditory signal.

The efficiency of detection is the ratio between the area of the detector and the area of the sphere of radiation. The ratio between these two increases proportionately to the square of the distance between them (Figure 3-1), according to the inverse square distance law. The

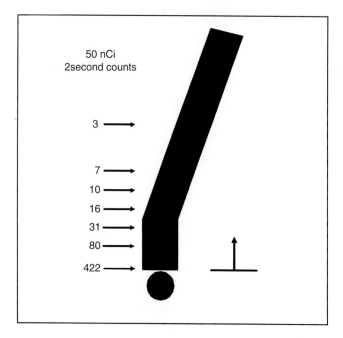

50 nCi
2second counts

3 ⟶

7 ⟶
10 ⟶
16 ⟶
31 ⟶
80 ⟶
422 ⟶

FIGURE 3-1. Probe over 50 nCi node (2-s count). Counts decrease proportionately to the square of the distance between the source and the detector. (From Schneebaum S et al. Clinical applications of gamma-detection probes—radioguided surgery. Eur J Nucl Med 1999;26(4 Suppl):S26–S35. Reprinted with permission.)

probe serves as a homing device by directing the surgeon to the tissue with the high-count rate.

The Neoprobe 1000 probe (Dublin, Ohio), as well as the later 1500 and 2000 models, have a special "squelch" mode character. This is a mathematical characteristic of the computer that calculates the mean count of a given point (5-second count) and the standard deviation (square root), and starts to emit a sound only when the count is 3 standard deviations above the mean count (denoting significantly higher radiation). This enables the surgeon to survey an area and be guided to the tissue with significantly higher radiation (9).

The surgeon carefully surveys the area in question, moving the probe slowly over the tissues. Most surgeons use the 3-point counting principle: 1) an in-vivo count is done; 2) the tissue is excised; and 3) an ex-vivo count is done, to verify that the right tissue was excised.

The bed of resection is then probed again to ascertain that no radioactive tissue was left behind. Table 3-1 describes several scenarios using this 3-point principle (10).

The rise of the gamma-detecting probe occurred with the clinical acceptance of the sentinel lymph node technique in tumors such as breast cancer. Sentinel node identification is usually done using an intradermal injection, which does not leave a high concentration of tracer in the blood pool; in radioimmunoguided surgery, the labeled monoclonal antibodies are injected intravenously, resulting in a long blood residence time and significant background, making target detection more challenging. If a low-energy radionuclide such as $^{125}$I were employed, there would be high tissue attenuation, improving the tumor-to-background ratio with good detector efficiency.

Preliminary studies were done to evaluate commercially available gamma-detecting probes for detecting the 511 keV gamma photons from $^{18}$F (11,12). These studies demonstrated that these probes can detect a source 1.7 to 4 cm from the maximal radiation source, but the sensitivity is low, and the ability to localize the radiation source is compromised (11). Furthermore, the side and back shielding of a gamma probe made of tungsten are a couple of millimeters thick and are only adequate for blocking low-energy gamma rays. Side shielding collimates the probe's field of view and thereby provides spatial resolution, but more shielding is required to stop high-energy gamma rays.

Essner et al. (13) tested such a probe, the IntraMedical Imaging (Los Angeles) prototype surgical probe, with high efficiency and effective side and back shielding for high-energy gamma rays (Figure 3-2). This probe's efficiency, the adequacy of shielding, and spatial resolution were determined by using a small (0.5-cm diameter) source of $^{18}$F. The $^{18}$F source was scanned using the probe at gradually increasing distances, and the count rates were recorded. The sensitivity of the probe at 1 cm distance was determined to be 100 counts per second (cps) per microcurie of $^{18}$F. A typical tumor weighing 0.5 g has a diameter of 0.5 cm and contains 0.5 µCi of FDG 1 hour after injection. Therefore, the probe records 50 cps when it is placed within 1 cm of such a tumor. This count rate is adequate to distinguish the tumor over a background that has 2 times less radioactive concentration (>3 standard deviations above back-

TABLE 3-1. The 3-point counting principle used with gamma-detecting probes.

| Scenario | In vivo | Ex vivo | Bed of resection | |
|---|---|---|---|---|
| 1 | + | + | − | Right tissue completely excised |
| 2 | + | − | + | Wrong tissue excised |
| 3 | + | + | + | Right tissue, not completely excised, additional tissue |
| 4 | + | − | − | Technical error resulting in high in-vivo count |

*Source:* Schneebaum S et al. Clinical applications of gamma-detection probes—radioguided surgery. Eur J Nucl Med 1999;26(4 Suppl):S26–S35. Reprinted with permission.

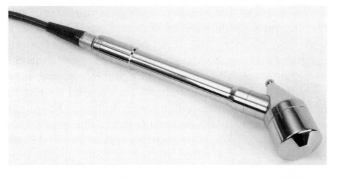

FIGURE 3-2. High-energy gamma-ray detecting probe (Intra-Medical Imaging, Los Angeles).

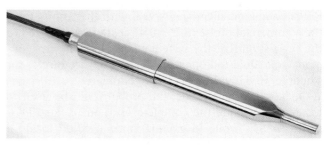

FIGURE 3-3. Beta-sensitive probe (IntraMedical Imaging, Los Angeles).

ground). Table 3-2 compares both gamma-detecting and PET probes.

## The Beta Probe

A beta-sensitive probe was created to circumvent the limitations of the traditional gamma probe (Figure 3-3). Because beta rays have a short depth of penetration in tissue (~1 mm), a beta-sensitive probe is not affected by the background gamma radiation. The positrons emitted by FDG-avid cancer cells can be used to detect milligram quantities of tumor when the probe is placed on the lesion. Phantom studies demonstrated that the beta probe is capable of finding tumors as small as a few milligrams or ~2 mm in diameter (14). These devices are optimized for detection of beta particles and have markedly less sensitivity for gamma or x-ray photons (14–18).

## The Dual Probe

Another development was suggested by Raylman (19), who tested a dual solid-state probe (probe detecting both beta and gamma rays). The detector unit of the intraoperative-probe system used in his study consisted of a stack of 2 ion-implanted silicon detectors separated by 0.5 mm. The system could be operated in 2 modes: beta-optimized, in which the difference between the signals from the 2 detectors was calculated to correct the beta signal for photon contamination; and photon-optimized, in which the signals were summed. Detection sensitivity and an index measuring beta detection selectivity were measured in both acquisition modes with the 3 different radionuclides: $^{18}$F, $^{99m}$Tc, and $^{111}$In. The gamma-ray detection sensitivity of the commercially available probe was measured with $^{99m}$Tc and compared with the results with a solid-state probe. The photon emissions (gamma rays and annihilation photons) produced by all 3 radionuclides were detected by the probe. In the beta-optimized acquisition mode, the greatest beta-detection sensitivity was achieved with $^{18}$F; photon sensitivity was greatest for measurements with $^{111}$In. The lowest detection sensitivities (beta and photon) were obtained with $^{99m}$Tc. In gamma-optimized mode, the greatest beta and photon sensitivities were achieved with $^{18}$F; the lowest were obtained with $^{99m}$Tc. The gamma-detection sensitivity measured with $^{99m}$Tc in gamma-mode (5.59 ± 0.41 cps/

TABLE 3-2. Features of gamma-detecting and positron emission tomography probes.

|  | Gamma detector | Positron emission tomography |
|---|---|---|
| Crystal | Cadmium telluride | Sodium iodide |
| Mode of injection | Intradermal | Intravenous |
|  | Intravenous, radioguided surgery |  |
| Shielding | Tungsten | Thicker side and back shielding |
|  | Millimeter thick |  |
| Time to surgery | 3–4 weeks (radioguided surgery) | 30–60 minutes |
|  | 2–24 hours (sentinel lymph node) |  |
| Use | Homing device (sentinel lymph node) | Margin of resection |
|  | Margin of resection (radioguided surgery) | Minute metastasis |
|  | Minute metastasis |  |
| Squelch | Needed | 1.5 ratio |
| Radionuclide | $^{99m}$Tc | $^{18}$F |
|  | $^{125}$I |  |

KBq) compared surprisingly well with the results from the commercial probe (8.75 ± 0.47 cps/KBq). This led to the suggestion that the system could allow the development of dual-radiopharmaceutical procedures—for example, FDG and $^{99m}$Tc-sulfur colloid.

Operated in beta-mode, the probe would be used to localize and guide the complete excision of the FDG-avid primary, while in gamma-mode it could locate a gamma-emitting radionuclide like $^{99m}$Tc. Indeed, a previous study using sham lesions and an anthropomorphic phantom demonstrated the potential of this system to localize tumor remnants after excision of the bulk tumor (15).

The commercially available Beta probe (IntraMedical Imaging, Los Angeles) has 2 detectors: 1 that predominantly detects positrons, and another that detects only gamma rays. Because gamma rays travel several centimeters in tissue, both detectors register counts emanating from distant tissues and not from the tissue under examination. Therefore, by subtracting the counts of the second detector from the first detector, the counts generated by positrons only are determined. Because positrons can travel only a couple of millimeters, this corrected count is an indication of local concentration of FDG within a couple of millimeters. The Beta probe's 2 detectors are not the same shape, and therefore do not have the same efficiency for gamma rays. Before subtracting from the first detector, the counts of the second detector should be multiplied by a weighting factor representing this difference in efficiency. This factor is stored in the system, and the result of the weighted subtraction, which is the pure positron count, is reported to the surgeon on-screen and updated each second.

Ultimately a hybrid gamma and beta device—for example the PET-Probe by IntraMedical Imaging—may be found to be best suited for intraoperative FDG localization, because the gamma probe could be used to identify tumors and the beta probe to evaluate surgical margins (13).

## Clinical Trials

### Gamma Detector Probes for Fluorine-18

Due to the high efficacy of FDG-PET, it was only a natural extension for investigators to use the gamma detector probes to identify FDG-avid tissue during surgery. In a study at Ohio State University, Desai et al. (20) investigated the feasibility of detection of FDG in tumor deposits using CdZnTe crystal (7 mm diameter, 2 mm thick). Fasted patients were given an IV bolus of FDG (4.0 to 5.7 mCi) 15 to 20 minutes prior to preparation for surgery. Catheterization and the diuretic furosemide were used to remove FDG activity from the bladder. The time from FDG injection to intraoperative probe data acquisition varied from 58 to 110 minutes. Using the gamma detector probe, they were able to detect in all patients background activity in normal tissues (aorta, colon, liver, kidney, abdominal wall, mesentery, and urinary bladder). The probe correctly identified single or multiple tumor foci in 13 out of 14 patients, as noted by an audible signal from the control unit (3 standard deviations above counts obtained from normal tissues). These tumor foci corresponded to regions of high FDG uptake, as seen on FDG-PET scans. The patient in whom the probe did not localize the lesion had a recurrent mucin-producing pseudomyxoma tumor consisting mainly of acellular, mucinous deposits. Ex-vivo gamma detector probe evaluations demonstrated significant tumor-to-normal adjacent tissue activity (audible signals in 6 out of 6 tumor samples tested). They concluded that this data demonstrate that tumors identified from preoperative, whole-body PET scans can be localized during surgery using a gamma probe detector and FDG.

Essner et al. (21) have performed a clinical trial evaluating the use of the gamma probe to detect FDG-avid solid malignancies. Eight patients with metastatic cancer (2 colon tumors and 6 melanomas) with a limited number of site of metastasis were enrolled. Each received a preoperative injection of 7 to 10 mCi of FDG. At surgery, the probe was used to detect radioactive counts from the known tumor sites (previous scan) and the adjacent normal tissue. Based on the results of the preoperative PET scans, 17 tumors were identified; 13 were resected, and 4 were found to be unresectable during surgery. Of the 17 tumors assessed in vivo, tumor-to-background ratio varied from 1.16 : 1 to 4.67 : 1 for the melanoma patients (13 tumors), and from 1.19 : 1 to 7.92 : 1 for the colon cancer patients (4 tumors).

Ratios were calculated from counts obtained from tumor and background sites simultaneously, to avoid bias in data related to the decay of $^{18}$F and the difference in counts from the onset of the procedure to more delayed counts (up to 4 hours later). Eight (62%) of the 13 melanoma metastases and 3 (75%) of the 4 colon cancer metastases met the criterion of a tumor-to-background ratio of at least 1.5 : 1. Analysis was also done according to the time of surgery. One patient had a tumor-to-background ratio of 1.19 : 1 when surgery was initiated within 30 minutes after injection of FDG. Count ratios ranged from 1.26 to 7.92 : 1 for tumors in which surgery was performed 30 to 60 minutes after injection of FDG. Seventy-five percent of these tumors met their criteria of a ratio of 1.5 : 1. Count ratios varied from 1.16 to 4.67 : 1, and 57% met their ratio criteria when surgery was performed from 60 to 180 minutes from injection of FDG.

The 13 resected tumors ranged in size from 0.60 to 8.2 cm. They found no relationship between the tumor size and the count ratios, although the smallest resected specimen had a count ratio of 2.9 : 1, suggesting that the probe was able to identify subcentimeter tumors from adjacent normal tissue. The lowest count ratio (1.16 : 1) was from a 2-cm melanoma metastasis, and the highest count ratio (7.92 : 1) was from a 4.5-cm colon cancer metastasis.

## Gamma Detector and Beta Probes

Zervos et al. (22) have tested both a gamma detector and a beta probe in a tumor "phantom". They used both probes in the operating room on 10 patients with recurrent colorectal cancer who had positive PET scans pre-operatively. They were able to identify all sites, with tumor-to-normal ratios of 1.6 beta and 1.5 gamma. All probe-positive tissue was histologically confirmed to be recurrent colon cancer.

Raylman also tested the feasibility of using a dual probe. He has suggested its use in breast cancer, acknowledging that FDG is perhaps the optimal choice for this purpose, given its good targeting to breast carcinoma (23). It has good beta-detection sensitivity for $^{18}$F with the probe in the beta-optimized mode. Switching the probe into the gamma-optimized mode, sentinel nodes in the axilla could also be localized during the same surgical procedure. This is possible thanks to the good detection sensitivity for 140 keV photons and the high concentration of sulfur colloid in sentinel lymph nodes (23) in spite of the presence of FDG in the patient.

In another study, the feasibility of using FDG in conjunction with a positron-sensitive intraoperative probe to guide breast tumor excision was also investigated (23). The ability to localize breast cancers in vivo was tested in a rodent model. Mammary rat tumors implanted in Lewis rats were examined after injection with FDG; these results were correlated with those of histologic analysis. Measurements of line-spread functions indicated that resolution could be maximized in a realistic background photon environment by increasing the energy threshold to levels at or above the Compton continuum edge (340 keV). At this setting, the probe's sensitivity was determined to be 58 and 11 cps/µCi for 3.18-mm and 6.35-mm diameter simulated tumors, respectively. Probe readings correlated well with histologic results: the probe was generally able to discriminate between tumor and normal tissue. This study indicates that surgery guided by a positron-sensitive probe warrants future evaluation in breast-conserving surgery of patients with breast cancer.

## Studies with Positron-Sensitive Probe

In a preliminary report presented at a meeting (24), Gulec et al. described the use of IntraMedical Imaging's PET probe in a prospective study of 35 patients to evaluate detection sensitivity and clinical utility. All patients had preoperative diagnostic, whole-body FDG-PET scans and computed tomography and/or magnetic resonance imaging of the suspected regions. The patients underwent surgical exploration using the PET-probe 1 to 4 hours after injection of 10 mCi of FDG on the day of surgery. The primary surgical indication was exploration of known or suspected recurrent metastatic disease (melanoma, 26; colon cancer, 3; breast cancer, 1; thyroid cancer, 1; lymphoma, 1; seminoma, 1; unknown primary, 1; sarcoidosis, 1). PET-Probe detected all FDG-PET image-positive lesions. The smallest detectable lesion was 0.5 cm. The anatomic locations of the lesions were the neck and supraclavicular (n = 5), axilla (n = 5), groin and deep iliac (n = 3), trunk and extremity subcutaneous (n = 3), abdominal and retroperitoneal (n = 17), and lung (n = 2). In 4 cases (11%), PET-Probe identified lesions that were not seen on PET images. In 5 cases (14%), PET-Probe detected surgically nonpalpable or visible lesions, 2 of which were under 1 cm. In 13 of 35 patients (37%), PET-Probe findings positively affected the intraoperative management by localizing the lesion in an anatomically difficult location, by identifying a lesion outside the planned resection limits, or by identifying residual disease post-resection. They concluded that the use of the PET-Probe improves the success of surgical exploration in selected indications.

## The Future of Positron-Guided Surgery

The use of PET-guided surgery is evolving. New PET probes are being created, with better detection capacities. Yamamoto et al. (25) reported the development of a positron probe with background rejection capacities. The probe uses a Phoswich detector composed of a plastic scintillator and a bismuth germanate (BGO) crystal, resulting in a spatial resolution of 11 mm full-width-at-half-maximum and a measured sensitivity for the $^{18}$F point source of 2.6 cps/KBq, 5 mm from the detector surface. The background count rate was less than 0.5 cps for a 20-cm diameter cylindrical phantom containing 37 MBq of $^{18}$F solution.

An endoscope that would enable radionuclide-guided endoscopy is another possibility for development (25). In addition, the initial use of a PET mammography device (26) and the known advantage of PET for detecting occult disease (27) are only the first steps in PET-guided breast surgery. These are just the start of exploration in this interesting field.

# References

1. Wahl RL, Hutchins GD, Buchsbaum DJ, et al. $^{18}$F-2-deoxy-2-fluoro-D-glucose uptake into human tumor xenografts. Feasibility studies for cancer imaging with positron-emission tomography. *Cancer.* 1991; 67:1544–1550.

2. Dienel GA, Cruz NF, Mori K, et al. Direct measurement of the lambda of the lumped constant of the deoxyglucose method in rat brain: determination of lambda and lumped constant from tissue glucose concentration or equilibrium brain/plasma distribution ratio for methyl glucose. *J Cereb Blood Flow Metab.* 1991;11:25–34.

3. Gorospe L, Raman S, Echeveste J, et al. Whole-body PET/CT: spectrum of physiological variants, artifacts and interpretative pitfalls in cancer patients. *Nucl Med Commun.* 2005;2 71–687.

4. Zervos EE, Badgwell BD, Burak WE Jr, et al. Fluorodeoxyglucose positron emission tomography as an adjunct to carcinoembryonic antigen in the management of patients with presumed recurrent colorectal cancer and nondiagnostic radiologic workup. *Surgery.* 2001;130:636–643.

5. Desai DC, Zervos EE, Arnold MW, et al. Positron emission tomography affects surgical management in recurrent colorectal cancer patients. *Ann Surg Oncol.* 2003;10:59–64.

6. Sweet WH. The use of nuclear disintegration in the diagnosis and treatment of brain tumor. *N Engl J Med.* 1951; 245:875–878.

7. Harvey WC, Lancaster JL. Technical and clinical characteristics of a surgical biopsy probe. *J Nucl Med.* 1981;22: 184–186.

8. Aitken DR, Hinkle GH, Thurston MO, et al. A gamma-detecting probe for radioimmune detection of CEA-producing tumors. Successful experimental use and clinical case report. *Dis Colon Rectum.* 1984; 27:279–282.

9. Thurston MO. Development of the gamma-detecting probe for radioimmunoguided surgery. In: Martin EW Jr, ed. *Radioimmunoguided Surgery (RIGS) in the Detection and Treatment of Colorectal Cancer.* Vol. 2. Austin: RG Landes; 1994:42–65.

10. Schneebaum S, Even-Sapir E, Cohen M, et al. Clinical applications of gamma-detection probes—radioguided surgery. *Eur J Nucl Med.* 1999;26(suppl):S26-S35.

11. Yasuda S, Makuuchi H, Fujii H, et al. Evaluation of a surgical gamma probe for detection of $^{18}$F-FDG. *Tokai J Exp Clin Med.* 2000;25:93–99.

12. Haigh PI, Glass EC, Essner R. Accuracy of gamma probes in localizing radioactivity: in-vitro assessment and clinical implications. *Cancer Biother Radiopharm.* 2000;15:561–569.

13. Essner R, Daghighian F, Giuliano AE. Advances in FDG PET probes in surgical oncology. *Cancer J.* 2002;8:100–108.

14. Daghighian F, Mazziotta JC, Hoffman EJ, et al. Intraoperative beta probe: a device for detecting tissue labeled with positron or electron emitting isotopes during surgery. *Med Phys.* 1994;21:153–157.

15. Raylman RR. A solid-state intraoperative probe system. *IEEE Trans Nucl Sci.* 2000; 47:1696–1703.

16. MacDonald LR, Tornai MP, Levin CS, et al. Small area, fiber coupled scintillation camera for imaging beta-ray distributions intraoperatively. *Proc SPIE: Int Soc Opt Eng.* 1996;2551:92–101.

17. Tornai MP, MacDonald LR, Levin CS, et al. Design considerations and initial performance of a 1.2 cm$^2$ beta imaging intraoperative probe. *IEEE Trans Nucl Sci.* 1996;43:2326–2335.

18. Tornai MP, Levin CS, MacDonald LR, et al. Development of a small area beta-detecting probe for intraoperative tumor imaging (abstract). *J Nucl Med.* 1995;36(suppl): 106p.

19. Raylman RR. Performance of a dual solid state intraoperative probe system with $^{18}$F, $^{99m}$Tc, and $^{111}$In. *J Nucl Med.* 2001;42:352–360.

20. Desai DC, Arnold M, Saha S, et al. Correlative whole-body FDG-PET and intraoperative gamma detection of FDG distribution in colorectal cancer. *Clin Positron Imaging.* 2000;3:189–196.

21. Essner R, Hsueh EC, Haigh PI, et al. Application of an [$^{18}$F]fluorodeoxyglucose-sensitive probe for the intraoperative detection of malignancy. *J Surg Res.* 2001;96:120–126.

22. Zervos EE, Desai DC, DePalatis LR, et al. $^{18}$F-labeled fluorodeoxyglucose positron emission tomography-guided surgery for recurrent colorectal cancer: a feasibility study. *J Surg Res.* 2001;97:9–13.

23. Raylman RR, Fisher SJ, Brown RS, et al. Fluorine-18-fluorodeoxyglucose-guided breast cancer surgery with a positron-sensitive probe: validation in preclinical studies. *J Nucl Med.* 1995;36:1869–1874.

24. Gulec SA, Daghighian F, Edwards K, et al. Clinical utility of PET-probe in oncologic surgery (abstract). *Ann Surg Oncol.* 2005;12(suppl):S10.

25. Yamamoto S, Matsumoto K, Sakamoto S, et al. An intraoperative positron probe with background rejection capability for FDG-guided surgery. *Ann Nucl Med.* 2005;19: 23–28.

26. Rosen EL, Turkington TG, Soo MS, et al. Detection of primary breast carcinoma with a dedicated, large-field-of-view FDG PET mammography device: initial experience. *Radiology.* 2005;234:527–534.

27. Pecking AP, Mechelany-Corone C, Bertrand-Kermorgant F, et al. Detection of occult disease in breast cancer using fluorodeoxyglucose camera-based positron emission tomography. *Clin Breast Cancer.* 2001;2:229–234.

# 4
# Gamma Ray Imaging Probes for Radioguided Surgery and Site-Directed Biopsy

Francesco Scopinaro and Alessandro Soluri

## Background

The imaging probe is a small field-of-view, portable, handheld, high-resolution gamma ray detector that aids the surgeon in finding specific targets either to be removed in the surgical field (such as sentinel lymph nodes or occult tumor lesions) or to be localized for transcutaneous needle biopsies (suspect lesions). High-resolution detectors can be defined as gamma cameras with spatial resolution better than 4 mm, which is the lower limit of the intrinsic resolution of Anger cameras. Radioguided surgery requires rapid and precise detection, as is generally (but not always) provided by simple probes with acoustic signaling, which will be referred to here as simple probes. Imaging probes are useful when intraoperative images help surgeons address small, sometimes deep, structures that have to be removed, and functional imaging also sometimes aids in precise guidance of a biopsy needle for x-ray-detected lesions. High-resolution images provided by imaging probes are useful in these instances, although some are not strictly surgical acts.

Confusion may sometimes arise regarding the terms. While imaging probe and handheld gamma camera are synonyms, handheld and portable (or mobile) detectors are not always the same. Detectors weighing about 1 kg or less can be held by the average man for the time necessary to achieve the required image—30 to 60 seconds, on average. However, those weighing 2 kg or more cannot be handled easily, and need some mechanical support that necessarily limits the camera movement. Finally, the term "mobile gamma camera" can also apply to a wheel-transported, conventional, regular-size camera, which obviously is not handheld.

As mentioned previously, high-resolution imaging is a prerequisite for any imaging probe. The development of high-resolution gamma imaging, as well as of imaging probes, has followed a limited number of basic technologies: an array of scintillation crystals coupled with a position-sensitive photomultiplier tube (PSPMT); an array of crystals coupled with photodiodes; or an array of semiconductor crystals, usually CdTe crystals, whose charge is directly read by dedicated electronics.

## History

The imaging probe is a rather young device, whose development began less than 10 years ago and which is still today produced as prototypes or small series. As stated previously, its development is closely tied to the development and technology of high-resolution gamma detectors.

The first handheld, high-resolution camera was patented by Soluri et al. in 1997 (1) and presented by Scopinaro and colleagues at the Mediterranean Congress of Nuclear Medicine "Radionuclides for Lymph Nodes" (Cyprus 1996) (2). It was called an imaging probe, and its field of view was slightly less than 1 square inch, similar to what is used today (Figure 4-1A). Its technology was of the crystal array-PSPMT type. Early valuable clinical results were obtained with imaging probes in the same year and presented at the 1999 congress of the European Association of Nuclear Medicine (Barcelona) (3). This device was built with CsI(Tl) crystal array-PSPMT technology, which was subsequently further developed by the same group (4–8). The term "imaging probe" was quickly adopted in the nuclear medicine community; in 1999, Hoffman et al. wrote an article on "intraoperative probes and imaging probes" (9).

Scopinaro et al. published the first series showing some interesting results on sentinel node detection (4) using this imaging probe, which had received some improvements on shielding, electronics, and software. Soluri et al. performed the first imaging probe-guided biopsies (6,10,11) of breast cancer with this prototype (Figure 4-1B), which had undergone further improvements based on clinical experience.

Gamma cameras based on crystal-photodiode coupling or on semiconductor crystals have often been

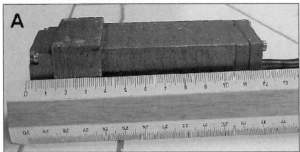
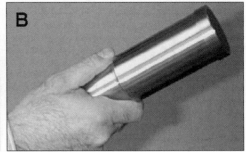
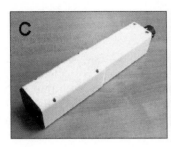
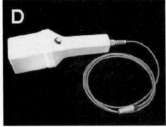
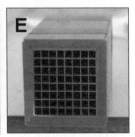

FIGURE 4-1. Evolution of the position-sensitive photomultiplier tube-based imaging probe, from 1999 to 2005. (A) The first 1-inch prototype, with a crystal matrix and hexagonal hole collimator. (B) The second prototype, with the same technique and faster electronics. (C) The present 1-inch prototype, showing a square-hole tungsten collimator with integrated crystals. (D) The present 2-inch prototype, with a square-hole tungsten collimator and integrated crystals. (E) Detail of the square-hole collimator.

classified as solid-state cameras. These technologies, studied previously for other detectors, have been developed for imaging probes since 2000. A small field-of-view portable camera based on CsI(Tl) crystals coupled with diodes was presented at the International Society for Optical Engineering in 2000 (Newport, RI) by MacDonald et al. and soon afterward tested by Narita et al. (12,13). Handheld cameras based on semiconductor crystal technology, mostly zinc cadmium telluride (ZnCdTe), started to be assembled as prototypes in 2001 (14–17). Although still quite heavy, these devices were ready for use in the operating room (sometimes requiring the help of a mechanical arm) and were tested on limited series of patients for sentinel lymph node detection (16). In 2002 Pitre et al., who had already studied solid-state cameras (18), used an interesting and probably cheap imaging probe (19) built with a continuous planar crystal, rather than a multicrystal array, coupled with a PSPMT. Pitre and colleagues reported some, although limited, results in sentinel lymph node detection.

In 2001, Soluri et al. patented the technology of crystals integrated into the collimator holes (20). Imaging probes built with this technology (Figures 4-1C, 4-1D, and 4-1E) exhibited much better resolution and sensitivity than the former ones, and had an important impact on several fields of radioguided surgery and biopsy, as well as in small animal imaging (21).

At present, more than 1 handheld camera for radioguided surgery has been developed. Diagnostic results are reported on small series, but related to several fields of applications of radioguided surgery. These results are consistent with the pioneer characteristics of diagnostic trials with new and often prototypal devices. The pioneering use of these new devices has suggested new fields for radioguided surgery (6,22,23) that should be explored more extensively.

## Device Characteristics

### Small Field-of-View Cameras Built with Scintillating Crystals and a Position-Sensitive Photomultiplier Tube

These cameras, among which is the first imaging probe, show a close relationship with intermediate field-of-view high-resolution cameras based on PSPMT, which began to be studied in the early 1990s (24–26) and continue to be explored today (27–29). Schematically, a multicrystal PSPMT gamma camera contains a collimator, an array of small crystals (30), a PSPMT, dedicated read-out electronics, and a dedicated computer.

The PSPMT accelerates the electrons (31) so that they generally remain in the position in which they were split by light beams coming from crystals on the bi-alkali cathode. A resistive chain collects charges at the anodes. Signals then undergo analog/digital conversion, and are processed and sent to the computer. Direct readout of anode charges is also possible: single anode readout generally gives more precise signals in comparison with the resistive chain (32,33). Energy tuning of these cameras can be precise, but the methods are complex.

Collimation is important: high resolution requires high counts per area unit, thus high transmission through the collimator. However, if collimator holes are too short, the depth of high resolution is a few centimeters. This effect is sometimes acceptable, but not always. Radioguided surgery can require detection of deep lesions—for example, an osteoid osteoma (22) can be more than 5-cm deep. Another problem lies with the shape of the holes: commonly available collimators have hexagonal holes, which do not fit well with the square section of crystals. Thus, photons passing through 1 hexagonal hole hit mainly 1, but also the neighboring crystals. This phenomenon worsens spatial resolution by creating a considerable blurring effect, and also decreases efficiency because of the dispersion of energy. Moreover, energy tuning is difficult (8). The most advanced Hamamatsu PSPMTs are square shaped, and are either 1 square inch or 4 square inches in size (31). Such small size creates technical problems that were much less important with the previous circular PSPMT with 3-inch or 5-inch diameters.

In every PSPMT, photo-multiplication is less efficient at the periphery than on the center. This means that the same radiation is revealed with a lower number of electrons at the periphery, thus as lower energy photons. It is difficult to multiply the final charge collected at the periphery for the exact gain. This effect is further enhanced by the inexact fit of the hexagonal collimator holes on square crystals. Moreover, when area decreases this effect is more important—missing 3 to 4 mm over 5 inches is less important than missing the same border over 1 inch. Of course, to enlarge the energy windows would decrease the precision of measurements and worsen spatial resolution.

The most advanced imaging probe built by Soluri and colleagues uses a new concept collimator with crystals integrated in the collimator holes. This patented collimator (20) is made with tungsten blades 100 to 200 μm thick, which form square holes covering the whole area. Crystals the same size as the holes are inserted into the holes themselves. This collimator overcomes several problems, completely avoiding crystal crosstalk and enhancing transmission even with rather long (25 mm) septa, which in turn maintain high resolution at more than 5 cm distance of the radioactive source from the detector (Figure 4-1E). Geometrical transmission is high; all the crystal area is covered and 86.32% of the PSPMT area is exposed (8). Moreover, energy tuning is more precise; a particular advantage of this collimator is that exact positioning of light coming from the crystals allows precise tuning of the dedicated readout electronics without a boundary effect, and effective use of the entire field of view (8).

Several other collimators have been developed for high-resolution devices based on crystal array and PSPMT, as well as for other devices. These include pinhole, multi-pinhole, and coded aperture collimators. In our opinion, pinhole collimators have too low transmission for radioguided surgery, which requires precise but also fast imaging. The family of coded aperture collimators is quite interesting, but a discussion of the theory and types of coded aperture collimators is beyond the scope of this overview. In principle, a possible advantage is the lack of fixed shielding on the part of the crystals: aside from the crystal-containing square hole collimator (8,20), every parallel hole collimator shields part of the crystal area, as discussed above. In principle, crystal irradiation with coded aperture collimators is homogeneous, or more so than with hexagonal holes on arrays of square crystals. However, a disadvantage is that the crystal irradiation has to be somehow "decoded." Coded aperture collimators have been used on small field of view cameras based on PSPMT mainly for small animal imaging (34).

## Handheld Cameras Based on Semiconductor Crystals

Some semiconductor devices for medical imaging (Figure 4-2) have been developed in the last decade (35). Most are based on cadmium telluride (CdTe) or zinc cadmium telluride (CdZnTe). Other semiconductors, such as those with GaAs crystals, are still in an experimental phase (36).

CdTe and CdZnTe are direct converters of photons to energy, with no light conversion. Because of this, there is no spread of light and corresponding crosstalk, as occurs with scintillating crystals. CdTe and CdZnTe crystal arrays show less peripheral problems than crystal array-PSPMT systems, with peripheral dead zones of about or less than 1 mm. Semiconductors allow better energy resolution than the majority of scintillating crystals, and small angle compton scattering can be rejected much more easily by semiconductors than by scintillators. Thus, devices based on junctional crystals can use collimators shorter than those required by scintillating crystals. The spectrometric ability of junction crystals compensates the poor addressing ability of short collimators. The latter property at least works for superficial sources. Coded aperture collimators also have been used on these detectors.

The major technical problems in the development of imaging systems are: 1) temperature instability, because temperature fluctuations cause total count variations; 2) the polarization phenomenon that can degrade energy resolution; 3) homogeneity of crystals; and 4) the complexity of the electronics.

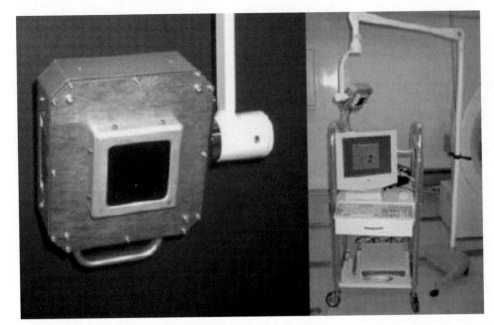

FIGURE 4-2. A typical ZnCdTe crystal camera. (Reprinted from Tsuchimochi M, Sakahara H, Hayama K, et al. A prototype small CdTe camera for radioguided surgery and other applications. Eur J Nucl Med Mol Imaging 2003;30(12):1605–14. With kind permission from Springer Science and Business Media.)

As with high-resolution cameras with scintillating crystals, semiconductor cameras are generally multicrystal cameras with 1.2 to 3 mm large elements, each provided with readout electronics. To form images, the electronic readout elements should be synchronised while showing homogeneous gain. Baumann recently described a CdTe camera (14), and Parnham a CdZnTe detector (37). A new prototype small CdTe gamma camera for radioguided surgery was reported by Tsuchimochi (15). This latter detector shows 32 cadmium telluride semiconductor arrays with a total of 1024 pixels (1.2 × 1.2 mm, 5 mm high), with application-specific integrated circuits (ASICs) and a tungsten collimator 10-mm long. Readout electronics consist of 8 ASICs, each with 128 channels to process an analog input signal from each CdTe pixel. The energy and position of the signals is digitized by analog-digital converters and transferred to a personal computer. Software controls the data acquisition. This detector shows 7.8% mean energy resolution at 140 keV and 1.5 mm spatial resolution. The camera's weight (described in 2003) was 2.7 kg—still heavy for a handheld camera, but suitable for use in surgery, if supported by a mechanical arm.

## Detectors Based on Crystal-Photodiode Matching

Digirad (Poway, CA) has developed a portable gamma camera, the 2020tc Imager, based on CsI(Tl) multicrystal scintillators and photodiode sensor (CsI(Tl)/PIN). The intrinsic energy resolution of this detector is about 10% FWHM, at 140 keV (13,38). Although CsI is a scintillating crystal, this type of detector is more similar to a semiconductor camera than to those using PSPMT. Photodiodes are fitted with each small CsI(Tl) crystal and directly convert light into electric charge. From a practical standpoint, each CsI(Tl)/PIN unit is thus somewhat similar to a semiconductor crystal. Readout electronics also show some similarities to semiconductors, and have similar problems. In principle, CsI(Tl)/PIN offers the advantages of semiconductor cameras, such as reduced peripheral dead zone and high energy resolution, and the benefits of the PSPMT.

## Experiences with Radioguided Surgery

As is characteristic of these types of pioneering diagnostic trials performed to validate prototypes, the studies have included only a limited number of patients.

### Sentinel Lymph Node Biopsy in Breast Cancer

The first validation of imaging probes generally occurs with sentinel lymph node biopsy, and this is the case with use of handheld gamma cameras in the operating room. Sentinel node biopsy is widespread and is performed using a variety of methods. Some groups perform lymphoscintigraphy with an Anger camera, followed by intraoperative node detection with a commercial probe fitted with acoustic signalling, while other teams confine themselves to only the latter procedure. Some groups will use vital dye techniques when radiocolloids miss the sentinel lymph node, whereas others fault the radiocolloid procedure for achieving variable rates of success and number of nodes identified. Thus, innovative methods would be welcomed.

After an initial learning stage, in 2000 Scopinaro et al. presented their first controlled trial with an imaging probe, in which the most interesting data were the reductions of the sentinel lymph node biopsy time (4) with use of the probe. This trial was carried out with the above-cited second-generation imaging probe. Similar studies by Schillaci et al. (39) and D'Errico et al. (40) with the same device confirmed Scopinaro's data. The data presented by Soluri et al. (41) with a third-generation imaging probe used in 50 cases not only further confirms that the same team of surgeons operates quicker when using an imaging probe, but also that the imaging probe detects the presence of a second node in a significantly higher number of patients than Anger camera lymphoscintigraphy plus conventional acoustic signaling detection. Finally, the same team used the imaging probe assisted by a laser beam pointer positioned on the detector's external shielding. The laser beam was guided by encoders and, once the nuclear physician had selected the "hot spot" on the computer, the laser beam indicated the hot spot site to surgeons after the imaging probe had been removed. The imaging probe-laser beam was used in operations on 5 patients using the radioguided occult lesion localization (ROLL) technique and sentinel lymph node biopsy (Figure 4-3), resulting in high effectiveness and precision. However, the procedure is quite complex and the use of robotised arms and laser pointers expensive (42,43).

Recently, Motomura et al. used the CsI(Tl)/PIN camera for sentinel node detection in 29 patients. In this experience, 1 node was identified by the Anger camera but not by their imaging probe, whereas 2 sentinel nodes were identified by the imaging probe alone, and not by the Anger camera (44).

In 2002, Pitre et al. (18) reported an interesting experience with their handheld camera based on a continuous NaI(Tl) crystal matched with a PSPMT. Their observations are comparable with those by Motomura et al. (44), in that some sentinel lymph nodes were only identified by the handheld camera and not by the Anger camera, and viceversa.

## Biopsy of Mammary Lesions

Weinberg and colleagues (45,46) proposed radioisotope guidance for breast cancer biopsy techniques. Soluri et al. performed the first radioguided biopsies of mammary lesions with an imaging probe in 2001 (6); just afterward, the same author mounted an imaging probe on a mammotome vacuum biopsy device and in 5 patients performed biopsies guided by $^{99m}$Tc-Sestamibi, after fusing the high-resolution radioisotope image with the stereotactic digital x-ray images. Shortly thereafter, the same researcher used this method to study new radiotracers and address the biopsy needle toward the region with the maximum uptake. He showed that in high-count mammotome samples, which correspond to high-count areas, the number of microvessels is significantly higher than in intermediate count samples of the same cancer; thus, the pathologist can use the radioisotope guide to find the most significant zone of the tumor to analyze. This result was achieved with both $^{99m}$Tc-Sestamibi and with the new tumor-seeking agent $^{99m}$Tc-bombesin (47).

In a third study by Di Santo and colleagues with the third-generation imaging probe, 10 women were submitted to radioguided biopsy; this short series confirmed previous diagnostic data obtained by Soluri et al. (6,47). The authors were also able to measure the target/background ratios of $^{99m}$Tc-Sestamibi and $^{99m}$Tc-bombesin obtained in vivo, with ex vivo counting of biopsy specimens (48). Unpublished experience by Soluri et al. now includes successful radioguided biopsies in 20 women with breast cancer.

## Thyroid and Parathyroid Surgery

Kitagawa and colleagues detected parathyroid glands with a portable detector made with semiconductor technology with full success in five cases (49).

Spanu et al. (50) used an imaging probe in localizing and characterizing small-size nodes in the thyroid that were not detected by the Anger camera, even when fitted with a pinhole collimator. The results were encouraging, but the study only involved 10 patients.

Studies on thyroid and parathyroid intraoperative high-resolution imaging are still preliminary, but at the moment show increasing interest, particularly from surgeons.

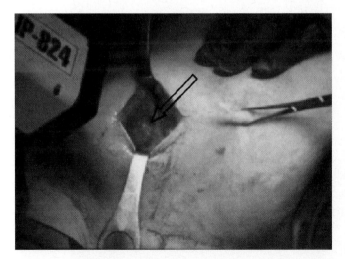

FIGURE 4-3. Surgery driven with an imaging probe, assisted by a laser beam pointer. The laser pointer continues to indicate the hot-spot site, even when the detector is moved away from the operation zone. The hot spot had been selected previously by a nuclear physician on the computer screen, when the imaging probe was in contact with the surgical wound.

## Bone Lesions

Excision of osteoid osteoma and detection of osteitis in patients with diabetic foot are the two main studies being conducted in this field with handheld high-resolution cameras.

Although the operation for osteoid osteoma is commonly called a biopsy, complete removal is mandatory to avoid recurrence and pain. Osteoid osteoma can be removed under radioguidance: the method is simple and cost effective, because the osteoid osteoma appears as a hot spot on the bone scan. Intraoperative imaging with a handheld, high-resolution camera was carried out by D'Errico and colleagues in 5 patients (22). This experience showed two definite advantages of imaging over acoustic signaling alone: 1) high-resolution imaging detects osteoid osteoma faster and much more clearly than acoustic signaling when osteoid osteoma is near radioactive sources, for example urine in the bladder; 2) high-resolution imaging clearly shows the presence of a double-nidus osteoid osteoma and is particularly useful in assessing complete resection (Figure 4-4).

Osteitis can pose an important clinical problem because of difficulties with antibiotic treatment. Early diagnosis and bone biopsy in the exact site of infection would be required. Soluri (51) and Scopinaro (23) used 2 different imaging probes in 10 patients with diabetic foot, who had been scheduled for surgery. Methods were complex; both authors used autologous leukocyte scans with early, intermediate, and late (20 to 24 hour) imaging, along with the imaging probe and Anger camera, and finally radioguidance with the imaging probe. Early osteitis of phalanges was present but not detected by the Anger camera in 4 patients. In both studies high-resolution imaging showed bone involvement in addition to soft tissue infection (not distinguished by imaging with the Anger camera) even before the operation; moreover, radioguidance was decisive for bone biopsy in 2 patients.

As mentioned previously, the method is complex, and the imaging probe had shown high precision and sensitivity, because of the low level of radioactivity present 24 hours after the administration of labeled leukocytes, which was minimal but nonetheless present.

## Conclusions

Since 1998, substantial technical progress has been made in the development of imaging probes and, more generally, high-resolution detectors. However, handheld high-

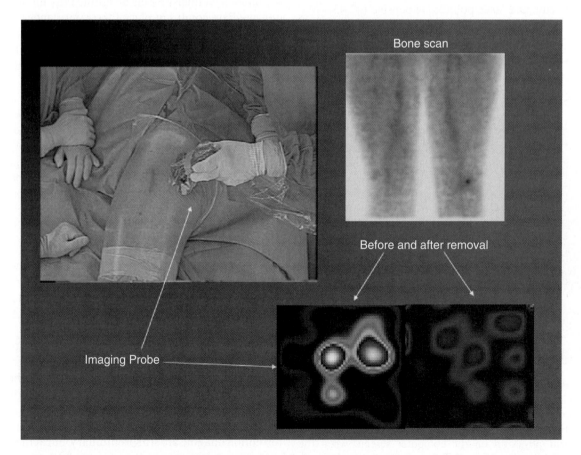

FIGURE 4-4. Excision of an osteoid osteoma. High-resolution scintigraphy with imaging probe shows 2 foci of osteoid osteoma, instead of the single focus shown by the bone scan (and by magnetic resonance and computed tomographic imaging).

resolution gamma cameras are not yet standardized and only recently have some cameras passed from prototypes to industrialized devices. Clinical studies are still in the form of pilot or feasibility studies. Scopinaro et al., who have the widest and most varied reports, have examined more than 100 cases so far, many of which have served to improve the detector.

The previously cited studies thus await validation of each method with multicentric studies on large cohorts of patients. If confirmed, the results obtained by investigators with different methods and differently designed devices will provide a valuable contribution to radioguided surgery. At present, imaging probes are complex detectors that promise to make radioguided surgery easier and more evidence-based. Moreover, use of these detectors will probably open new fields of interest for radioguided operations.

# References

1. Soluri A, et al, Italian National Research Council (CNR). Miniaturized gamma camera with very high spatial resolution. Italian patent RM97A000233. April 23, 1997; US patent 6 242 744 B1 del. June 5, 2001.
2. Scopinaro F, Di Luzio E, Pani R, et al. Sentinel node biopsy in breast cancer: use of an imaging probe. In: Limouris GS, Shukla SK, Biersack HJ. *Radionuclides for Lymph Nodes.* Athens: Mediterra Publishers; 1999: 60–65.
3. Scopinaro F, Pani R, Pellegrini R, Soluri A, De Vincentis G, Monteleone F. The imaging probe: a miniature gamma camera for sentinel node biopsy and radioimmunoguided biopsy. *Eur J Nucl Med.* 1999;26:96.
4. Scopinaro F, Pani R, Soluri A, et al. Detection of sentinel node in breast cancer: pilot study with the imaging probe. *Tumori.* 2000;86:329–331.
5. Soluri A, et al, Italian National Research Council (CNR). Miniaturized gamma camera with very high spatial resolution. US patent 6 242 744 B1. June 5, 2001.
6. Soluri A, Scafè R, Capoccetti F, et al. Imaging probe for breast cancer localization. *Nucl Instrum Methods A.* 2003;497:114–121.
7. Scopinaro F, Massa R. Role and perspectives of scintimammography. 2003;497:14–20.
8. Soluri A, Massari R, Trotta C, et al. New imaging probe with crystals integrated in the collimator's square holes. *Nucl Instrum Methods.* 2005;554:331–339.
9. Hoffman EJ, Tornai MP, Janecek M, Patt BE, Iwanczyk IS. Intraoperative probes and imaging probes. *Eur J Nucl Med.* 1999;26:913–935.
10. Soluri A, Scafe R, Falcini F, et al. New localization technique for breast cancer biopsy: mammotome guidance with imaging probe. *Tumori.* 2002;88:S37–S39.
11. Soluri A, Falcini F, Sala R, et al. Mammotome breast cancer biopsy: combined guide with x-ray stereotaxis and imaging Probe. *Nucl Instrum Methods A.* 2003;497: 122–128.
12. MacDonald LR, Bradly EP, Iwanczyk JS, et al. High-resolution handheld gamma camera. Medical application of penetrating radiations. *Proceedings SPIE.* 2000:4508–4512.
13. Narita H, Kawaida Y, Ooshita T, et al. Evaluation of efficiency of a multi-crystal scintillation camera Digirad 2020c imager using a solid state detector. *Kaku Igaku.* 2001;38: 355–362.
14. Baumann E, Bruin NM, Ijbema T, Fougeres P, Teule GJ. A prototype: pixelized small imaging CdTe probe for intraoperative use. *J Nucl Med.* 2001;42(suppl):203P.
15. Tsuchimochi M, Sakahara H, Hayama K, et al. A prototype small CdTe gamma camera for radioguided surgery and other imaging applications. *Eur J Nucl Med Mol Imaging.* 2003;30:1605–1614.
16. Abe A, Takahashi N, Lee J, et al. Performance evaluation of a handheld, semiconductor (CdZnTe)-based gamma camera. *Eur J Nucl Med Mol Imaging.* 2003;30:805–811.
17. Scheiber C. New developments in clinical applications of CdTe and CdZnTe detectors *Nucl Instrum Methods Phys Res A.* 1996;380:385–391.
18. Pitre S, Menard L, Charon Y. A high-resolution handheld gamma camera for cancer surgery. *J Nucl Med.* 2001; 42(suppl):202P.
19. Pitre S, Menard L, Richard M, Solal M, Garbai JR, Charon Y. A handheld imaging probe for radio-guided surgery: physical performance and preliminary clinical experience. *Eur J Nucl Med Mol Imaging.* 2003;30:339–343.
20. Soluri A, et al, Italian National Research Council (CNR). High spatial resolution scintigraphic device having collimator with integrated crystals. Italian patent RM2001A000279. May 23, 2001; US patent 6 734 430 B2. May 11, 2004.
21. Scopinaro F, Paschali E, Di Santo G, et al. Bombesin receptors and transplanted stem cells in rat brain: high-resolution scan with $^{99m}$Tc BN1.1. *Nucl Instrum Methods Phys Res A.* 2006;568:525–528.
22. D'Errico G, Rosa MA, Soluri A, et al. Radioguided biopsy of osteoid osteoma: usefulness of imaging probe. *Tumori.* 2002;88:S30–S32.
23. Scopinaro F, Capriotti G, Di Santo G, et al. High-resolution mini gamma camera for diagnosis and radioguided surgery in diabetic foot infection. *Nucl Instrum Methods.* 2006;569:269–272.
24. Pani R, Scopinaro F, Pellegrini R, Soluri A, Depaola A. Very high-resolution gamma camera based on position sensitive photo-multiplier. *Physica Medica.* 1993;9:233–236.
25. Scopinaro F, De Vincentis G, Pani R, et al. $^{99m}$Tc MIBI uptake in green plants. *Nucl Med Commun.* 1994;15:905–915.
26. Pani R, Pergola A, Pellegrini R, et al. New generation position sensitive PMT for nuclear medicine imaging. *Nucl Instrum Methods Phys Res A.* 1997;392:319–323.
27. Pani R, De Vincentis G, Scopinaro F, et al. Dedicated gamma camera for single photon emission mammography (SPEM). *IEEE Trans Nucl Sci.* 1998;45: 3127–3133.
28. Scopinaro F, Pani R, De Vincentis G, Soluri A, Pellegrini R, Porfiri LM. High-resolution scintimammography improves the accuracy of technetium-99m methoxyisobutylisonitrile scintimammography: use of a new, dedicated gamma camera. *Eur J Nucl Med.* 1999;26: 1279–1288.

29. Loudos GK, Nikita KS, Giokaris ND, et al A 3D high-resolution gamma camera for radiopharmaceutical studies with small animals. *Appl Radiat Isot.* 2003;58:501–508.

30. Blazek K, De Notaristefani F, Maly P, et al. YAP multi-crystal gamma camera prototype. *IEEE Trans Nucl Sci.* 1995;42:1474–1482.

31. Hamamatsu Photonics KK, Electron Tube Center. R8520-00-C12 Data Sheet, Technical Notes B-21, (2000).

32. Barone LM, Blazek K, Bollini D, et al. A detector for submillimeter gamma cameras. *Nucl Phys B.* 1995;44:729–733.

33. Pani R, Pellegrini R, Soluri A, et al. Eight-inch diameter PSPMT for gamma ray imaging. *IEEE Nucl Sci Symposium Med Imaging Conf Abstr.* 1997;131:1654–1658.

34. Garibaldi F, Accorsi R, Cinti MN, et al. Small animal imaging by single photon emission using pinhole and coded aperture collimation. *IEEE Trans Nucl Sci.* 2005;52:573–579.

35. Mori I, Takayama T, Motomura N. The CdTe detector and its imaging performance. *Ann Nucl Med.* 2001;15:487–494.

36. Bertolucci E, Maiorino M, Mettiver G, Montesi MC, Russo P. Preliminary test of an imaging probe for nuclear medicine using hybrid pixel detectors. *Nucl Instrum Methods Phys Res A.* 2002;487:193–201.

37. Parham KB, Grosholz J, Davies RK, Vydrin S, Cupec CA. Development of a CdZnTe-based small field of view gamma camera. *Proc 46th Annual Meeting SPIE.* 2001;4508:173.

38. Patt BE, Iwanczyk JS, Tornai MP, Hoffmann EJ, Rossington C. High-resolution CsI(Tl)/ Si-PIN detector for breast imaging. *IEEE Trans Nucl Sci.* 1998;45:2126–2131.

39. Schillaci O, D'Errico G, Scafè R, et al. Sentinel node detection with imaging probe. *Tumori.* 2002;88:S32–S35.

40. D'Errico G, Scafè R, Soluri A, et al. One-inch field of view imaging probe for breast cancer sentinel node location. *Nucl Instrum Methods Phys Res A.* 2003;497:105–109.

41. Soluri A, Massari R, Trotta C, et al. Small field of view, high-resolution, portable gamma camera for axillary sentinel node detection. *Nucl Instrum Methods Phys Res.* 2006;569:273–276.

42. Soluri A. Radioguided surgery and open biopsy with real time laser profile and high-resolution scintigraphy co-registration. *Eur J Nucl Med.* 2004;31:S404.

43. Sala R, Zappa E, Manzoni S, Soluri A. Image-guided stereo biopsy. *Proc IMEKO, IEEE, SICE 2nd International Symposium on Measurement, Analysis and Modeling of Human Functions, 1st Mediterranean Conference on Measurement.* Genoa, Italy: 2004:267–272.

44. Motomura K, Nogonuchi A, Hashizume T, et al. Usefulness of a solid state gamma camera for sentinel node identification in patients with breast cancer. *J Surg Oncol.* 2005;89:12–17.

45. Weinberg IN, Berg WA, Pani R, Scopinaro F, Bakale G, Adler LP. Methodology for combining x-ray and metabolic images of nonpalpable primary breast cancers. *Eur J Nucl Med.* 1997;24:881.

46. Weinberg IN, Pani R, Pellegrini R, et al. Small lesion visualization in scintimammography. *IEEE Trans Nucl Sci.* 1997;44:1398–1402.

47. Soluri A, De Vincentis G, Varvarigou AD, Spanu A, Scopinaro F. $^{99m}$Tc [$^{13}$Leu] bombesin and a new gamma camera, the imaging probe, are able to guide mammotome biopsy. *Anticancer Res.* 2003;23:2139–2142.

48. Di Santo G, Archimandritis S, Soluri A, et al. High-resolution scintigraphy and $^{99m}$Tc Bombesin are able to guide mammotome biopsy and to detect lymph node invasion. *Nucl Instrum Methods Phys Res A.* 2006;569:171–174.

49. Kitagawa W, Shimizu K, Kumita S. Radioguided parathyroidectomy for primary hyperparathyroidism combined with video-assisted surgery using the solid state multi-crystal gamma camera. *J Surg Oncol.* 2002;80:173–175.

50. Spanu A, Soluri A, Scopinaro F, et al. A new radioisotopic procedure in small-size thyroid nodule detection: a preliminary study. *Eur J Nucl Med Mol Imaging.* 2003;30:S358.

51. Soluri A, Massari R, Trotta C, et al. High-resolution gamma camera and $^{99m}$Tc [HMPAO] leukocytes for diagnosis of infection and radioguided surgery in diabetic foot. *G Chir.* 2005;26:246–250.

# 5
# Radiation Protection in Radioguided Surgery

Edwin C. Glass and Wendy A. Waddington

The human population has always been exposed to low levels of ionizing radiation. Naturally occurring radioactive substances are present in all living organisms and in the environment, and ionizing radiation from space showers the planet continuously in the form of cosmic rays. The greatest single contribution to natural low-level radiation, however, is from radon, which accounts for more than half of ambient low-level radiation. Other sources are found in rocks and soil, as well as radioactive elements trapped in the body, such as $^{40}K$.

Since the discovery of x-rays by Roentgen in 1895, an additional source of radiation has evolved: medical applications. Medical radiation now contributes a significant portion—approximately 15%—of the total radiation exposure of the human population.

## Biological Effects of Radiation

When x-rays, gamma rays, or radioactive particles, such as alpha or beta particles, are stopped by tissue, their energy is deposited in the tissue. This deposition of energy generates free radicals in the tissue, which can alter biomolecules such as proteins and gene segments. Short-term cellular damage may ensue, or in the longer term, genetic alterations can occur that are manifest in the progeny of the irradiated cell lines.

Tissue damage induced by ionizing radiation is usually classified as either deterministic or stochastic. Deterministic effects are those that are predictably related to the dose of radiation received, such as sunburn from sun exposure—the longer one is out in the sun, the worse the sunburn. A threshold dose may exist for these effects, below which the effect does not occur (e.g., cataract formation resulting from radiation exposure). Stochastic effects, on the other hand, are probabilistic, and may or may not occur. The probability of their eventual occurrence, but not the severity, is related to the dose. An example of stochastic effect in this same context would

be the development of actinic skin cancer, where the likelihood of developing skin cancer is related to the amount of sun exposure, but where the "severity" of the cancer is not related to the dose.

## Measurement and Units of Radiation

The literature on radiation exposure from medical procedures can be confusing, even for persons who are classified as radiation workers. This is in part because of the differing terminologies used by writers. An Internet search for "radiation exposure from chest x-rays" yields hundreds of websites, with dozens of different units and quantities of radiation exposure from even this common, relatively standardized procedure.

Principal among the reasons for such confusion are the different units used to quantify radiation exposure. This chapter focuses on exposures measured only in body tissue, and not in the air or other materials. Three terms are commonly encountered here: tissue dose, equivalent dose, and effective dose.

First, tissue dose is expressed in standard international (SI) units of grays (Gy), or alternatively, in the United States, in special units of rads (1 joule/kilogram = 1 gray = 100 rad). It expresses the amount of energy deposited in tissue when radiation energy is absorbed within that tissue. Second, equivalent dose is determined by multiplying the radiation dose absorbed (in rads or grays) by weighting factors based on the type of radiation (e.g., x-rays or gamma rays, alpha particles, neutrons, etc.). To distinguish this quantity from tissue dose, the equivalent dose is expressed in Sieverts (Sv), although within the United States, this is still defined in rems. This holds true even if the radiation weighting factor is equal to 1, in which case the tissue dose and equivalent dose are numerically equal. Third, effective dose is determined by adding the weighted equivalent doses for all the organs in the body, applying another weighting factor for each organ that reflects its relative sensitivity to the effects of radiation. Because of the scattering of radiation in the body, as well as distribution throughout the body in the case of internal radioactive materials, the effective dose always encompasses a weighted sum of doses to all organs in the body.

Determinations of effective dose usually are expressed either as effective dose or as effective dose equivalent. Both terms represent the dose to the whole body, considering weighting factors for individual organs based on their relative radiosensitivities, but they use different organ risk-weighting factors. More recent factors for calculating effective doses were proposed and released in International Commission on Radiological Protection 60 (1990).

Effective dose is also expressed in the same units as equivalent dose (Sieverts or, within the United States, rems), but the expressions have distinct meanings. These units all have standard derivative terms, such as mrem (1/1000 of 1 rem), $\mu$Sv (1 millionth of 1 Sv), etc. Sieverts are the standard international units of measurement.

Readers also encounter quantities of radioactive materials expressed in units of either millicuries (mCi) or megabecquerels (MBq). Both express the number of atoms that decay per unit time. A becquerel is defined as a unit of radioactivity equal to the rate of 1 radioactive decay per second. A curie was historically defined as the radioactivity present within 1 gram of $^{226}$Ra, one of the first radionuclides isolated.

How are the units related? For x-rays and gamma rays, 1 rad of energy absorbed in tissue gives 1 rem of equivalent dose to that tissue. Similarly, 1 gray gives 1 Sievert of equivalent dose. Various units in the literature are related, as shown in Table 5-1. In medical literature dealing with radiation exposures from intraoperative procedures, these terms will be variously encountered and often intermingled.

The differences between equivalent dose, expressed in mrem or mSv, and effective dose, also expressed in the same units, should be considered. If a computed tomographic (CT) scan of the head is performed, the head will receive the highest dose of radiation, and the other parts of the body will receive lesser amounts, with the tissue doses falling off from the head toward the feet. However, to consider the net overall dose to the body and the potential overall risk to the individual, the concept of effective dose is introduced. Effective dose considers not only the scatter of radiation from one area to another,

but also the relative tissue volumes and their sensitivities. These considerations allow radiation exposures of different types to be compared in a somewhat standard fashion. In the case of the head CT, the effective dose, which is also measured in, say, mSv, will be significantly less than the equivalent dose to the head, even though both are expressed in the same terms of mrem or mSv.

Similarly, when a radiocolloid is injected into tissue, the local equivalent dose to that tissue is much higher than the effective dose to the body as a whole. When surgeons manipulate radioactive tissue, their hands will receive more radiation than their body as a whole. Persons with higher levels of concern about radiation doses usually choose to express the higher equivalent dose, whereas those who seek to downplay the doses, such as vendors of radiation-producing machinery or radiopharmaceuticals, will detail exposures as a dose to the whole body or effective dose. In best practice, both figures should be expressed, but that is not often done. In the case of a CT scan of the head, for example, the eyes receive equivalent doses of approximately 20 to 50 mSv, but the effective dose would be approximately 5 mSv (1).

The reason for using effective dose as a measure of the radiation dose received is that by weighing the individual organ doses according to their relative radiosensitivity and then summing them, the magnitude of the effective dose will be proportional to the total risk to the person arising from the stochastic effects to which all the individual organs are subject, specifically for induction of cancer. Thus, the radiation risk arising from a pelvic CT, barium swallow, radionuclide myocardial perfusion study, and a radionuclide thyroid scan may all be compared directly and objectively through their effective doses. The risk to a particular organ, however—such as the increment in risk for breast cancer from a CT scan of the chest—is better represented by the equivalent dose to that organ.

## Natural Background Radiation

Natural background radiation exposure is generally considered to be delivered to the whole body. Background doses range approximately 2.5 to 3.0 mSv (250–300 mrem) per year (Figure 5-1). This exposure results from terrestrial sources, radon that escapes from the earth into the air we breathe, and cosmic sources. Persons living at higher altitudes experience exposures in the higher range because of lessened atmospheric protection for cosmic radiation.

In addition, individuals living in some mountainous areas experience higher levels of ambient radiation because of naturally occurring radon and other unstable substances that are more prevalent in the rocks and soil of certain parts of the world. Extremely wide varia-

TABLE 5-1. Common units of radiation measurement.

| | |
|---|---|
| 1 Gy = 100 rads | 1 rad = 0.01 Gy = 1 cGy |
| 1 Sv = 100 rem | 1 rem = 0.01 Sv = 10 mSv |
| 1 mSv = 100 mrem | 1 mrem = 0.01 mSv = 10 microSv |
| 1 microSv = 0.1 mrem | 1 mCi = 37 MBq; 1 MBq = 0.027 mCi |

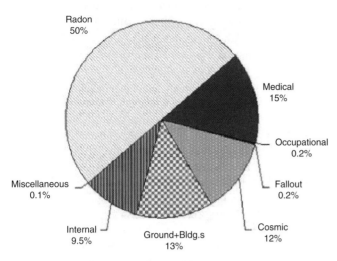

Average annual dose (2005) to the U.K. population 2.7 mSv

Radon 50%

Medical 15%

Occupational 0.2%

Fallout 0.2%

Miscellaneous 0.1%

Internal 9.5%

Ground+Bldg.s 13%

Cosmic 12%

FIGURE 5-1. Radiation dose to the public within the United Kingdom. (Adapted from Watson SJ, Jones AL, Oatway WB, Hughes JS. Ionising Radiation Exposure of the UK Population: 2005 Review. Health Protection Agency, HPA-RPD-001.) Available at: http://www.hpa.org.uk/radiation/publications/hpa_rpd_reports/2005/hpa_rpd_001.pdf. Accessed January 7, 2007.)

tions—by factors of 10 or more—in the prevailing level of natural background radiation have been measured across the planet; in some isolated locations defined by their uranium or radon-rich geology, radiation exposure levels may reach or even exceed a few hundred mSv per annum (2). Nevertheless, no increase in risk has been identified with these higher levels of exposure, and no differential levels of risk have been correlated with this wide geographic variability.

By comparison to these levels of natural exposure, examples of exposures from common medical tests are: chest x-ray (2 views), 0.02 to 0.12 mSv (2–12 mrem); CT of body, 8 to 20 mSv (800–2000 mrem); $^{99m}$Tc-Sestamibi cardiac scan, 8 to 25 mSv (800–2500 mrem) (1,3). These exposures vary considerably, depending on factors that are particular to the study. In the case of CT, settings employed for tube current, the number of slices acquired, and many other factors significantly affect the dose to the patient. With scans using $^{99m}$Tc, the radiation dose increases in proportion to the amount of $^{99m}$Tc injected in the patient. Tobacco smokers also receive additional radiation exposure from radioactive substances inhaled in smoke.

## Limitation and Control of Radiation Doses

Radiation is used in medical environments to gather information about patients and disease processes. In general, the use of more radiation gives more information: for example, clearer, more diagnostic images in nuclear medicine and CT. However, to control this tendency, limits are set on radiation burdens for the patient, and statutory limits are also placed on permissible exposures for personnel classified as medical radiation workers. Additionally, the concept of "As Low As Reasonably Achievable" (ALARA) stands as an overriding principle that constrains radiation use. These principles dictate prudence in the medical uses of radiation, with the aim of optimizing radiation usage in consideration of patient care, economic and environmental concerns, worker safety, and other factors.

Facilities and institutions that make use of radioactive materials need to be licensed. This is done to control the receipt, possession, use, transfer, and disposal of licensed material, and to ensure that the user is fully trained in the safe and appropriate use of the material. The licensee is responsible for using the material in such a manner that the total dose to an individual (including doses resulting from licensed and unlicensed radioactive material, and from radiation sources other than background radiation) does not exceed legislated standards for protection against radiation. In the United States, these regulations are set forth in 10 CFR§ 20.

## Role of Radiation Safety Personnel and Institutional Policy

The policies and procedures for handling radioactive materials, including injectable tracers or radioactive tissue specimens, must be developed in conjunction with the radiation safety officer at each institution licensed to use radioactive materials. The procedures adopted at each institution must fall within the scope of their licensure. In the United States, the radiation safety officer has the overall responsibility for: 1) developing safety procedures; 2) monitoring and minimizing exposure risk to all personnel; and 3) determining whether, where, and when surveys and measurements of radioactivity should be used. This person is also responsible for training the staff in surgery, pathology, environmental management, nuclear medicine, and other areas with respect to radiation safety issues. In the United Kingdom, the radiation protection advisor has a similar role. The procedures should consider and encompass all stages in the acquisition, handling, processing, distribution, and eventual decay and disposal of radioactive materials. Each service and laboratory should set forth rules for the safe handling of radioactive materials, including $^{99m}$Tc-labeled tissue specimens and procedures for managing radioactive patients. These procedures will vary among institutions, because of the different demands for patient care, regulations, patient populations, and staff expectations.

## Limits for the General Public

The total effective dose (ed) to individual members of the public from an operation licensed to use radioactive materials should not exceed 1 mSv (0.1 rem = 100 mrem) in a year (Canada, EU, and United States). In the United States, public areas with ambient exposure rates below 2 mrem per hour (20 µSv/hr) do not require restricted access or designation as radiation areas (10 CFR § 20.1301). In the UK, the corresponding level is 0.5 µSv/hr.

## Limits of Exposure for Radiation Workers

Workers are classified as radiation workers according to statutory limits. When employees can reasonably be expected to receive over certain amounts of radiation exposure in the course of their work in a defined period of time, they are classified as radiation workers. In the United States, these limits are defined in 10 CFR § 20.1502 and 10 CFR § 20.1201.

An adult employee in the United States is classified as a radiation worker if the person can be expected to receive more than 10% of the amounts permitted annually for radiation workers in the course of employment. The annual limits for radiation workers in the United States are: 1) a total effective dose equivalent being equal to 5 rem (0.05 Sv); 2) a sum of the equivalent deep-dose and the committed equivalent dose to any individual organ or tissue, other than the lens of the eye, being equal to 50 rem (0.5 Sv); 3) an equivalent dose of 15 rem (0.15 Sv) to the lens of the eye; and 4) a shallow equivalent dose of 50 rem (0.5 Sv) to the skin of the whole body or the skin of any extremity. These amounts do not include other exposure the person might incur from background radiation, medical administrations, exposure to individuals administered radioactive material and released under 10 CFR § 35.75, voluntary participation in medical research programs, and the licensee's disposal of radioactive material into sanitary sewerage in accordance with 10 CFR § 20.2003. Adults whose exposure is likely to exceed these 10% threshold levels should be classified as radiation workers, receive appropriate training in radiation safety, and be monitored with personal dosimetry devices.

In the EU, any member of the public receiving a whole body radiation dose greater than the 1 mSv annual limit should be defined as a radiation worker, and the following annual dose limits then apply: 1) a whole-body effective dose of 20 mSv (0.02 Sv or 2 rem); 2) an equivalent dose to the lens of the eye of 150 mSv (15 rem); 3) or an equivalent dose to an extremity of the body (e.g., hands)

of 500 mSv (50 rem). The employer is additionally required to make all reasonable efforts to reduce a worker's dose to below a "classification level" set at three-tenths of any of these limits; if this is not possible, then the worker must be subject to increased health surveillance, among other requirements.

To safeguard the unborn, special (lower) exposure limits and restrictions are placed on workers who declare themselves to be pregnant. In the United States, these are defined in 10 CFR § 20.1208. These limits vary between nations, but it is important that personnel involved in sentinel node or other procedures requiring radioactive materials be cognizant of the applicable restrictions. They should use the expertise of their local radiation safety personnel to ensure compliance. This entails badge monitoring on the abdomen, and might entail changes in work assignments. The risk of exposure due to possible contamination must also be assessed and minimized—for example, such as that caused by an accident during the administration of the radiolabeled tracer.

In general, several studies have confirmed the theoretical calculated predictions that under normal working conditions, staff members in pathology, courier, and environmental care are not likely to reach prevailing threshold dose limits requiring their designation as a radiation worker in any country mentioned previously. These considerations are addressed in greater detail in the following sections.

## Estimating Radiation Exposure from Radioisotopes

Exposure from a source of radiation will increase in direct proportion to the strength of the source and the duration of exposure. As distance from a focal source of radioactivity increases, the exposure rate diminishes in proportion to the inverse square of the distance. The pattern of drop-off for larger, more disseminated sources of activity—such as in a patient—does not mirror this rule exactly, but it follows its characteristics sufficiently well enough to be used as good general guidance.

The strengths of the emissions from most common radionuclides are known, and several are presented in Table 5-2. The units of these constants are presented in 3 forms in the table. To estimate exposure, multiply the rate constant by the dose and time of exposure, and divide by the square of the distance. For example, the exposure from 20 MBq of $^{99m}$Tc at 2 meters for 2 hours would be: $(0.021 \times 20 \text{ MBq} \times 2 \text{ hours})/(2 \text{ meters} \times 2 \text{ meters}) = 0.21$ microGy.

This method can be refined when radioactive decay, attenuation, scattered radiation, and other factors are

TABLE 5-2. Exposure rate constants[†], half lives, and gamma energies.

| Isotope | mR×m²/(mCi-hr) | μGy-m²/(MBq-hr) | mR-ft²/(mCi-hr) | Half life | Gamma ray emission (keV) |
|---|---|---|---|---|---|
| $^{99m}$Tc | 0.078 | 0.021 | 0.84 | 6 hours | 140 |
| $^{201}$Tl | 0.047 | 0.013 | 0.51 | 3.04 days | 72 |
| $^{131}$I | 0.217 | 0.059 | 2.34 | 8.04 days | 364 |
| $^{123}$I | 0.16 | 0.043 | 1.72 | 13 hours | 159 |
| $^{111}$In | 0.32 | 0.086 | 3.44 | 2.8 days | 173, 247 |
| $^{11}$C | 0.591 | 0.160 | 6.36 | 20 minutes | 511 (β⁺) |
| $^{18}$F | 0.573 | 0.155 | 6.17 | 108 minutes | 511 (β⁺) |

[†]Reported values will vary slightly depending on method of measurement

β⁺ = positron decay

also being considered (4). Nevertheless, the simple approach outlined above can be useful as a radiation safety tool for generating upper-limit estimates of exposure.

## Radiation Exposure of Surgeons from Sentinel Lymph Node Procedures

Several issues should be considered regarding exposure of surgical staff to radiation. Since exposure is proportional to the time exposed, and decreases as the inverse square of distance from the source of the radioactivity, the highest calculated and measured doses are to the surgeon's hands. Doses to the surgeon's torso are lower by about an order of magnitude, and exposures of other staff, including assistant surgeons, anesthesia staff, and nurses in the operating room are lower by another order of magnitude (Table 5-3).

Exposure rates generally decrease as the inverse square of distance from the source of radioactivity in the patient. Accordingly, persons at a distance of more than 1 meter will not receive measurable amounts of radioactivity during even a 3-hour sentinel lymph node procedure. The exposure rate constant for $^{99m}$Tc (Table 5-2) is: 0.021 microSv × meter × meter/(MBq-hr). Therefore, the potential exposure to a worker from a 3-hour procedure at a distance of 1 meter from a patient with a 30 MBq dose injected would be: 0.021 × 30MBq × 3 hours/(1 meter × 1 meter) = 1.89 microSv (= 0.189 mrem).

Assuming a caseload of 100 cases per year, this would yield cumulative exposures of 189 microSv or 0.189 mSv (18.9 mrem).

Most available commercial badges for radiation monitoring have lower limits of detection of approximately 10 to 100 microSv (1–10 mrem). Thus, these potential exposures at 1 meter for 100 cases are well below the annual dose levels of 5 mSv (500 mrem) mandated for consideration of classification as a radiation worker in the United States (10 CFR § 20.1201 and 10 CFR § 20.1502). These exposures are also below the annual dose limits for the general public of 1 mSv (100 mrem) in the United States, as discussed previously and detailed in 10 CFR § 20.1301, and as required in Europe (EU) and Canada.

However, surgeons stand next to the patient's side, and their gloved hands are in close proximity to the foci of deposition of $^{99m}$Tc (or other) tracers. Surgical gloves offer protection from radioactive contamination of the surgeon's skin, but do not shield the 140 keV emissions from $^{99m}$Tc. Hence, surgeons receive significantly higher exposures than other surgical and anesthesia staff, and their hands in particular receive the highest doses.

It is instructive to consider surgeons' exposure first from a theoretical or calculated perspective, with subsequent discussion of documentations of exposures in the literature. The exposure rate constants of $^{99m}$Tc or other radioisotopes (see Table 5-2) can be used to calculate worst-case or other potential exposures under many different clinical scenarios. Actual radiation levels are almost always lower than the values calculated using

TABLE 5-3. Calculated estimates of exposures (microSv).

| | Hands | Surgeon, torso | Other Personnel |
|---|---|---|---|
| Distance (cm) | 2.5 cm | 30 cm | 100 cm |
| Short procedure (30 minutes) | 311 (31 mrem) | 4.32 | 0.39 |
| Long procedure (5 hours) | 3 108 (311 mrem) | 43.2 | 3.885 |
| General public, annual | Not applicable | 1000 (100 mrem) | |
| Level for classification as radiation worker (US) | 50,000 (5000 mrem) | 5000 (500 mrem) | |

TABLE 5-4. Reported radiation exposures.

| Author | Surgeon hands Equivalent dose microSv | Surgeon body Effective dose microSv | Pathologist Equivalent dose microSv |
|---|---|---|---|
| Waddington (13) | 90 | 0.34 | surgeon |
| Miner (6) | 94 | NR | NR |
| Mitsui (26) | 35 | 1.84 | 3.78 |
| De Kanter (9) | 18–61 | 8.2 | 0.4 |
| Brenner (27) | 42–420 | 1.8–18 | 22/hr (hands) |
| | 350 (35 mrem) | | 186 (18.6) hands |
| Stratmann (5) | per hr | 13.3 (1.33 mrem) per hr | 3.4 (0.34) torso |

Legend:
NR—not recorded

these rate constants, because many photons pass through the fingers, and some also pass through the torso (although most 140 keV photons are absorbed in the torso). Only absorbed photons impart energy—and accordingly, potential molecular damage—to tissue. It is also important to assign a realistic duration for the operative procedure. Stratmann et al. documented operating times of 30 minutes and 300 minutes for sentinel lymph node radiolocalization procedures for breast cancer and head and neck cancers, respectively (5).

Assuming a distance of 2.5 cm. ($2.5 \times 10^{-2}$ meters), operating times of 5 hours (300 minutes), with the surgeon's hands in close proximity for 50% of this time, and a dose of 37 MBq (1 mCi), the predicted dose to the fingers could be estimated as follows: from Table 5-2, the gamma exposure rate constant for $^{99m}$Tc is 0.021 microSv $\times$ meter $\times$ meter/(MBq-hr). The dose to the fingers would be: $0.021 \times 37$ MBq $\times 5$ hours $\times 50\%/(2.5 \times 10^{-2} \times 2.5 \times 10^{-2}) = 3108$ microSv $= 3.108$ mSv $= 310.8$ mrem. At 30 cm, the estimated torso dose would be $0.021 \times 37$ MBq $\times 5$ hours$/(0.3 \times 0.3) = 43.2$ microSv $= 0.0432$ mSv (4.32 mrem). For a 30-minute procedure, the exposures would be 10% of the values for 5 hours, or 0.31 mSv (31 mrem) to the hands and 4.32 microSv ($0.00432$ mSv $= 0.432$ mrem) to the torso. The results are presented in Table 5-3.

These calculated values should be regarded as upper-limit estimates, because they do not consider radioactive decay from the time of the injection to the operative procedure, attenuation of radiation within the patient, reduction of the radioactivity present after resection, variable fractional times when the hands are more distant from the radioactive tissue, and other factors that tend to mitigate the dose actually imparted to the surgeon.

From Table 5-3, it is apparent that a surgeon in the UK performing more than 200 cases per year (note: 200 = 1000 μSv per year/5 μSv per 30-minute procedure) could potentially exceed the threshold for classification as a radiation worker, and therefore require training and monitoring by the radiation safety officer. However, several recent studies have directly addressed the issue of exposures with measurements and other calculations, and the results from several of them are summarized in Table 5-4. Note that measured exposures are of the same order of magnitude as those predicted by calculations using exposure rate constants, but that actual exposures are lower than those predicted by these worst-case calculations.

Clearly then, 3 of the principal determinants of radiation exposure are: 1) the amount of radioactivity present in vivo at the time of the operative procedure, 2) the duration of the exposure to the source of radiation, and 3) the distance of the body, or body part under consideration, from the source of radiation.

The doses of radioactivity employed in sentinel lymph node procedures are small compared with those used in many other nuclear medicine procedures. Typical administered activities range from 10 to 45 MBq (0.3 to 1.2 mCi) of $^{99m}$Tc. By comparison, the typical activity of $^{99m}$Tc employed for a radionuclide bone scan is approximately 740 MBq (20 mCi).

Surgery duration obviously affects radiation exposure. Radiation exposures to surgeons of 10 and 2 mrem (0.1 and 0.02 mSv) have been reported for sentinel lymph node procedures for breast cancer and melanoma (6), respectively; higher values are reported for the same surgery for head and neck cancers, due to the significantly longer durations of these procedures (5).

Thus, most surgeons would not be expected to reach levels of exposure that would require them to be classified as radiation workers, although this consideration must be qualified depending on workload and case mix. Many are already monitored, however, because of their intraoperative use of x-ray or fluoroscopic devices.

## Radiation Exposure to Staff Other Than Surgeons

Personnel more distant from the patient receive significantly less radiation exposure than the surgeon, usually less than 1 microSievert per case. From Table 5-3, for example, assuming 1 microSv exposure per case and 300 cases per year (300 microSv dose), the subject would not reach the 1 mSv (1000 microSv) limit allowed for the general public in EU, Canada, and the United States. Hence, these individuals would not qualify as radiation workers. Notwithstanding, many personnel in the surgical suite wear radiation monitoring badges for other reasons, usually because they work in areas where x-ray-generating machines are used for other types of surgery, such as orthopedic procedures.

Other individuals who have casual or brief exposures as they pass by or briefly transport specimens, such as couriers and miscellaneous workers in pathology, experience inconsequential exposures. Nevertheless, these individuals should be informed if their work involves repeated exposures, so that their exposures remain low.

## Radiation Exposure to Pathology Staff Working with Radioactive Specimens

Since pathology staff members usually handle tissue specimens for shorter times than surgeons do, radiation exposures to their hands and torso are lower than those of surgeons [7–9]. Given the considerations, calculations, and reports discussed previously for sentinel node specimens, staff in pathology would not meet criteria for classification as radiation workers within the United States, and therefore do not require personal monitoring devices. In other countries the criteria for classification differ, but it is extremely unlikely that a pathology staff member handling such samples would receive an exposure to radiation that would require the person to be designated as a radiation worker.

## Transportation of Radioactive Tissue

Couriers should be informed if they are asked to transport radioactive specimens. However, their levels of exposure from specimens involved in sentinel node procedures are not usually sufficient to warrant their classification as radiation workers.

Tissues transported to other institutions require labeling and shipment according to restrictions on public transport of radioactive materials. In the United States, the labeling of packages containing radioactive materials is required by the Department of Transportation (DOT) if the amount and type of radioactive material exceed the limits for an excepted quantity or article, defined as 0.002 µCi/gm under DOT regulations 49 CFR §173.403 (m) and (w) and §173.421–425.

As an example of the situation within EU, the UK legislation restricts the transportation of radioactive materials by road vehicle to those persons who have been formally trained in the safe transport of these goods. In the case of $^{99m}$Tc, quantities of less than 4000 MBq that are transported within a suitable container and with a surface dose rate of less than 5 µSv/hr (for which the use of shielding should not normally be necessary) and bearing accompanying documentation are defined as "excepted packages." Packages whose radioactive specimen contains a total activity of less than 10 MBq, or an activity concentration of less than 100 Bq/gm, are not regarded as radioactive for the purposes of transportation. Transport "within an establishment . . . not involving the use of public roads," or by foot, even across a public highway, is exempt from these regulations.

## Cryotome Specimens

If frozen sections are employed during surgery, such as to evaluate nodal status, some contamination of the equipment used for sectioning the tissue results [6]. The quantity of this contamination is minimal in the case of sentinel node procedures, and universal biohazard precautions, which are applicable for the cryotome, are thought to be sufficient for addressing this low level of contamination [6,10]. Nevertheless, some might prefer to employ a separate cryotome for radioactive specimens [11], to use removable linings for each case, or to clean the cryotome after any use involving potentially radioactive specimens, with subsequent segregation and disposal of shavings and cleaning wipes as radioactive specimens.

## Processing Radioactive Specimens

Usually, at least a portion of the tissue resected during sentinel node studies using radioactive materials will be radioactive. Depending on the delay after injection and many other factors, roughly 90% to 99% of the injected dose will remain as a quasi-focal source of activity in the vicinity of the primary tumor or injection site, and from 1% to 10% of the radioactive colloid will have migrated to the regional nodal basins. Thus, the greatest proportion of the administered activity remains effectively "fixed" in situ at the injection site. Because these specimens are radioactive, appropriate policies and procedures must be established in cooperation with the radiation safety officer at each institution. All personnel involved in the handling, transportation, processing, and storage of radioactive specimens should be informed of these policies, and their training should be documented. They must be aware that the specimens are radioactive and therefore require special handling.

Calculations suggest that exposure rates near the surface of sentinel node tissue specimens would be in the range of 1 to 20 μSv/hr (12), and dose equivalent rates of 0.1 to 18 μSv/hr have been measured and reported (3). These exposures fall off rapidly with distance, however, as per the inverse square of distance law.

Some laboratories withhold processing of radioactive specimens for 1 to 3 days to allow for decay of $^{99m}$Tc, but in view of the predicted and documented low exposures to personnel in pathology, this has been debated, since it can delay patient care (11). After histologic sections are taken, segregation of radioactive specimens until they are no longer considered radioactive is easily implemented, without interfering with patient care. If delays for decay are employed, patients should be advised of this before surgery.

Labeling sealed containers containing radioactive specimens as radioactive may or may not be required, depending on the activity of radiation administered and the interval between injection and operative resection, applicable legislative limits, and local institutional policies. In general, tissues transported outside of an institution (e.g., to another medical center) will mandate more stringent labeling requirements than those transported within a single institution and building, for example, down the hall from the operating room to the pathology section. As each institution performing radioguided surgery establishes policies with their radiation safety officers, it is imperative that the transportation of specimens be addressed in view of applicable regulations.

## Radiation Exposure to the Patient

$^{99m}$Tc is unstable and decays to $^{99}$Tc by a process of isomeric transition, with a half-life of approximately 6.02 hours. When this occurs, the 140 keV gamma ray photon is emitted and travels outside the atom. This photon is the basis for the use of $^{99m}$Tc as an external tracer; at this gamma energy, 50% of photons are able to pass through a layer of approximately 50 mm of soft tissue. The 140 keV photons can be detected by radiosensitive probes in surgery, and they can be visualized by gamma cameras to allow preoperative and intraoperative imaging of the migration of the $^{99m}$Tc-labeled colloid for localization.

Radiation that escapes the patient confers no dose to the patient, but it can confer a dose to others, for example via the 140 keV photons of $^{99m}$Tc. However, radiation that does not escape the patient confers radiation exposure to the patient. In addition to the 140 keV photon, the decay process liberates several other low-energy emissions—conversion electrons, Auger electrons, and low-energy x-rays—that essentially are completely absorbed within the patient. These low-energy emissions contribute significantly to the local absorbed dose in the tissues

(4), although they do not contribute to the radiation received by others from the patient because these emissions do not escape from the patient. The distribution of radiation doses throughout the body depends on the distribution of the radiopharmaceutical (Figures 5-2 and 5-3).

Since the majority of the injected dose remains at the injection site in breast lymphoscintigraphy (Figures 5-2B and 5-3), with only at most 10% migrating to the sentinel lymph node (12), the maximal localized radiation dose at the injection site itself will be considerable (40–150 rem or 0.4–1.5 Sv) (13–15). Tissue doses in this range have been found to be associated with an increased incidence of breast cancer in Japanese women after exposure to the atomic bombings at Nagasaki and Hiroshima (16,17), although the conditions of exposure after the bombings are not directly comparable to those resulting from sentinel node studies. This concern is most relevant when the area of tracer injection and diffusion in the breast is not completely resected, which is frequent. Despite the potential for local radiation to the breast reaching levels

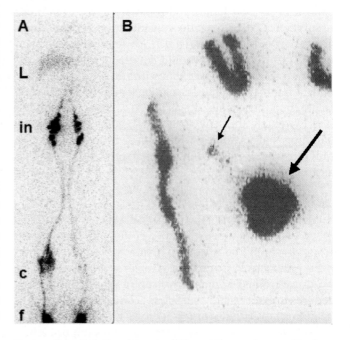

FIGURE 5-2. Relative doses to different tissues from radiopharmaceuticals depend on tracer localization. (A) Whole body lymphoscintigram 2 hours following bipedal injection of $^{99m}$Tc filtered sulfur colloid. Localization of tracer demonstrates that the tissues receiving the greatest radiation dose are the injection sites in the feet (f), the inguinal nodes (in), and the liver (L), with some retention in the right calf (c). (B) Lymphoscintigram of a right breast, demonstrating significant retention of tracer within the breast (thick arrow), with quantitatively minimal migration to sentinel nodes (small arrow). The shoulder and neck are also outlined in the image.

FIGURE 5-3. Sentinel lymph node images of the left breast, obtained using $^{99m}$Tc nanocolloid. The left panels show lymphoscintigraphic images without body outlines. The right panels show images with body outlines obtained using an external transmission shadow source. Transmission image data is included for landmarking. Retention of tracer is seen at the intradermal, peri-areolar injection site (large arrow), and a single sentinel node is seen superior and lateral to this (small arrow), with a smaller amount of tracer in the node. LAO = left anterior oblique; Em = emission.

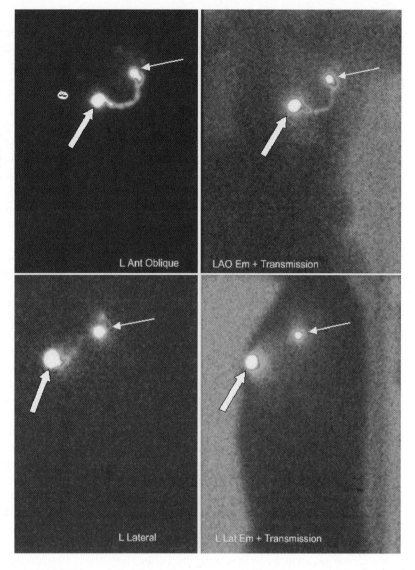

associated with small increases (less than 1%) in the likelihood of radiation-induced carcinogenesis, this likelihood would be at least 1 order of magnitude below the likelihood of recurrent breast cancer at or near the site of the primary tumor, which roughly ranges from 5% to 22% after breast conservation surgery (18). Furthermore, a significant proportion of patients receive a 50 Gy course of external beam radiotherapy to the affected breast. Hence, the risk/benefit considerations weigh strongly in the direction of performing the studies, but prudence dictates the use of the lowest administered activity of radiolabeled colloid possible that permits a strong likelihood of obtaining an accurate localization of the sentinel node(s). For same-day studies, a dose of 10 to 20 MBq is usually sufficient (19). When localization is performed the day after injection, a higher dose of 40 to 70 MBq may be needed, because of the decay of $^{99m}$Tc that occurs overnight (20,21). Other localization tests result in different biodistributions of tracer, but with dif-ferent relative radiation doses throughout the body (Figure 5-2A).

## Disposal of Radioactive Materials

Proper disposal of radioactive materials is an immense and complex topic, but in general, radioactive materials may be disposed of: 1) by transfer to an authorized recipient, 2) by decay in storage, 3) by release in effluents in sanitary sewage, or 4) by incineration, especially clinical waste. Each of these methods is subject to national and local governance, and again, policies for sentinel node procedures must be established with the local radiation safety personnel. Of these 3 methods, decay in storage usually provides the most efficacious approach for sentinel lymph node procedures. The half-life $^{99m}$Tc is 6.02 hours. Storage for 10 to 12 half-lives (60 to 75 hours, or 2.5 to 3 days) is usually sufficient to allow the materials from sentinel lymph node procedures to be classified as nonradioactive (6), but this broad general rule must be checked if concentrated and/or very active waste items are considered. Often, activity limits for the classification of an item of waste as nonradioactive are quoted in Bq/gram. Thus, the concentration of activity within an item, such as in a bag or bin, is a key factor, and specific lower limits will apply in certain countries (for example, the UK) for disposal of clinical waste by incineration with respect to those prevailing for disposal by landfill/burial. Labels indicating radioactivity should be removed from containers or waste at the time of disposal, and these labels should be destroyed. The materials can then be classified as nonradioactive.

Two types of radioactive materials should be considered: radioactive surgical waste (e.g., sponges, swabs, and other absorbent materials), and radioactive tissue specimens. It has been documented (12) that surgical swabs used in a patient who has undergone a sentinel lymph node procedure may absorb up to 22% of the administered colloidal activity from the injection site if the tissue at this site is surgically exposed during the operating procedure, as is the case when an intradermal injection sited immediately above a small lesion is coupled with the local excision of that lesion. Conversely, when the injection site is left undisturbed, e.g., if a mastectomy is performed, this situation does not arise.

Using radiation survey meters, contamination of surgical sponges and other materials used in the handling of radioactive tissues is frequently documented. It is therefore advisable to monitor these materials for contamination, and if contaminated, the trash should be clearly labeled as "not for disposal" and held for decay-in-storage behind shielding, or in a suitable, safe location of low occupancy, such as in a storeroom. After that, the waste materials can be handled as nonradioactive waste would be, and any labels destroyed.

Radioactive tissue specimens should be stored in an area separate from those for nonradioactive specimens. Lead shielding of this separate storage area may not be mandated by radiation safety personnel, but it is easy to set up and helps segregate the tissue specimens. After 10 half lives (2.5 days for $^{99m}$Tc), tissue specimens from sentinel node studies can be regarded as nonradioactive.

larger doses of $^{99m}$Tc, however, without careful consideration of their physical and biologic properties.

Table 5-2 presents exposure rate constants, expressed in 3 different units, and half-lives of several different radioisotopes used for presurgical and intraoperative localization studies, in addition to $^{99m}$Tc. When radiopharmaceuticals are used for localization after intravenous injections, the injected doses of radioactivity are considerably larger, by about an order of magnitude, than those employed for direct tissue injection in sentinel lymph node studies. These higher doses, combined with the higher emission constants of several of the other radioisotopes (Table 5-2), can significantly increase potential exposure to staff and patients. The external exposures to staff relative to those from $^{99m}$Tc can be roughly approximated from data in Table 5-2. For example, at 1 hour after injection the potential (calculated) exposure rate to surgical staff from a patient receiving 185 MBq (5 mCi) $^{18}$F-fluorodeoxyglucose (FDG) for tumor localization would be about 25 times greater than that from a patient given a 37 MBq (1 mCi) dose of $^{99m}$Tc for a sentinel lymph node procedure. Due to various mitigating influences, however, actual documented exposure rates from $^{18}$F-FDG have exceeded those from $^{99m}$Tc sentinel node procedures by factors closer to 5 to 10 (22).

In addition, policies established for small doses of $^{99m}$Tc cannot be extended to other radiopharmaceuticals used in different dosages, and for other purposes. The physical, chemical, and biological properties of each agent employed must be considered. When other radiopharmaceuticals and/or other quantities of radioactivity are adopted for intraoperative uses, the processes for the acquisition, handling, processing, distribution, and eventual decay and disposal of radioactive materials should be reconsidered. For example, the use of intravenous tumor-localizing radiopharmaceuticals in millicurie doses (22–24) or oral radioiodine for localizing thyroid cancer would require reconsideration of the safety issues addressed in this chapter. This could be performed as a useful exercise using $^{18}$F-FDG as a tracer for intraoperative tumor localization, for example, reviewing the considerations presented here regarding exposure to personnel, specimens (handling, processing, transportation, and storage), and waste disposal.

## Radiation Exposure from Radioisotopes Other Than $^{99m}$Tc

As discussed previously, radiation exposures to personnel from submillicurie doses of $^{99m}$Tc for sentinel lymph node procedures is low. This conclusion should not be extended to the use of other radiopharmaceuticals and

## Conclusion

Although this chapter presents many of the issues, considerations, and some recommendations for the use of radionuclides for intraoperative localization of sentinel lymph nodes, these suggestions should not be regarded as final or absolute. Regulatory constraints vary considerably among governances, and a single chapter on this topic cannot provide guidelines that would be universally relevant. Instead, the processes discussed should be individualized and adapted for the procedures and practices within each institution, based on the considerations presented here. Before introducing this technique at an institution, advice should be sought from local radiation safety personnel to ensure that all regulatory requirements are met. Surgical procedures that use radioactive materials are best implemented as a multidisciplinary effort involving personnel from surgery, pathology, nuclear medicine, and radiation safety.

## References

1. Rehani MM, Berry M. Radiation doses in computed tomography. The increasing doses of radiation need to be controlled. *BMJ.* 2000;320:593–594.
2. Ghiassi-nejad M, Mortazavi SMJ, Cameron JR, Niroomand-rad A, Karam PA. Very high background radiation areas of Ramsar, Iran: preliminary biological studies. *Health Phys.* 2002;82:87–93.
3. Colgan TJ, Booth D, Hendler A, McCready D. Appropriate procedures for the safe handling and pathologic examination of technetium-99m-labelled specimens. *CMAJ.* 2001;164:1868–1871.
4. Smith EM. Dose estimation techniques. In: Rollo FD, ed. *Nuclear Medicine Physics, Instrumentation, and Agents.* St. Louis: Mosby; 1977:513–543.
5. Stratmann SL, McCarty TM, Kuhn JA. Radiation safety with breast sentinel node biopsy. *Am J Surg.* 1999;178:454–457.
6. Miner TJ, Shriver CD, Flicek PR, et al. Guidelines for the safe use of radioactive materials during the localization and resection of the sentinel lymph node. *Ann Surg Oncol.* 1999;6:75–82.
7. Radiation Safety Advisory 99-1. State of California Department of Health Services; 1999.
8. Veronesi U, Paganelli G, Viale G, et al. Sentinel lymph node biopsy and axillary dissection in breast cancer: results in a large series. *J Natl Cancer Inst.* 1999;91:368–373.
9. De Kanter AY, Arends PP, Eggermont AM, Wiggers T. Radiation protection for the sentinel node procedure in breast cancer. *Eur J Surg Oncol.* 2003;29:396–399.
10. Turner RR, Giuliano AE, Hoon DSB, Glass EC, Krasne DL. Pathologic examination of the sentinel node for breast carcinoma. *World J Surg.* 2001;25:798–805.
11. Fitzgibbons PL, LiVolsi A. Recommendations for handling radioactive specimens obtained by sentinel lymphadenectomy. *Am J Surg Pathol.* 2000;24:1549–1551.
12. Waddington WA, Keshtgar MR, Taylor I, Lakhani SR, Short MD, Ell PJ. Radiation safety of the sentinel lymph node technique in breast cancer. *Eur J Nucl Med.* 2000;27:377–391.
13. Glass EC, Basinski JE, Krasne DL, Giuliano AE. Radiation safety considerations for sentinel node techniques. *Ann Surg Oncol.* 1999; 6:10–11.
14. Bronskill MJ. Radiation dose estimates for interstitial radiocolloid lymphoscintigraphy. *Semin Nucl Med.* 1983;13:20–25.
15. Glass EC, Essner R, Giuliano AE. Sentinel node localization in breast cancer. *Semin Nucl Med.* 1999; 28:1–13.
16. Wanebo CK, Johnson KG, Sato K, Thorslund TW. Breast cancer after the exposure to the atomic bombings of Hiroshima and Nagasaki. *N Engl J Med.* 1968;279:667–671.
17. Kohn HI, Fry RJM. Radiation carcinogenesis. *N Engl J Med.* 1984;310:504–511.
18. Huston TL, Simmons RM. Locally recurrent breast cancer after breast conservation. *Am J Surg.* 2005;189:229–235.
19. Cody HS III, Borgen PI. State-of-the-art approaches to sentinel node biopsy for breast cancer: study design, patient selection, technique, and quality control at Memorial Sloan-Kettering Cancer Center. *Surg Oncol.* 1999;8:85–91.
20. Gray RJ, Pockaj BA, Roarke MC. Injection of Tc99m-labeled sulfur colloid the day before operation for breast cancer sentinel node mapping is as successful as injection the day of operation. *Am J Surg.* 2004;188:685–689.
21. Babiera GV, Delpassand ES, Breslin TM, et al: Lymphatic drainage patterns on early versus delayed breast lymphoscintigraphy performed after injection of filtered Tc99m sulfur colloid in breast cancer patients undergoing sentinel lymph node biopsy. *Clin Nucl Med.* 2005;30:11–15.
22. Griff M, Berthold T, Buck A: Radiation exposure to sonographers from fluorine-18-FDG PET patients. *J Nucl Med Technol.* 2000;28:186–187.
23. Raylman RR, Fisher SJ, Brown RS, Ethier SP, Wahl RL. Fluorine-18-fluorodeoxyglucose-guided breast cancer surgery with a positron-sensitive probe: validation in preclinical studies. *J Nucl Med.* 1995;36:1869–1874.
24. Kuhn JA, Corbisiero RM, Buras RR, et al: Intraoperative gamma detection probe with presurgical antibody imaging in colon cancer. *Arch Surg.* 1991;126:1398–1403.
25. Chandra R. Physical characteristics of some radionuclides of interest in nuclear medicine. In: *Nuclear Medicine Physics.* 5th edition, appendix A. New York: Lippincott Williams & Wilkins; 1998:157–159.
26. Mitsui Y. Paper presented at: Second International Sentinel Node Conference; December 1–4, 2000; Santa Monica, CA.
27. Brenner W, et al. Paper presented at: Second International Sentinel Node Conference; December 1–4, 2000; Santa Monica, CA.

# 6
# Training and Credentialing for Radioguided Surgery

Eric D. Whitman

New medical technology, whatever the form, places stress on our health care delivery system. Many technologies, such as laparoscopic surgery, require the surgeon and the operating room team be trained on and adapt to new devices and techniques. Other technologies, such as immunohistochemistry or other advanced diagnostic capabilities, demand new techniques or new personnel in the laboratory or pathology department, which often can be outsourced initially until the necessary expertise is acquired by staff or otherwise available locally. Radioguided surgery is perhaps unique in that it demands adoption of new techniques, technologies, and procedural guidelines across multiple disciplines. As such, it is not just the surgeons, radiologists, or pathologists who must adapt to this new technology; a successful radioguided surgical program must have the cooperation and focus of these hospital departments (1).

This cooperation must be enforced by the hospital, through rigorous quality assurance and peer review processes. Specifically, individual physicians, regardless of specialty, must be trained adequately to perform their portion of the procedure. The hospital medical staff is responsible for credentialing these physicians, to certify that they have met the standards necessary to undertake this procedure. The medical staff is also responsible for reviewing the performance of all 3 components of a radioguided surgical program, to ensure that the local public is receiving a level of care consistent with published national standards and milestones. If not, the appropriate hospital staff committee must review specific cases to identify the process or individual that must change to raise the quality of care.

Unfortunately, effective training and credentialing for new surgical technology remain elusive goals for medical institutions, most of whom struggle to keep up with the constant influx of new technology for the operating room and other parts of the hospital (2). This chapter describes potential solutions to this problem, based on the recent historical experience with radio-guided surgical programs as well as other surgical technologies and procedures.

## Training

The training requirements for a radioguided surgical program primarily revolve around the surgeons (3). For specialists in nuclear medicine, the lymphoscintigraphy is a procedure that had been performed prior to the introduction of radioguided surgery (4,5), although perhaps not as frequently. This procedure has not changed much, and in general the purchase of new equipment is not necessary for most institutions. The only real change for these physicians may be an increased demand on their nuclear medicine resources. This demand is accompanied by specific time constraints, since many surgeons perform lymphoscintigraphy immediately before a scheduled surgery. Understandably, scintigraphic procedures are designed to obtain the best possible image, but this may conflict with the needs of the surgeon and the operating room to get the patient back to the holding area in time to complete the scheduled surgery.

Similarly, the pathology department typically does not require additional personnel, technology, or training for a radioguided surgical program. The only exception may be at a small pathology department that does not have in-house immunohistochemistry available, but there are many reference laboratories available that can rapidly provide immunohistochemical testing, if needed. Thus, from a pathology perspective, the only change is the adoption of an evolving standard of care for the pathologic evaluation of sentinel lymph nodes, which is inherently different from the historically accepted evaluation of other lymph node specimens (i.e., step sectioning and immunohistochemistry as necessary) (6,7). Again, this does not require additional training for pathologists, merely an evaluation of the published medical literature from leading radioguided surgical centers and adoption of those (already known but potentially not yet used) laboratory operating procedures.

Surgeons, however, will require additional training. As with laparoscopic surgery, when radioguided surgery first began to be used frequently, in the mid- to late 1990s, the majority of surgeons who wished to use this technique were already out of residency training and in clinical practice. The sudden and pressing need for surgical training in a new technique and technology was met by the creation of several Continuing Medical Education (CME) accredited courses that would periodically train a group of surgeons in this technology (8). Interestingly, for both laparoscopic surgery and radioguided surgery, within a few years there was no longer a need for frequent occurrences of the majority of these courses, once a critical mass of surgeons had been trained. Since then, residency programs have trained the majority of the other surgeons in this practice today, as part of their standard training. Other surgeons already in clinical practice learned through periodic updates and/or courses provided by the American College of Surgeons or other educational bodies, or underwent a local training/mentoring process by a more experienced partner or associate.

As sentinel lymph node biopsy was rapidly adopted for both melanoma and breast cancer, this posed an interesting and perplexing problem for the organizers of large multicenter studies: Since so many surgeons were trained after residency, without any nationally applied standards, how could multicenter study organizers ensure that the same procedures and processes were being followed at each institution?

This was effectively addressed by the National Surgical Adjuvant Breast Project (NSABP) B32 trial, a randomized phase III clinical trial to compare sentinel node biopsy to conventional axillary dissection in clinically node-negative breast cancer (9). As a requirement for a surgeon's participation in the trial, there was a pre-randomization training phase overseen by a core group of experienced surgical trainers. This included a training manual, site visit, and follow-up of 5 pre-randomization sentinel lymph node biopsy procedures. In each case, surgeons who registered to participate in the trial were provided with a comprehensive training manual and assigned a core trainer surgeon. The training manual included sections on surgery, pathology, and quality assurance. At the time of the site visit, the core trainer instructed the newly participating surgeon in sentinel lymph node surgery intraoperatively. Training was also provided in other components of sentinel node care, including pathology and nuclear medicine. Each participating surgeon was required to perform a minimum of 5 training cases that included both sentinel lymph node biopsy as well as a mandatory completion of an axillary node dissection. The data from these 5 cases were then reviewed by the principal investigator. Once protocol compliance, source documentation, and data accuracy were confirmed, the surgeon was allowed to begin to randomize cases to full axillary node dissection versus sentinel lymph node biopsy on the clinical trial. Failure to successfully complete the first 5 pre-randomization cases could result in extension of the training phase for that surgeon and institution.

The results of this training program have been separately published (9). Overall, 132 of 187 surgeons (70.6%) completed training and were approved to randomize patients after the minimum 5 cases. The remaining 55 surgeons (29.4%) required more than 5 training cases. The authors found that ongoing case-by-case feedback resulted in a higher initial compliance rate than delaying the review until the full complement of 5 training cases had been performed and made it more likely that surgeons would meet the requirements to begin to randomize patients after only 5 cases. Regardless of their success with the initial 5 cases, all surgeons eventually were able to follow the protocol and complete the necessary case report forms with a high compliance rate.

Efforts such as this, which were similarly pursued by other multicenter sentinel lymph node studies (3,10), along with the efforts of residency training programs, have resulted in a large cohort of motivated, well-trained surgeons who are able to perform radioguided surgery at institutions with fairly standardized procedural techniques. However, the need still exists, although less intensely than that of 5 to 10 years ago, for extramural training programs in radioguided surgery. Surgeons who might require this training may be: those who finished surgical residency before 1995 and only recently were interested or able to perform radioguided surgery at their hospital; those who trained in specialties other than general surgery but now as part of their practice require sentinel lymph node biopsy proficiency (i.e., plastic surgery or otolaryngology); or those who require additional training or evidence of having taken a specific course in radioguided surgery for credentialing purposes at their hospital.

The requirements for radioguided surgical training have not changed substantially since the courses were first introduced (on a much more frequent basis) 5 to 10 years ago. A typical 1- to 2-day course might include the following topics:

- Surgical techniques: melanoma (sentinel lymph node); breast cancer (sentinel lymph node); other skin cancers (sentinel lymph node); radioguided surgery in general, including parathyroidectomy, tumor localization, or other procedures.
- Nuclear medicine.
- Pathologic examination: melanoma; breast cancer, including touch prep.
- Observation of live surgical cases.
- Animal laboratory of sentinel node biopsy (optional).

The effect of advanced technology on training courses cannot be ignored in this context. Many courses can now offer live videoconferencing from the operating room, which enables students to remotely observe a case. Other hands-on instructional modalities are also possible (11).

From a practical standpoint, most surgeons currently in practice will not require formal training in radioguided surgery in the future. In addition, it is reasonable to expect that all general surgical residency training programs will provide their trainees with an adequate level of instruction and experience in radioguided surgery. Therefore, what kind of training program in radioguided surgery is best suited to meet the future needs of our health care system? Future radioguided surgical training programs will need to focus more on re-training, quality assurance, and peer review. Hospitals must continue to monitor the progress of newer health care technology, such as radioguided surgery, once it is initially implemented. Regardless of the form this evaluation takes, in some cases inadequate quality of care will be identified, and training programs must exist for this eventuality. These courses may take the form of a nationally identified team of mentoring surgeons, who could be dispatched by the American College of Surgeons or a similar agency to assist the requesting facility with evaluation and improvement of a radioguided surgical program. This assistance could include more intensive case review by experts, on-site examination of equipment and facilities, and/or intraoperative surgical mentoring. Alternatively, third-party payors may demand external review of radioguided surgical programs to assess their quality and potentially designate "centers of excellence" for enhanced reimbursement by the payors. In both of these situations, with a less formalized schedule than that previously required for the CME courses, training programs would be indispensable.

The demand for future training programs in radioguided surgery may also center on the need to provide clinicians and hospitals with information that will aid in the logistic aspects of initiating and maintaining a radioguided surgical clinical service. These materials and information may include sample protocol documents (for new radiosurgery programs), consent forms, data collection sheets, database program files, potential press releases, and letters to referring physicians. Essentially, this could also be described as providing the clients of a radioguided surgical training program with the necessary business plan for a successful program.

In summary, radioguided surgery in the United States has progressed to the point where multiple, frequent training courses are no longer necessary. However, ongoing training in surgical technique remains important for surgical residents. Future training programs may focus more on the needs of the hospital institution and/or the third-party payor.

# Credentialing

Credentialing is the process by which a hospital and its medical staff grant permission for a physician to practice medicine within that institution. For surgeons, credentialing extends the general concept of permission to practice medicine to a list of specifically requested surgical procedures that the surgeon can perform at that hospital.

The analogy between the rapid adoption of laparoscopic general surgical techniques and the more recent implementation of radioguided surgery is also appropriate when discussing hospital credentialing. In both cases, new technology and creative surgical perspectives combined to create a set of revolutionary surgical procedures. After training, which was inconsistent and incompletely regulated, surgeons would return to their institutions in various stages of readiness to perform radioguided—or earlier, laparoscopic—surgery. Yet the hospitals themselves were ill-prepared to regulate the performance of these new surgical procedures, particularly since (in many cases) the majority of their surgical staff was not yet trained to perform them.

Different policies were developed at individual institutions (12,13), but it was inherently difficult to limit performance of these new procedures as they rapidly became the standard of care. Hospitals were unwilling to take the chance of losing a valuable market share if they hindered surgical progress. The surgeons who did not initially receive training but were already in practice soon recognized that competency in these new procedures was essential to maintaining any level of clinical involvement in those areas. Unfortunately, in laparoscopy the largely unregulated rush to become laparoscopic surgeons resulted in a higher incidence of cholecystectomy-related complications, particularly bile duct injuries (14). In response, most hospitals established minimal criteria to allow surgeons to perform this surgery, and in New York state a law was passed defining the training and experience necessary for a surgeon to be allowed to perform laparoscopic surgery. However, despite these precautions, in a recent study the incidence of bile duct injury was 2.5 to 4 times higher after laparoscopic cholecystectomy than in the open cholecystectomy era (14).

The issues with radioguided surgery are somewhat more complex, because the surgery itself is probably less morbid, or with less morbid potential, than the comparison between laparoscopic and open cholecystectomy. Presently, radioguided surgery is used primarily to stage malignancies, so that errors in technique when performing these procedures might have a delayed adverse outcome, measured in years rather than days. Patients could develop unexpected recurrences months or years after surgery, if it was performed inappropriately or with poor quality. These patients might otherwise have received different therapy for their cancers, with resulting life-threatening and/or medicolegal implications.

There are few, if any, consistent policies and procedures for credentialing radioguided surgery/sentinel lymph node biopsy—or for that matter, any new surgical technology. However, the following elements appear consistently in various policies, and are unquestionably relevant:

1. Adequate and appropriate overall or "general" training in a relevant surgical specialty. This takes the form of the surgeon being board-certified or board eligible. It is important that the requesting surgeon has adequate experience and insight to deal with any potential unforeseen complications of the new surgical procedure or technology.

2. Specific training or relevant prior experience in the requested surgical procedure. This could either be proof of training and experience during surgical residency, a certificate proving attendance at a specific radioguided surgery course, or a case log proving extensive experience with the new technology at another hospital. Ideally, this should be accompanied by a letter from the administrative chief of surgery at the outside hospital, verifying the surgeon's case numbers and general competence.

3. Surgeons applying for credentialing in radioguided surgery (or for any newer or advanced surgical procedure) must specifically request privileges to do these surgeries in whatever format is appropriate for that hospital institution (i.e., surgical procedure checklist). This creates a Joint Commission on Accreditation of Healthcare Organizations (JCAHO) mandated paper trail that documents the intention of the applicant surgeon to perform a specific case. Obviously, to receive this credentialing following the request, the surgeon must have proved adequate training or prior experience. However, the request itself is essential for the credentialing process.

4. The surgeon must be observed, mentored, or otherwise evaluated through the first series of cases performed. There are two major questions involved with this process. The first is which surgeon or surgeons at a given hospital institution are capable of evaluating this new technology. Can it be someone who is not necessarily familiar with the technology, but is otherwise an outstanding clinical surgeon? Or must it be someone with extensive knowledge and experience with the new procedure? If there is no such person at the hospital, must an outside mentor be retained from another institution? The second major issue is the length of time or number of cases for this observation/mentoring/evaluation process. Although this varies from institution to institution, it is probably best to evaluate a surgeon on a new technology for a minimum of 3 to 5 cases, but no more than 10 cases. However, this number could be extended if the surgeon

shows continued poor quality outcomes. Some literature suggests that radioguided surgery may require up to 25 to 30 cases before the surgical skill and the outcomes plateau (15), but this number is noted to be unrealistic in other publications, particularly as the new surgical procedure or technology becomes the community standard of care and is demanded by the general public (as happened with both laparoscopic surgery and sentinel node biopsy) (10). The experience with the NSABP B-32 trial suggests that 5 cases is a reasonable number to achieve consistent results in the majority of cases with a new surgical technology (9). For most surgeons, it is probably not necessary to extend the case number beyond 5, and this could even be shortened to 2 or 3 cases, if someone has extensive prior experience at other institutions.

5. Regardless of the number of cases, what is most important in evaluating a surgeon's competence to perform a new surgical technique or to use a new surgical technology is a comprehensive and thorough prospective quality review of at least the first 5 to 10 cases performed by that surgeon. Note that this is separate and discrete from mentoring or observation at the time of surgery; this is a postoperative chart review done to ensure that quality care has been provided. This initial chart evaluation could be further used if the institution preferred to give initial "provisional" privileges and then upgrade that to "full" privileges after the initial case review.

These criteria apply to surgeons who wish to perform radioguided surgery. Credentialing here is much less relevant to radiologists and pathologists, since in almost all cases the skills and techniques required of them in a radioguided surgery program are a pre-existing part of their clinical practice.

## Performance Improvement

Once physicians have been trained and have credentials to perform radioguided surgery, their clinical actions and outcomes must be monitored and critiqued as part of an overall quality control or performance improvement program. Currently, most data, experience, and case volume are in sentinel lymph node biopsy, typically for breast cancer and melanoma. Therefore, the performance measures and criteria are best defined for these procedures, and not for other radioguided surgical procedures. Table 6-1 describes a potential performance improvement report card for sentinel node biopsy, as assessed by the institution with attention to the actions of individual departments and physicians.

Like credentialing, performance improvement and peer review are the responsibility of both the hospital and the medical staff. At present, tracking and reporting

TABLE 6-1. Quality criteria for sentinel lymph node biopsy.

| Item | Definition | Expected normal value | Responsible party |
|---|---|---|---|
| Failure rate | % patients in whom a sentinel lymph node is not identified | 0–5% (9,15,17) | Surgeon, nuclear physician |
| Positivity rate | % patients with sentinel lymph lymph node positive for metastasis | 20–30%* (1,7,9) | Surgeon, pathologist |
| Recurrence rate | % patients developing recurrent disease | 0–10% (16)* | Surgeon, pathologist |
| Late operating room start | Delay in operating room case start time | Varies by hospital | Nuclear physician, surgeon |
| Time | Time to perform lymphoscintigraphy | Varies by hospital | Nuclear physician |
| Surgical complications (varies) | | Varies (20) | Surgeon |

Legend:
N/A—not applicable
*Varies by case mix, i.e. relative risk level of cancers treated

the quality of outcomes is not used to index or alter reimbursement, but this may change. These "pay-for-performance" proposals will mandate the active monitoring of surgical outcomes; this monitoring likely will be crucial for future hospital and clinician reimbursement for any new technologies or procedures, and may also apply to newer procedures already in clinical practice, such as radioguided surgery. The first step in implementing a performance improvement program for radioguided surgery is to establish standards expected of all clinicians involved with the program: surgeons, specialists in nuclear medicine, and pathologists. Clinicians or departments that do not meet the standards would then be referred to the peer review system for evaluation of any deficiency and initiation of any necessary corrective action(s).

Most of the performance improvement standards apply to some extent to all the specialists involved with radioguided surgery programs. For example, clinicians are expected to keep current on the relevant medical literature for radioguided surgery and their particular clinical practice. These efforts can be assisted by interaction with peers at tumor boards, grand rounds, CME courses, or journal clubs. Likewise, clinicians must monitor their clinical outcomes, as they apply to their particular practice and specialty.

Several specific outcome measurements should be recorded for sentinel node biopsy (16). First, one must measure the rate of successful identification and biopsy of sentinel nodes for each patient (detection rate, identification rate, or success rate), defined as the percentage of all patients planned to receive the procedure who successfully have a sentinel node identified and sent to pathology. The converse measurement is the failure rate, or the percentage of cases in which the surgeon is unable to identify and biopsy a sentinel node. In plotting learning curves for sentinel node biopsy, Cox and colleagues identified several interesting relationships between failure rate and number of cases, both individual and institutional (17,18). Individual surgeons were assessed by plotting the failure rate versus the sequential cumula-

tive case volume. This was found to vary considerably from surgeon to surgeon, even among those with extensive experience. Overall, at their institution about 25 cases were required to consistently move a surgeon below the 10% failure rate threshold, while about 50 were necessary to reach the 5% failure rate threshold, although these case numbers were highly variable (15). Although it is difficult to know exactly what failure rate threshold is acceptable for any given surgeon—especially as data suggest that some surgeons are more likely to achieve a lower failure rate more quickly than others—it is nonetheless important for these data to be plotted for each surgeon performing this procedure. Moreover, the institutional case failure rate should be plotted as well. If the overall failure rate remains high even after several dozen cases have been performed, this suggests a breakdown in either surgical technique or nuclear medicine (injection or imaging) technique. Failure rate for sentinel node biopsy is not a quality outcome that applies to pathology.

Another data-monitoring relationship explored by Cox and colleagues was a comparison between the monthly frequency of cases, expressed as the surgical volume index or SVI, as opposed to the cumulative number of cases (17). In this analysis, surgeons performing fewer than 3 sentinel node biopsy procedures per month had a lower overall success rate than those performing more than 6 per month. A logistic regression model was calculated and predicted that the failure rate for a surgeon performing his or her first case would be about 16%, which was predicted to decrease to less than 2% when the SVI reached 13. This translates into an estimated 18% decrease in the odds of failure for each unit increase in SVI (17). This curve can also be applied to an institution, as a similar assessment for the success and quality of both the surgical program and nuclear medicine/imaging program.

When sentinel node biopsy first was applied to melanoma and breast cancer, a false-negative rate was assessed (7,19), defined as the percentage of cases where the sentinel node does not contain metastatic disease but non-sentinel nodes do have evidence of metastasis. This can only be measured if all patients are receiving mandatory completion lymph node dissection. The current standard of care for select cases of melanoma and breast cancer allows performance of a sentinel lymph node biopsy without mandatory completion node dissection; node dissection is reserved for those cases where definite metastatic disease is found in the sentinel node. This evolution of the standard of care makes it impossible to directly measure the false-negative rate; it can only be assessed through indirect means. Patients who develop recurrent disease, particularly in the regional lymph node basin where the sentinel lymph nodes were originally biopsied, presumably had a false-negative sentinel lymph node biopsy. These recurrence rate data can be compared to historical standards, and a higher-than-expected recurrence rate should warrant further review of the sentinel node biopsy program. This quality outcome applies to the surgeons who are responsible for biopsying the tissue (i.e., lymph node) and the pathologists who analyze it.

Thus, as an institution, the main sentinel lymph node biopsy outcome data to be monitored are the technical/procedural success rate and the long-term clinical recurrence (i.e., cancer treatment failure) rate. The involved clinical specialties must also track quality indicators specific to their component of a radioguided surgical program. These quality indicators reflect on both the clinical quality or accuracy of the procedure itself, and on the effect of a physician's or department's actions on the efficiency and consistency of the hospital's radioguided surgical program.

Nuclear physicians also should be evaluated for their ability to work within the constraints of the operating room schedule, particularly if the sentinel lymph node biopsy cases are typically scheduled with same-day lymphoscintigraphy. The most straightforward way to track this data is for the operating room to record the frequency of start-time delays due to extended time in the nuclear medicine suite for lymphoscintigraphy. In addition, the nuclear physicians should record the amount of time it takes to perform a lymphoscintigraphy, from the time of injection to the final image acquisition sequence, as a function of the location of the melanoma or breast cancer. For melanoma, this would be head and neck versus truncal versus extremity; for breast cancer, this would be measured as a function of the primary cancer's quadrant of the breast. Evaluation of this data and release of the information to the operating room and surgeons will improve the scheduling efficiency of these cases. Also, these 2 time variables are important for the hospital's cost structure, to minimize any procedural delays that may result in increased employee overtime expenses. Delays also may contribute to lower patient satisfaction with the hospital and its physicians, which may eventually negatively impact a hospital's financial performance.

Finally, pathologists are responsible for maintaining their clinical practice in line with what is best described as an evolving clinical standard of care to evaluate sentinel nodes for cancer (6). As the standards are published in the literature, pathologists must update their biopsy protocol accordingly. They must maintain internal quality of care audits on their immunohistochemistry program, as they would for any other type of biopsy. If frozen section analysis of sentinel nodes is undertaken, they should monitor their work for any discrepancies, whether false-negative or false-positive findings; a high rate of either of these adverse quality outcomes, relative to the published medical literature, should prompt a team discussion of the benefits of frozen section analysis at that particular institution. The pathology department, along with the other involved clinicians, should monitor the positivity rate, or the overall percentage of patients who have pathologically involved sentinel nodes. Significant deviation of the positivity rate from nationally published results suggests a quality issue in either the ability of the surgeon to successfully identify the sentinel node, or the pathologic evaluation of the sentinel nodes.

Mariani et al. have summarized prior literature concerning training in radioguided surgery as a team rather than as individual specialties involved in such combined effort (20).

## Peer Review

Like the credentialing and performance improvement processes, peer review is undertaken by the hospital and its medical staff to ensure that a high quality of care is maintained, and to efficiently and effectively intervene if inadequate quality is documented. The exact structure of a hospital's peer review committee or process is beyond the scope of this chapter; but as it specifically pertains to a radioguided surgical program, a hospital's peer review process should be prepared to periodically assess the quality of the radioguided surgical program. This is done through review of the performance improvement criteria described above. Inadequate performance in these areas should trigger formal discussion, review, and potential action to correct the deficiency. The support of the medical staff and the hospital administration for the peer review process and its potential actions is indispensable.

Specific surgical complications of sentinel lymph node biopsy are most typically wound seroma or fluid collection, and wound infection. The occurrence rate of these complications has been reported in various studies, as noted in Table 6-1 (16,21). Other, less common complications that may occur include lymphedema, vascular injury, nerve injury, or others (21).

In addition, there are standard complications of any surgical procedure that are mandated by national quality organizations as being subject to automatic peer review. These include unscheduled readmission to the hospital less than 31 days after surgery, unplanned return to the operating room in the postoperative period, death less than 48 hours after surgery, cardiac or respiratory arrest, or an unplanned admission when initially scheduled for outpatient surgery.

## Summary

As with any new technology, proper training and logical, well-documented credentialing standards are essential to the safe and clinically prudent implementation of radioguided surgical programs. The lessons learned during the advent of laparoscopic cholecystectomy, where the incidence and type of operative biliary complications changed from the "open" era, should be built upon to prevent similar occurrences with radioguided surgery, particularly since most applications developed to date involve the treatment of malignancies, where adverse outcomes may not become clinically apparent for months or years.

Now that a critical mass of clinical practitioners is adequately trained, the issue of training physicians in radioguided surgery has become less significant. Of more importance is a rational credentialing process that takes into account prior experience and/or training and provides for strict and mandatory mentoring, observation, and review of initial cases for both the institution and the individual surgeons. Institutions should track the performance of their radioguided surgical program in several outcome measurements, particularly technical success/failure rates and eventual cancer recurrence rates. Within each department, there are specific performance criteria that should be recorded as well, which reflect on both the clinical quality and accuracy of care and diagnostic testing provided and the hospital's overall efficiency and cost structure. Finally, measurement of these outcomes would be irrelevant if they were not acted upon by an efficient and empowered peer review process.

As radioguided surgery is adopted for more and more clinical indications, it is hoped that the suggestions in this chapter will enable our health care system to avoid many of the pitfalls experienced with the rapid adoption of laparoscopic surgery more than 10 years ago. We further hope that the programs implemented today for radioguided surgery might also apply to the next revolutionary new technology.

## References

1. Reintgen D, Albertini J, Berman C, et al. Accurate nodal staging of malignant melanoma. *Cancer Control.* 1995;405–414.
2. Reintgen D. The credentialing of American surgery. *Ann Surg Oncol.* 1997;4:99–101.
3. Wilke LG. Training and mentoring surgeons in lymphatic mapping. *Semin Oncol.* 2004;31:333–337.
4. Uren RF, Howman-Giles RB, Thompson JF, et al. Lymphoscintigraphy to identify sentinel lymph nodes in patients with melanoma. *Melanoma Res.* 1994;4:395–399.
5. DeCicco C, Cremonesi M, Chinol M, et al. Optimization of axillary lymphoscintigraphy to detect the sentinel node in breast cancer. *Tumori.* 1997;83:539–541.
6. Turner RR, Ollila DW, Krasne DL, Giuliano AE. Histopathologic validation of the sentinel lymph node hypothesis for breast carcinoma. *Ann Surg.* 1997;226:271–278.
7. Reintgen D, Cruse CW, Wells K, et al. The orderly progression of melanoma nodal metastases. *Ann Surg.* 1994;220:759–767.
8. Bass SS, Cox CE, Reintgen DS. Learning curves and certification of breast cancer lymphatic mapping. *Surg Clin N Am.* 1999;8:497–509.
9. Harlow SP, Krag DN, Julian TB, et al. Prerandomization surgical training for the National Surgical Adjuvant Breast and Bowel Project (NSABP) B-32 Trial. *Ann Surg.* 2005;241:48–54.
10. Reintgen D, Modarelli C, Cox C. The training of surgeons in America. *Ann Surg Oncol.* 2001;8:1–2.
11. Dunnington GL. A model for teaching sentinel lymph node mapping and excision and axillary lymph node dissection. *J Am Coll Surg.* 2003;197:119–121.
12. Cox CE, Pendas S, Cox JM, et al. Guidelines for sentinel node biopsy and lymphatic mapping of patients with breast cancer. *Ann Surg.* 1998;227:645–653.
13. Kuehn T, Bembenek A, Decker T, et al. A concept for the clinical implementation of sentinel lymph node biopsy with breast carcinoma with special regard to quality assurance. *Cancer.* 2004;103:451–461.
14. Strasberg SM, Hertl M, Soper NJ. An analysis of the problem of biliary injury during laparoscopic cholecystectomy. *J Am Coll Surg.* 1995;180:101–125.
15. Cox CE, Bass SS, Boulware D, Ku NK, Berman C, Reintgen DS. Implementation of new surgical technology: outcome measures for lymphatic mapping of breast carcinoma. *Ann Surg Oncol.* 1999;6:553–561.
16. Yee VSK, Thompson JF, McKinnon JG, et al. Outcome in 846 cutaneous melanoma patients from a single center after a negative sentinel node biopsy. *Ann Surg Oncol.* 2005;12:429–439.
17. Cox CE, Salud CJ, Cantor A, et al. Learning curves for breast cancer sentinel lymph node mapping based on surgical volume analysis. *J Am Coll Surg.* 2001;193;593–600.
18. Dupont E, Cox C, Shivers S, et al. Learning curves and breast cancer lymphatic mapping: institutional volume index. *J Surg Res.* 2001;97:92–96.
19. Shivers S, Cox C, Leight G, et al. Final results of the Department of Defense Multicenter Breast Lymphatic Mapping Trial. *Ann Surg Oncol.* 2002;9:248–255.
20. Mariani G, Moresco L, Viale G, et al. Radioguided sentinel lymph node biopsy in breast cancer surgery. *J Nucl Med.* 2001;42;1198–1215.
21. Wrightson WR, Wong SL, Edwards MJ, et al. Complications associated with sentinel lymph node biopsy for melanoma. *Ann Surg Oncol.* 2003;10:676–680.

# Part II
## Sentinel Lymph Nodes

# 7
# The Anatomy and Physiology of Lymphatic Circulation

Preya Ananthakrishnan, Giuliano Mariani, Luciano Moresco, and Armando E. Giuliano

The lymphatic system is formed by a network of vessels, nodes, and specialized organs that are vital in maintaining both localized and systemic immunity. Lymph nodes are the first place where lymphocytes are exposed to foreign antigens, leading to the production and dissemination of antigen-specific T lymphocytes and plasma cells. By delivering immunocompetent cells to sites where they are needed through the lymph, locally initiated immunity becomes generalized (1).

Lymph is also responsible for collecting protein and fluid from the interstitial spaces and returning them to the vasculature (2). Other substances including red blood cells and bacteria are also cleared through the lymphatics; blood and benign epithelial cells can be seen in sentinel lymph nodes after breast biopsies (3). In addition, fat is absorbed from the intestine and transported through lacteals in the lymph to the systemic circulation through the thoracic duct. After trauma, sepsis, and burns, systemic mediators are carried from the intestine to the circulation through the mesenteric lymph (4). Protein and fluid are returned from the cellular environment back into the circulation through 2 routes: from collecting lymphatics to the thoracic duct into the subclavian vein, and through extensive lymphovenous connections between peripheral lymphatic vessels and peripheral veins (5).

## Embryology

The lymphatic system originates as buds from the venous system and is lined by venous endothelium (6). Paired lymphatic sacs are present in the neck and lumbar areas of the developing fetus by the sixth week of gestation. The right lymphatic bud comes from the right jugular venous sac, and it is the basis of the lymphatic drainage of the heart and lungs (except bilateral pulmonary lower lobes and the left upper lobe.) The left jugular venous

sac becomes the thoracic duct, from which the lymphatics of the esophagus, thoracic aorta, and upper segments of the left lung originate. A retroperitoneal lymph sac and developing cisterna chyli are present by the eighth week of gestation. Lymphatic channels follow the growth of arteries toward the periphery by a process of endothelial sprouting, by which the tip of the lymphatic lobule extends forward (7). Eventually, the right and left lymphatic ducts merge at the level of the fourth to sixth thoracic vertebrae and empty into the junction of the left subclavian and internal jugular veins. The lymphatic system also remains connected to the venous system through peripheral lymphovenous connections.

Lymph nodes develop in the fetus as foci of lymphocyte aggregates after the formation of the lymphatic network. Lymph nodes change with time—at birth they do not contain germinal centers. Germinal centers develop after age 2 months, are well formed by age 2 years, and continue to grow through puberty. Lymph nodes become smaller and undergo fatty degeneration with advancing age, although they remain relatively constant in number throughout life (6).

Though they have a common embryologic origin, the lymphatic system differs from the venous system in that there are more lymphatics throughout the body than veins, and the lymphatics have a greater number of valves. In addition, lymphatic walls are much thinner than those for veins, and there is a great deal of variation in their caliber (6).

Components of the fully developed lymphatic system include primary lymphoid organs, where precursors to both B and T lymphocyte cell lines differentiate, as well as secondary or peripheral lymphoid organs. Primary lymphoid organs include the thymus and bone marrow, while secondary lymphoid tissues include the lymph nodes, spleen, Peyer patches, tonsils, and conjunctiva of the eye. Unencapsulated lymphoid tissue, called mucosa-associated lymphoid tissues, exists in the walls of the alimentary, respiratory, reproductive, and urinary tracts as well as the skin (1).

## Histology

The lymphatic system is composed of lymphatic capillaries, deeper collecting lymph vessels, lymph nodes, lymphatic trunks, and terminal lymphatic vessels that drain into the venous circulation (8). An extensive lymph capillary network travels in the superficial dermis as well as in the mucosa lining the gastrointestinal and respiratory tracts. The capillaries drain into deeper collecting vessels, which are stronger and larger caliber channels.

Structurally, the lymphatic capillaries are lined by a single layer of continuous endothelial cells. The capillaries lack an underlying basement membrane, which makes the passage of molecules between cells possible. Overlapping interendothelial junctions function as valves that facilitate unidirectional permeability (from the interstitial space into the lymphatic capillaries) (9). Larger particles are transported through the endothelium through pinocytosis (6). The small lymphatic capillaries contain no muscle cells; however, actin-like filaments have been described within the endothelial cell lining that appear to regulate cell shape and permeability (10). Lymphatic capillaries have the capacity to expand in response to physiologic need, but may also become obstructed in the face of inflammation or malignancy. This extensive capillary network is present in every organ of the body except bone marrow, the central nervous system, muscle, and liver lobules (11).

The superficial plexus of lymphatic capillaries in the dermis drains into valved channels in the deep dermis and subdermal tissues. Larger collecting lymph channels travel with the vasculature to the deep fascia, and these collecting lymph channels drain into lymph nodes (11). In general, the collecting lymph trunks can be found superficial to the veins (6). In contrast to the lymphatic capillaries, the larger lymphatic channels contain smooth muscle within their walls which contracts to propel the forward movement of lymph (9). These larger lymph channels have an outer coat consisting of longitudinal connective tissue fibers along with elastic fibers, a middle coat of circular smooth muscle, and an inner coat of longitudinal fibrils with an endothelial lining (9). Larger vessels drain primarily to lymph nodes.

The movement of lymph throughout this extensive network is due to several factors. An osmotic pressure gradient exists between the interstitium and the lymphatic capillaries, causing the capillaries to fill (10). Muscular contractions of the larger lymphatic channels cause forward lymph flow, and backflow is prevented by the numerous valves, which are present every 2 to 3 mm (6). External pressures, including arterial pulsation and respiration, also facilitate forward lymph flow. Compression of the muscles surrounding lymph vessels and changes in limb position also contribute to forward movement of lymph (12).

## Lymph Nodes

Lymph nodes are discrete structures comprised of lymphoid tissue, lymphatic vessels, a single artery and vein, and a supporting structural framework of fibrous connective tissue. They vary in size, ranging from 2 to 3 mm to 3 or 4 cm, and are round or oval in shape. Each node has multiple afferent lymphatic vessels that penetrate at different points along the convex side of the nodal capsule, and the lymph exits at the concave side of the node through efferent channels in the hilum (1).

Lymph flows into the afferent lymphatic channels to the peripheral or marginal sinus of the node, which is a space within the inner periphery filled with lymph (Figure 7-1). The marginal sinus contains a retinaculum, which serves to anchor large antigens such as cancer cells and infectious agents. Lymph then extravasates from this sinus and slowly travels through the central portion of the node. Initial contact between foreign material and the immune system takes place within the lymph node parenchyma in zones rich in B or T lymphocytes. Primary follicles, or aggregates of B lymphocytes, are adjacent to the peripheral sinus. The paracortex, or T lymphocyte–rich zone, lies between the primary follicles. The medulla (deep to the cortex) contains plasma cells. The medullary sinuses come together to form the efferent channel in the hilum that travels with the nodal blood supply, through which the lymph exits the lymph node (11).

Both the lymph exiting the node and the venous blood exiting the node contain activated lymphocytes, including B and T cells for the production of antibodies and cytotoxic T cells. Activated lymphocytes then reach the systemic circulation, ensuring immunocompetence (13). From the lymph nodes, the efferent lymph channels join to form terminal collecting ducts that drain into large lymphatic trunks, which in turn drain into the blood circulation.

While the primary flow of lymph is through the node, antigenic agents may also enter the lymph node through the blood via the arteries entering the lymph node hilum (14). This provides a means for these substances to reach the germinal centers directly from the circulation. It should be noted, however, that numerous lymphaticovenous connections exist that allow bypass of regional lymph nodes (5).

Lymph nodes are widely distributed throughout the body and are the most easily accessible part of the lymphoid system. Due to their accessibility, lymph nodes are frequently evaluated by needle or surgical biopsy for

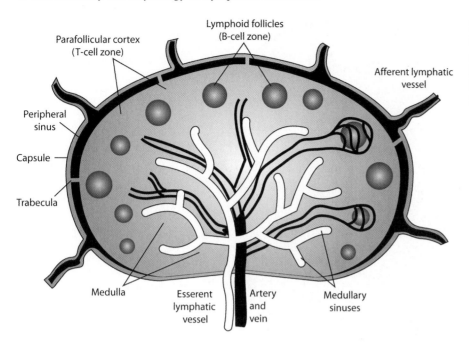

Parafollicular cortex
(T-cell zone)

Lymphoid follicles
(B-cell zone)

Peripheral
sinus

Capsule

Trabecula

Medulla

Esserent
lymphatic
vessel

Artery
and
vein

Medullary
sinuses

Afferent lymphatic
vessel

FIGURE 7-1. Schematic diagram illustrating the blood and lymphatic supply of a lymph node. (Cotran RS, *Robbins Pathologic Basis of Disease*, 1999. Reprinted with permission from Elsevier.)

diagnosis of lymphoreticular disorders and malignancy. Lymph nodes are in constant dynamic interaction with their environment, and their shape and size may change in response to the substances they encounter. They are prone to inflammation during infection and obstruction in the face of metastatic disease (15).

Lymph nodes also change and respond to stimuli in the absence of clinical disease. Antigenic stimulation may cause primary follicles within the node to enlarge and develop germinal centers. The degree of morphologic change depends on the inciting factor and the intensity of the subsequent immune response. Significant insults or infections produce enlargement of nodes and can leave residual scarring.

It is unclear whether lymph nodes regenerate after removal or regional lymph node dissection. Animal studies have suggested that regeneration of lymph nodes occurs in the young but not in adults (6). While it is unknown whether lymph nodes regenerate, it has been shown in animal models that lymphatic channels have a remarkable capacity to regenerate within days of severing them.

## Imaging Techniques

Various techniques for studying the lymphatic system have evolved over time. In the early 20th century, oil colors dissolved in turpentine were injected into fresh cadaver specimens. In the 1930s, the contrast agent Thorotrast was introduced for postmortem injection of lymphatics; the Thorotrast precipitated after specimens were fixed, and then radiographs were obtained illustrating the lymphatic network. In vivo injection materials,

including blue dyes, were also introduced in the 1930s. The radiologic imaging of lymphatics by directly injecting contrast material into them is known as lymphangiography, and it has been an ongoing method of study for regional nodes (6).

Imaging of the lymphatic system has evolved from imaging of the lymph vessels themselves through lymphangiography, to cross-sectional imaging including x-ray transmission computed tomography (CT) and magnetic resonance imaging (MRI). These imaging modalities provide a morphologic assessment of shape, size, and patterns of contrast enhancement, which are used as diagnostic guides for the presence of disease (16). Newer imaging modalities, including positron emission tomography (PET), evaluate tumor metabolism in lymph using a radioactive tracer (2-$^{18}$F-2-desoxy-D-glucose) that is consumed by cells in proportion to glucose utilization (malignant and inflammatory cells consume more glucose than normal tissue). PET scanning is based on the principle that tumor cells metabolize more glucose compared to normal tissue, providing a functional assessment of nodal status. Currently, multimodality imaging techniques, including fusion PET-CT, are being investigated to assess the functional status of a lymph node in addition to precise anatomic information (17).

## Regional Anatomy of the Lymphatic System

In general, the naming of lymph node groups follows several patterns. Nodes are named according to the associated vasculature, as many nodal groups are adjacent to a prominent blood vessel or vessel branch. Nodes

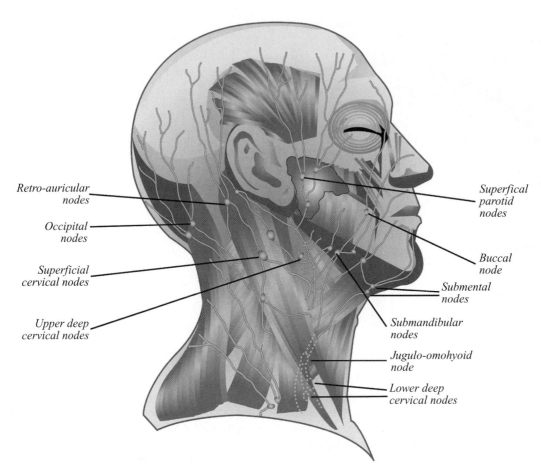

*Retro-auricular nodes*

*Occipital nodes*

*Superficial cervical nodes*

*Upper deep cervical nodes*

*Superfical parotid nodes*

*Buccal node*

*Submental nodes*

*Submandibular nodes*

*Jugulo-omohyoid node*

*Lower deep cervical nodes*

FIGURE 7-2. Superficial lymph nodes and lymphatic vessels of the head and neck. (Gray H. *Gray's Anatomy*, 38e, 1995, reprinted with permission from Elsevier.) (See Color Plate.)

also can be designated according to adjacent or related organs, or general topographic location may figure in the naming, such as the axillary nodes or inguinal nodes (18).

## Head and Neck

There is marked variation in the lymphatic drainage of the head and neck, with extensive interconnection between the lymphatic channels and even drainage to the contralateral side. The scalp has afferents that drain into multiple regional lymph node basins, including the submental, submandibular, facial, parotid, postauricular, and occipital groups. The scalp can be divided into the frontal zone, which drains into the preauricular parotid nodes, and the parietal zone, which drains into the postauricular nodes (which continue efferently into the lateral internal jugular nodes). The occipital zone of the scalp drains to the internal jugular or spinal accessory chains (19).

The face above the commissure of the lip and anterior to the pinna of the ear drains to the parotid nodes (Figure 7-2, see Color Plate). The face inferior to the commis-

sure of the lip drains to the cervical nodal basin. The ear drains to the parotid and submandibular nodes. The forehead, upper half of the ear, anterior wall of the external acoustic meatus, zygoma, and lateral vessels from the eyelids drain to the superficial parotid nodes anterior to the tragus. The auricle, floor of the meatus, and skin over the angle of the mandible drain to the superficial cervical nodes. The lower lip, external nose, cheeks, upper lip, and mucous membranes of the lips and cheeks drain to the submandibular nodes. The central part of the lower lip, buccal floor, and lingual apex drain to the submental nodes (11).

The parotid basin consists of the extraglandular and intraglandular nodes. The extraglandular nodes include the preauricular and infra-auricular nodes, which receive afferents from the lateral and frontal scalp, the external auditory canal, the upper lid and lateral aspect of the lower lid, the nose, and the upper lip and malar regions. The intraglandular nodes are along the facial vein, between the superficial and deep lobes of the parotid gland. These nodes drain the lateral aspect of the eyelids, the conjunctiva, the eustachian tube, and the tympanic membrane (19).

The roof of the nasopharynx contains the pharyngeal tonsils, which are collections of lymphoid tissue in the pyriform fossae and in the lymphoid ring of Waldeyer. The posterior pharyngeal wall drains to the jugulodigastric, midjugular, jugulo-omohyoid, and retropharyngeal nodes. There is extensive lymphatic drainage of the hypopharynx into the midjugular, jugulo-omohyoid, and retropharyngeal lymph node basins. The nasopharyngeal region drains into the jugulodigastric nodal chain or the posterior triangle. The nasal cavity and paranasal sinuses drain into the retropharyngeal lymph nodes (11).

The larynx is divided into the supraglottic, glottic, and subglottic regions. The supraglottic larynx has copious lymphatic drainage extending anteriorly to the pre-epiglottic space and laterally to the midjugular and paratracheal lymph nodes. The glottic region, which contains the vocal cords, has a paucity of lymphatic drainage. The subglottic larynx drains into the cervical lymph node basins.

The skin of the neck can be divided by the posterior border of the sternocleidomastoid muscle up to the earlobe into an anterior and a posterior portion. The anterior skin generally drains into the internal jugular chain, while the posterior skin drains into the spinal accessory chains (19).

Traditionally, cervical lymph nodes comprise 5 levels. Level I contains the submental and submandibular lymph nodes. Level II incorporates the upper jugular chain, including the jugulodigastric nodes. Level III includes the middle jugular chain (between the digastric muscle superiorly, and the omohyoid muscle inferiorly.) Level IV contains the lower jugular chain (below the omohyoid muscle,) and level V includes the posterior triangle, or spinal accessory chain lymph nodes (11).

The thyroid gland drains primarily to the tracheal, pretracheal, and paratracheal groups of nodes, as well as directly into the thoracic duct. In addition, the superior pole can drain into the superior group of internal jugular nodes, while the inferior pole may drain into the mid- and lower internal jugular nodes.

## Thorax

The lung has an extensive network of lymphatic drainage, divided into pulmonary lymph nodes and mediastinal lymph nodes. The pulmonary nodes consist of intrapulmonary or segmental nodes that mark the points of division of segmental bronchi as well as the pulmonary artery bifurcation. Lobar nodes lie along the upper, middle, and lower lobe bronchi. The interlobar nodes, situated in the angles formed by the bifurcation of the main bronchi into lobar bronchi, drain all the pulmonary lobes of the corresponding lung. Hilar nodes are positioned along the main bronchi (20).

The mediastinal nodes consist of 3 main groups: anterior mediastinal (brachiocephalic), posterior mediastinal, and the tracheobronchial groups. The anterior mediastinal or brachiocephalic nodes are anterior to the aortic arch and brachiocephalic veins, and drain the heart, pericardium, thymus, thyroid gland, and lateral diaphragm. The posterior mediastinal nodes are located behind the pericardium and drain the esophagus, posterior pericardium, diaphragm, and possibly the left lobe of the liver. This nodal group drains efferently directly into the thoracic duct or into the tracheobronchial nodes (11).

The tracheobronchial group is comprised of the tracheal, superior tracheobronchial, inferior tracheobronchial, bronchopulmonary, and pulmonary nodal basins. The tracheal nodes drain the trachea and upper esophagus and receive afferents from the subgroups of the tracheobronchial nodes. Efferents from the tracheal nodes form the right and left bronchomediastinal trunks, after joining with the parasternal and anterior mediastinal nodal trunks. The right and left bronchomediastinal trunks usually drain into the junction of the internal jugular and subclavian veins on their respective sides, but may occasionally drain into the thoracic duct (20).

The thoracic duct is the largest lymphatic channel draining all the lymph from below the diaphragm and the left half of the thorax, as well as the left side of the head and neck and the left upper extremity. It forms from the confluence of the right and left abdominal trunks, which drain the abdominal aortic lymph nodes and occasionally form a cisterna chyli. The thoracic duct ascends through the thorax to the right of the vertebral column, passes posterior to the aortic arch, and travels to the left of the esophagus into the neck. It then loops over the left subclavian artery to empty into the junction of the left internal jugular and subclavian veins. The thoracic duct has tributaries that include the confluence of lymph trunks, the anterior mediastinal, internal mammary, internal jugular, tracheobronchial, subclavian, and transverse cervical trunks. The lymphatic drainage on the right side is variable, and may include lymph trunks from the right thorax and mediastinum that drain into the right internal jugular and subclavian vein junction. Occasionally, the right jugular trunk, right subclavian trunk, and right bronchomediastinal trunk merge to form the right lymphatic duct, which empties into the right internal jugular and subclavian vein junction (11).

The pleura contains lymphatic vessels in both the visceral and parietal layers. The deeper tissues of the thoracic wall drain into parasternal internal thoracic nodes along the internal thoracic artery. Intercostal nodes receive deep lymphatic vessels from the posterolateral aspects of the chest wall and the breast. The thoracic surface of the diaphragm contains lymphatic channels that drain to the parasternal nodes. The upper esophagus drains to the deep cervical nodes, the thoracic portion drains to the posterior mediastinal nodes, and the abdominal portion drains to the left gastric nodes.

## Stomach, Duodenum, and Pancreas

Gastric lymphatics follow the vascular distribution and are extensively interconnected (Figure 7-3, see Color Plate). Malignant gastric nodal involvement often spreads to nodal groups well beyond the area of primary drainage. The primary drainage of the proximal lesser curvature is to the left gastric nodes near the gastroesophageal junction, which have both superior and inferior subgroups. Lymph from both the stomach and abdominal esophagus is collected in these nodes, which then drain into the celiac group of preaortic nodes. The proximal greater curvature drains into splenic nodes as well as

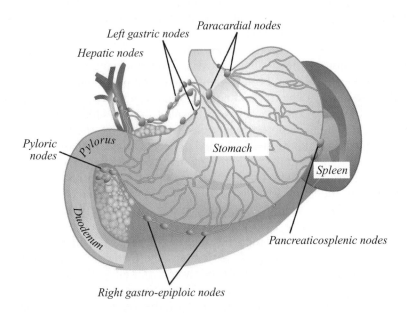

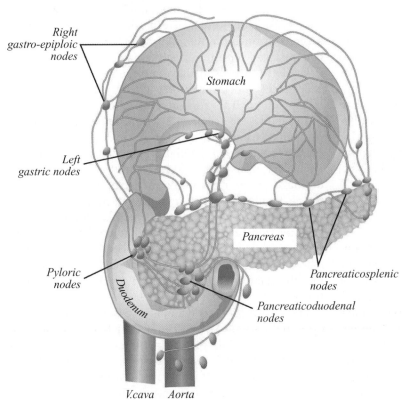

FIGURE 7-3. Lymphatic drainage of the stomach, duodenum, and pancreas. (Gray H. *Gray's Anatomy*, 38e, copyright 1995, reprinted with permission from Elsevier.) (See Color Plate.)

right gastroepiploic nodes that are found in the greater omentum along the pyloric side of the greater curvature. The right gastroepiploic nodes drain into the pyloric nodal basins. The gastric fundus and body drain into the pancreaticosplenic nodes along lymphatic channels accompanying the short gastric and left gastroepiploic vessels (21).

The pyloric nodes consist of suprapyloric and infrapyloric basins, which are located near the bifurcation of the gastroduodenal artery in the angle between the first and second portion of the duodenum. These drain the pylorus, the first portion of the duodenum, and the right gastroepiploic nodes. The pyloric nodes drain into the celiac nodes. Valves within the lymphatic channels direct lymph from the right part of the stomach to the lesser curvature, and from the left part of the stomach to the greater curvature. The remainder of the duodenum is drained by lymphatics traveling anteriorly and posteriorly in the groove between the pancreatic head and the duodenum. These duodenal channels drain efferently into the hepatic and preaortic nodes around the origin of the superior mesenteric artery (11).

Lymphatic drainage of the pancreas generally follows venous drainage. Superior nodes drain the anterior and superior upper half of the pancreas, while inferior nodes along the inferior margin of the head and body drain the anterior and posterior lower half. Anterior nodes located inferior to the pylorus drain the anterior surface of the head of the pancreas. Posterior nodes in the groove between the pancreas and duodenum drain the posterior surface of the pancreatic head. Posterior nodes are also found along the common bile duct and in the aorta at both the origin of the celiac and superior mesenteric arteries. The tail of the pancreas drains into splenic nodal basins (11).

## Small Bowel

The small bowel is important in the maintenance of immune function, since the large surface area of the small bowel mucosa provides a potential portal of entry for bacteria and pathogens. The small bowel contains a secretory immune system that produces antibodies that resist bacterial proliferation, neutralize viruses, and minimize the transluminal penetration of toxins (Figure 7-4).

Antigens from the intestinal lumen that cross the mucosal barrier initially contact specialized cells called microfold (M) cells, which overlie lymphoid nodules (11). These M cells are specialized to take up and transport antigen, by taking antigen in at the luminal surface and transferring it to the intraepithelial regions at their base, where T cells and antigen-presenting cells are present. Lymphoblast production of immunoglobulin A is initiated after interacting with the antigen presented

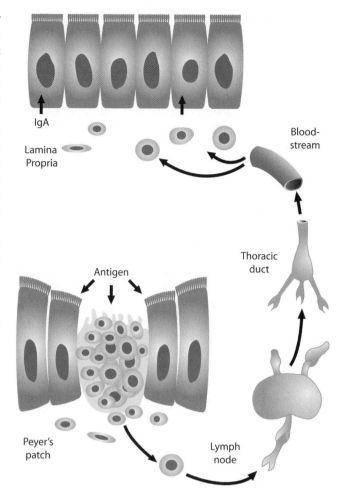

FIGURE 7-4. Schematic representation of the pathways involved in the secretory immune system. Lymphocytes in Peyer patches encounter antigens in the gut lumen and migrate to regional lymph nodes and to the bloodstream via the thoracic duct. In the blood, they travel back into the lamina propria of the gut and develop into plasma cells that secrete IgA and are released into the gut lumen. (Schwartz, *Principles of Surgery*, 1999, used by permission of the McGraw-Hill Companies.)

by the M cells. The primed lymphoblasts then migrate to the regional lymph nodes. These antigen-primed lymphoblasts are carried into the systemic circulation, thereby enabling a localized immune response to disseminate and become a systemic response. They are eventually returned to the intestine and distributed in the lamina propria (22).

There are 3 groups of mesenteric nodes. The first is located in close proximity to the intestinal wall along the terminal branches of the jejunal and ileal arteries. The second group is found among the looping and primary branches of the arteries. The third juxtaarterial group is situated along the upper trunk of the superior mesenteric artery (11).

## Colon and Rectum

Lymphatic drainage of the colon and rectum also parallels the arterial distribution (Figure 7-5, see Color Plate). The ascending and transverse colon drain into nodes along the right and middle colic arteries and their branches. These drain efferently into the superior mesenteric nodes. The descending and sigmoid colon drain into nodes along the left colic artery, entering the paraaortic nodes at the origin of the inferior mesenteric artery (23).

The colonic mucosa has no lymphatics, so superficial cancers that do not extend to the submucosa cannot metastasize via lymphatic channels. The submucosa and muscularis mucosa have lymphatic channels that run circumferentially around the lumen. Lymph nodes may be categorized as epicolic (on the bowel wall and the appendices epiploicae), paracolic (along the inner margin of the bowel), intermediate (along the named mesenteric arteries), and main (along the superior and inferior mesenteric arteries). Tumor involvement of the circumferential lymphatics may result in the classic annular constricting lesion (11).

The ascending and transverse colon are drained by nodes along the branches of the right colic and middle colic arteries, and into the superior mesenteric nodal basin. The descending and sigmoid colon drain into channels along the left colic vessels, with efferents into the paraaortic nodes at the level of the inferior mesenteric artery.

The lymphatic drainage of the rectum also corresponds to the blood supply. The upper and middle rectum initially drain to pararectal nodes, then to inferior mesenteric nodes. The lower rectum follows the superior rectal artery and drains into the inferior mesenteric nodal basin; it can also drain laterally along the middle and inferior rectal arteries, posteriorly along the middle sacral artery, or anteriorly through the rectovesicular or rectovaginal septum. These channels drain to the iliac and then periaortic nodes. The anal canal above the dentate line drains to the inferior mesenteric nodes via the superior rectal lymphatics, or laterally to the hypogastric nodes; below the dentate line, it is drained primarily by the inguinal nodes (11).

## Liver and Spleen

The liver has an extensive superficial subserosal plexus in the capsule, as well as channels accompanying the hepatic artery and portal vein. Hepatic nodes vary both

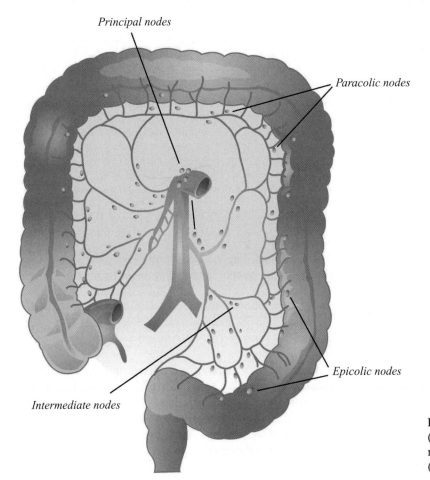

FIGURE 7-5. Lymph nodes of the colon. (Gray H. *Gray's Anatomy*, 38e, copyright 1995, reprinted with permission from Elsevier.) (See Color Plate.)

in location and in number. Nodal groups are located along the hepatic arteries, bile duct, lesser omentum, and the junction of the cystic and common bile ducts; they drain not only the liver, but also the stomach, duodenum, liver, gallbladder, bile ducts, and pancreas. The hepatic nodes drain efferently to the celiac nodal basin. Some lymph flows directly from the liver into the thoracic duct through the coronary and right triangular ligaments, which contain lymph channels draining directly into the thoracic duct without any intervening nodes (24).

The spleen's lymphatic channels travel with the splenic artery, along the posterosuperior aspect of the pancreas. In addition, nodes are located in the gastrosplenic ligament. Splenic nodes also drain afferents from the stomach and pancreas, and these channels drain efferently into the celiac nodes.

## Urinary Tract and Reproductive Tract

The kidney lymphatics drain through the hilar trunks in the region of the renal artery and vein. The surrounding perinephric fat contains capsular lymphatics that carry afferents from the perinephric tissue and adrenals to the lateral aortic nodal plexus. The lateral aortic nodes travel along both sides of the aorta, terminating in a lumbar trunk on each side. The ureter has segmental drainage to preaortic and caval nodes. The bladder drains to the perivesicular, hypogastric, and preaortic nodes.

In men, the prostate and seminal vesicles send afferents to the obturator nodes, external/internal/common iliac nodes, and then to the preaortic nodes. The penis and urethra drain to the superficial and deep inguinal nodes, and then to the external and internal iliac nodes.

The testis drains to the preaortic nodes in the region of the kidney via channels that ascend adjacent to the spermatic cord and travel with the testicular vessels (11).

In women, the ovaries have lymphatic drainage that follows the ovarian vessels to the lateral aortic and preaortic nodes. The uterus and cervix drain to external iliac, internal iliac, rectal, sacral, obturator, and gluteal nodes. The upper portion of the uterus drains primarily to the lateral aortic and preaortic nodes, as well as the external iliac nodes. The cervix is drained along the round ligament to the superficial inguinal nodes. The vaginal vessels drain to the internal and external iliac nodes. The vulva and perineal skin drain to the superficial inguinal nodes, while the clitoris and labia minora drain to the deep inguinal nodes.

## Breast

The breast drains to lymph nodes at several different sites (25,26). The axilla is the main site, draining most of the breast lymph (Figure 7-6). Lymph vessels within the breast include those within the gland in interlobular spaces, paralleling the milk ducts. There is an intricate subareolar plexus draining the skin over the middle of the breast, as well as the nipple and areola; however, it is controversial whether it provides drainage for the breast parenchyma. Some believe this plexus collects lymph from the parenchymal lymphatics and transports it to the axilla, and this has led to the use of subareolar injections to localize the sentinel lymph node (25). There is also a network on the posterior surface of the breast parallel to the deep fascia in the retromammary space, which drains efferently into the axilla, the internal

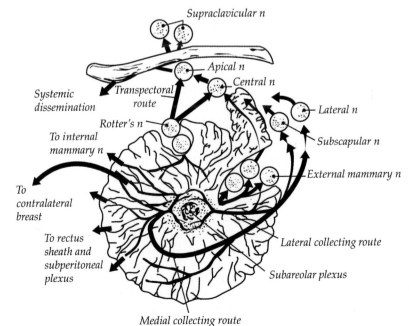

FIGURE 7-6. Routes of lymphatic drainage of the breast. (Bland, Copeland, *The Breast*, 3e, Vol 1, 2004. Reprinted with permission from Elsevier.)

mammary chain, or the parasternal nodes. The deeper thoracic structures drain into the parasternal, intercostal, or diaphragmatic nodes.

The axillary nodes consist of 3 groups defined by their relationship to the pectoralis minor muscle. Level I axillary nodes are located lateral to the pectoralis minor muscle and include the external mammary group, which runs parallel to the lateral thoracic artery and drains the lateral breast. The subscapular group is parallel to the subscapular vessels and drains the lower posterior neck, posterior trunk, and posterior shoulder. The lateral axillary vein group is situated on the anteriormost aspect of the latissimus dorsi and contains the largest number of nodes in the axilla. The axillary vein group, comprising 4 to 6 nodes medial or posterior to the axillary vein, receives most of the drainage from the upper extremity (11).

Level II axillary nodes are the central nodes, posterior to the pectoralis minor muscle in the axillary fat. These central nodes may receive lymph directly from the breast, but also receive afferents from the level I nodal groups.

Level III nodes are medial to the pectoralis minor muscle, and are the highest and most medial nodal group. The level III nodal group drains the other axillary groups and merges with vessels from the subclavicular groups to form the subclavian trunk.

An accessory route of lymphatic drainage for the breast is through the Rotter nodes, which lie between the pectoralis major and pectoralis minor muscles. The transpectoral channels originate in the retromammary plexus and penetrate the pectoralis major muscle, to travel with the thoracoacromial vessels and terminate in the level III nodal group. The retropectoral pathway drains the superior and medial aspects of the breast and also ends in the level III nodal group (27).

Central and medial lymphatics of the breast travel medially parallel to the arterioles to the internal mammary nodal chain. The right internal mammary chain drains efferently into the right lymphatic duct, while the left internal mammary group drains efferently into the thoracic duct. Rarely, the upper inner portion of the breast may drain directly to the supraclavicular nodes. Ipsilateral supraclavicular metastases are no longer considered stage IV disease (28).

## Extremities

Regional lymphatics of the limbs are usually located on their flexor aspect. The upper extremities are drained to the axillary nodes. The arm contains superficial lymphatic vessels in the subcutaneous tissue, which follow the median vein of the forearm to the antecubital area. They then travel proximally and through the deep fascia at the anterior axillary fold to enter the lateral axillary lymph nodes. The lateral forearm follows the cephalic

vein to the level of the deltoid tendon, and then to the lateral axillary nodes. The deep tissues of the arm drain along channels along the radial, ulnar, interosseous, and brachial neurovascular bundles, also ending in the lateral axillary nodes. The epitrochlear or supratrochlear node is located above the medial condyle of the humerus adjacent to the basilic vein. The deltopectoral lymph nodes are situated adjacent to the cephalic vein below the clavicle. The deltopectoral nodes drain directly into the subclavicular or level III axillary nodal basin (11).

The lower extremity similarly has deep lymphatic channels accompanying the major vessels (anterior tibial, posterior tibial, peroneal, popliteal, and femoral). The deep vessels from the foot and leg travel to the popliteal nodes, but may also run directly to the femoral nodes (Figure 7-7, see Color Plate). The deep vessels of the thigh drain to the deep inguinal nodes. The gluteal and ischial regions drain to the internal and external iliac nodes (29).

The groin has 2 contiguous node-bearing areas: superficial and deep inguinal nodes. The superficial nodes are

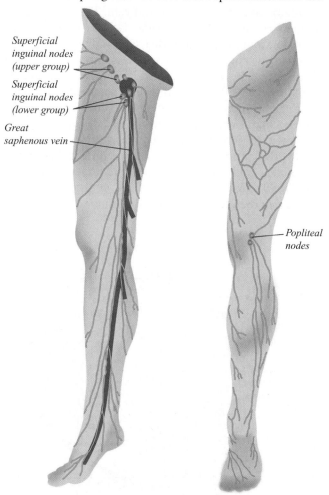

*Superficial inguinal nodes (upper group)*

*Superficial inguinal nodes (lower group)*

*Great saphenous vein*

*Popliteal nodes*

FIGURE 7-7. Lymphatic drainage of the superficial tissues of the lower extremity. (Gray H. *Gray's Anatomy*, 38e, copyright 1995, reprinted with permission from Elsevier.) (See Color Plate.)

found within the femoral triangle and drain the external genitalia, inferior anal canal, perianal region, lower abdominal wall, and the uterine vessels. In addition, the lower extremity drains primarily to the superficial inguinal nodes. The deep inguinal nodes are located medial to the femoral vein above the inguinal ligament, along the iliac and obturator vessels. The deep nodes receive lymphatics from the femoral vessels, the penis or clitoris, and efferents from the superficial inguinal nodes; they drain into the external iliac nodes (29).

## Pathophysiology of Lymph Node Metastases

In the 19th century, Virchow postulated that a substance is eluted by a primary tumor that travels to the regional nodal basin and produces secondary foci of tumors (14). His contemporaries established that tumor cells disseminate through the lymphatic system, leading to nodal and distant metastatic disease. There are 2 methods of tumor spread through lymphatics. The first is permeation, in which the cancer cells directly invade lymphatic vessels and grow in continuity along their lumen until they reach the lymph nodes (6). The second and more common method of spread is by metastasis, in which cancer cells travel through lymphatic vessels as tumor emboli (Figure 7-8) (30). Historically, radical lymph node dissections were incorporated into cancer operations to include resection of the organ of origin with en bloc removal of the intervening lymphatics and regional lymph nodes (6).

Factors affecting lymph node metastases include both anatomic and mechanical forces. Anatomic factors start within the primary tumor itself, in which a dynamic

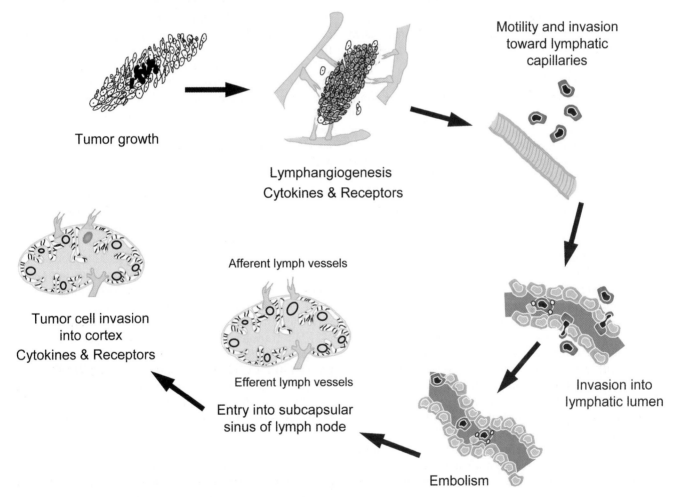

**Tumor growth**

**Lymphangiogenesis Cytokines & Receptors**

**Motility and invasion toward lymphatic capillaries**

**Tumor cell invasion into cortex Cytokines & Receptors**

Afferent lymph vessels

Efferent lymph vessels

**Entry into subcapsular sinus of lymph node**

**Invasion into lymphatic lumen**

**Embolism**

FIGURE 7-8. As the tumor enlarges and secretes lymphangiogenic cytokines, new lymphatics grow toward the edge of the tumor. Intratumoral lymphangiogenesis may occur. Tumor cells invade the extracellular matrix and move toward the lymphatic capillaries. Malignant cells invade into the lymphatic lumen and follow the lymphatic stream into the sentinel lymph node. Tumor cells enter the node through the subcapsular sinus, and then invade the cortex of the lymph node and proliferate and metastasize to other lymph nodes. (Nathanson, SD, Insights into the mechanisms of lymph node metastasis. Cancer 2003;98(2):413–423, used with permission.)

interaction between intratumoral and peritumoral forces takes place. Interstitial fluid pressure within the tumor increases as the tumor grows in size. Cells from the growing tumor break through and invade the extracellular matrix, driven by an interstitial fluid pressure gradient (with pressure lower in the extracellular matrix). In addition, hydrostatic pressure differences lead to tumor cell movement toward peritumoral lymphatic capillaries. The tumor cells then essentially embolize through the lymphatic system (30).

Tumor cells are pushed along the external surface of the endothelium on the lymphatic capillaries by fine cytoplasmic processes. As the interstitium swells, anchoring filaments pull the intercellular junctions open, which allows the tumor cells to enter the lumen through these gaps. The junctions close when the pressure outside the lymphatic capillaries decreases, which prevents backflow into the interstitium. Some tumor cells can adhere to the endothelium and locally invade through the surrounding tissues, causing intransit metastases or localized areas of tumor cell growth. Most tumor cells travel singly or in clusters through the lymphatic channels and deposit in the regional lymph nodes (30).

Tumor cells enter the sentinel lymph node through afferent channels into the peripheral subcapsular sinus, where they are initially caught in a retinaculum within the sinus, which acts as a matrix to anchor antigenic substances including cancer and infectious cells (14). As they multiply, the tumor cells grow through the walls of the sinus and into the parenchyma of the lymph node. The entire node may eventually be replaced by disease. The tumor cells can then permeate the capsule of the node and invade surrounding tissues, causing the node clinically to become fixed and firm. With extensive malignant lymph node involvement, lymph flow may be blocked, causing diversion or reversal of lymph flow. This can precipitate new emboli traveling in different directions through the lymphatic system (30).

Not all metastatic tumor cells cause lymph node infiltration. Metastatic tumor cells may be destroyed by physiologic or immune processes within the node, may remain within the node without progressive growth, or may grow within the node to become a metastatic deposit (31). Metastatic cancer cells within the lymph node serve as an indicator of the ability of cancer cells to metastasize from the primary tumor site. Patients may have lymph node metastases but never develop systemic disease. The number of lymph node metastases has been shown to relate to the future development of systemic disease (32).

Metastatic cancer cells appear to attach to the lymphatic metastatic site via specific interactions between the tumor cell and endothelial or lymph node structural element receptors (30). Once the tumor cells attach, to remain viable they have to evade possible immune system rejec-tion as well as produce angiogenic factors that are essential for growth. Organ-specific metastases have also been demonstrated in animal models (33). Metastatic tumor cells have been harvested in animal models that metastasize preferentially to the liver, lung, or lymph nodes. Tumor cells that lodge and grow in lymph nodes may not have the ability to proliferate in other organs (34).

Ongoing research indicates that there is a complex relationship between the tumor cells and the microenvironment in which it lodges in the host (35). In metastatic melanoma, cell lines highly metastatic to lymph nodes have been shown to express high levels of the integrin receptor alpha$_v$beta$_3$ molecule, which binds preferentially to vitronectin as opposed to fibronectin (36). In addition, synthesis of vitronectin in the lymph node is upregulated in the presence of tumor cells (37). This indicates that not only does the regulation of adhesion molecules change in the tumor cell environment, but the lymph node may also become favorable to tumor cells by upregulating receptors. Immunosuppressive products of tumor cells also have been demonstrated in melanoma cell lines that suppress lymph node activity (38).

Tumors actively interact with the lymphatics by inducing lymphangiogenesis, or the development of new lymphatics from host vessels (39). This promotes the entry of tumor cells into the lymphatic vessels and their subsequent transport to lymph nodes. Histologic studies have shown an increase in lymphatics at the periphery of growing tumors, as lymphangiogenesis appears to accompany angiogenesis (40). It is still unclear whether intratumoral lymphatics are present, since the lymphatic vessels noted within tumors may be related to normal host tissue that has been invaded by tumor (41). Manipulation of lymphangiogenesis factors may represent a potential avenue for therapy of malignant tumors.

Some molecular markers help distinguish lymphatic endothelial cells from blood vessel endothelial cells. Vascular endothelial growth factor receptor-3 is a receptor tyrosine kinase restricted to lymphatic endothelial cells (42). In transgenic mice, the tumor-secreted cytokine VEGF-C has been shown to induce lymphatic vessel hyperplasia (40). In addition, podoplanin and PROX-1 are receptors found only on lymphatic endothelial cells (43, 44). The gene Prox1 is expressed in a population of endothelial cells that gives rise to the lymphatic system (45).

Chemokine factors are also thought to affect lymphatic metastases (46). Chemokines are chemoattractant cytokines that bind to cell surface receptors and initiate cell-signalling pathways through G-protein–coupled receptors. They orchestrate the movement of various cells to specific anatomic sites and are involved with regulation of lymphocyte and phagocyte directional movement. Several studies indicate that both chemokines and their receptors play an important role in the metastatic destination of malignant cells (46–48).

# Lymph Node Dissections

Lymph node dissections have been an essential part of the surgical treatment of malignancy. Reasons to perform regional lymph node dissections include obtaining regional control, staging, and perhaps improving survival. In the past, radical resections included removal of the tumor, intervening lymphatics, and regional lymph nodes. Regional lymph nodes were believed to serve as a filter that functioned as a temporary barrier to the further spread of tumor cells; it was thought that if the affected nodes could be removed before the systemic spread of the tumor, progression of metastases to systemic disease could be halted (14).

Rather than acting as a filter, the lymph node is now understood to act as an antigen recognition station that allows tumor cells to either pass through or remain within the node through specific interactions between the tumor cells and the lymph node (14). However, the question of whether a lymph node metastasis serves as a nidus of tumor that can disseminate, or whether nodal involvement is merely indicative of overall metastatic potential, remains unanswered.

The sentinel lymph node concept is based on the idea that the afferent lymphatic channel draining a primary tumor goes first to the "sentinel" node, and this lymph node will be the most likely to harbor metastasis, if present. This concept was first tested by Cabanas in the 1970s (49), then revisited by Morton in an animal model and then validated in melanoma patients (50). Subsequently, beginning in 1991, it was validated for axillary evaluation in breast cancer patients by Giuliano et al. at the John Wayne Cancer Institute and reported in 174 patients using a vital dye (Figure 7-9) (51). Current techniques for sentinel lymph node evaluation include dye-directed lymphatic mapping, isotope-based radiolocalization, and most commonly a combination of dye and radioisotope localization. The relatively new technique of sentinel lymph node biopsy spares patients the morbidity of a radical lymph node dissection if the sentinel node is unaffected, while still obtaining valuable prognostic information.

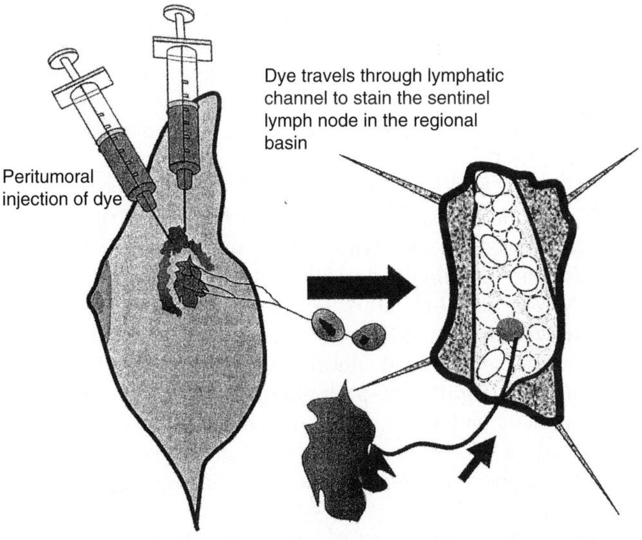

The sentinel lymph node also appears to play a key part in host immunity against the tumor (52). Tumor-suppressor cell activity has been demonstrated in the draining lymph nodes from breast cancer, with downregulation of antigen-presenting cells in the paracortex and modulation of paracortical dendritic cells and T cells (53). This immune activity has been demonstrated in sentinel and not in nonsentinel lymph nodes, indicating that the sentinel node has a unique role in the host immune response. In addition, regional lymph nodes have demonstrated the capability to destroy tumor cells (54).

There are marked variations in lymphatic metastases (55). Contralateral lymph node involvement is also possible in breast cancer as well as melanoma. This is more likely in the setting of a previous regional lymph node dissection on the ipsilateral side of the tumor or obstruction of the primary drainage basin by metastases, but contralateral drainage is possible in any circumstance. In addition, there is also a possibility of retrograde or more peripheral lymphatic spread of tumor; in this case, the flow of lymph is thought to be reversed despite the presence of the numerous valves in the lymphatic network. Reversal of flow is attributed to blockage of lymph flow along normal routes by lymph node metastases, causing retrograde embolization of tumor cells.

FIGURE 7-9. Schematic diagram of blue dye transit from primary breast tumor to the sentinel node. (Bland, Copeland, *The Breast*, 3e, Vol 1, 2004, Reprinted with permission from Elsevier.)

## References

1. Aster J, Kumar V. White cells, lymph nodes, spleen, and thymus. In: Cotran RS, Kumar V, Collins T. *Robbins Pathologic Basis of Disease*. Philadelphia: WB Saunders; 1999:644–686.
2. Shields JW. Lymph, lymph glands, and homeostasis. *Lymphology*. 1992;25:147–153.
3. Bleiweiss IJ, Nagi CS, Jaffer S. Axillary sentinel lymph nodes can be falsely positive due to iatrogenic displacement and transport of benign epithelial cells in patients with breast carcinoma. *J Clin Oncol*. 2006;24:2013–2018.
4. Deitch Ea, Xu D, Kaiser VL. Role of the gut in the development of injury and shock-induced SIRS and MODS: the gut-lymph hypothesis, a review. *Front Biosci*. 2006;11:520–528.
5. Yaghoobian J, Markowitz H, Pinck L. Venolymphatic communication. *Lymphology*. 1982;15:178–180.
6. Haagensen CD. *The Lymphatics in Cancer*. Philadelphia: WB Saunders; 1972.
7. Yoffey JM, Courtice F. *Lymph, Lymphatics, and the Lymphomyeloid Complex*. London: Academic Press; 1970.

8. Foster RS Jr. General anatomy of the lymphatic system. *Surg Oncol Clin N Am.* 1996;5:1–13.

9. Schmid-Schonbein GW. Microlymphatics and lymph flow. *Physiol Rev.* 1990;70:987–1021.

10. Aukland K, Reed RK. Interstitial-lymphatic mechanisms in the control of extracellular fluid volume. *Physiol Rev.* 1993;73:1–78.

11. Bannister LH. Haemolymphoid system. In: *Gray's Anatomy.* London: Churchill Livingstone; 1999:1417–1450.

12. Olszewski W, Engeset A, Jaeger PM, Sokolowski J, Theodorsen L. Flow and composition of leg lymph in normal men during venous stasis, muscular activity, and local hyperthermia. *Acta Physiol Scand.* 1977;99:149–155.

13. Butcher EC, Picker LJ. Lymphocyte homing and homeostasis. *Science.* 1996;272:60–66.

14. Gervasoni JE, Taneja C, Chung MA, Cady B. Biologic and clinical significance of lymphadenectomy. *Surg Clin N Am.* 2000;80:1631–1673.

15. Van der Valk P, Meijer CJ. The histology of reactive lymph nodes. *Am J Surg Pathol.* 1987;11:866–882.

16. Luciani A, Itti E, Rahmouni A, Meignan M, Clement O. Lymph node imaging: basic principles. *Eur J Rad.* 2006; 58:338–344.

17. Veit P, Ruehm S, Kuehl H, Stergar H, Mueller S, Bockisch A, et al. Lymph node staging with dual-modality PET/CT: enhancing the diagnostic accuracy in oncology. *Eur J Rad.* 2006;58:383–389.

18. Gabella G. Cardiovascular system. In: *Gray's Anatomy.* London: Churchill Livingstone; 1999:1604–1626.

19. Lin D, Franc BL, Kashani-Sabet M, Singer M. Lymphatic drainage patterns of head and neck cutaneous melanoma observed on lymphoscintigraphy and sentinel lymph node biopsy. *Head and Neck.* 2006;28:249–255.

20. Mountain CF, Dresler CM. Regional lymph node classification for lung cancer staging. *Chest.* 1997;111:1718–1723.

21. Maruyama K, Gunven P, Okabayashi K, Sasako M, Kinoshita T. Lymph node metastases of gastric cancer. *Ann Surg.* 1989;210:596–602.

22. Evers BM, Townsend CM, Thompson JC. Small intestine. In: Schwartz SI. *Principles of Surgery.* New York: McGraw-Hill; 1999:1217–1264.

23. McDaniel KP, Charnsangavej C, Dubrow RA, Varma DGK, Granfield CAJ, Curley SA. Pathways of nodal metastasis in carcinomas of the cecum, ascending colon, and transverse colon: CT demonstration. *AJR.* 1993;161: 61–64.

24. Magari S. Hepatic lymphatic system: structure and function. *J Gastroenterol Hepatol.* 1990;5:82–93.

25. Chung M, Cady B. Selective management of the axilla in minimally invasive and small invasive ductal carcinoma. In: Bland KI, Copeland EM. *The Breast: Comprehensive Management of Benign and Malignant Disorders.* Vol 2. St. Louis: Elsevier; 2004:1031–1039.

26. Grube BJ, Giuliano AE. Lymphatic mapping and sentinel lymphadenectomy for breast cancer. In: Bland KI, Copeland EM. *The Breast: Comprehensive Management of Benign and Malignant Disorders.* Vol 2. St. Louis: Elsevier, 2004:1041–1079.

27. Tanis PJ, Niewig OE, Valdes Olmos RA, Kroon BR. Anatomy and physiology of lymphatic drainage of the breast from the perspective of sentinel node biopsy. *J Am Coll Surg.* 2001;192:399–409.

28. Singletary SE, Allred C, Ashley P, et al. Revision of the American Joint Committee on Cancer staging system for breast cancer. *J Clin Oncol.* 2002;20:3628–3636.

29. Pflug JJ, Calnan JS. The normal anatomy of the lymphatic system in the human leg. *Br J Surg.* 1971;58:925–30.

30. Nathanson SD. Insight into the mechanisms of lymph node metastasis. *Cancer.* 2003;98:413–423.

31. Weiss L. The pathobiology of metastasis within the lymphatic system. *Surg Oncol Clin N Am.* 1996;5:15–24.

32. Kryj M, Maciejewski B, Withers HR, Taylor JM. Incidence and kinetics of distant metastases in patients with operable breast cancer. *Neoplasm.* 1997;44:3–11.

33. Brodt P. Adhesion mechanisms in lymphatic metastasis. *Cancer Metastasis Rev.* 1991;10:23–32.

34. Brodt P, Reich R, Moroz LA, Chambers AF. Differences in the repertoires of basement membrane degrading enzymes in two carcinoma sublines with distinct patterns of site-selective metastasis. *Biochim Biophys Acta.* 1992;1139:77–83.

35. Liotta LA, Kohn LC. The microenvironment of the tumor-host interface. *Nature.* 2001;411:375–379.

36. Nip J, Shibata H, Loskutoff DJ. Human melanoma cells derived from lymphatic metastases use integrin-3 to adhere to lymph node vitronectin. *J Clin Invest.* 1992;90:1406–1413.

37. Reilly JT, Nash JRG. Vitronectin (serum spreading factor): its localizations in normal and fibrotic tissue. *J Clin Pathol.* 1988;41:1269–1272.

38. Hoon DS, Bowker R, Cochran AJ. Suppressor cell activity in melanoma-draining lymph nodes. *Cancer Res.* 1987;47: 1529–1533.

39. Lymboussaki A, Achen MG, Stacker SA, Alitalo K. Growth factors regulating lymphatic vessels. *Curr Top Microbiol Immunol.* 2000;251:75–82.

40. Jeltsch M, Kaipainen A, Joukov V, Meng X, Lakso M, Rauvala H, et al. Hyperplasia of lymphatic vessels in VEGF-C transgenic mice. *Science.* 1997;276:1423–1425.

41. Padera TP, Kadambi A, diTomaso E, Carreira CM, Brown EB, Boucher Y, et al. Lymphatic metastasis in the absence of functional intratumor lymphatics. *Science.* 2002;296: 1883–1886.

42. He Y, Kozaki K, Karpanen T, Koshikawa K, Yla-Herttuala S, Takahashi T, et al. Suppression of tumor lymphangiogenesis and lymph node metastasis by blocking vascular endothelial growth factor receptor 3 signaling. *J Natl Cancer Inst.* 2002;94:819–825.

43. Breiteneder-Geleff S, Soleiman A, Kowalski H. Angiosarcomas express mixed endothelial phenotypes of blood and lymphatic capillaries: podoplanin as a specific marker for lymphatic endothelium. *Am J Pathol.* 1999;154:385–394.

44. Banerji S, Ni J, Wang SX. LYVE-1, new homologue of the CD-44 glycoprotein, is a lymph-specific receptor for hyaluronan. *J Cell Biol.* 1999;144:789–801.

45. Wigle JT, Oliver C. PROX-1 function is required for development of the murine lymphatic system. *Cell.* 1999;98:769–778.

46. Baglioni M. Chemokines and leukocyte traffic. *Nature.* 1998;392:565–568.

47. Springer TA. Traffic signals for lymphocyte recirculation and leukocyte migration: the multistep paradigm. *Cell.* 1994;76:301–314.

48. Muller A, Homey B, Soto H. Involvement of chemokine receptors in breast cancer metastasis. *Nature.* 2001;410: 50–56.

49. Cabanas RM. An approach for the treatment of penile carcinoma. *Cancer.* 1977;39:456–466.

50. Wong J, Cagle L, Morton D. Lymphatic drainage of the skin to a sentinel lymph node in a feline model. *Ann Surg.* 1991;214:637–641.

51. Giuliano AE, Kirgan DM, Guenther JM, Morton DL. Lymphatic mapping and sentinel lymphadenectomy for breast cancer. *Ann Surg.* 1994;220:391–398.

52. Cochran AJ, Morton DL, Stern S, Lana AM, Essner R, Wen D. Sentinel lymph nodes show profound down-regulation of antigen-presenting cells of the paracortex: implications for tumor biology and treatment. *Mod Pathol.* 2001;14:604–608.

53. Huang RR, Wen DR, Guo J, Giuliano AE, Nguyen M, Offodile R, et al. Selective modulation of paracortical dendritic cells and T-lymphocytes in breast cancer sentinel lymph nodes. *Breast J.* 2000;6:225–232.

54. Hoon DSB, Korn EL, Cochran AJ. Variations in functional immunocompetence of individual tumor-draining lymph nodes in humans. *Cancer.* 1987;47:1740–1744.

55. O'Toole GA, Hettiaratchy S, Allan R, Powell BW. Aberrant sentinel nodes in malignant melanoma. *Br J Plast Surg.* 2003;53:415–417.

# 8

# The Role of Lymph Node Staging for Clinical Decision Making in Patients with Solid Cancers

Fausto Badellino, Ilaria Pastina, Elisa Borsò, Sergio Ricci, H. William Strauss, and Giuliano Mariani

The treatment of solid tumors is based on consideration of the 3 most important biologic factors affecting prognosis: 1) local extension of malignant tissue, 2) lymphatic dissemination, and 3) hematogenous spread. Currently, the TNM classification system of malignant tumors, periodically updated by the International Union Against Cancer (UICC) (1) and the American Joint Committee on Cancer (AJCC) (2), is used to describe the tumor status of a patient. The "TNM" acronym indicates that the staging system takes into account the local extent of the primary "tumor," its dissemination to locoregional lymph "nodes," and the presence of distant "metastases." Staging is intended to: 1) estimate the "life cycle" of a tumor; 2) assess the location and extent of malignant disease; 3) estimate the prognosis, risks of recurrence, and risks of mortality; 4) plan treatment (local and systemic therapy); 5) correlate anatomy and pathology with outcomes of disease and treatment; 6) unify reporting of clinical trials, and 7) increase knowledge of cancer biology.

The TNM system, originally developed about 50 years ago, defines a common, internationally accepted classification system for epithelial and connective tissue tumors at 44 anatomic sites (1,2). Specific criteria are described to define the locoregional extension of the primary tumor and the involvement of regional lymph nodes, and to identify distant metastases.

Radionuclide studies have been used for more than 50 years to demarcate the extent of tumor involvement. The neurosurgeon Sweet used beta detectors in the operating room to identify the tumor margins (3). This was followed by anecdotal reports by Pochin from London and Müller from Zurich, who used Geiger counters connected to needle probes to detect [131]I in residual thyroid tissue in patients undergoing thyroidectomy.

Despite this auspicious beginning, it was another 40 years before intraoperative radionuclide techniques became part of mainstream clinical care. An additional development that helped advance the field was radioimmunoscintigraphy, which in turn led to radioimmuno-

guided surgery. Surgeon Martin Jr., helped design a handheld gamma probe to detect residual/recurrent colorectal cancer during surgical exploration of the abdomen using anti-carcinoembryonic antigen (anti-CEA) monoclonal antibody (B72.3) labeled with [125]I (4). Use of the probe improved staging by searching for micro- and macroscopic tumor residues (indicated as R1 and R2, respectively). The intraoperative probe technology was particularly useful in identifying micrometastases and isolated tumor cells in lymph nodes, which is difficult when relying only on standard histologic procedures (hematoxylin and eosin, or H&E, staining). Combining use of the probe in the operating room for specific node identification with immunohistochemistry and molecular biology-based techniques (such as the polymerase chain reaction, or PCR) (5) greatly improves sensitivity in the detection of metastatic involvement of lymph nodes. These procedures modify tumor stage, often resulting in upstaging (6). While lymph node mapping and especially sentinel lymph node biopsy are invasive, they can spare the patient unnecessary aggressive node dissections.

Radioguided sentinel lymph node biopsy has become a standard surgical procedure. Proposed initially for penile cancer, it has been extended to melanoma and breast cancer, supplemented by vital or fluorescent dyes (7) administered at the time of sentinel node harvest. A number of studies are underway to determine the value of sentinel lymph node mapping in tumors affecting the head and neck, upper aerodigestive tract, thyroid, salivary glands, lungs, stomach, uterus, external genitalia, prostate, colorectal, and others (Table 8-1).

Effective radioguided sentinel lymph node biopsy requires a team consisting of the surgeon, a nuclear physician, and a pathologist (8) to optimize the technique of radioisotope and dye injection, the site of injection, the modality of sentinel lymph node identification (by color and radioactivity counting), excision and handling of the sentinel lymph node, and histology. The team must agree

TABLE 8-1. Intraoperative clinical applications of the gamma probe in different oncologic indications.

| Indication of | Tumor type | Clinical utility |
|---|---|---|
| Sentinel lymph node by intra- or peritumoral administration of $^{99m}$Tc-colloids | Breast cancer | ++ |
| | Melanoma | + |
| | Skin cancer | ++ |
| | Penile/vulvar cancer | ++ |
| | Colon cancer | ± |
| | Lung cancer | ± |
| | Head and neck cancer | ± |
| Tumor deposits by tumor-seeking agents (monoclonal antibodies, $^{99m}$Tc-sestamibi) | Colon cancer | ± |
| | Ovarian cancer | − |
| | Breast cancer | − |
| | Medullary thyroid cancer | + |
| | Melanoma | − |
| | Neuroblastoma | ± |
| | Parathyroid adenoma | ++ |
| Bone abnormalities by $^{99m}$Tc-diphosphonate | Osteoid osteoma | ++ |
| | Bone lesions suspected for bone metastasis | ++ |
| Occult tumors by intratumoral administration of an isotope tracer | Occult breast cancer | ++ |

Legend:
++ = proven clinical value
+ = may be of clinical value
± = clinical relevance insufficiently evaluated
− = proven not to be of clinical value
Source: Adapted from Ell PJ, Gambhir SS, eds. *Nuclear Medicine in Clinical Diagnosis and Treatment*. Vol 1. Edinburgh: Churchill-Livingstone; 2004:217–227, with permission from Elsevier.

on specific issues that include the site of radiocolloid injection (e.g., in case of breast cancer intratumoral, peritumoral, intradermal, or subareolar) (9,10), as well as the type and size of the radiocolloid particles, which are known to affect both the velocity of migration of radiocolloids and their retention pattern in the nodes (11).

Although the techniques work, false-negative cases (i.e., a sentinel lymph node free from metastatic involvement in the presence of other lymph nodes that are found to be metastatic at histology) occur with small but significant frequency. In addition, different distributions of the radiotracer and the vital dye in the nodal basin continue to occur in about 15% of cases. In a recent editorial, Goit (12) addresses the biological variables that possibly cause these events (13).

The sensitivity of immunohistochemistry and sentinel lymph node biopsy has led to the identification of small tumor cell clusters (i.e., <0.2 mm). It is unclear if these isolated tumor cells have the potential to produce metastatic disease (e.g. proliferation or stromal reaction) or invade blood vessel walls and sinusoid spaces in a lymph node.

The most recent revision of the TNM system (1,2), based on results from several large-scale studies and consensus conferences (14–17), suggests classifying the histopathologic status of sentinel lymph node(s) as: 1) "pNX(sn)" when no data are available; 2) "pN0(sn)" when the sentinel lymph node was analyzed and found to be free from metastasis, or 3) "pN1(sn)" when the sentinel

lymph node was analyzed and found to harbor metastasis. In particular, isolated tumor cells are not to be taken into account (especially if identified with molecular biology techniques); thus a lymphatic basin where only isolated tumor cells were detected is classified as pN0, and there is no reason for upstage migration (Table 8-2).

TABLE 8-2. Example of correct notation for staging of isolated tumor cells and micrometastases.

| Lymph node biopsy | Histologic finding | Size of lesion* | Notation |
|---|---|---|---|
| | 1 node IHC positive | 0.1 mm | pN0 (sn) (i+) |
| SLND | 1 node H&E positive | 0.1 mm | pN0 (sn) |
| SLND | 1 node IHC positive | 1.0 mm | pN1mi (sn) (i+) |
| SLND | 1 node H&E positive | 1.0 mm | pN1mi (sn) |

Legend:
*Isolated tumor cells are defined as metastatic lesions no larger than 0.2 mm in diameter. Micrometastases are defined as metastatic lesions between 0.2–2.0 mm diameter. Metastatic cell deposits seen with immunohistochemical staining alone are considered to be equivalent to those seen on standard H&E staining.
H&E—hematoxylin and eosin staining
IHC—immunohistochemistry
SLND—sentinel lymph node dissection
Source: Data from and used with permission of the American Joint Committee on Cancer (AJCC), Chicago, Illinois. The original source for this material is the AJCC Cancer Staging Manual, Sixth Edition (2002) published by Springer-New York, www.springeronline.com.

# Radioguidance and Staging in Tumors

## Melanoma

Sentinel lymph node biopsy is accepted worldwide as the method of choice to stage regional lymph nodes in patients with melanoma, even at unexpected/abnormal draining sites (which have a frequency of about 5%) (18). Because there are often many nodes (radioactive and/or colored), it is difficult to establish which are the true sentinel lymph nodes. In the Sunbelt Melanoma Trial of 1,184 patients, it was found that sometimes the most radioactive lymph node was negative for metastatic involvement, whereas other, less radioactive lymph nodes were metastatic (13.1% of cases) (19). It appears reasonable therefore to recommend resection and histologic analysis of all "blue" nodes and nodes with radioactivity count rates greater than 10% of the ex-vivo count rate of the node with the greatest radioactivity. This approach should reduce the risk of false-negative biopsies.

Another issue concerns the reliability of the histologic analysis of the node. A consensus is emerging that frozen section and H&E staining alone have too low a sensitivity for clinical use, since they demonstrate metastasis in less than 50% of the lymph nodes that actually harbor melanoma cells (20). Additional analysis with step sections and immunohistochemical staining increases the sensitivity.

Radioguided surgery is particularly useful in patients with melanomas that are located in the perineum, since lymph drainage is clinically ambiguous. These lesions may drain to nodes in the groin, iliac, and obturator regions, as demonstrated by lymphoscintigraphy (21,22).

Regional lymph node metastases (N1 to N3) define stage III disease and are cardinal prognostic variables for patients with cutaneous melanoma. In 580 patients whose sentinel lymph nodes (identified using dye and lymphoscintigraphy) were found to be free from metastasis, the status of the sentinel node was the single most powerful prognostic factor after Breslow thickness (23,24). Since patients with melanomas <1.0 mm thick rarely have nodal disease (25), sentinel node biopsy is not commonly performed in this group, but should be considered when negative prognostic features such as ulceration or Clark level IV to V invasion are present (26). For patients with melanomas that are >1 mm thick, sentinel node staging can be considered for prognostic purposes, and to evaluate eligibility for clinical trials and the need for adjuvant therapy. Accurate staging can identify patients whose risk of recurrence is sufficiently high to justify adjuvant systemic treatment.

## Breast Cancer

The sixth edition of the TNM classification system introduced important changes in the classification of regional nodes in breast cancer, specifically: 1) modifying the role of metastatic involvement for lymph nodes of the internal mammary chain; 2) including again the supraclavicular lymph nodes (whose metastatic involvement is now defined as N3 and no longer as M1); and 3) adopting the definition of clinical apparent metastases for internal mammary nodes on the basis of imaging and physical examination (with the exclusion of lymphoscintigraphy). Micrometastases in lymph nodes (0.2–2 mm) are classified as pN1, and the parameters include the number of metastatic nodes (up to 3, between 4 and 9, or more than 10 involved, respectively) and the simultaneous presence of metastases in the axillary, and/or the internal mammary chain, and/or the supraclavicular lymph nodes (1,2).

According to the new classification, staging of the axilla can be based on either axillary dissection or sentinel lymph node biopsy. In the first instance, resection of the first level lymph nodes (lower axilla) is required for histopathologic classification. The specimen usually contains 6 or more lymph nodes; if less than 6 nodes are examined and they are negative for metastatic involvement, the classification is pN0.

In the case of sentinel lymph node biopsy, if only the sentinel node is resected and examined (without total axillary dissection), this factor is reported with a specific notation, for example pN1(sn). Although some investigators have reservations about this approach (27), the revised TNM classification recognizes that sentinel lymph node biopsy (including both lymphoscintigraphic mapping and intraoperative gamma probe detection) plays an important role in the care of patients with breast cancer. Nevertheless, consideration should be paid to some limiting factors of the procedure, such as partial lymphatic drainage to the internal mammary chain (in about 17% of the cases, if the radiocolloid is injected peritumorally), depending on the location of the primary tumor within the breast (28).

It is unclear whether lymphatic mapping and sentinel lymph node biopsy should be performed in patients with ductal carcinoma in situ. By definition, an in-situ breast cancer should not yet have invaded the lymphatic channels, yet foci of microinfiltration can be observed at extensive histopathology of some resected cancers that had been defined as in situ before resection (29). Another issue concerns the possibility of predicting metastases in nonsentinel nodes, when the sentinel lymph node is positive for metastasis (an event reported to occur in about 50% of the cases) (30). A confounding variable in patients treated with neoadjuvant chemotherapy before surgery is fibrosis of the lymphatic channels, which can raise the rate of false-negative sentinel lymph node biopsies in up to 33% of cases (31).

It is generally agreed that the combined use of a dye and radiotracer yields better identification rates (32,33).

The intraoperative analysis of the excised sentinel lymph node using "touch imprints" is fast, convenient, and highly sensitive for detecting tumor cells in the lymph node (34). On the other hand, staging of a residual tumor (R0, R1, R2) is not influenced if a marginal, apical, or sentinel node is metastatic (35).

Preoperative lymphoscintigraphy has become the standard of practice in breast cancer patients to detect nonaxillary sentinel lymph nodes (such as those of the internal mammary chain, as well as those located in the supraclavicular, subclavicular, and interpectoral regions, or the lateral and medial intramammary lymph nodes).

One prognostic factor is the number of positive axillary lymph nodes, based on at least a level I or II axillary dissection and a detailed histologic evaluation. As the number of involved lymph nodes rises, relapse rates increase and survival rates decrease. A second important factor is tumor size. Other factors such as patient age, hormone receptor status, and HER2/neu status are of lesser importance than node status and tumor size. Historical information suggests that patients with negative lymph nodes have a 60% to 75% 10-year disease-free survival, whereas those with positive lymph nodes have a 25% to 30% 10-year disease-free survival. The 1998 result of the Early Breast Cancer Trialists' Collaborative Group (EBCTCG) demonstrated a proportional reduction in the risk of relapse and death in node-positive and node-negative disease for patients treated with adjuvant therapy. However, proportional risk reductions translate into larger absolute benefits for higher risk patients with node-positive disease than for lower risk patients with node-negative disease. While the absolute benefit of treating node-positive patients with chemotherapy is large enough to warrant the potential risks, it is reasonable to wonder whether the same is true for patients with node-negative disease (36).

## Head and Neck Cancers

The usefulness of sentinel lymph node biopsy in tumors of the thyroid (37,38), salivary glands, or squamous cell cancers of the head and neck is still not established. It is clear that lymphoscintigraphic mapping identifies bilateral draining basins, suggesting nodal sites that can be sampled for staging, leading to selective nodal dissection or conservative management (39–41). In the neck, there are about 200 lymph nodes, with many separate anatomic structures adjacent to one another, so often the primary tumor and draining lymph nodes are in close proximity. On the other hand, elective neck dissection reveals lymph node metastases in an average 30% of clinically N0 patients, so in about 70% of patients this operation is unnecessary. Even the most advanced nuclear medicine imaging method, positron emission tomography (PET,

which is useful for detecting local recurrences), is largely ineffective for evaluating tumor status of the sentinel lymph node(s), as well as of the second-echelon and contralateral nodes (42). Thus, lymphoscintigraphic mapping holds promise for guiding surgery, although larger trials and further experience (with longer follow-up studies) are necessary before radioguided sentinel lymph node biopsy becomes the standard of care for planning treatment (43,44). Different figures have been reported for clinically occult metastatic involvement of sentinel lymph node(s) identified under radioguidance: 21% of oropharyngeal cancer, 34% of squamous cell cancers of the tongue, and 34% and 45% respectively of oral and tongue cancers (45). However, in a series of 41 patients with primary head and neck cancers, radioguided sentinel lymph node identification failed in 3/9 patients with metastatic lymph nodes (46).

At the Tenth International Congress on Oral Cancer in April 2005 (Crete), investigators reported >95% negative predictive value for sentinel lymph node biopsy, suggesting that elective neck dissection should become clinical routine only in those patients with a metastatic sentinel lymph node (47). It was also noted that sentinel lymph node biopsy improves surgical staging, especially for patients with tumors located on the midline or crossing the midline, and allows better pathologic staging. Sentinel node biopsy can modify the prognostic assessment and is helpful for selecting patients for adjuvant therapies and/or more aggressive treatment protocols (48). In contrast to melanoma, here intraoperative frozen-section histopathology seems to be more reliable, since only 4 of 48 patients with metastatic involvement of the sentinel lymph node were missed on frozen-section analysis (49). Advances in molecular biology techniques (based on 1-step reverse-transcriptase polymerase chain reaction) also make it possible to detect metastases within an intraoperative timeframe (50). Lymphoscintigraphy is greatly improved when single photon emission computed tomography (SPECT) images are recorded and when the technique is used in combination with ultrasonography (51). Furthermore, lymphoscintigraphic mapping of the sentinel node can reduce the rate of complications (52), especially those related to unnecessary modified radical neck dissection (53). There was general consensus on the feasibility and usefulness of lymphoscintigraphic mapping for sentinel node identification and radioguided biopsy, leading to discovery of micrometastases in clinically N0 oral and oropharyngeal cancers (54–57).

Head and neck cancers are associated with a 20% to 30% incidence of occult cervical lymph node metastases, even with a clinically negative examination. These observations have led to the generally accepted need for elective lymph node neck dissection as part of standard surgical management (58,59). Patients who did not undergo elective dissection were more likely to present with more advanced neck disease when disease recurred than those who opted for prophylactic lymph node dissection. The presence of lymph node metastases dictates the use of combination surgery and postoperative external radiation therapy. Surgery alone is reserved for those situations in which only a single lymph node is involved and where there is no extension of disease beyond the lymph node capsule.

## Gastrointestinal Tract

Both blue dye and radiocolloids are used for lymph node mapping and identification of the sentinel node in patients with cancer of the gastrointestinal tract. Interstitial injection is performed either submucosally around the tumor (during endoscopy prior to surgery) or subserosally (during open or laparoscopic surgery) (60–62).

In esophageal cancer, a close correlation has been found between the number of sentinel lymph nodes (identified with the use of $^{99m}$Tc-labeled rhenium sulphide), lymph node status, pathologic stage, and the number of metastatic nodes (63). Sentinel lymph node biopsy is especially useful in minimally invasive surgery (64). Lymph nodal status is the most powerful prognostic factor in esophageal cancer, and accurate staging is necessary to distinguish potentially curable patients from those with local advanced disease. Although esophagectomy remains the standard of care in early-stage tumors (stage I, IIA), its role is being questioned in patients with locally advanced disease (stage IIB, III) because of the generally poor outcomes following surgical resection alone. The overall 5-year survival rate for patients with esophageal cancer is 20% to 25% (60% to 70% for patients with stage I disease, 5% to 10% for patients with stage III disease).

In Japan, the high incidence of gastric cancer has led to evaluation of sentinel lymph node biopsy for patients with this type of tumor. The standard treatment for early cases is gastrectomy with en-bloc lymph node dissection. Lymphatic mapping has disclosed unexpected/aberrant sites of drainage, thus guiding surgeons to perform a regional dissection approach tailored to the individual patient. Both conventional histochemistry and molecular biology techniques have been applied in the search for micrometastatic involvement of the sentinel lymph node(s) (65,66). Management of gastric cancer depends upon complete resection of the primary tumor and extensive en-bloc lymph node dissection, but as yet there is no consensus on whether more extensive dissection (D2) improves survival compared with less aggressive surgery. Several studies have demonstrated that lymph node dissection limited to the D1 level understages 60% to 75% of patients, compared to a D2 dissection (67). The

number of lymph nodes containing metastasis is an accurate predictor of clinical outcome: patients with more than 15 positive lymph nodes have an unfavorable outcome, comparable to those with distant metastatic disease. Furthermore, the 5-year survival rate ranges from 78% for patients with superficial tumors and negative lymph nodes (stage IA), to 7% to 8% for patients with metastatic N2 nodes or with distant metastases (stages IIIB and IV). In patients with lymph node metastases in the resected specimen, disease recurrences and cancer-related deaths are at least 70% to 80%. Recent meta-analyses suggest that adjuvant systemic treatment may confer a small but clinically significant improvement in survival (68,69), with the benefit to node-positive patients being greater than for node-negative patients (70).

Aberrant lymph drainage leading to modification of the intended surgical approach can be identified as well in 5% to 8% of patients with colorectal cancer. Lymphatic mapping and sentinel lymph node analysis performed with molecular biology techniques can detect micrometastases in up to 14% of the cases, identifying a subgroup of patients who can benefit from adjuvant chemotherapy. In a study of 492 consecutive patients (401 with colon cancer, 91 with rectal cancer), the overall success rate for radioguided sentinel lymph node identification was 97.8%, with most of the failures occurring in rectal cancers (8.8% of the cases, versus 0.7% for colon cancer), most likely due to local submucosal lymphatic fibrosis induced by neoadjuvant radiation therapy administered prior to surgery (71). The overall accuracy rate for predicting lymph node metastases was 95.4% (with 89.3% sensitivity), while the overall incidence of skip metastasis was 10.9%.

A minimum number of lymph nodes must be assessed for accurate staging of patients with colorectal cancer, as nodal status (the number of nodes resected and the presence of micrometastases) is crucial for planning treatment after primary surgery (72). Inadequate retrieval and assessment of sentinel lymph nodes is associated with worse outcome (e.g., in stage II patients) (73). Although lymph node mapping per se (either with blue dye or radiocolloids) does not generally modify the surgical procedure (which usually follows a standardized approach), it does identify the crucial node(s) to be submitted to extensive analysis with sophisticated laboratory techniques searching for micrometastases. Adjuvant chemotherapy is performed in the positive cases. The lymphotropic agents are most frequently injected subserosally during open surgery, with a specificity approaching 100% when using the blue dye (74), and during laparoscopic procedures (75). Submucosal injection is generally performed during endoscopy prior to surgery, and the use of radiocolloids is increasing (76).

The potential advantages of lymphatic mapping for patients with colorectal cancers and malignant polyps

(77) are less obvious than for those with breast cancer or melanoma, and the procedure is generally performed in strictly controlled clinical trials. Nevertheless, for colorectal cancer the simplest and most widely applied prognostic feature is the presence of lymph node metastases in the surgical resection specimen. Accurate staging of regional lymph nodes is critical not only for its prognostic relevance, but also for the therapeutic implications. While the 5-year survival rate for patients with stage I or II colorectal cancer is approximately 80%, those with metastatic lymph nodes have an approximately 50% 5-year survival. Furthermore, the presence of lymph node metastases represents the primary indication for adjuvant chemotherapy, whose therapeutic benefits have largely been proved (78,79). In stage II (node-negative disease with the primary tumor through the muscle wall) or stage III (metastatic involvement of regional lymph nodes) rectal cancer, adjuvant chemotherapy plus concurrent radiation therapy is based on clinical observations of the high incidence of pelvic recurrences and on the significant morbidity associated with local recurrences observed following surgery alone.

## Urogenital Cancers

In cancers of the bladder and prostate preoperatively staged as N0, the optimal extent of regional lymph node dissection is under debate. Preliminary reports indicate that in bladder cancer it is possible to map the sentinel lymph node even outside of the obturator fossa. If this lymph node is metastatic, nodes from the obturator fossa must be dissected and removed. Nevertheless, further study is required to elucidate all the clinical and surgical implications of sentinel lymph node biopsy. Similar considerations apply to prostate cancer, as the extent of lymph node dissection might be guided by the metastatic status of the sentinel lymph node, especially if it is found in unexpected, extraregional locations.

For testicular cancer, lymphatic mapping is still in a very early phase of clinical experience. However, for penile cancer (a typical tumor of the midline, in which bilateral lymphatic drainage is the rule) sentinel lymph node biopsy may spare unnecessary bilateral (heavy) groin lymph node dissection, a surgical procedure with a heavy burden of morbidity and side effects, and at the same time result in considerable improvement of the quality of life.

Interesting studies have been published on sentinel lymph node biopsy in patients with vulvar or cervical cancers (80–82), where lymphatic mapping is performed with blue dye and/or radiocolloids during either open or laparoscopic surgery. In a multicenter study of 232 patients, the identification rate of the sentinel lymph node ranged from 15% to 100%, and was not affected by preoperative neoadjuvant chemotherapy. Intraoperative lymphatic mapping with sentinel node biopsy may affect the care management of patients with these tumors, leading to more accurate detection of lymph node metastases and reduced postoperative morbidity (in case a lymphatic basin assessed as free from metastases based on sentinel lymph node findings is not submitted to extensive lymph node dissection). The success rate in sentinel lymph node identification is generally high, and the status of the node plays an important role in the selection of more or less aggressive therapeutic approaches (83). Nevertheless, before definite evidence is accumulated, "it can be stated only that such procedure may permit a reduction in the amount of surgery" (84).

Regional lymph node status is a major prognostic factor for the therapeutic strategy of gynecologic malignancies. Early cervical cancer is treated with surgery and/or radiotherapy; surgery consists of radical hysterectomy and pelvic lymphadenectomy. However, metastasis in pelvic lymph nodes is found in only 15% of the women with stage Ib cervical cancer (85,86), and thus the vast majority of these patients does not benefit from a surgical treatment associated with considerable morbidity (nerve and vessel damage, lymphedema) (87). As in other applications of surgical oncology, sentinel lymph node biopsy could represent a definite advantage to select women for whom lymphadenectomy is really necessary.

Similar considerations also apply to patients with vulvar cancer, a condition in which the status of the regional lymph nodes is crucial for therapeutic decision-making. Standard treatment includes bilateral inguino-femoral lymphadenectomy, but this surgery is associated with high rates of short-term and long-term morbidity, and only 10% to 26% of the patients with vulvar cancer have inguinal metastases. Therefore, the majority of early-stage patients unnecessarily undergo overtreatment (i.e., lymphadenectomy with an ensuing negative impact on quality of life). Sentinel lymph node biopsy could ensure accurate lymph node staging as a prerequisite to implement less aggressive treatments, especially in patients with early vulvar cancer (88).

## Conclusions

Regional lymphatic mapping with sentinel lymph node biopsy is becoming increasingly important in clinical oncology. This procedure can improve lymph node staging and guide the subsequent treatments (systemic neoadjuvant and adjuvant chemotherapy, radiation, and surgery), especially for melanoma, breast cancer, and squamous cell carcinoma of the vulva (and penis). In the sixth edition of the TNM classification system of malignant tumors (1,2), the status of the sentinel lymph node is specifically included in the staging of regional lymph nodes for patients with breast cancer or malignant cutaneous melanoma.

Large-scale single-institution and multicenter trials are being conducted concerning both the clinical and technological aspects of the procedure. Among the latter worth noting are the development of cordless gamma probes for easier handling during surgery (89) and the semi-conductor or solid-state miniature gamma camera, which can overcome some limitations of the non-imaging gamma probe, in particular to avoid leaving residual sentinel lymph nodes in the surgical bed (90).

Global interest in this topic became evident with the establishment of the International Sentinel Node Society in Yokohama in 2002, during the Third International Sentinel Node Congress. This scientific association's stated goals are: 1) to promote the concept of the sentinel lymph node in the scientific and medical community and to stimulate its use; 2) to foster an interdisciplinary interchange of knowledge; 3) to hold periodical international meetings; 4) to conduct educational activities and increase professional skills; 5) to stimulate clinical and laboratory research; and 6) to encourage and facilitate collaborative clinical trials. During the society's recent congress in Los Angeles (December 3–6, 2004), experts from around the world (surgeons, nuclear medicine specialists, pathologists, and medical oncologists) gathered to discuss the many different aspects of this topic. The interest of the international oncologic community in sentinel lymph node biopsy and other forms of radioguided surgery has also been demonstrated by the growing space devoted to such topics in "organ-oriented" meetings focusing on different solid cancers.

## References

1. *TNM Classification of Malignant Tumors (UICC)*. 6th edition. New York: Wiley-Liss; 2002.
2. Greene FL, Page DL, Fleming ID, et al. *AJCC Cancer Staging Manual*. 6th edition. New York: Springer; 2002.
3. Sweet WH. The uses of nuclear disintegration in the diagnosis and treatment of brain tumor. *N Engl J Med.* 1951;245:875–887.
4. Martin EW Jr, Hinkle GH, Tuttle S, et al. Intraoperative radioimmunodetection of colorectal tumors with a hand-held radiation detector. *Am J Surg.* 1985;150:672–675.
5. Onishi A, Nakashiro K, Mihara M, et al. Basic and clinical studies on quantitative analysis of lymph node micrometastasis in oral cancer. *Oncol Rep.* 2004;11:33–39.
6. Reintgen DS, Cruse WE, Wells K. The next revolution in general surgery. *Ann Surg Oncol.* 1999;6:125–126.
7. Shintani S, Mihara M, Nakahara Y, et al. Lymph node metastases of oral cancer visualized in live tissue by green fluorescent protein expression. *Oral Oncol.* 2002;38:664–669.
8. Sampath S, Temple CLF, Temple W. Precision handling of sentinel node. *J Surg Oncol.* 2003;84:176–177.
9. Mariani G, Moresco L, Viale G, et al. Radioguided sentinel lymph node biopsy in breast cancer surgery. *J Nucl Med.* 2001;42:1198–1215.
10. Shen P, Glass EC, Di Fronzo LA, Giuliano AE. Dermal versus intraparenchymal lymphoscintigraphy of the breast. *Ann Surg Oncol.* 2001;8:241–248.
11. Hodgson N, Zabel P, Mattar AC, et al. A new radiocolloid for sentinel node detection in breast cancer. *Ann Surg Oncol.* 2001;8:133–137.
12. Goit DG. The "true" sentinel lymph node: in search of an operational definition of a biological phenomenon. *Ann Surg Oncol.* 2001;8:187–189.
13. Nathanson SD. Insights into the mechanism of lymph node metastasis. *Cancer.* 2003;98:413–423.
14. Schwartz GF, Giuliano AE, Veronesi U. Consensus Conference Committee. Proceedings of the consensus conference on the role of sentinel lymph node biopsy in carcinoma of the breast. *Cancer.* 2002;97:2542–2551.
15. International Breast Cancer Consensus Conference. Image-detected breast cancer: state of the art diagnosis and treatment. *Breast J.* 2002;8:70–76.
16. Jacub JW, Pendas S, Reintgen DS. Current status of sentinel lymph node mapping and biopsy. Facts and controversies. *Oncologist.* 2003;8:59–69.
17. Lagios MD. Clinical significance of immunohistochemically detectable epithelial cells in sentinel lymph node and bone marrow in breast cancer. *J Surg Oncol.* 2003;83:1–4.
18. Sumner WE 3rd, Ross MI, Mansfield PF, et al. Implications of lymphatic drainage to unusual sentinel lymph node sites in patients with primary cutaneous melanoma. *Cancer.* 2002;95:354–360.
19. McMasters KM, Reintgen DS, Ross MI, et al. Sentinel lymph node biopsy for melanoma: how many radioactive nodes should be removed? *Ann Surg Oncol.* 2001;8:192–197.
20. Tanis PJ, Boom RPA, Schraffordt Koops H, et al. Frozen section investigation of sentinel node in malignant melanoma and breast cancer. *Ann Surg Oncol.* 2001;8:222–226.
21. Strobbe LJA, Jonk A, Hart AAM, et al. The value of Cloquet's node in predicting melanoma nodal metastases in the pelvic lymph node basin. *Ann Surg Oncol.* 2001;8:209–214.
22. Gallino G, Maccauro M, Belli F, et al. Detection of clinical occult lymph node metastases by lymphoscintigraphy and sentinel node biopsy in anorectal melanoma patients. *Ospedali d'Italia—Chirurgia.* 2003;9:257–259.
23. Reintgen D, Rapaport D, Tanabe KK, Ross M. Lymphatic mapping and sentinel node biopsy in patients with malignant melanoma. *J FL Med Assoc.* 1997;84:188–193.
24. Gershenwald JE, Thompson W, Mansfield PF, et al. Multi-institutional melanoma lymphatic mapping experience: the prognostic value of sentinel lymph node status in 612 stage I or II melanoma patients. *J Clin Oncol.* 1999;17:976–983.
25. Bleicher RJ, Essner R, Foshag LJ, Wanek LA, Morton DL. Role of sentinel lymphadenectomy in thin invasive cutaneous melanomas. *J Clin Oncol.* 2003;21:1326–1331.

26. Balch CM, Buzaid AC, Soong SJ, et al. Final version of the American Joint Committee on Cancer staging system for cutaneous melanoma. *J Clin Oncol.* 2001;19:3635–3648.

27. Theriault RL. Commentary on the revision of the American Joint Committee on Cancer staging system for breast cancer. In: *ASCO Educational Book.* 2003:575–580.

28. Byrd DR, Dunnwald LK, Mankoff DA, et al. Internal mammary lymph node drainage patterns in patients with breast cancer documented by breast lymphoscintigraphy. *Ann Surg Oncol.* 2001;8:234–240.

29. McMasters KM, Chao C, Wong SL, et al. Sentinel lymph node biopsy in patients with ductal carcinoma in situ—a proposal. *Cancer.* 2002;95:15–20.

30. Weiser MR, Montgomery LL, Tan LK, et al. Lymphovascular invasion enhances the prediction of nonsentinel node metastases in breast cancer patients with positive sentinel nodes. *Ann Surg Oncol.* 2001;8:145–149.

31. Buchholz TA, Hunt KK, Whitman GJ, et al. Neoadjuvant chemotherapy for breast cancer–multidisciplinary considerations of benefits and risks. *Cancer.* 2003;98:1150–1160.

32. Munakata S, Aihara T, Morino H, Takatsuka Y. Application of immunofluorescence for intraoperative evaluation of sentinel lymph nodes in patients with breast carcinoma. *Cancer.* 2003;98:1562–1567.

33. Ikeda T, Jinno H, Kitagawa Y, Kitajima M. Emerging patterns of practice in the implementation and application of sentinel node biopsy in breast cancer patients in Japan. *J Surg Oncol.* 2003;84:173–175.

34. Aihara T, Munakata S, Morino H, et al. Comparison of frozen section and touch imprint cytology for evaluation of sentinel lymph node metastases in breast cancer. *Ann Surg Oncol.* 2004;11:747–750.

35. Wittekind C, Compton CC, Greene FL, Sobin LH. TNM residual tumor classification revised. *Cancer.* 2002;94:2511–2516.

36. Early Breast Cancer Trialists' Collaborative Group (EBCTCG). Effects of chemotherapy and hormonal therapy for early breast cancer on recurrence and 15-year survival: an overview of the randomized trials. *Lancet.* 2005;365:1687–1717.

37. Fukui Y, Yamakawa T, Taniki T, et al. Sentinel lymph node biopsy in patients with papillary thyroid carcinoma. *Cancer.* 2001;92:2868–2874.

38. Wiseman SM, Hicks WL Jr, Chu QD, Rigual NR. Sentinel lymph node biopsy in staging of differentiated thyroid cancer: a critical review. *Surg Oncol.* 2002;11:137–142.

39. McMasters KM. Sentinel lymph node biopsy: beyond melanoma and breast carcinoma. *Cancer.* 2003;97:2134–2136.

40. Delgado R, Kraus D, Coit DG, Busam KJ. Sentinel lymph node analysis in patients with sweat gland carcinoma. *Cancer.* 2003;97:2279–2284.

41. Bogner PN, Fullen DR, Lowe L, et al. Lymphatic mapping and sentinel lymph node biopsy in the detection of early metastasis from sweat gland carcinoma. *Cancer.* 2003;97:2285–2289.

42. Hyde NL, Prvulovich E, Newman L, et al. A new approach to the pre-treatment assessment of the N0 neck in oral squamous cell carcinoma: the role of sentinel node biopsy and positron emission tomography. *Oral Oncol.* 2003;39:350–360.

43. Greenberg JS, El Naggar AK, Mo V, Roberts D, Myers JN. Disparity in pathological and clinical lymph node staging in oral tongue carcinoma. Implications for therapeutic decision making. *Cancer.* 2003;98:508–515.

44. Ross GL, Shoaib T, Soutar OS, et al. The First International Conference on sentinel node biopsy in mucosal head and neck cancer and adoption of a multicenter trial protocol. *Ann Surg Oncol.* 2002;9:406–410.

45. Pitman KT, Ferlito A, Devaney KO, et al. Sentinel lymph node biopsy in head and neck cancer. *Oral Oncol.* 2003;39:343–349.

46. Akmansu H, Oguz H, Atasever T, et al. Evaluation of sentinel nodes in the assessment of cervical metastases from head and neck squamous cell carcinomas. *Tumori.* 2004;90:596–599.

47. Stoeckli SJ. Sentinel node biopsy–methodology and results of validated studies [abstract]. *Oral Oncol.* 2005;1(suppl):54.

48. Thompson R. Determining the clinical place of sentinel node biopsy in head and neck squamous cell carcinoma [abstract]. *Oral Oncol.* 2005;1(suppl):54.

49. Zbaren P. Sentinel node biopsy–is fine sectioned frozen section analysis followed by immediate neck dissection a reliable concept? *Oral Oncol.* 2005;1(suppl):54–55.

50. Thompson R. Determining the clinical place of sentinel node biopsy in head and neck squamous cell carcinoma [abstract]. *Oral Oncol.* 2005;1(suppl):54.

51. Sorensen JA, Thomsen JB, Krogdahl A. Sentinel lymph node and attenuation corrected SPECT imaging in patients with oral squamous cell carcinoma [abstract]. *Oral Oncol.* 2005;1(suppl):89.

52. Thomsen JB, Grube P, Sorensen JA. Lymphatic mapping with tomography in oral cancer: image technique, projection and observer reliability [abstract]. *Oral Oncol.* 2005;1(suppl):91.

53. Longo F, Manola M, Villano S, Ionna F. Effectiveness of sentinel node technique in oral cancer [abstract]. *Oral Oncol.* 2005;1(suppl):89.

54. Rigual N, Douglas W, Wiseman S, et al. Sentinel lymph node biopsy: a dependable tool for staging squamous cell carcinoma of the oral cavity [abstract]. *Oral Oncol.* 2005;1(suppl):89.

55. Cizmarevic B, Lanisnik B, Didanovic V. Results of sentinel node examination with frozen section in patients with oral cavity and oropharyngeal carcinoma [abstract]. *Oral Oncol.* 2005;1(suppl):89–90.

56. Vigili MG, Tartaglione G, Rahimi S, et al. Lymphoscintigraphy and radioguided sentinel node biopsy in oral squamous cell carcinoma: preliminary report of same day protocol [abstract]. *Oral Oncol.* 2005;1(suppl):90.

57. Gallegos-Hernandez JF, Pichardo-Romero P, Hernandez-Hernandez D, et al. The number of sentinel nodes identified as prognostic factors in mucosal oral cavity epidermoid cancer [abstract]. *Oral Oncol.* 2005;1(suppl):90.

58. Vandenbrouck C, Rancho-Garnier H, Chassange D, et al. Elective versus therapeutic radical neck dissection in

epidermoid carcinoma of the oral cavity. Results of a randomized clinical trial. *Cancer.* 1980;46:386–390.

59. Lydiatt DD, Robbins KT, Byers RM, Wolf PF. Treatment of stage I and II oral tongue cancer. *Head Neck.* 1993; 15:308–312.

60. Catarci M, Guadagni S, Zaraca F, et al. Prospective randomized evaluation of preoperative endoscopic vital staining using CH-40 for lymph node dissection in gastric cancer. *Ann Surg Oncol.* 1998;5:580–584.

61. Chin PL, Medejros J, Schwarz RE. Use of sentinel lymph node in metastases of gastrointestinal malignancies. A word of caution. *J Surg Oncol.* 1999;71:239–242.

62. Saha S, Wiese D, Badin J, et al. Technical details of sentinel lymph node mapping in colorectal cancer and its impact on staging. *Ann Surg Oncol.* 2000;7:120–124.

63. Kato H, Miyazaki T, Nakajima M, et al. Sentinel lymph nodes with Technetium-99m colloidal rhenium sulfide in patients with esophageal carcinoma. *Cancer.* 2003;98:932–939.

64. Natsugoe S, Matsumoto M, Okumura H, et al. Initial metastatic, including micrometastatic, sites of lymph nodes in esophageal squamous cell carcinoma. *J Surg Oncol.* 2005;89:6–11.

65. Nakajo A, Natsugoe S, Ishigami S, et al. Detection and prediction of micrometastases in the lymph nodes of patients with pN0 gastric cancers. *Ann Surg Oncol.* 2001;8:158–162.

66. Morgagni P, Saragoni L, Follis S, et al. Lymph node micrometastases in patients with early gastric cancer: experience with 139 patients. *Ann Surg Oncol.* 2001;8:170–174.

67. Bunt AMG, Hermans J, Smit VT. Surgical/pathologic stage migration confounds comparisons of gastric cancer survival rates between Japan and Western countries. *J Clin Oncol.* 1995;13:19–25.

68. Mari E, Floriani I, Tinazzi A, et al. Efficacy of adjuvant chemotherapy after curative resection for gastric cancer: a meta-analysis of published randomized trials. A study of GISCAD (Gruppo Italiano per lo Studio dei Carcinoma dell'Apparato Digerente). *Ann Oncol.* 2000;11:837–843.

69. Giani L, Panzini I, Tassinari D, et al. Meta-analysis of randomized trials of adjuvant chemotherapy in gastric cancer. *Ann Oncol.* 2001;12:1178–1180.

70. Earle CC, Maroun JA. Adjuvant chemotherapy after curative resection for gastric cancer in non-Asian patients: revisiting a meta-analysis of randomized trials. *Eur J Cancer.* 1999;35:1059–1064.

71. Saha S, Dan AG, Bilchic A, et al. Mechanism of failure and skip metastasis in sentinel lymph node mapping for colorectal cancers. *Ann Surg Oncol.* 2005;12(suppl):142.

72. Cserni G, Vinih-Hung V, Burzkowsky T. Is there a minimum number of lymph nodes that should be histologically assessed for a reliable nodal staging of T3N0M0 colorectal carcinomas? *J Surg Oncol.* 2002;81:63–69.

73. Law CHL, Wright FC, Rapanos TH. Impact of lymph node retrieval and pathological ultra-staging on the prognosis of stage II colon cancers. *J Surg Oncol.* 2003;84: 120–126.

74. Roseano M, Scaramucci M, Ciutto T, et al. Sentinel lymph node mapping in the management of colorectal cancer: preliminary report. *Tumori.* 2003;89:412–416.

75. Wood TF, Saha S, Morton DL, et al. Validation of lymphatic mapping in colorectal cancer: in vivo, ex vivo and laparoscopic techniques. *Ann Surg Oncol.* 2001;8:150–159.

76. Nastro P, Sodo M, Dodaro CA, et al. Intraoperative radiochemoguided mapping of sentinel lymph node in colon cancer. *Tumori.* 2002;88:352–353.

77. Andreoni B, Crosta C, Bianchi PP, et al. La strategia del linfonodo sentinella nel trattamento dei polipi maligni del colon-retto. *Proc 106th Congress Italian Society of Surgery,* vol. I. Roma: Pozzi Editore; 2004:93–114.

78. Moertel CG, Fleming TR, MacDonald JS, et al. Levamisole and fluorouracil for adjuvant therapy of resected colon carcinoma. *N Engl J Med.* 1990;322:352–358.

79. Andrè T, Boni C, Mounedji-Boudiaf L, et al. Oxaliplatin, fluorouracile, and leucovorin as adjuvant treatment for colon cancer. *N Engl J Med.* 2004;350:2343–2351.

80. Levenback C, Burke TW, Gershenson DM, et al. Intraoperative lymphatic mapping for vulvar cancer. *Obst Gynecol.* 1994;84:163–167.

81. De Hullu JA, Hollema H, Piers DA, et al. Sentinel lymph node procedure is highly accurate in squamous cell carcinoma of the vulva. *J Clin Oncol.* 2000;18:2811–2816.

82. Barranger E, Grahek D, Cortez A, et al. Laparoscopic sentinel lymph node procedure using a combination of patent blue and radioisotope in women with cervical carcinoma. *Cancer.* 2003;97:3003–3009.

83. Barranger E, Darai E. Sentinel lymph nodes [letter]. *Cancer.* 2003;98:2524–2525.

84. Covens A. Sentinel lymph nodes. What have we learned and where will it lead us? *Cancer.* 2003;97: 2945–2947.

85. Michel G, Morice P, Castagne D, et al. Lymphatic spread in stage Ib and II cervical carcinoma: anatomy and surgical implications. *Obstet Gynecol.* 1998;91:360–363.

86. Sakuragi N, Satoh C, Takeda N, et al. Incidence and distribution pattern of pelvic and paraaortic lymph node metastasis in patients with stages IB, IIA, and IIB cervical carcinoma treated with radical hysterectomy. *Cancer.* 1999;85:1547–1554.

87. Lecuru F, Taurelle R. Transperitoneal laparoscopic pelvic lymphadenectomy for gynecologic malignancies. Technique and results. *Surg Endosc.* 1998;12:1–6.

88. Rouzier R, Haddad B, Dubernard G, et al. Inguinofemoral dissection for carcinoma of the vulva: effect of modifications of extent and technique on morbidity and survival. *J Am Coll Surg.* 2003;196:442–450.

89. World of Medicine USA, Inc. Cordless gamma finder. *General Surgery News.* 2003;30:47.

90. Motomura K, Noguchi A, Hashizume T, et al. Usefulness of a solid state gamma camera for sentinel node identification in patients with breast cancer. *J Surg Oncol.* 2005;89: 12–17.

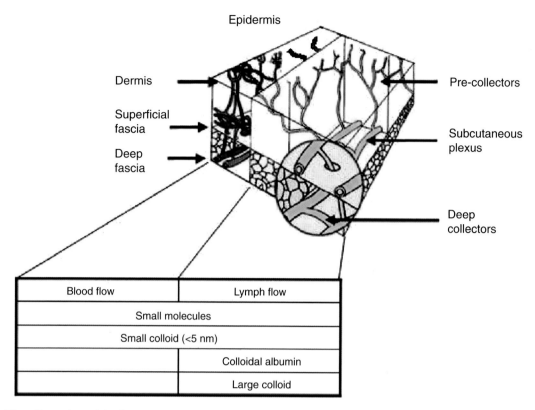

FIGURE 1-3. The effect of particle size on the colloid clearance pathway. Blood is represented in red and blue, and the lymphatic vessels in yellow.

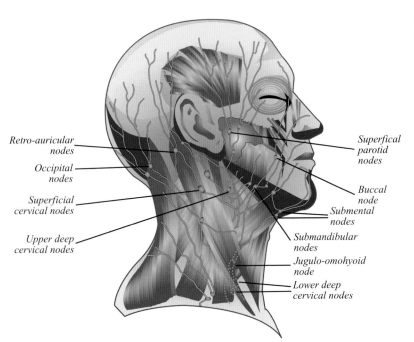

FIGURE 7-2. Superficial lymph nodes and lymphatic vessels of the head and neck. (Gray H. *Gray's Anatomy*, 38e, copyright 1995, reprinted with permission from Elsevier.)

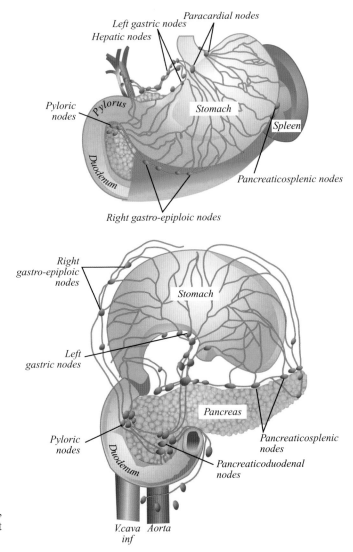

FIGURE 7-3. Lymphatic drainage of the stomach, duodenum, and pancreas. (Gray H. *Gray's Anatomy*, 38e, copyright 1995, reprinted with permission from Elsevier.)

FIGURE 7-5. Lymph nodes of the colon. (Gray H. *Gray's Anatomy*, 38e, copyright 1995, reprinted with permission from Elsevier.)

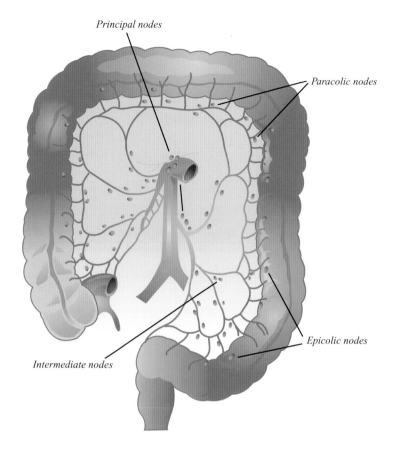

*Principal nodes*

*Paracolic nodes*

*Epicolic nodes*

*Intermediate nodes*

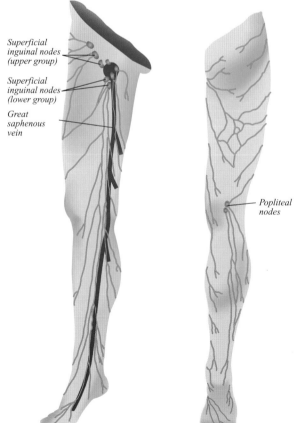

*Superficial inguinal nodes (upper group)*

*Superficial inguinal nodes (lower group)*

*Great saphenous vein*

*Popliteal nodes*

FIGURE 7-7. Lymphatic drainage of the superficial tissues of the lower extremity. (Gray H. *Gray's Anatomy*, 38e, copyright 1995, reprinted with permission from Elsevier.)

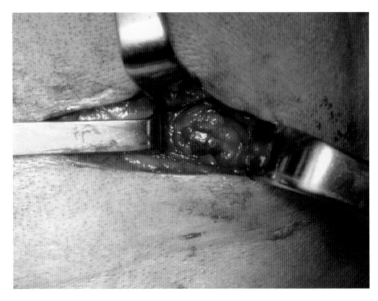

FIGURE 12-3. Intraoperative identification of the sentinel node (colored by blue dye). (Dr. Franco Ionna, G. Pascale National Cancer Institute of Naples, Italy. Used by permission.)

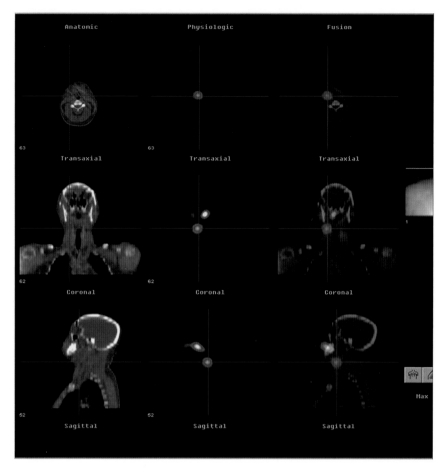

FIGURE 12-7. Lymphoscintigraphic images obtained using a SPECT/CT gamma camera for better anatomic localization of the sentinel node.

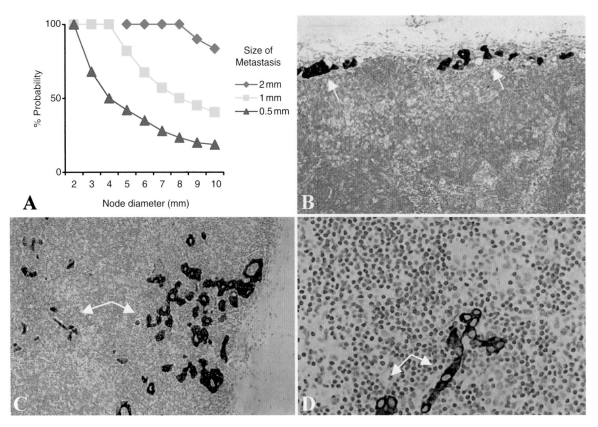

FIGURE 19-1. (A–B) Distribution patterns of metastases in sentinel lymph nodes of patients with breast cancer. Metastases are highlighted by their cytokeratin immunoreactivity. Tumor cells are present in peripheral sinus (A, arrows), the outer cortex (B, arrows), and medulla (C, arrows). The probability of sampling such metastases as a function of their size is illustrated in (A). (B–D). Avidin-biotin complex immunoperoxidase staining. (Original magnification: (A), ×40; (B), ×100; (C), ×200). (A, Wilkinson and Hause, 1974 (23). Used by permission.)

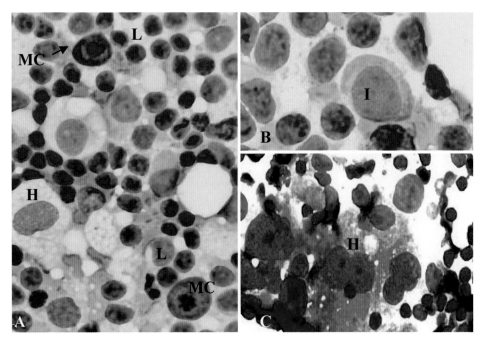

FIGURE 19-3. Normal cytology of sentinel lymph node constituents. Note lymphocytes of different size (L), histiocytes (H), immunoblasts (I), and mast cells (MC). Diff-Quik stain. (A–C, original magnification ×400).

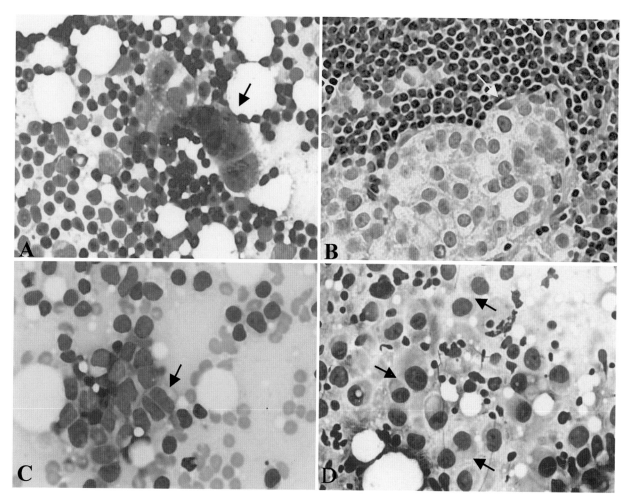

FIGURE 19-4. Cytological patterns of breast cancer metastases. Note cohesive group (A, arrow) and corresponding morphology in permanent section (B), rare (C, arrow) and diffuse (D, arrows) single cell pattern. A, C, and D. Diff-Quik stain (original magnification ×400). B. Hematoxylin and eosin stain (original magnification ×200).

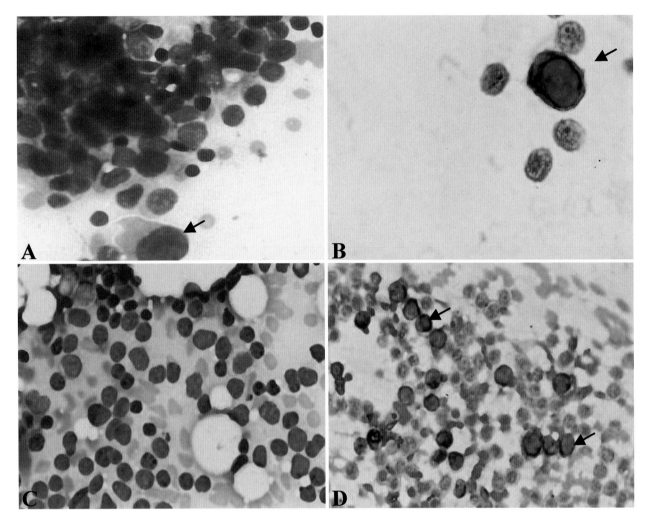

FIGURE 19-5. Cytokeratin expression in cytological imprints from sentinel lymph nodes with an occasional but cytologically evident metastatic tumor cell in a patient with ductal carcinoma (A, arrow), or with frequent but inconspicuous tumor cells in a patient with lobular carcinoma (C, arrow). Note sensitive visualization of tumor cells after application of rapid intraoperative immunocytokeratin staining (B and D, arrows). A and C. Diff-Quik stain. B and D. Avidin-biotin-complex immunoperoxidase. (All original magnifications are ×400.)

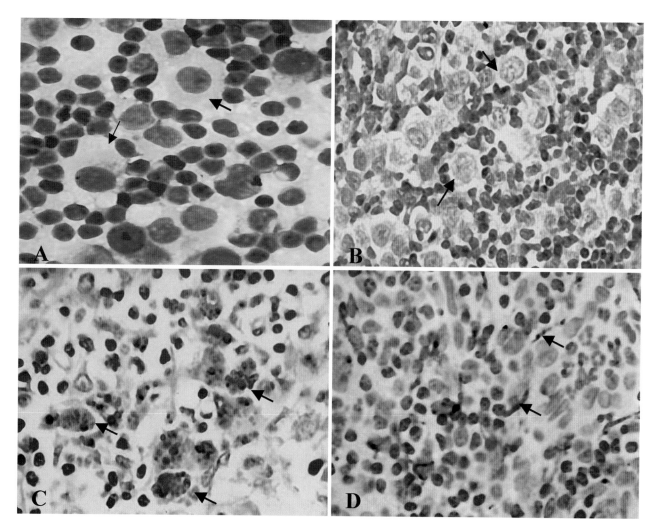

FIGURE 19-6. Histiocytes (A–C, arrows) and dendritic cells (D, arrows) in sentinel lymph nodes. These cells may rarely be a source of diagnostic dilemma due to their overall epithelial-like morphology, especially when in aggregates, or to nonspecific immunoreactivity for cytokeratin (C and D). A. Diff-Quik stain. B. hematoxylin and eosin stain. C–D. Avidin-biotin-complex immunoperoxidase. (All original magnifications are ×400.)

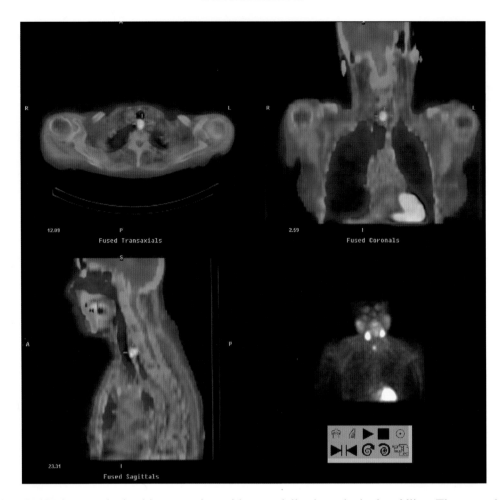

FIGURE 23-2. SPECT/CT images obtained from a patient with primary hyperparathyroidism, about 2 hours after the intravenous administration of $^{99m}$Tc-sestamibi. The lower right panel shows the anterior planar projection of the head and chest, where physiologic uptake in the myocardium and salivary glands is clearly visible; in addition, the parathyroid adenoma is clearly shown as an area of persistent tracer uptake located caudally along the body midline. The upper left, upper right, and lower left panels show the SPECT/CT fusion images, respectively in the transaxial, coronal, and sagittal planes. Both the transaxial and the sagittal sections clearly demonstrate the location of the parathyroid adenoma posteriorly to the trachea, thus providing to the surgeon useful preoperative information for planning the most adequate approach.

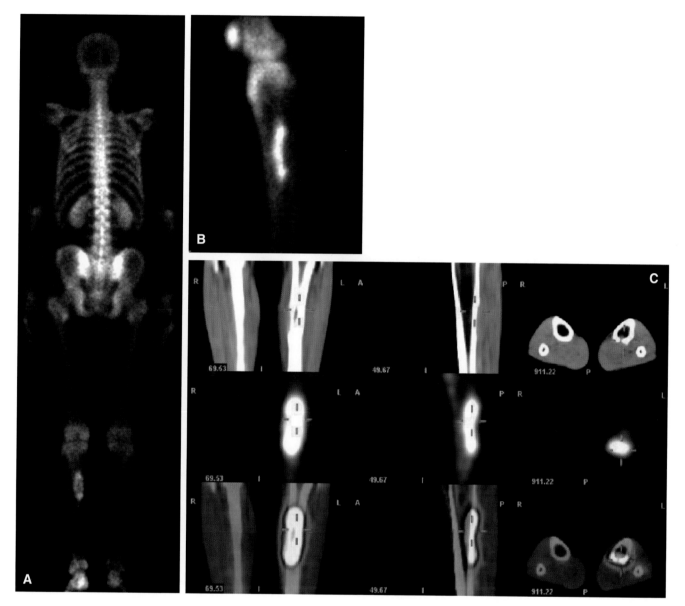

FIGURE 27-1. In a 56-year-old man, an unusual presentation of a single metastatic lesion at the diaphyseal portion of the left tibia from a previously unnoticed breast cancer. The posterior view of the $^{99m}$Tc-labeled methylene diphosphonate whole-body scan (A) shows a quite large area of increased uptake with a doughnut-type pattern (peripheral rim of increased uptake with central area of decreased uptake) that the left lateral spot view (B) demonstrates to be located posteriorly in the diaphyseal portion of the left tibia. There is also alteration in the longitudinal profile of the bone, suggesting possible extension to adjacent soft tissue. A SPECT-CT examination (panel C) better demonstrates the boundaries of the lesion in the 3 standard reconstruction planes (coronal, sagittal, transversal). The CT images (upper row) show important erosion of cortical bone in the posterior aspect of the left tibia and extension of the lesion also to adjacent soft tissue. The fusion images (bottom row) elucidate anatomic correspondence between the structural abnormality and the pattern of abnormal uptake of the bone-seeking radiopharmaceutical. Left, center, and right columns in panel C depict, respectively, the coronal, sagittal, and transverse section planes for the CT (upper row), the SPECT (middle row), and the fusion images (bottom row).

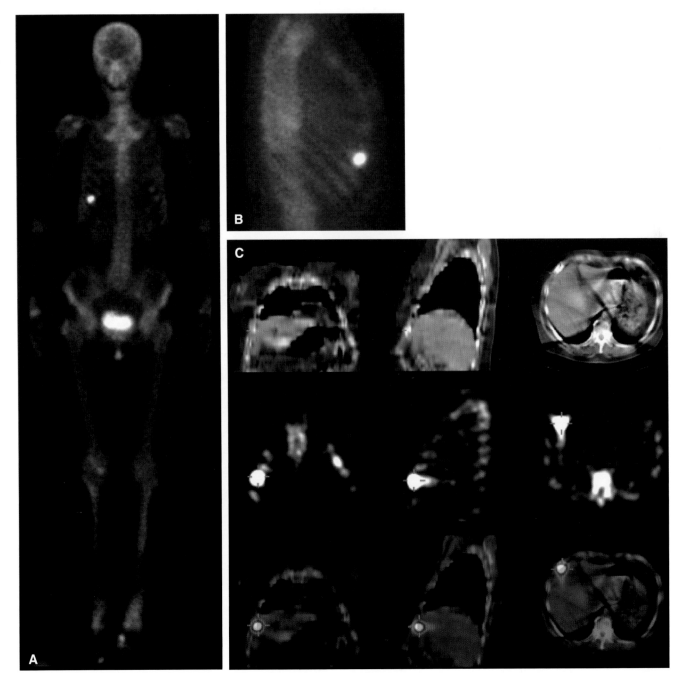

FIGURE 27-2. Markedly increased uptake of ⁹⁹ᵐTc-labeled methylene diphosphonate in the anterior portion of the tenth right rib in a 53-year-old woman, well delineated both in the whole-body scan (A) and in the right lateral spot view of the chest (B). A SPECT-CT examination (C) clearly demonstrates close topographic correlation of the rib lesion with the liver underneath the ribcage, especially in the fusion images (lower row of panel C). Such anatomic relations should be taken into account when planning biopsy of the bone lesion in the rib. Left, center, and right columns in panel C depict, respectively, the coronal, sagittal, and transverse section planes for the CT (upper row), the SPECT (middle row), and fusion images (bottom row).

# 9
# Sentinel Lymph Node Biopsy in Patients with Breast Cancer

Charles E. Cox, John M. Cox, Giuliano Mariani, Caren E.G. Wilkie, Laura B. White, Samira Khera, and Danielle M. Hasson

## Historical Background

The term "sentinel node" was first used by Gould et al. in 1960 to describe the first node in the drainage pathway of a malignant tumor (1). In 1977, Cabanas proposed that sentinel lymph nodes could be removed and evaluated to determine the need for complete lymph node dissection in penile carcinoma (2). Landmark studies by Norman et al. in the early 1990's redefined Sappey's line physiologically and demonstrated the necessity of lymphoscintigraphy to accurately assess nodal basins in truncal and head and neck melanoma (3,4). Morton and colleagues then observed that preoperative lymphoscintigraphy demonstrated a single lymph node receiving drainage from the primary melanoma (5,6). Alex et al. and Krag et al. reported the use of a handheld gamma probe to identify sentinel lymph nodes following lymphoscintigraphy in both melanoma and breast cancer patients (7,8). Giuliano demonstrated that blue dye accurately identified the sentinel lymph node in 174 breast cancer patients (9,10). The early sentinel node mapping experience using single agents was associated with 65% to 70% accuracy rates (7–9), and in 1996 Albertini et al. described a combination technique that improved the success rate of sentinel node localization to 92% (11).

As the technique of sentinel lymph node biopsy was refined and developed for melanoma and breast cancer, the remaining task was to prove equivalence or superiority when compared to conventional nodal dissection. The incidence of lymphedema and intercostal brachial nerve symptoms was clearly less with sentinel lymph node biopsy (12,13), but the primary oncological issue was staging equivalence. Since the earliest studies of sentinel lymph node mapping in melanoma demonstrated the reliance upon immunohistochemical techniques to validate and improve mapping accuracy, investigators who recognized this significance applied immunohistochemistry technology with cytokeratin staining to breast cancer sentinel lymph nodes.

Initial controversy surrounding immunohistochemistry evaluation of sentinel nodes was based upon conflicting reports suggesting that micrometastatic disease did not influence clinical outcome, and that the technology was too expensive and clinically superfluous for routine use.

Up-to-date, in-depth discussion of the issues and controversies surrounding pathological analysis of sentinel lymph nodes is presented in Chapters 18, 19, and 20 of this book, including different modalities of intraoperative analysis and advanced techniques based on molecular biology.

As techniques and histological analysis have evolved for sentinel lymph nodes, the emphasis has not been on enhanced detection of metastatic disease and consequent lowering of the false-negative rate. Rather, the primary focus has been on operator inexperience and the clinical relevance of micrometastatic nodal disease. There is a defined learning curve for the performance of sentinel lymph node biopsy, and experience decreases failure to identify a sentinel node and lowers the false-negative rates.

The accuracy, reliability, and low morbidity of this technique offer many advantages over conventional axillary dissection in clinically negative breast cancer patients, and it is the current standard of care in the United States based upon the frequency of performance for breast cancers treated at the parent institutions of the National Comprehensive Cancer Network (14).

Mariani et al. have summarized in 2001 state of the art in radioguided biopsy of the sentinel lymph node for breast cancer (15). More recent guidelines and reviews have updated the field, which encompasses an ever-growing body of literature dealing with several aspects of the procedure, from technical modalities to immediate and long-term clinical implications (16–21).

TABLE 9-1. Worldwide experience with sentinel lymphadenectomy: blue dye versus radiocolloid detection.

| Technique | Number of patients | Success rate (%) | False-negative rate (%) |
|---|---|---|---|
| Blue dye | 1435 | 78 | 7.2 |
| Radiocolloid | 1126 | 83 | 6.6 |
| Combination | 2185 | 90 | 6.1 |

*Source:* Cox C, et al. (23). Reprinted with permission.

## Technical Considerations of Lymphatic Mapping

The ability to perform lymphatic mapping and sentinel lymphadenectomy requires coordinated efforts from surgeons, specialists in nuclear medicine, pathologists, and operating room staff. In experienced centers, this technique is highly successful (22). Table 9-1 shows the average results of many authors in their experience with sentinel lymphadenectomy using blue dye only, radiocolloid only, or the combination of both as the localization technique (23).

## Agents for Lymphatic Mapping

The type of dye and/or radioactive tracer used by breast surgeons for lymphatic mapping varies. Regardless of which type of dye and/or radioactive tracer is used, there is a similar success rate in finding the sentinel node(s) (Table 9-1) (23). By far the most common dye used is blue dye, either Lymphazurin 1% or Patent Blue V dye. Less commonly used dyes include methylene blue, indigo carmine, and indocyanine green. The most common isotope used is $^{99m}$Tc, but a wide array of carrier particles may be used in sentinel node mapping. In the United States, the only registered radiopharmaceutical for lymphoscintigraphy is $^{99m}$Tc-sulfur colloid. Other agents used are colloidal particles of human albumin, antimony sulphide colloid, tin colloid, and cysteine-rhenium colloid. According to a recent meta-analysis of the worldwide experience with sentinel lymphadenectomy using blue dye only, radiocolloid only, or both, the success rate was increased when both techniques were used in combination (23).

The 2 agents referred to in mapping literature are trademarked as Lymphazurin and Patent Blue V dye. Biochemically, these are essentially the same agents. Lymphazurin 1% (isosulfan blue) is a sterile aqueous solution in a phosphate buffer made with pyrogen-free sterile water to yield a final pH of 6.8–7.4. Following injection, isosulfan blue is selectively picked up by the lymphatic vessels, rendering them a bright blue color that makes them easily discernible from surrounding tissues. Up to 10% of the injected dose of Lymphazurin is excreted unchanged in the urine within 24 hours. The remaining 90% is presumably excreted through the biliary route.

Lymphazurin 1% (isosulfan blue) has demonstrated a 1.5% incidence of localized allergic reactions. Localized swelling at the site of administration and mild hives of the hands, abdomen, and neck have been reported within several minutes following drug administration.

In a series of more than 7000 patients, approximately 1% demonstrated allergic reactions to isosulfan blue. This has been manifested by an initial wheal reaction at the injection site, followed by the development of blue hives scattered about the ipsilateral axilla, neck, groin, and other intertriginous areas. Generally these have responded to intravenous Benadryl and cleared rapidly. It is advisable to observe the patient for at least 30 to 60 minutes following the administration of isosulfan blue, since severe or delayed anaphylactic reactions may occur. In our own series of 7000 mapping cases, there have been 5 anaphylactic cases, for an incidence of 1/1400 (0.07%), in which the patient had a dramatic fall in blood pressure about 30 minutes following blue dye injection. These patients responded to the prompt administration of intravenous epinephrine for titration of blood pressure with fluid resuscitation, Benadryl, and occasionally, Solu-Medrol. One case of death due to anaphylactic reaction following injection with the dye is said to have occurred in the northeastern United States (Table 9-2). In a large prospective study of the American College of Surgeons Oncology Group, the incidence of anaphylaxis was 0.1% among 5500 patients (24).

The admixture of isosulfan blue with local anesthetics in the same syringe prior to administration results in an immediate precipitation of the drug complex. Similar precipitation of $^{99m}$Tc-sulfur colloid occurs with the mixture of these 2 compounds. Mixing agents with each other, or with local anesthetics, should be avoided. Local anesthetics and/or $^{99m}$Tc-sulfur colloid should be administered using separate syringes and at separate time intervals.

Patients should be warned about the excretion of the blue dye: it will rapidly appear in the urine and will also be excreted in the fecal material through the biliary tract. The blue dye staining of the superficial tissues of the breast will disappear quickly, but there may be some residual staining up to 6 months later. Occasionally, the patient will have a profound and moribund blue hue to the skin over the entire body, especially if bilateral mappings are performed in a fair-skinned patient of small stature; this resolves overnight, and positive reassurance is helpful to the patient.

A combination of $^{99m}$Tc-labeled sulfur colloid and Lymphazurin blue dye has been shown to be most effective for identification of the sentinel lymph node for the practicing surgeon (25), but either technique appears to

TABLE 9-2. Sentinel lymph node mapping techniques in breast cancer.

| Method of Detection | Description | Success rate (%) |
|---|---|---|
| *Dye* | | |
| Overall | | 78 |
| Lymphazurin (isosulfan) Blue | Used in most Western countries. No local toxicity, mild hypersensitivity reactions uncommon and self-limited, anaphylaxis rare. Aqueous. Penetrates lymphatic vessels in breast parenchyma more easily than indigo carmine. | |
| Patent V Blue | Used in Europe. Similar to Lymphazurin. There are cases of anaphylaxis documented, although not sufficient to contraindicate the use of Patent Blue. | |
| Methylene Blue | Less expensive than Lymphazurin. Readily available. Safe but only used by a few surgeons. No hypersensitivity reactions reported. Localized reactions due to extravasation of dye include cutaneous and subcutaneous tissue necrosis and necrotic abscesses. | |
| Indocyanine Green | Used in Japan. Popular diagnostic agent and readily available. Rare side effects. No allergic reactions observed. | |
| Indigo carmine (blue) | Used in Japan. Aqueous. A dye used for a classical urination test using ureterocystoscopy. | |
| *Radioisotope ($^{99m}$Tc)* | | |
| Overall | | 83 |
| Sulfur Colloid | Does not affect outcome if filtered or unfiltered. | |
| Albumin Colloid | Advantage of smaller particle size than sulfur colloid with easier lymphatic migration. It has a more neutral pH with less pain on injection and does not require filtration, thereby minimizing radiation exposure to technologists. | |
| Antimony Trisulfide Colloid | Able to visualize sentinel nodes in the internal mammary chain as well as in the axillary node group. Excellent properties for lymphoscintigraphy. | |
| Tin Colloid | Used in Japan. | |
| Cysteine-Rhenium Colloid | Similar as albumin colloid | |
| Stannous Phytate | Used in Japan. | |
| Rhenium Sulfate | Used in Japan. | |
| *Combination* | | 90 |

be successful at experienced centers. Chapter 1 of this book describes the various types of $^{99m}$Tc-labeled colloids employed for lymphoscintigraphic mapping and for intra-operative guidance with the handheld gamma probe during sentinel lymph node biopsy.

Despite remarkable disparities in the technique of radiocolloid injection (type of radiocolloid, dose injected and volume of the injectate, site of injection, timing of lymphoscintigraphy prior to surgery and intraoperative detection), radioguidance results in consistently high success rates for the identification of the sentinel lymph node. The radiocolloid injection, usually performed by a nuclear medicine specialist, should be done 1 to 8 hours prior to axillary exploration, with the optimal injection time 2 to 3 hours before the operation. Some authorities even inject the day before. At the Moffitt Cancer Center, approximately 200 to 2000 µCi of radiolabeled sulfur colloid is diluted to 6 mL as the injectant, and given in 1 mL aliquots, intraparenchymally at the tumor margin, periareolar, or intradermal locations. Other groups, and especially those employing the smaller particle radiocolloid $^{99m}$Tc-nanocolloidal albumin rather than $^{99m}$Tc-sulfur colloid, inject smaller volumes of the tracer (150 µL aliquots), whichever is the preferred route of administration (peritumoral, subdermal over the cutaneous

projection of the tumor, or peri- sub-areolar) (see review in ref. 15). The consistently high success rate in identifying the sentinel lymph node despite such diverse routes of interstitial injection of the radiocolloid (and of the dye) suggests that lymphatic drainage of the entire breast towards the axilla basically follows a common route to a single sentinel lymph node or to a limited number of sentinel nodes (26,27). This conclusion is consistent with prior observations on the central role of the Sappey's periareolar plexus in lymphatic drainage of the breast (28) (see also Figure 7-6). In this regard, recent popularity of the subareolar route of radiocolloid injection (29–31) is supported also by the consideration that this approach would overcome limitations to sentinel lymph node biopsy in patients with multicentric or multifocal breast cancer.

Although lymphoscintigraphy is not routinely performed at some cancer centers, most authorities in the field agree that such preoperative imaging constitutes an essential component of radioguided biopsy of the sentinel lymph node in patients with breast cancer (32–34). In fact, lymphoscintigraphy can detect unexpected patterns of aberrant lymphatic drainage that would often go undetected if relying only on intraoperative gamma probe guidance. In this regard, the application of a more

TABLE 9-3. Sentinel lymphadenectomy injection sites and their associated success rates.

| Injection Site | Number of patients | Success rate (%) | False-negative rate (%) |
|---|---|---|---|
| Subareolar | 76 | 99 | 0 |
| Peritumoral | 1055 | 89 | 8.6 |
| Dermal/intradermal | 775 | 98 | 6.5 |
| Subdermal | 510 | 96 | 7.2 |

*Source:* Cox C. et al. (23). Reprinted with permission.

recent imaging technique based on hybrid equipment (SPECT-CT) may actually help in better guiding the surgeon to the site of the sentinel lymph node(s), as the images also include detailed information on depth of the sentinel node within tissues (35).

Lymphazurin blue dye is injected prior to beginning the operation. The dye can be injected intraparenchymally or given subdermally in the subareolar region; unless the injected area is to be excised, intradermal injection should be avoided due to permanent tattooing (Table 9-3). Again, this is followed by 5 minutes of intermittent manual breast massage. With the aid of the blue channel, a handheld gamma probe is then used to locate and surgically removal the sentinel lymph node.

The pathologist may examine the sentinel lymph node intraoperatively, using either imprint cytology methods or frozen section. If either of these modalities reveals cancer within the node, a complete axillary lymph node dissection should be performed. The pathologist later examines the removed negative sentinel lymph nodes using H&E staining. If positive, no further exam is required. When initial H&E screen is negative, cytokeratin staining may be routinely performed. A complete axillary node dissection should be conducted if either of these modalities reveals the presence of metastases within the sentinel lymph node. The care for the patient with micrometastases or isolated tumor cells within the node is more controversial. The likelihood of nonsentinel node or additional nodal metastases when the sentinel node has micrometastases only is about 10% to 15%; if the sentinel node has isolated tumor cells, the likelihood is less than 5% (36). Some authorities do not advocate completion node dissection in these instances. An algorithm has been proposed to predict the presence of nonsentinel node metastases after a sentinel node biopsy to aid the surgeon and patient in the selection of further treatment options. Axillary radiation may be an effective alternative to complete axillary lymph node dissection, but lacks the staging information obtained with surgery.

## Procedure

The following procedural protocol is based on a breast sentinel lymph node task-specific checklist provided by the American College of Surgeons Oncology Group for surgeons being trained, mentored, and evaluated in sentinel lymphadenectomy. This checklist is for surgeons learning how to perform sentinel lymph node biopsies, and was derived using a modified Delphi technique. Experts were asked to provide a list of how they performed sentinel node biopsy, along with videos of their performance of the technique. An educational consulting group, employed by the study group, then reviewed the tapes and validated the list. The list was resubmitted to the experts for final review and approval. Expert groups validated the checklist through observing and grading both novice and expert sentinel node surgeons. The procedure is as follows:

1. Patient selected has a disease appropriate for mapping (based on a review of the exam, imaging studies, and past history).

2. The timing of the operation is appropriate for radionuclide injection (>30 minutes for same day or next day).

3. The patient must be clinically node negative.

4. The surgeon must have an intraoperative pathology plan.

5. The surgeon must review the radionuclide injection procedure.

6. The patient is positioned correctly on the operating room table.

7. The surgeon injects the blue dye correctly (peritumoral or subareolar).

8. The breast should be massaged for 5 minutes.

9. The "hot spot" must then be marked on axilla prior to incision.

10. The incision is selected beneath the axillary hairline.

11. The clavipectoral fascia is identified.

12. Dissection is directed to blue and/or "hot" lymph nodes (a properly excised node is any blue node or any "hot" node with an ex-vivo radioactivity count ratio of sentinel lymph node to nonsentinel lymph node of 10:1, an in-vivo radioactivity count ratio of sentinel lymph node to background of 3:1, or both).

13. The probe must be used appropriately to assess potential sentinel nodes.

14. Sentinel nodes are removed with ligature/clip of lymphatic channels as appropriate for the size of lymphatics/vessels.

15. A 10-second ex-vivo count or peak instantaneous count must be obtained on each removed node.

16. Lymph nodes are appropriately labeled for the pathologist.

17. The axilla is reevaluated for "hot" and/or blue nodes.

18. All nodes with counts greater than 10% of hottest sentinel lymph nodes are removed.

19. The surgeon then palpates the axilla prior to closing the incision.

## Extras

1. The surgeon should preoperatively review the lymphoscintigram, if it was done, and develop an operative plan based on these findings.
2. A careful examination is conducted near the lateral thoracic vein if no sentinel lymph nodes are identified.
3. A full axillary node dissection is performed if no sentinel lymph nodes are identified or a sentinel lymph node is positive.

(Procedure section from Cox C, et al. (23) Reprinted with permission from Springer.)

## General Guidelines

In the care of the breast cancer patient, clinical evaluation of the axilla is a primary role of the surgeon, and identification of lymph node metastases is the main goal of axillary surgery. In the face of these new mapping technologies, it is important not to abandon good clinical judgment. A dilated blue lymphatic channel ending abruptly in a palpably firm lymph node is a positive sentinel node and should be removed. Nodes must continue to be evaluated in light of their clinical appearance and palpable abnormality (37).

It should be noted that, as experience continues to accumulate, initial absolute and relative contraindications for sentinel lymph node biopsy (irrespective of radioguidance alone or combined with blue dye) are continuously been challenged and are actually reduced. Thus, the field is still evolving, and conditions such as prior biopsy, prior breast and axillary surgery, prior neoadjuvant chemotherapy in locally advanced disease, tumor size, multicentric/multifocal disease, and even pregnancy now require careful evaluation on a patient-by-patient basis that in most cases results in application of the procedure (especially if performed under radioguidance) (38–44).

## Lumpectomy and Sentinel Node Biopsy

Certain situations can add a level of difficulty to the sentinel lymph node biopsy with lumpectomy. If the tumor lies in the upper outer quadrant, lesional injection can add to axillary background counts ("shine through"). In these cases, it may be better to have the patient injected with the radiocolloid the night before surgery. Some studies have shown higher false-negative rates with radiocolloid injection in the upper outer quadrant (45). Subareolar injection may be done for tumors high in the upper outer quadrant. Several studies (46–48) have demonstrated that mapping failures, when analyzed, were primarily associated with 2 comorbid factors: age and obesity (48).

In the analysis of multiple factors, these 2 factors have emerged as the only ones that could not be modified to reduce the failure rate. Thus, surgical skill, injection techniques, massage, appropriate dyes, colloidal particle size, adequate and well-calibrated instrumentation, careful pathologic analysis, and experience may and still do lead to mapping failures. An assessment tool in the form of a nomogram predicts the likelihood of failure based upon age and body mass index. The large ACOSOG prospective study showed that among 5500 patients, age, obesity, and surgeon experience were the factors associated with sentinel lymph node biopsy failure.

## Mastectomy

Patients undergoing mastectomy can often be mapped through 1 incision. The sentinel node incision may be done at any point during the procedure. Some authorities make a small axillary incision at the start of the mastectomy to identify a sentinel node. When the breast is reflected laterally, the surgeon needs to be aware of the variation of shine-through coming from a different direction. With the breast reflected medially, the shine-through comes from the posterior direction. Skin-sparing mastectomies can be accomplished through a single incision; however, the entire procedure may be performed through a breast and axillary incision (49,50).

## Learning Curves, Operative Experience, and Volume of Practice

Mapping success rates and accuracy must be evaluated to determine the success of lymphatic mapping. Success reflects the ability to identify the sentinel lymph node; accuracy is the false-negative rate, defined as the proportion of patients who have axillary metastases and a negative sentinel lymph node. These 2 pieces of information are necessary to provide adequate quality control of lymphatic mapping, and they should be tracked at every institution to validate results and compare them to established series. Surgeons with appropriate training should be able to map with 85% success rate and with no more than 1 false-negative case in their first 10 patients with metastatic disease.

Recommendations that require the surgeon to perform 30 cases of sentinel lymph node biopsy followed by completion axillary lymph node dissections allow for initial learning curve adjustments. Once these results are analyzed and an 85% success rate is achieved, with 1 or fewer false negative cases, then a complete axillary lymph node dissection is carried out only in the face of a positive sentinel lymph node. Failure to map may be a function of surgical skill, or nuclear medicine injection methodology, or the pathologic evaluation of the sentinel lymph node.

**Total mapping failure 4/'94 to 7/'04**

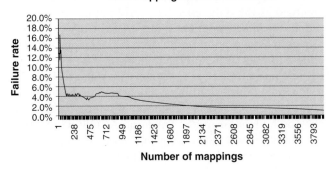

FIGURE 9-1. Sentinel node mapping learning curve, from the H. Lee Moffitt Cancer Center Series, April 94 to July 2004. The success rate was 98.9%. (Modified from Dupont EL, Cox CE, Shiever S. Learning curves and breast cancer. Breast Diseases 2002;12(4):420. Reprinted with permission from IOS press.)

By calculating learning curves for surgeons training to perform a new procedure, evidence-based techniques are established that allow feedback (Figure 9-1). This is important for several reasons. Quality monitoring and outcomes measurement are rapidly becoming the standards by which surgery is measured. This methodology provides a framework for meeting these standards (51–58).

## Special Situations in Lymphatic Mapping

### Internal Mammary Nodes

According to recent studies, 2% to 29% of patients who receive a sentinel lymphadenectomy will map to at least 1 internal mammary node, and 10% to 14% of those patients who map to the internal mammary area, will have at least 1 internal mammary node positive (59). In all lymphatic mapping cases, the internal mammary locations should be thoroughly evaluated, especially in the second and third parasternal interspaces (60). Radio-guided excision may be accomplished by separating the fibers of the pectoralis major muscle and dividing the intercostal muscles at the parasternal location. Careful localization and delicate dissection will result in the uneventful removal of the internal mammary node/s. Following removal, marking the location with a small surgical clip will allow radiographic localization, should the node return positive on final pathology.

Impeccable care must be taken during the dissection to avoid entering the pleural space, which could result in a pneumothorax. If this occurs, the patient is treated with intraoperative pleural aspiration and postoperative observation until the resolution of the pneumothorax.

If an internal mammary node cannot be safely removed, an intraoperative clip can be placed at the site of the node, the patient can be scanned or x-rayed postoperatively (60), and the location of the internal mammary node can be tattooed for later radiation. If the internal mammary node is positive upon final pathological evaluation, then radiation is given to the internal mammary node chain. In contrast, a negative internal mammary node would obviate the need for radiation in at least 86% of the cases (60). Identification of the internal mammary sentinel node is not routinely performed at most cancer centers. An involved internal mammary sentinel node without axillary involvement is seen in only 3% to 5% of cases. Internal mammary recurrences are a rare clinical problem, and the role of internal mammary radiotherapy is unclear. Prior to excising an internal mammary sentinel node, consideration should be given to the clinical relevance of knowing the status of the internal mammary nodes.

Figure 9-2 shows disease-free survival for patients who have positive internal mammary nodes alone. A patient with a positive internal mammary node has an equivalent disease-free survival to that of a patient with only axillary node involvement (61).

### Ductal Carcinoma In Situ

Ductal carcinoma in situ (DCIS) is by definition a local disease and does not metastasize. Treatment emphasizes local control, which should equal cure. Lymphatic mapping should have no role in a disease where axillary metastasis occurs in less than 1% of patients and long-term survival is almost 100% (62). Consensus reports on

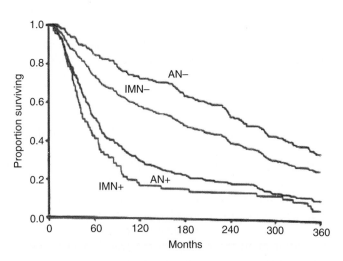

FIGURE 9-2. Overall survival curves for axillary node involvement (node negative [AN−] and node positive [AN+]) and for internal mammary node involvement (node negative [IMN−] and node positive [IMN+]). (Veronesi et al. [61]. Reprinted with permission from Elsevier.)

TABLE 9-4. Invasive cancer found at definitive surgery for ductal carcinoma in situ (DCIS).

| Institution and reference | Number of patients with DCIS | Number of cases positive for invasive ductal carcinoma (%) |
|---|---|---|
| Moffitt (66) | 675 | 66 (10) |
| Brigham and Women's (79) | 289 | 40 (14) |
| European Institute of Oncology (80) | 244 | 31 (13) |
| Ohio State University (81) | 89 | 10 (11) |
| Yale University (82) | 59 | 17 (29) |
| Stanford University (83) | 54 | 8 (15) |

DCIS dating to 1989 espoused that axillary evaluation was not further recommended in DCIS (63–65).

The increased use of sentinel lymph node biopsy for staging breast cancer and its low morbidity compared with axillary dissection has renewed interest in axillary staging for patients with DCIS (66). DCIS represents a heterogeneous group of lesions, and percutaneous image-guided core biopsies will miss 10% to 29% of invasive cancers in cases diagnosed as DCIS (67). Regardless of biopsy method, the final pathologic diagnosis may be wrong (see Tables 9-4 and 9-5) (62,66,67). At the H. Lee Moffitt Cancer Center in Tampa, FL, in our own series of 675 patients, 613 had a biopsy diagnosis of DCIS and 55 (9%) were upstaged, while 62 had a biopsy diagnosis of DCIS with microinvasion and 11 (18%) were upstaged. The factor associated with a higher incidence of upstaging DCIS to invasive carcinoma is high grade (13% of patients with grade III biopsy histology were upstaged to invasive cancer) (66).

Based on current data, we recommend sentinel lymph node biopsy in patients who are undergoing mastectomy for DCIS, those who have DCIS with microinvasion, those who have high-grade DCIS at the time of core biopsy, and those who have a mass and or extensive microcalcifications on mammography (66). These findings have been validated by a recent study at the University of Texas MD Anderson Cancer Center (68). There is a greater risk for invasive carcinoma at the time of definitive resection in high-risk patients with DCIS. Sentinel lymph node biopsy is an important diagnostic tool with low morbidity. Most of the positive nodes involved micrometastases detected only by cytokeratin immunohistochemistry. Lymph node micrometastases associated with invasive breast cancer are a well-known phenomenon, but their prognostic significance is debatable. The finding of micrometastatic disease on immunohistochemistry analysis is of little consequence in patients with a final diagnosis of DCIS (69).

In conclusion, the points are as follows:

1. No data emanating from retrospective reviews of tumor registry data of DCIS will answer the question of whether to map patients with a preoperative diagnosis of DCIS.

2. Careful review of the biopsy literature for concordance of biopsy to final diagnosis is the key to the decision of sentinel lymph node biopsy in DCIS.

3. Sentinel lymph node biopsy carries minimal morbidity.

4. Cytokeratin-positive disease alone (N0i+) in the presence of a final diagnosis of DCIS requires no axillary dissection and carries no adverse prognostic significance; chemotherapy in this situation is contraindicated.

## Prophylactic Mastectomy

A prophylactic mastectomy is an operation that removes the entire breast, the nipple areolar complex, and the tail of Spence to prevent a subsequent cancer in that breast. In selected patients, prophylactic mastectomy has become a widely accepted alternative to routine close surveillance. The reasons for this procedure may include 1 or

TABLE 9-5. Underestimation* in patients with a diagnosis of ductal carcinoma in situ (DCIS).

| DCIS identified by | Invasive cancer found by number (%) |
|---|---|
| *Initial Pathologic Interpretation* | *Pathologic re-review* |
| Fisher et al. (84) | 17/790 (2%) |
| Bijker et al. (88) | 27/863 (3%) |
| *14 gauge ALCBB* | *Surgical excision* |
| Darling et al. (79) | 14/67 (21%) |
| Jackman et al. (85) | 76/373 (20%) |
| *14 gauge DVABB* | *Surgical excision* |
| Darling et al. (79) | 8/47 (17%) |
| Jackman et al. (85) | 38/348 (11%) |
| *11 gauge DVABB* | *Surgical excision* |
| Darling et al. (79) | 18/175 (10%) |
| Jackman et al. (85) | 69/605 (11%) |
| *Core biopsy* | *Surgical excision or mastectomy* |
| Cox et al. (67) | 44/310 (14%) |
| Morrow et al. (86) | 13/90 (14%) |
| *Surgical biopsy* | *Surgical excision or mastectomy* |
| Cox et al. (87) | 19/343 (6%) |
| Morrow et al. (86) | 9/61 (7%) |
| *Surgical or core biopsy* | *Mastectomy* |
| Cox et al. (87) | 19/653 (3%) |
| Morrow et al. (86) | ns (12%) |
| *Mastectomy** | *Positive sentinel lymph node biopsy* |
| Cox et al. (87) | 11/61 (18%) |

Legend:
ALCBB—automated large-core breast biopsy
DVABB—directional vacuum-assisted breast biopsy
ns—not stated
*The proportion of patients with a DCIS diagnosis found on definitive surgery to have invasive cancer
**Patients with a final pathologic diagnosis of DCIS (no invasion found in the mastectomy specimen)

more of the following: histological risk factors, such as lobular carcinoma in situ; a positive family history; breast cancer gene test (BRCA-1/BRCA-2) positive diagnoses; cosmesis symmetry with a contralateral mastectomy for carcinoma; and/or cancer phobia. Currently, the main indications are the genetic mutations linked to breast cancer (70).

Premenopausal patients with a strong family history of breast cancer will most likely require genetic counseling to determine their personal risk, recurrence risk, and risk to family or offspring.

Patients with a strong history of breast cancer, who have a lesion treatable with lumpectomy, may receive a lumpectomy with sentinel lymph node biopsy and subsequent genetic screening. If diagnosed as BRCA-1/BRCA-2 positive following the lumpectomy and sentinel lymph node biopsy, the patient may choose to not receive radiation but may get a bilateral mastectomy and reconstruction perhaps with oophorectomy. The BRCA-negative patient may receive radiation to the breast alone. Dupont et al. demonstrate that up to 5% of prophylactic mastectomies harbor occult cancer, and patients with a history of carcinoma have an increased risk of 0.5% to 1% per year of developing a contralateral breast cancer (70).

Mapping patients with prophylactic mastectomy is built upon a few basic premises (70). First, mapping may help avoid the incidence of inadvertent axillary node removal in a prophylactic mastectomy, which is approximately 15%. Second, lymph node mapping may eliminate the need for total axillary dissection if cancer is detected in the prophylactic breast when the sentinel node is negative. Third, sentinel lymph node mapping may detect occult nodal disease prior to the detection of disease in the breast. As a result of lymphatic mapping and sentinel lymphadenectomy, patients with unsuspected primary breast cancer can be spared the potential risks and long-term morbidity of a complete axillary node dissection. If mapping is not performed at the time of prophylactic mastectomy and a breast cancer is detected, a second operative procedure may be required. Some studies have shown that the absence of known disease in the breast does not preclude the presence of occult disease in the axilla (70,71). The practice of mapping is a logical extension of the prophylactic procedure, but is likely to benefit few patients.

## Implants and Reduction Mammoplasty

With the ever-increasing popularity of breast augmentation and reduction mammoplasty, the question of whether patients can be mapped following these procedures has become important. Lymphatic mapping conducted at the H. Lee Moffitt Cancer Center on more than 50 patients with prior breast augmentation proved to be 100% successful. Despite these favorable results,

good clinical judgment by the attending surgeon is imperative. When a patient undergoes a breast reduction, the inferior pedicle technique causes the least disruption of lymphatic flow to the axillary basin. However, difficulty in mapping can arise when the tumor is located within the pedicle flap region (at 5 to 7 o'clock). This is especially true in patients with recent reductions. Augmentation mammoplasty seems to have no effect on sentinel lymph node biopsy success rates. However, axillary incisions may decrease success rates. Several studies have shown that cosmetic breast surgery does not eliminate the ability to perform successful mapping. However, depending on the location of the tumor and the technique of implant placement, cosmetic surgery can possibly jeopardize the mapping success rate (72–78).

## Consensus Guidelines

In January 2005, the Ninth Conference on Primary Therapy of Early Breast Cancer in St Gallen, Switzerland, compiled consensus guidelines on the treatment of breast cancer (89). Highlights of these guidelines include:

- Nodal status remains the most important risk factor, underscoring the importance of accurately assessing the nodal basin with mapping.
- Micrometastases, although recognized to have prognostic relevance, are not recommended to be used in treatment choice or risk allocation.
- For DCIS, sentinel lymph node biopsy is unnecessary, with several exceptions. Exceptions include when invasive cancer cannot be definitively excluded, or if mastectomy is planned.
- Two new prognostic categories for risk assessment were added: overexpression or amplification of the HER2/neu gene; and peritumoral vessel invasion, especially lymphovascular.
- Endocrine responsiveness was stressed as the most important selection factor for adjuvant chemotherapy, and these patients are divided into 3 groups: endocrine responsive; endocrine response uncertain; and endocrine non-responsive.

## Comments

The consensus implications for selective use of sentinel lymph node biopsy in DCIS highlight some of the statistically significant criteria that were identified in an H. Lee Moffitt Cancer Center study (90). With an approximate 20% upstaging in patients originally diagnosed with DCIS via core biopsy (90), this group should also be considered for selective sentinel lymph node biopsy. An additional study by the University of Texas MD Anderson Cancer Center shows a similar upstaging among the core biopsied group (approximately 30%) (91) and validates selective lymph node biopsy for this group.

The prognostic significance of micrometastases, although not yet a factor in systemic treatment according to the above consensus guidelines, has brought some notable findings. Although themselves not significant detriments to survival, their presence in the sentinel node has signaled a 12% to 15% chance of finding further macrometastases (92–94) in the nodal basin. For this reason, completion dissection is recommended for this subset of patients.

## References

1. Gould EA, Winship T, Philbin PH, Kerr HH. Observations on a "sentinel node" in cancer of the parotid. *Cancer.* 1960;13:77–78.
2. Cabanas RM. An approach for the treatment of penile carcinoma. *Cancer.* 1977;39:456–466.
3. Norman J, Cruse CW, Espinosa C, et al. Redefinition of cutaneous lymphatic drainage with the use of lymphoscintigraphy for malignant melanoma. *Am J Surg.* 1991;162:432–437.
4. Norman J Jr, Cruse W, Ruas E, et al. The expanding role of lymphoscintigraphy in the management of cutaneous melanoma. First Place Winner: Conrad Jobst award. *Am Surg.* 1989;55:689–694.
5. Morton DL, Wen DR, Foshag LJ, Essner R, Cochran A. Intraoperative lymphatic mapping and selective cervical lymphadenectomy for early-stage melanomas of the head and neck. *J Clin Oncol.* 1993;11:1751–1756.
6. Morton DL, Wen DR, Wong JH, et al. Technical details of intraoperative lymphatic mapping for early stage melanoma. *Arch Surg.* 1992;127:392–399.
7. Alex JC, Krag DN. Gamma-probe guided localization of lymph nodes. *Surg Oncol.* 1993;2:137–143.
8. Krag DN, Weaver DL, Alex JC, Fairbank JT. Surgical resection and radiolocalization of the sentinel lymph node in breast cancer using a gamma probe. *Surg Oncol.* 1993;2:335–339.
9. Giuliano AE, Kirgan DM, Guenther JM, Morton DL. Lymphatic mapping and sentinel lymphadenectomy for breast cancer. *Ann Surg.* 1994;220:391–398.
10. Giuliano AE. Sentinel lymphadenectomy in primary breast carcinoma: an alternative to routine axillary dissection. *J Surg Oncol.* 1996;62:75–77.
11. Albertini JJ, Lyman GH, Cox C, et al. Lymphatic mapping and sentinel node biopsy in the patient with breast cancer. *JAMA.* 1996;276:1818–1822.
12. Swenson KK, Nissen MJ, Ceronsky C, Swenson L, Lee MW, Tuttle TM. Comparison of side effects between sentinel lymph node and axillary lymph node dissection for breast cancer. *Ann Surg Oncol.* 2002;9:745–753.
13. Burak WE, Hollenbeck ST, Zervos EE, Hock KL, Kemp LC, Young DC. Sentinel lymph node biopsy results in less postoperative morbidity compared with axillary lymph node dissection for breast cancer. *Am J Surg.* 2002;183:23–27.
14. Carlson RW, Anderson BO, Bensinger W, et al. NCCN practice guidelines for breast cancer. *Oncology (Williston Park, NY).* 2000;14:33–49.
15. Mariani G, Moresco L, Viale G, et al. Radioguided sentinel lymph node biopsy in breast cancer surgery. *J Nucl Med.* 2001;42:1198–1215.
16. Chagpar AB, McMasters KM. Sentinel lymph node biopsy for breast cancer: from investigational procedure to standard practice. *Expert Rev Anticancer Ther.* 2004;4:903–912.
17. Aarsvold JN, Alazraki NP. Update on detection of sentinel lymph nodes in patients with breast cancer. *Semin Nucl Med.* 2005;35:116–128.
18. Thompson JF, Uren RF, Scolyer RA, Stretch JR. Selective sentinel lymphadenectomy: progress to date and prospects for the future. *Cancer Treat Res.* 2005;127:269–287.
19. Lyman GH, Giuliano AE, Somerfield MR, et al. American Society of Clinical Oncology guideline recommendations for sentinel lymph node biopsy in early-stage breast cancer. *J Clin Oncol.* 2005;23:7703–7720.
20. James TA, Edge SB. Sentinel lymph node in breast cancer. *Curr Opin Obstet Gynecol.* 2006;18:53–58.
21. Kim T, Giuliano AE, Lyman GH. Lymphatic mapping and sentinel lymph node biopsy in early stage breast carcinoma: a metaanalysis. *Cancer.* 2006;106:4–16.
22. Giuliano AE, Jones RC, Brennan M, et al. Sentinel lymphadenectomy in breast cancer. *J Clin Oncol.* 1997;15:2345–2350.
23. Cox C, Furman B, White L, et al. Selective sentinel lymphadenectomy for breast cancer. In: Leong S, Kitagawa Y, Kitajima M (eds). *Selective Sentinel Lymphadenectomy for Human Solid Cancer.* Series: Cancer Treatment and Research Vol. 27 [Series editor: Rosen ST]. New York: Springer; 2005:77–104.
24. Wilke LG, McCall LM, Posther KE, et al. Surgical complications associated with sentinel lymph node biopsy: results from a prospective international cooperative group trial. *Ann Surg Oncol.* 2006;13:491–500.
25. Edwards MJ, Whitworth P, Tafra L, et al. The details of successful sentinel lymph node staging for breast cancer. *Am J Surg.* 2000;180:257–261.
26. Chao C, Wong SL, Woo C, et al. Reliable lymphatic drainage to axillary sentinel lymph nodes regardless of tumor location within the breast. *Am J Surg.* 2001;182:307–311.
27. Zavagno G, Rubello D, Franchini Z, et al. Axillary sentinel lymph node in breast cancer: a single lymphatic pathway drains the entire mammary gland. *Eur J Surg Oncol.* 2005;31:479–484.
28. Grant RN, Tabah EJ, Adair EE. The surgical significance of the subareolar lymph plexus in cancer of the breast. *Surgery.* 1953;33:71–78.
29. Klimberg VS, Rubio IT, Henry R, et al. Subareolar versus peritumoral injection for location of the sentinel node. *Ann Surg.* 1999;229:860–864.
30. Tuttle TM, Colbert M, Christensen R, et al. Subareolar injection of $^{99m}$Tc facilitates sentinel lymph node identification. *Ann Surg Oncol.* 2002;9:77–81.
31. Krynyckyi BR, Kim CK, Shafir MK, et al. Breast cancer and its management: the utility and technique of lymphoscintigraphy. In: Freeman LM, ed. *Nuclear Medicine Annual, 2003.* Philadelphia: Lippincott Williams & Wilkins; 2003;131–169.

32. Kim SC, Kim DW, Moadel RM, et al. Using the intraoperative hand held probe without lymphoscintigraphy or using only dye correlates with higher sensory morbidity following sentinel lymph node biopsy in breast cancer: a review of the literature. *World J Surg Oncol.* 2005:3:64.

33. Goyal A, Newcombe RG, Mansel RE, et al. Role of routine preoperative lymphoscintigraphy in sentinel node biopsy for breast cancer. *Eur J Cancer.* 2005;41:238–243.

34. Goyal A, Mansel RE. Does imaging in sentinel node scintigraphic localization add value to the procedure in patients with breast cancer? *Nucl Med Commun.* 2005;26:845–847.

35. Lerman H, Metser U, Lievshitz G, Sperber F, Shneebaum S, Even-Sapir E. Lymphoscintigraphic sentinel node identification in patients with breast cancer: the role of SPECT-CT. *Eur J Nucl Med Mol Imaging.* 2006; 33:329–337.

36. Giuliano AE, Dale PS, Turner RR, et al. Improved axillary staging of breast cancer with sentinel lymphadenectomy. *Ann Surg.* 1995;222:394–401.

37. Schwartz GF, Giuliano AE, Veronesi U. Consensus Conference Committee. Proceedings of the consensus conference on the role of sentinel lymph node biopsy in carcinoma of the breast. *Breast J.* 2002;8:126–138.

38. Luini A, Galimberti V, Gatti G, et al. The sentinel node biopsy after previous breast surgery: preliminary results on 543 patients treated at the European Institute of Oncology. *Breast Cancer Res Treat.* 2005;89:159–163.

39. Mamounas EP, Brown A, Anderson S, et al. Sentinel node biopsy after neoadjuvant chemotherapy in breast cancer: results from national Surgical Adjuvant Breast and Bowel Project Protocol B-27. *J Clin Oncol.* 2005;23:2694–2702.

40. Heuts EM, van der Ent FW, Kengen RA, van der Pol HA, Hulsewe KW, Hoofwijk AG. Results of sentinel node biopsy not affected by previous excisional biopsy. *Eur J Surg Oncol.* 2006;32:278–281.

41. Tanaka Y, Maeda H, Ogawa Y, et al. Sentinel node biopsy in breast cancer patients treated with neoadjuvant chemotherapy. *Oncol Rep.* 2006;15:927–931.

42. Tausch C, Konstantiniuk P, Kugler F, Reitsamer R, Roka S, Postlberger S, Haid A. Sentinel lymph node biopsy after preoperative chemotherapy for breast cancer: findings from the Austrian Sentinel Node Study Group. *Ann Surg Oncol.* 2006 May 24; [Epub ahead of print].

43. Knauer M, Konstantiniuk P, Haid A, et al. Multicentric cancer: a new indication for sentinel node biopsy—a multi-institutional validation study. *J Clin Oncol.* 2006; 24:3374–3380.

44. Pandit-Taskar N, Dauer LT, Montgomery L, St Germain J, Zanzonico PB, Divgi CR. Organ and fetal absorbed dose estimates from $^{99m}$Tc-sulfur colloid lymphoscintigraphy and sentinel node localization in breast cancer patients. *J Nucl Med.* 2006;47:1202–1208.

45. Krag D, Weaver D, Ashikaga T, et al. The sentinel node in breast cancer—a multicenter validation study. *N Engl J Med.* 1998;339:941–946.

46. Morrow M, Rademaker AW, Bethke KP, et al. Learning sentinel node biopsy: results of a prospective randomized trial of 2 techniques. *Surgery.* 1999;126:714–720.

47. Ng PC, Chua AC, Lannin DP, et al. Age and surgeon experience: the only significant factors contributing to sentinel lymph node mapping failure in breast cancer. *Soc Surg Oncol* [abstract]. 1999.

48. Cox CE, Dupont E, Whitehead GF, et al. Age and body mass index may increase chance for failure in sentinel lymph node biopsy for women with breast cancer. *Breast J.* 2002;8:88–89.

49. Cunnick, GH, Mokbel K. Skin-sparing mastectomy. *Am J Surg.* 2004;188:78–84.

50. Simmons RM, Hollenbeck ST, LaTrenta GS. Two-year follow-up of areola-sparing mastectomy with immediate reconstruction. *Am J Surg.* 2004;188:403–406.

51. Veronesi U, Paganelli G, Viale G, et al. A randomized comparison of sentinel-node biopsy with routine axillary dissection in breast cancer. *N Engl J Med.* 2003;349:546–553.

52. Torrenga H, Fabry H, van der Sijp JR, van Diest PJ, Pijpers R, Meijer S. Omitting axillary lymph node dissection in sentinel node negative breast cancer patients is safe: a long term follow-up analysis. *J Surg Oncol.* 2004;88:4–7.

53. Veronesi U, Galimberti V, Mariani L, et al. Sentinel node biopsy in breast cancer: early results in 953 patients with negative sentinel node biopsy and no axillary dissection. *Eur J Cancer.* 2005;41:197–198.

54. Sanjuan A, Vidal-Sicart S, Zanon G, et al. Clinical axillary recurrence after sentinel node biopsy in breast cancer: a follow-up study of 220 patients. *Eur J Nucl Med Mole Imaging.* 2005;32:932–936.

55. Smidt ML, Janssen CM, Kuster DM, et al. Axillary recurrence after a negative sentinel node biopsy for breast cancer: incidence and clinical significance. *Ann Surg Oncol.* 2005;12:29–33.

56. Fuhrman GM, Gambino J, Bolton JS, Farr G, Jiang X. 5-year follow-up after sentinel node mapping for breast cancer demonstrates better than expected treatment outcomes. *Am Surg.* 2005;71:564–569.

57. Carlo JT, Grant MD, Knox SM, et al. Survival analysis following sentinel lymph node biopsy: a validation trial demonstrating its accuracy in staging early breast cancer. *BUMC Proc.* 2005;18:103–107.

58. de Kanter AY, Menke-Pluymers MM, Wouters MW, et al. 5-year follow-up of sentinel node negative breast cancer patients. *Eur J Surg Oncol.* 2006;32:282–286.

59. Dupont EL, Salud CJ, Peltz ES, et al. Clinical relevance of internal mammary node mapping as a guide to radiation therapy. *Am J Surg.* 2001;182:321–324.

60. Cox CE, Salud CJ, Harrinton MA. The role of selective sentinel lymph node dissection in breast cancer. *Surg Clin North Am.* 2000;80:1759–1777.

61. Veronesi U, Marubini E, Mariani L, et al. The dissection of internal mammary nodes does not improve the survival of breast cancer patients. Thirty-year results of a randomized trial. *Eur J Cancer.* 1999;35:1320–1325.

62. Cody HS, Van Zee KJ. Point: Sentinel lymph node biopsy is indicated for patients with DCIS. *J Natl Compr Cancer Netw.* 2003;1:199–206.

63. Rutgers E. Controversies surrounding the use of sentinel node approaches in breast cancer: sentinel node and DCIS.

Presentation at the Sentinel Lymph Node Consensus Conference. Los Angeles; December 2004.

64. van Dongen JA, Fentiman IS, Harris JR, et al. In-situ breast cancer: the EORTC consensus meeting. *Lancet.* 1989;2:25–27.

65. Schwartz GF, Finkel GC, Garcia JC, et al. Subclinical ductal carcinoma in situ of the breast. Treatment by local excision and surveillance alone. *Cancer.* 1992;70:2468–2474.

66. Wilkie C, White L, Dupont E, et al. An update of sentinel lymph node mapping in patients with ductal carcinoma in-situ. *Am J Surg.* 2005;190:563–566.

67. Cox CE, Jakub JW. Can ductal carcinoma in situ be distinguished from invasive carcinoma before definitive surgery? *Breast Dis Year Book Q.* 2003;14:128–131.

68. Yen TW, Hunt KK, Ross MI, et al. Predictors of invasive breast cancer in patients with an initial diagnosis of ductal carcinoma in situ: a guide to selective use of sentinel lymph node biopsy in management of ductal carcinoma in situ. *J Am Coll Surg.* 2005;200:516–526.

69. El-Tamer M, Chun J, Gill M, et al. Incidence and clinical significance of lymph node metastasis detected by cytokeratin immunohistochemical staining in ductal carcinoma in situ. *Ann Surg Onc.* 2005;12:254–259.

70. Dupont EL, Kuhn MA, McCann C, Salud C, Spanton JL, Cox CE. The role of sentinel lymph node biopsy in women undergoing prophylactic mastectomy. *Am J Surg.* 2000;180:274–277.

71. Lopez MJ, Porter KA. The current role of prophylactic mastectomy. *Surg Clin North Am.* 1996;76:231–242.

72. O'Hea BJ, Hill AD, El-Shirbiny AM, et al. Sentinel lymph node biopsy in breast cancer: initial experience at Memorial Sloan-Kettering Cancer Center. *J Am Coll Surg.* 1998;186:423–427.

73. Mertz L, Mathelin C, Marin C, et al. Subareolar injection of 99m-Tc sulfur colloid for sentinel nodes identification in multifocal invasive breast cancer. *Bull Cancer.* 1999;86:939–945.

74. Bass SS, Cox CE, Ku NN, Berman C, Reintgen DS. The role of sentinel lymph node biopsy in breast cancer. *J Am Coll Surg.* 1999;189:183–194.

75. Smith LF, Cross MJ, Klimberg VS. Subareolar injection is a better technique for sentinel lymph node biopsy. *Am J Surg.* 2000;180:434–437; discussion 437–438.

76. Tafra L, Lannin DR, Swanson MS, et al. Multicenter trial of sentinel node biopsy for breast cancer using both technetium sulfur colloid and isosulfan blue dye. *Ann Surg.* 2001;223:51–59.

77. Kern KA. Sentinel lymph node mapping in breast cancer using subareolar injection of blue dye. *J Am Coll Surg.* 1999;189:539–545.

78. Boolbol SK, Fey JV, Borgen PI, et al. Intradermal isotope injection: a highly accurate method of mapping in breast carcinoma. *Ann Surg Oncol.* 2001;8:20–24.

79. Darling ML, Smith DN, Lester SC, et al. Atypical ductal hyperplasia and ductal carcinoma in situ as revealed by large-core needle breast biopsy: results of surgical excision. *Am J Roentgenol.* 2000;175:1341–1346.

80. Veronesi U; European Institute of Oncology. Sentinel node biopsy in early breast cancer. Presented at the World Congress on Sentinel Node Biopsy. Yokohama, Japan; November 15–18, 2002.

81. Burak WE, Owens KE, Tighe MB, et al. Vacuum-assisted stereotactic breast biopsy: histologic underestimation of malignant lesions. *Arch Surg.* 2000;135:700–703.

82. Lee CH, Carter D, Philpotts LE, et al. Ductal carcinoma in situ diagnosed with stereotactic core needle biopsy: can invasion be predicted? *Radiology.* 2000;217:466–470.

83. Jackman RJ, Nowels KW, Rodriguez-Soto J, et al. Stereotactic, automated, large-core needle biopsy of nonpalpable breast lesions: false-negative and histologic underestimation rates after long-term follow-up. *Radiology.* 1999;210:799–805.

84. Fisher ER, Costantino J, Fisher B, et al. Pathologic findings from the National Surgical Adjuvant Breast Project (NSABP) Protocol B-17. Intraductal carcinoma (ductal carcinoma in situ). The National Surgical Adjuvant Breast and Bowel Project Collaborating Investigators. *Cancer.* 1995;75:1310–1319.

85. Jackman RJ, Burbank F, Parker SH, et al. Stereotactic breast biopsy of nonpalpable lesions: determinants of ductal carcinoma in situ underestimation rates. *Radiology.* 2001;218:497–502.

86. Morrow M, Venta L, Stinson T, et al. Prospective comparison of stereotactic core biopsy and surgical excision as diagnostic procedures for breast cancer patients. *Ann Surg.* 2001;233:537–541.

87. Cox CE, Nguyen K, Gray RJ, et al. Importance of lymphatic mapping in ductal carcinoma in situ (DCIS): why map DCIS? *Am Surg.* 2001;67:513–519.

88. Bijker N, Peterse JL, Duchateau L, et al. Risk factors for recurrence and metastasis after breast-conserving therapy for ductal carcinoma-in-situ: analysis of European Organization for Research Treatment of Cancer Trial 10853. *J Clin Oncol.* 2001;19:2263–2271.

89. Goldhirsch A, Glick JH, Gelber RD, et al. Meeting highlights: international expert consensus on the primary therapy of early breast cancer 2005. *Ann Oncol.* 2005;16:1569–1583.

90. Wilkie C, White L, Dupont E, et al. An update of sentinel lymph node mapping in patients with ductal carcinoma in-situ. *Am J Surg.* 2005;190:563–566.

91. Yen TW, Hunt KK, Ross MI, et al. Predictors of invasive breast cancer in patients with an initial diagnosis of ductal carcinoma in situ: a guide to selective use of sentinel lymph node biopsy in management of ductal carcinoma in situ. *J Am Coll Surg* 2005;200:516–526.

92. Cox CE, Cox JM, Riker AI, et al. Significance of sentinel lymph node micrometastasis on survival for patients with invasive breast cancer. Presented at the San Antonio Breast Cancer Symposium. San Antonio; December 2005.

93. Teng S, Dupont E, McCann C, et al. Do cytokeratin-positive-only sentinel lymph nodes warrant complete axillary lymph node dissection in patients with invasive breast cancer? *Am Surg.* 2000;66:574–578.

94. Jakub JW, Diaz NM, Ebert MD, et al. Completion axillary lymph node dissection minimizes the likelihood of false negatives for patients with invasive breast carcinoma and cytokeratin positive only sentinel lymph nodes. *Am J Surg.* 2002;184:302–306.

# 10
# Sentinel Lymph Node Biopsy in Cutaneous Melanoma

Jeffrey E. Gershenwald, Roger F. Uren, Giuliano Mariani, and John F. Thompson

## Background

In a landmark paper published in 1992, Morton et al. (1) described the technique of lymphatic mapping and sentinel lymph node biopsy in melanoma and set in motion a series of changes that has led to a paradigm shift in the identification of nodal metastases in this disease. Using this approach, the specific lymph node or nodes in a regional nodal basin that are the first to receive the afferent lymphatic drainage from a primary cutaneous melanoma—the sentinel nodes—are identified and removed. Since this approach limits the size of the surgical specimen submitted for evaluation (i.e., fewer nodes), the sentinel lymph node(s) can be subjected to a more thorough pathological analysis to assess the presence of disease. The likelihood of identifying patients who harbor microscopic metastases, and thus may be offered early therapeutic lymph node dissection and adjuvant therapy, is improved. Since its introduction, the technique of lymphatic mapping and sentinel lymph node biopsy has been refined (2–4) and validated (1–8). Methods to more intensely assess the histologic status of the sentinel lymph node, including serial sectioning and immunohistochemistry (9–13) have been developed and refined to enhance identification of occult nodal disease. More recently, molecular techniques such as reverse transcriptase–polymerase chain reaction (RT-PCR) analysis (14–19) are also being explored for their role in enhancing the detection of sentinel lymph node metastases.

Lymphatic mapping and sentinel node biopsy offer clinicians an accurate and minimally morbid technique for identifying patients with occult nodal disease. Although questions remain regarding which primary melanoma lesions are associated with sufficient metastatic risk to warrant these procedures, and whether all patients with microscopic metastatic disease should be offered complete lymph node dissection (currently the standard of care for patients with a positive sentinel lymph node), lymphatic mapping and sentinel lymph node biopsy have had a profound impact on the identification of nodal disease in the contemporary clinical melanoma practice.

In this chapter, lymphatic mapping and sentinel lymph node biopsy for invasive cutaneous melanoma are discussed.

## Evolution of Lymphatic Mapping and Sentinel Node Biopsy

Historically, the surgical treatment of clinically negative regional lymph nodes in patients with melanoma has been controversial. Although the majority of patients presenting with invasive cutaneous melanoma have clinically negative nodal basins, many harbor occult regional lymph node metastases. Some surgeons have chosen to dissect regional lymph nodes in patients who are at increased risk for nodal basin metastasis, even when the nodes appear clinically normal (elective lymph node dissection), whereas others perform lymphadenectomy only in cases of clinically evident nodal metastases (therapeutic lymph node dissection). Advocates of the former argue that patients with clinically negative, histologically positive lymph nodes at elective lymph node dissection have a better chance for survival (50% to 60%) than do those in whom clinically apparent metastases develop in the regional lymph nodes during follow-up (15% to 35%) (20–24).

Although all prospective randomized clinical trials have failed to show any benefit to routine elective lymph node dissection, data from the World Health Organization (WHO) Melanoma Group Trial #14 and the Intergroup Melanoma Surgical Trial suggest that some

Portions of this chapter are reprinted from Gershenwald JE, Aloia TA. Management of early stage melanoma. Curr Probs Surg 2005;42(7):468–534. Reprinted with permission from Elsevier.

subgroups might benefit from this procedure (24–27). Results from the WHO elective lymph node dissection trial indicate that patients with truncal melanoma >1.5 mm thick and microscopic nodal disease in the elective lymph node dissection treatment arm had improved overall survival compared with patients in whom palpable adenopathy developed after wide excision of the primary melanoma alone (26). Patients enrolled in the Intergroup Melanoma Surgical Trial who had 1–2 mm and non-ulcerated primary tumors also had a survival benefit with elective lymph node dissection (27).

On the other hand, a policy advocating elective lymph node dissection in all patients with melanomas >1 mm and in those with ulcerated melanomas would expose more than half of these patients who do not harbor occult metastases to a procedure with significant morbidity and potential disability. Although the survival advantage of elective lymph node dissection over observation in selected patients is an important finding, it is difficult to recommend a procedure with significant risks of morbid complications to a broad group of melanoma patients when only 20% to 30% would be found to harbor metastatic nodes in clinically negative basins.

The technique of lymphatic mapping and sentinel lymph node biopsy has subsequently been proposed as a minimally invasive procedure for identifying the approximately 20% of patients who harbor occult microscopic disease (1,28). Over the past 15 years, this technique has gained increasing acceptance and has been substantially refined (2–4) and validated (1–8,29–32). Accurate lymphatic mapping using lymphoscintigraphy is vital to the success of sentinel lymph node biopsy, as it can locate all sentinel lymph nodes, whether they lie in standard node fields or in unexpected sites. Methods to more intensely assess the histologic status of the sentinel node, including serial sectioning and immunohistochemistry (9–13), have been developed and refined to enhance identification of occult nodal disease. Recently, molecular techniques such as RT-PCR analysis (14–19,33,34) are being investigated to aid in detection of sentinel lymph node metastases.

In its current form, the technique of lymphatic mapping and sentinel node biopsy is both accurate and safe. Numerous studies have found that sentinel lymphadenectomy accurately identifies the node or nodes most likely to contain disease, if any are involved (35–39). According to these studies, the procedure has a low false-negative rate (<4%), with a predictive value of a negative sentinel node that approaches 99% in the most recent ones reported (32,37,40). Other studies have confirmed the validity of sentinel lymphadenectomy as a staging procedure (3–5,28,32,41). At the same time, the sentinel lymph node biopsy technique is associated with a low morbidity (42,43). There are substantially fewer postoperative complications after sentinel lymph node biopsy compared with elective lymph node dissection (44), and the rate of lymphedema, pain, numbness, and loss of active range of motion are lower when compared with a full anatomic dissection (43,45,46).

Some authors have suggested that dissection of the regional nodal basin—either by sentinel lymph node biopsy or complete lymphadenectomy—increases the risk of in-transit metastases (47,48). They hypothesize that dissection disturbs lymph flow, leading to deposition of metastatic cells in the intervening lymphatic vessels. A critical analysis of the data, however, provides compelling evidence that neither sentinel node biopsy nor completion node dissection in sentinel lymph node-positive patients increases the incidence of in-transit metastases. In a recent review of 2,018 patients with primary melanomas at least 1-mm thick treated over a 10-year period at the Sydney Melanoma Unit (Royal Prince Alfred Hospital, Camperdown, Australia), there was no significant difference in the rate of in-transit metastases between patients treated with wide local excision alone (4.9%) and those treated with wide local excision and sentinel lymph node biopsy (3.6%) (49). Since the 2 groups were similar in terms of median tumor depth, rate of ulceration, and Clark level, these data strongly support the concept that early nodal intervention has little impact on the natural history of in-transit metastases. In a separate study of 1,395 patients from the University of Texas M.D. Anderson Cancer Center, patients with a positive sentinel lymph node biopsy had a significantly higher rate of in-transit metastases (12%) than those with a negative one (3.5%) (50,51). Taken together, these data, recently corroborated in a study at the John Wayne Cancer Institute in Santa Monica (52), indicate that biology—and not surgical technique—establishes the risk of in-transit metastases (50).

# The Goals and Benefits of Regional Lymph Node Treatment

The goals of surgical regional nodal therapy are: 1) pathological regional lymph node staging, 2) regional disease control, and 3) potential cure of stage III disease. The role of lymphatic mapping and sentinel lymph node biopsy in each of these areas will be discussed.

## The Role of Sentinel Lymph Node Biopsy in Melanoma Regional Lymph Node Staging

Recently the prognostic significance of the pathological status of the sentinel lymph node has been convincingly demonstrated. Gershenwald et al. (5) showed that sentinel lymph node status was the most significant independent clinicopathologic prognostic factor with respect to

TABLE 10-1. Average five-year survival rates (percent ± standard error of the mean) for patients with stage III tumors (nodal metastases), stratified by number of metastatic nodes, ulceration, and tumor burden.

| Melanoma ulceration | Microscopic | | | Macroscopic | | |
|---|---|---|---|---|---|---|
| | 1 node | 2–3 nodes | >3 nodes | 1 node | 2–3 nodes | >3 nodes |
| Absent | 69 ± 3.7 (n = 252) | 63 ± 5.6 (n = 130) | 27 ± 9.3 (n = 57) | 59 ± 4.7 (n = 122) | 46 ± 5.5 (n = 93) | 27 ± 4.6 (n = 109) |
| Present | 52 ± 4.1 (n = 217) | 50 ± 5.7 (n = 111) | 37 ± 8.8 (n = 46) | 29 ± 5.0 (n = 98) | 25 ± 4.4 (n = 109) | 13 ± 3.5 (n = 104) |

Legend:
n—number of patients
*Source:* Balch et al. (53), by permission from the American Society of Clinical Oncology.

survival, even when primary tumor thickness and ulceration status were included in the analysis. In an updated analysis of 1,487 patients who underwent sentinel lymph node biopsy (median tumor thickness 1.5 mm) (Gershenwald, unpublished data), the 5-year survival rate for patients with positive sentinel lymph nodes was 73.3%, compared with 96.8% for patients with negative sentinel nodes. Several other multivariate regression analyses have confirmed that regional lymph node status is the most powerful predictor of recurrence and survival (5,27,53–56), even among patients with thick melanomas (32,54,57,58). According to a recent analysis of the American Joint Committee on Cancer (AJCC) database, 5-year survival rates for stage III disease range from 69% for patients with a non-ulcerated melanoma and only 1 microscopically positive lymph node, to 13% for patients with ulcerated primary tumors and clinically evident nodal disease with more than 3 pathologically involved nodes (Table 10-1) (53).

In the revised AJCC staging system, tumor burden in the regional nodal basins is an important predictor of survival (53,59,60). Both the number of positive nodes (53,61) and their extent of disease (macroscopic versus microscopic) are significant predictors (53). Interestingly, recent data indicate that the extent of sentinel lymph node microscopic tumor burden is an important predictor of survival in patients with stage III melanoma as determined by sentinel lymph node biopsy (61–64).

Tumor burden will likely be important as accurate microscopic staging of sentinel lymph node becomes even more widespread and patients are better stratified on the basis of microscopic tumor burden into similar-risk subgroups. As our understanding of the significance of microscopic nodal tumor burden is refined, clinical decisions regarding the need for and extent of further surgery or adjuvant therapy may also be based on the extent of microscopic nodal tumor burden.

Since the histologic status of the sentinel lymph node is the dominant independent predictor of survival in clinically node-negative patients with melanoma (5,27,32,53–58), identifying the predictors of sentinel lymph node metastasis has been the subject of intense investigation. Knowledge of the factors associated with a positive sentinel lymph node is necessary for appropriate patient counseling regarding treatment options and possible outcomes. In the analysis conducted by the AJCC's Melanoma Task Force, which validated the recently published revisions to the melanoma staging system, clinical and primary tumor factors that independently predicted worse survival included (in descending order of importance) greater tumor thickness, the presence of primary tumor ulceration, older age, axial location of the primary tumor, higher Clark level, and male gender (see Table 10-2).

Tumor thickness and ulceration are the dominant independent AJCC factors predictive of sentinel lymph node metastasis in patients with clinically negative regional lymph nodes (Table 10-3) (65–68). Therefore, it is not surprising that the incidence of sentinel lymph node metastasis increases with the AJCC T category. In 1 large series, 4% of patients with tumors less than or equal to 1-mm thick (T1) had positive sentinel lymph nodes, while as many as 44% of patients with tumors thicker than 4 mm (T4) had positive sentinel lymph nodes (30). Similarly, the presence of ulceration is a strong predictor of sentinel lymph node metastases; when patients are stratified solely according to this factor, those with ulcerated tumors have a higher incidence of sentinel lymph node metastases (35%) than do patients

TABLE 10-2. Multivariate analysis of prognostic factors for predicting sentinel lymph node metastases (n = 1351).

| Prognostic factor | OR | 95% CI | p-value |
|---|---|---|---|
| Tumor thickness | 3.42 | 2.54–4.61 | <0.0001 |
| Ulceration | 2.21 | 1.57–3.13 | <0.0001 |
| Age > 50 years | 1.81 | 1.31–2.51 | 0.0003 |
| Axial location | 1.45 | 1.05–2.02 | 0.026 |
| Clark level IV/V | 1.34 | 0.94–1.92 | 0.107 |
| Male gender | 1.09 | 0.78–1.52 | 0.629 |

Legend:
OR—odds ratio
CI—confidence intervals
*Source:* Rousseau et al. (30), Revised American Joint Committee on Cancer staging criteria accurately predict sentinel lymph node positivity in clinically node-negative melanoma patients. Ann Surg Oncol 2003;10:569–74. Reprinted with permission.

TABLE 10-3. The effect of ulceration on sentinel lymph node metastases for a given tumor thickness (n = 1375).

| Tumor Thickness (mm) | Total patients (%) | Positive sentinel lymph node | | | | | |
|---|---|---|---|---|---|---|---|
| | | All (%) | Not ulcerated | | Ulcerated | | p-value* Ulcerated vs not |
| | | | (%) | AJCC Stage[†] | (%) | AJCC Stage[†] | |
| <1.00 | 28 | 4 | 3 | IA | 16 | IB | 0.026 |
| 1.01–2.00 | 38 | 12 | 11 | IB | 22 | IIA | 0.007 |
| 2.01–4.00 | 23 | 28 | 25 | IIA | 34 | IIB | 0.115 |
| >4.00 | 11 | 44 | 33 | IIB | 53 | IIC | 0.021 |
| All patients | 100 | 17 | 12 | | 35 | | <0.0001 |

*Fisher's exact test for each tumor thickness group
[†]Stage groupings calculated using tumor thickness and ulceration data only
Source: Rousseau et al. (30), Revised American Joint Committee on Cancer staging criteria accurately predict sentinel lymph node positivity in clinically node-negative melanoma patients. Ann Surg Oncol 2003;10:569–74. Reprinted with permission.

with non-ulcerated lesions (12%) (30). When patients are stratified by both ulceration and tumor thickness, persons with ulcerated primary lesions are more likely to have positive sentinel lymph nodes than those without evidence of ulceration (30). This pattern provides a useful paradigm for preoperative patient counseling. Recently other factors, including high mitotic index, tumor drainage to multiple nodal basins, and younger patient age, have also been shown to increase sentinel lymph node positivity rates (30,67,69–72).

Primary tumor cellular mitotic rate is a compelling candidate for a tumor-related factor with prognostic significance. It was first identified by Salman and colleagues, who reported that for patients with melanoma >0.75-mm thick, those with a mitotic index >5 had a worse prognosis (73). Subsequently, other groups have found similar relationships between mitotic rate/index and survival (74). In the largest review to date, a Sydney Melanoma Unit analysis of 3,661 patients found that the prognostic value of mitotic rate surpassed that of ulceration, and was second only to Breslow thickness (70,71). Most recently, Sondak and colleagues have reported that, in a cohort of patients undergoing sentinel lymphadenectomy, along with age and Breslow thickness, the number of mitoses per square millimeter in the primary tumor was strongly predictive of regional nodal metastases (69). Given this data, some melanoma centers have used mitotic rate as a relative indication of sentinel lymph node biopsy in patients with thin invasive cutaneous melanoma (69,75).

Vertical growth phase (VGP) is a pathological description of melanoma cell alignment characterized by a small expansile nodule of vertically aligned infiltrating melanoma cells, which form dominant nests within the papillary dermis that are larger than any nest within the epidermis or surrounding dermis. VGP is a feature of nodular melanoma, but may also occur in other growth types. Many pathologists feel that the presence of a VGP is synonymous with the ability of a melanoma to form metastases (76); patients whose tumors demonstrate VGP have a higher rate of regional nodal metastases

(77). Thus, frequently the presence of VGP is used to justify a more aggressive approach to staging. As with regression, it is a relative indication for sentinel lymphadenectomy in patients with thin melanoma.

## The Role of Sentinel Lymph Node Biopsy in Regional Disease Control

For patients with both microscopic and macroscopic regional nodal metastasis, complete lymphadenectomy can provide effective control of regional disease and local palliation. Until recently, the impact of sentinel lymph node biopsy on regional control was unclear. In 2000, Gershenwald et al. (63) showed that regional nodal control is not compromised by previous sentinel lymph node biopsy in patients with melanoma. Recurrence in the previously dissected nodal basin was observed in only 10% of patients who had undergone successful lymphatic mapping and sentinel node biopsy, and none had it in the mapped regional nodal basin as the sole site of recurrence. Overall, these low rates of in-basin recurrence compare favorably with those observed after formal lymphadenectomy in patients who have clinically evident nodal disease (9% to 36%) and are similar to the in-basin failure rates of patients who have undergone elective lymph node dissection with proven microscopic disease (63,78–82).

## Prediction of Nonsentinel Lymph Node Involvement

Several studies have demonstrated that sentinel lymph nodes will be the first regional basin nodes to contain metastasis (1,3–5,35,83,84), and thus the nodes' pathological status reflects that of the regional basin. If the sentinel node lacks metastasis, other regional lymph nodes are unlikely to contain disease, and a completion lymphadenectomy is not necessary. If, however, the sentinel lymph node contains metastatic tumor cells, the effectiveness of sentinel node biopsy in regional basin control is dependent on the addition of a completion nodal dissection.

With the widespread use of lymphatic mapping and sentinel node biopsy, in most clinically node-negative patients who actually have nodal metastases, the metastases are microscopic. Current standard clinical practice for such patients includes completion lymph node dissection, as this strategy improves regional disease control and may provide a survival benefit (26). However, additional positive nonsentinel lymph nodes are identified in only 8% to 33% of completion lymphadenectomy specimens (4,5,35,68,83–89), suggesting that a subset of patients with microscopic nodal disease may not benefit from completion dissection after a positive sentinel lymph node biopsy. Understanding which factors predict additional nonsentinel lymph node disease in patients with positive sentinel lymph nodes may allow better selection of those who may benefit from completion dissection, and spare patients at "minimal" risk from the morbidity of a completion lymph node dissection.

In one study, the presence of a thick and/or ulcerated primary tumor in patients with a positive sentinel node predicted involvement of nonsentinel nodes at completion lymph node dissection (88). Other reports, however, have failed to identify clinicopathologic variables that accurately predict the subset with additional disease in the nodal basin (90,91). In a recent study of 232 patients who had completion lymph node dissection after the discovery of positive sentinel nodes (61), 18.5% had additional nonsentinel lymph node disease in the lymphadenectomy specimen. The extent of microscopic tumor burden in the sentinel node(s) was examined to see whether it could be a predictor of nonsentinel lymph node involvement. Interestingly, all markers of tumor burden were significant predictors of the presence of nonsentinel lymph node disease, which suggests that selection of patients for completion lymph node dissection may be based, at least in part, on this factor. Other recent studies have demonstrated that micromorphometric features of the sentinel lymph node metastasis predict nonsentinel node involvement (68,83,84,88,89,92–94). Further study in this area using larger multi-institutional data sets is warranted.

The completion lymph node dissection specimen is not routinely histologically assessed in the same fashion as the sentinel lymph node (95). Therefore, additional disease in the completion nodal specimen may go undetected with standard histologic techniques, and could represent a potential source of subsequent recurrence if it is not removed. Because recurrences are difficult to treat surgically and may contribute to significant morbidity, completion dissections performed for microscopic disease provide the potential for improved regional control and thus lend support to the sentinel lymph node

approach. Although less than one-fifth of patients with a positive sentinel lymph node will have additional melanoma detected by routine histology in the nonsentinel nodes, a completion lymphadenectomy remains the standard of care for patients with a positive sentinel lymph node.

## The Role of Sentinel Lymph Node Biopsy in Potential Cure

At present, the contribution of sentinel lymph node biopsy to survival is unclear. There is some early evidence that patients staged by sentinel lymphadenectomy have a longer overall survival than those staged by either clinical examination or elective lymph node dissection (96), but determination of the precise benefit of sentinel lymphadenectomy, with or without completion node dissection, awaits publication of the results from ongoing clinical trials including the Multicenter Selective Lymphadenectomy Trial I (MSLT).

The MSLT, initiated by the John Wayne Cancer Institute, opened to accrual in 1994. Eligibility criteria included primary cutaneous melanoma of Breslow thickness $\geq 1$ mm, or Clark level IV or V with any Breslow thickness. Patients were randomly assigned to lymphatic mapping/sentinel lymph node biopsy (LM/SNB) or nodal observation, with a $60:40$ distribution of wide excision/(LM/SNB) to wide excision alone. Preoperative lymphoscintigraphy was performed. The sentinel lymph node was serially sectioned and examined histologically at 4 levels and immunohistochemically (S-100 protein and HMB-45 monoclonal antibody) at 2 levels. Patients with a positive sentinel lymph node subsequently underwent completion lymphadenectomy.

This trial was designed to assess whether a selective approach to regional lymphadenectomy, limiting complete nodal dissection to those with occult disease in the sentinel lymph node, confers a survival benefit for patients over those in whom wide excision of the primary with observation of the regional nodal basin was performed.

This trial reached target accrual in 2002: 797 patients were assigned to wide excision only, and 1,204 patients to wide excision and lymphatic mapping/sentinel lymph node biopsy (LM/SNB). The third of 5 planned analyses was completed in October 2004 at a median follow-up of 54 months; preliminary data was recently presented (97). Five-year disease-free survival was 78% with LM/SNB, versus 73% with wide excision only (p = 0.01; HR 0.74). Sentinel node tumor status was the most important factor for 5-year survival of LM/SNB patients: survival was 88% for 944 node negative patients, versus 71% for 215 node positive (p < 0.0001, log rank). Nodal metastases were identified in 215 (19%) LM/SNB patients; nodal recurrence developed in 142 (18%) wide excision only patients. Five-year survival was significantly higher after immediate complete nodal dissection for node positive patients, than delayed complete nodal dissection for clinical nodal recurrence (71% versus 55%; p = 0.0033, log rank; p = 0.0077, Cox multivariate). From this data, the authors concluded that sentinel node status is the most important prognostic factor in early-stage melanoma, and that LM/SNB allows early and accurate detection of occult nodal metastases. In addition, disease-free and melanoma-specific survival rates are significantly higher after immediate complete nodal dissection for occult nodal metastases than after delayed complete nodal dissection for clinical nodal recurrence.

## Evolution of Pathological Analysis

Historically, histologic assessment of lymph nodes has involved conventional hematoxylin and eosin (H&E) examination. Because of the tremendous interest in the sentinel lymph node biopsy technique and, in particular, because this technique produces a specimen that contains fewer lymph nodes than that from a formal lymph node dissection, there has been an evolution in the approach to assessing sentinel lymph node pathological status.

Pathologists have traditionally examined the multitude of lymph nodes from lymphadenectomy specimens by submitting the node and examining 1 H&E-stained section from each paraffin block. This approach is the standard of care for pathological evaluation of formal lymphadenectomy specimens, regardless of the type of neoplasia. With the advent of the sentinel lymph node biopsy technique, however, an average of approximately 2 lymph nodes per nodal basin are submitted for pathological review, rather than the 10 to 35 nodes per basin typically found in a formal lymph node dissection specimen. With fewer lymph nodes to analyze, the pathologist can focus on those nodes at highest risk—the sentinel lymph nodes—and this makes a much more detailed examination of the tissue possible.

This technique facilitates the application of a more intense investigative process that uses serial sectioning, immunostaining, or both, and it has become the standard approach in most melanoma centers (98–100). More recently, molecular techniques such as reverse transcriptase-polymerase chain reaction (RT-PCR) have been used in assessing sentinel lymph nodes to detect submicroscopic disease that might not be detectable by conventional histologic methods. The clinical significance of H&E negative, immunohistochemistry negative, and RT-PCR positive nodes is under investigation. These data were recently formally published for the subset of patients with intermediate thickness melanoma.

(Reference Morton DL, Thompson JF, Cochran AJ et al. Sentinel-node biopsy or nodal observation in melanoma. N Eng J Med 2006 Sept;355(13):1307–17. Erratum in: N Eng J Med. 2006 Nov;355(18):1994.)

## Intraoperative Assessment of the Sentinel Lymph Node

During the early development of the sentinel lymph node technique, immediate frozen-section analysis was often used for histologic analysis (1). Intraoperative pathological assessment of the sentinel lymph node could identify individuals with microscopic regional nodal (i.e., stage III) disease, who would then undergo concomitant lymphadenectomy under a single anesthetic. Unfortunately, multiple studies have shown that intraoperative pathological assessment of the sentinel lymph nodes in patients with melanoma has a low sensitivity, among other reasons due to the inferior quality of frozen sections when compared with permanent sections (101–105). When a frozen-section specimen prepared from a lymph node is less than a complete section, most often the subcapsular sinus is omitted, which is the portion of the node most likely to contain occult tumor cells (13,106). This may explain why frozen-section analysis may fail to identify metastases greater than 2 mm in diameter in up to 30% of patients (61,62,107,108). There is also concern that frozen-section analysis may result in the loss of informative tissue, because diagnostic tissue may be lost as the block is cut. The sensitivity of imprint cytology compared with that of paraffin-embedded permanent sections also appears to be low (109), but this approach may represent a useful initial diagnostic strategy for intraoperative assessment of patients with a grossly suspicious sentinel lymph node when concomitant completion lymphadenectomy is considered.

In summary, routine intraoperative sentinel lymph node frozen-section or imprint cytologic assessment has a low sensitivity. Frozen-section analysis is also potentially harmful, because it can destroy diagnostic tissue, and should not be performed routinely on sentinel lymph nodes in patients with melanoma. However, if intraoperative assessment of the sentinel lymph node suggests gross involvement, imprint cytology or a limited frozen-section analysis may be appropriate to confirm the diagnosis, so that concomitant completion lymphadenectomy can be performed, provided that this approach has been discussed before surgery with the patient.

## Beyond Conventional Histologic Analysis: Step Sectioning and Immunohistochemistry

One reason for recurrence in a basin that previously yielded a negative sentinel node is pathological miss, where the true sentinel lymph node is identified but the pathological examination misses the micrometastasis. Data from several studies suggest that the failure to use specialized pathological techniques represents an important explanation of understaging the nodal basin, and of subsequent nodal basin recurrence, after otherwise successful lymphatic mapping and sentinel node biopsy (9,12,13,15,35). An estimated 5% to 15% of metastatic nodes may be missed with H&E alone (5,13,37,98,99,110,111), and as a result, 2 techniques have been instituted to facilitate a more intense histologic evaluation of sentinel lymph nodes: step-sectioning and immunohistochemical staining of the node. When used together, they can double the yield of positive dissections (112,113). The limiting step—determining the number of sections to be cut, stained, and examined—remains expensive, time-consuming, and controversial (114), so a balance between maximum detection rate and technical feasibility is required. Despite the added expense, most groups now consider some combination of immunohistochemistry and serial sectioning with H&E to be an essential diagnostic tool (99,100,115–117). A detailed discussion of their important input is beyond the scope of this chapter, so the reader is referred to recent reviews (29) and to Chapter 18 of this book.

## Molecular Detection of Submicroscopic Disease

Identification of isolated melanoma cells or oligocellular deposits remains difficult with histopathologic and immunohistochemical examination of the sentinel lymph node, and depends on the section of the sentinel lymph node being examined. A possible alternative to this tedious examination is a molecular-based diagnostic approach, such as RT-PCR, which here is used to detect tumor-specific messenger RNA (mRNA) in sentinel node tissue (14,18,118,119). The RT-PCR-based techniques provide enhanced sensitivity to lymphatic mapping and sentinel lymph node biopsy in the detection of occult regional metastases. Use of RT-PCR is based on the hypothesis that molecular evidence of metastatic disease can be obtained by identifying mRNA for melanoma-specific markers; in this way, a sentinel lymph node can be subjected to molecular staging for identification of submicroscopic metastatic disease (14,16,18,118,120–122). Several melanocyte-associated genes have been identified as potential targets for molecular-based assessment of sentinel lymph nodes, and a number of RT-PCR primer sets have been developed to amplify and detect melanoma tumor cell mRNA in regional lymph nodes and peripheral blood. These include primers that amplify tyrosinase, gp100, MART-1, and MAGE-3, among others.

Preliminary data suggest that the prognosis of patients with a sentinel lymph node that is RT-PCR positive, but negative by histology or immunohistochemistry, is worse than that of patients who have negative results by both techniques. Bostick et al. (123) reported that patients with sentinel lymph nodes that were histopathologically melanoma-free but positive by multiple-mRNA marker RT-PCR were at an increased risk of recurrence, compared with those with sentinel lymph nodes that were positive for fewer mRNA markers. Li et al. (124) also reported an increase in recurrence and death rates in a cohort of patients with a sentinel lymph node that was positive for disease by RT-PCR detection alone. The recurrence rate for histologically negative and RT-PCR-negative patients was only 1.6%, compared with 10.1% for histologically negative but RT-PCR-positive patients. The prognostic significance of a negative sentinel lymph node by RT-PCR has been recently corroborated. Ribuffo et al. (19) reported that no patient with RT-PCR-negative nodes developed a recurrence, and that the prognostic significance of RT-PCR-negative nodal status was independent of Breslow tumor thickness. Furthermore, in an independent study by the Pisa group, RT-PCR positivity of the sentinel lymph node in patients with negative conventional pathology (H&E staining plus immunohistochemistry) identified persons with intermediate prognosis in terms of disease-free survival from among patients for whom conventional pathology and molecular analysis were either both negative (best prognosis) or both positive (worse prognosis). Concerning overall survival, prognosis of patients with RT-PCR sentinel lymph node positivity alone was equally poor as that for patients with sentinel lymph node positivity to both analyses (34). A comprehensive overview of the results obtained by various groups with molecular analysis of sentinel lymph nodes in patients with melanoma is reported in Table 10-4, while a comprehensive meta-analysis of studies including over 4000 patients is described in a recent article (119).

Although these preliminary findings, which are intriguing by demonstrating that RT-PCR-based sentinel lymph node diagnostics may be able to identify subsets of patients at higher risk of recurrence within the histologically negative sentinel lymph node group, the true clinical significance is still unknown. Critics of this data cite that most studies addressing this question have short follow-up times and do not compare RT-PCR with current standard histologic techniques. Most recently, Kammala and colleagues have shown that for 112 patients (Histo+/PCR+: 15 patients; Histo-/PCR+: 58 patients; Histo-/PCR-: 39 patients) with a longer median follow-up of 67 months, there was no difference in recurrence rates between the Histo-/PCR+ (24%) and the Histo-/PCR- (15%) groups (P = 0.25) (33). These data suggest that judgment on the value of RT-PCR staging should be reserved until larger studies with median follow-up intervals of at least 5 years are reported (e.g., the Sunbelt Melanoma Trial in the United States and Canada).

TABLE 10-4. Review of literature on the correlation of sentinel lymph node status evaluated by conventional histopathology and by molecular markers with recurrences in patients with melanoma.

| Author (year) | Patients (n) | Molecular marker(s) | Median follow-up (months) | Recurrences | | |
|---|---|---|---|---|---|---|
| | | | | PATH+/PCR+ (%) | PATH–/PCR+ (%) | PATH–/PCR– (%) |
| Shivers (1998) | 114 | Tyr | 28 | 14/23 (61) | 6/47 (13) | 1/44 (2) |
| Bostick (1999) | 72 | MM§ | 12 | 5/16 (31) | 3/20 (15) | 0/35 (0) |
| Li (2000) | 233 | Tyr | 20 | 18/49 (36.7) | 12/115 (10) | 1/64 (1.6) |
| Blaheta (2000) | 116 | Tyr | 19 | 10/15 (67) | 9/36 (25) | 4/65 (6) |
| Rimoldi (2003) | 57 | MM§§ | 36 | 6/16 (38) | 3/19 (16) | 2/22 (9) |
| Goydos (2003) | 175 | Tyr | 34 | 17/34 (50) | 14/68 (21) | 0/73 (0) |
| Kammula (2004) | 112 | Tyr | 42* | 8/15 (53) | 8/18 (14) | 0/39 (0) |
| | | | 67** | 10/15 (67) | 14/68 (24) | 6/39 (15) |
| Romanini (2005) | 124 | Tyr MART-1 | 30 | 14/23 (60) | 5/16 (31) | 8/85 (9.4) |

Legend:
PATH––conventional histopathology negative
PATH+—conventional histopathology positive
PCR––reverse transcriptase polymerase chain reaction negative
PCR+—reverse transcriptase polymerase chain reaction positive
Tyr—tyrosinase
MM§—multiple markers (Tyr, MART-1, MAGE-3)
MM§§—multiple markers (Tyr, Melan-A/MART-1)
* Early follow-up
** Late follow-up
Source: Romanini A, Manca G, Pellegrino D, et al. Molecular staging of the sentinel lymph node in melanoma patients: correlation with clinical outcome. Ann Oncol 2005;16(11):1832–1840. Reprinted by permission of Oxford University Press.

## Practice Guidelines for Lymphatic Mapping and Sentinel Lymph Node Biopsy

Candidates for this approach include patients with clinically node negative stage I and II melanoma who are at risk for occult nodal disease. In general, patients with a diagnosis of primary cutaneous melanoma are offered this procedure if their tumor is at least 1.0-mm thick or, if less than 1.0-mm, is at least Clark level IV or ulcerated, and there is no evidence of metastatic melanoma in regional lymph nodes and distant sites as determined by physical examination and staging evaluation (chest x-ray and lactate dehydrogenase levels) (5,31,125). Strong consideration for sentinel lymphadenectomy is selectively given to patients whose thin melanomas demonstrate regression or vertical growth phase (77), or which have a positive deep biopsy margin (126). Recently, several groups have offered sentinel lymph node biopsy to patients whose thin primary tumors have a high mitotic rate, as this has been reported to be a strong predictor of sentinel lymph node positivity (69,70,75,89). Patients with thick melanoma (>4 mm) are also offered this approach (54,57,58). Regardless of primary melanoma thickness, all patients undergo wide local excision of the primary melanoma, with margins appropriate for tumor thickness, at the same time as the sentinel lymph node biopsy.

## Technical Considerations of Sentinel Lymphadenectomy

Success of the sentinel lymphadenectomy technique involves the integration of several disciplines—nuclear medicine, surgery, and pathology. The modern sentinel node technique consists of 3 main components: 1) preoperative cutaneous lymphoscintigraphy to identify and mark the location of sentinel lymph nodes, whether in standard node fields or in unexpected sites; 2) intraoperative localization and excisional biopsy of sentinel nodes in all regional nodal basins at risk as shown by lymphoscintigraphy, vital blue dye, and $^{99m}$Tc-labeled colloid accompanied by intraoperative use of the handheld gamma probe; and 3) careful pathological evaluation of the sentinel nodes. Using the combined approach, successful identification of the sentinel lymph node can be expected in more than 98% of cases.

### Preoperative Lymphoscintigraphy

The goals of preoperative cutaneous lymphoscintigraphy are (8,125,127–137):

• To provide an accurate map of the lymphatic drainage from the primary melanoma site, thus revealing the precise surface location of all true sentinel lymph nodes, the number at each location, and their depth from the skin.

- To identify the regional nodal basins at risk in patients whose primary melanoma arises in a region of ambiguous nodal drainage (trunk, and head and neck locations).
- To identify patients with distal upper or lower extremity melanomas who may have sentinel nodes located in the epitrochlear or popliteal nodal basins, respectively.
- To identify in-transit or ectopically located sentinel nodes (e.g., scapular lymph nodes) located outside of the normal anatomic landmarks that define the named regional nodal basins, including the cervical, axillary, inguinal, epitrochlear, and popliteal basins.

We recommend that all patients with melanomas who are considered for sentinel lymph node biopsy receive preoperative lymphoscintigraphy. This is necessary in the trunk and the head-and-neck region, since multiple node fields may drain in these areas and contralateral flow is not uncommon. Unexpected drainage to the triangular intermuscular space or over the shoulder to neck nodes will also be detected in back melanomas, when present. In the distal upper and lower limb, lymphoscintigraphy is needed to identify epitrochlear and popliteal drainage, respectively; in the upper arm, it can identify sentinel lymph nodes above the axilla in the neck, especially in level V. Even in the thigh, lymphoscintigraphy is useful to identify drainage to deep iliac or obturator nodes present in some patients. It can also identify interval nodes in any part of the body.

Lymphoscintigraphy begins with a 2- or 4-point intradermal injection of $^{99m}$Tc-labeled colloid using a 25- or 27-gauge needle. The injections should be given within a couple of millimeters of the excision biopsy scar around the center of the scar that represents the site of the original melanoma. Injections should not be given at the ends of a long excision biopsy scar, as this may cause nodes to be radiolabeled that did not originally drain the melanoma site. Between 10 and 40 MBq is given per injection, depending on whether surgery is planned for the same day or the day after the lymphoscintigraphy. The choice of radiocolloid is beyond the scope of this discussion, but usually it is determined by what tracer is available locally, and includes $^{99m}$Tc-sulfur colloid in the United States, $^{99m}$Tc-nanocolloid of albumin in Europe, $^{99m}$Tc-stannous colloid in Japan, and $^{99m}$Tc-antimony sulfide colloid in Australia and Canada. Following radiotracer injection, dynamic images at 1 frame per minute are usually acquired over the injection site for 10 minutes, with further early imaging performed for 5 to 10 minutes over the draining node fields. Anterior (or posterior) and lateral views are obtained as necessary. Delayed imaging is performed 1 to 2 hours later, again in the anterior/posterior and lateral projections to define the precise location of all sentinel lymph nodes. Examples of variable

patterns of lymphatic drainage visualized by lymphoscintigraphy are shown in Figures 10-1 to 10-4.

The surface location of each sentinel lymph node should be marked on the skin with an indelible marker, and a small point tattoo of carbon black is useful for later follow-up, especially if the sentinel nodes are not later removed. Skin marking should always be performed with the patient in the same position to be used at surgery. The depth of the sentinel lymph node from the skin should also be recorded, to aid in its speedy surgical removal. Although images obtained in patients whose primary melanoma is remote from the regional nodal basin are often easily interpreted, it may be difficult to discern discrete lymphatic drainage patterns in patients whose melanomas are close to potential regional nodal basins. This is especially a problem in the head and neck and around the shoulder; in these instances, multiple views are helpful in maximizing the ability to document drainage to the regional nodal basin.

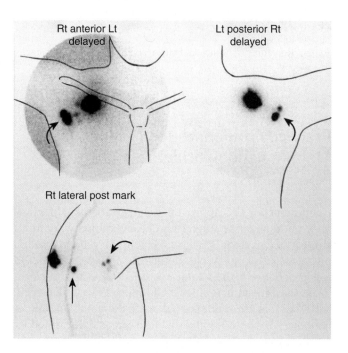

FIGURE 10-1. Lymphoscintigraphy delayed scans performed in the anterior, posterior, and right lateral projections after intradermal injection of $^{99m}$Tc-antimony sulfide colloid in a patient with a melanoma excision biopsy site on the upper back, to the right of midline. In the anterior and posterior views (top panels), activity is seen in what appears to be 2 sentinel lymph nodes in the right axilla (curved arrow). The right lateral view, however, clearly shows a bright sentinel lymph node (vertical arrow) in the right triangular intermuscular space, just to the deep fascia of the back posterior to the axilla (bottom panel). There are also 2 sentinel lymph nodes in the right axilla (curved arrow). If lateral views are not acquired in back melanomas, these sentinel nodes will be missed, as they are obscured by activity in the axillary nodes on the anterior and posterior views.

FIGURE 10-2. Dots mark the skin sites of melanomas that included drainage to a sentinel lymph node in the triangular intermuscular space.

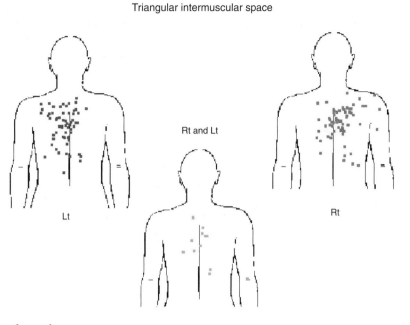

Sometimes, the radiocolloid does not migrate from the injection site. This is more common in older patients, and when the melanoma is on the head, neck, or shoulder area. It also may occur when lymphoscintigraphy is performed soon after a diagnostic biopsy. Gentle massage over the injection site for 5 minutes usually ensures migration of the tracer to a sentinel node. If the biopsy was recent, a further attempt to find sentinel lymph nodes with follow-up lymphoscintigraphy may be performed after waiting an additional week, to allow for healing and resolution of any inflammation that may have developed. Rarely, failure of the radiocolloid to migrate may be due to subcutaneous rather than intradermal injection, especially in patients with thin skin. Alternatively, if a 27-gauge needle is used, an epidermal

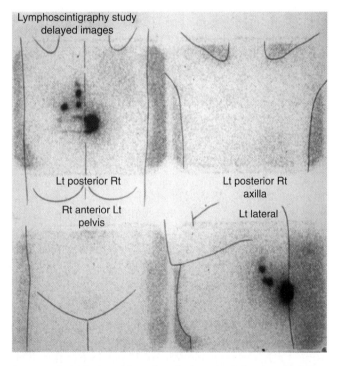

FIGURE 10-4. Delayed lymphoscintigraphy following the intradermal injection of $^{99m}$Tc-antimony sulphate colloid in a patient with a melanoma site on the posterior loin, just to the right of midline. The tracer has passed across the midline and through the posterior body wall to sentinel nodes in the left retroperitoneal and paravertebral region, with no drainage at all to either axilla or groin. A metastasis here would be locoregional disease, not systemic metastasis. (From Uren RF, Hoefnagel CA. Lymphoscintigraphy. In: Thompson JF, Morton DL, Kroon BBR (eds), Textbook of Melanoma. London: Martin Dunitz; 2004, pp 339–364. Reproduced by permission of Taylor & Francis Books UK.)

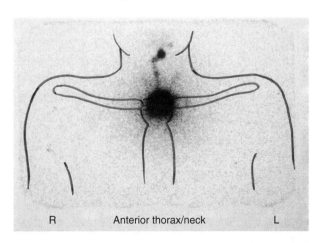

FIGURE 10-3. Dynamic phase lymphoscintigraphy following the intradermal injection of $^{99m}$Tc-antimony sulfide colloid in a patient with melanoma above the sternal notch. The summed 10-minute dynamic phase shows a single lymphatic collector vessel passing up the neck to a sentinel lymph node.

injection may result, and there are no lymphatics in the epidermis. Lymphoscintigraphy may be re-attempted in these patients as well. Table 10-5 shows the variable patterns of drainage from different sites of the primary melanoma to lymphatic basins, as observed in over 3000 consecutive patients.

## Intraoperative Considerations

Beginning as early as 1994, centers began performing lymphatic mapping and sentinel lymphadenectomy using both a vital blue dye and $^{99m}$Tc-labeled colloid detected using a handheld gamma probe. If surgery cannot be performed on the same day as the lymphoscintigraphy or the day after, then radiocolloid can be injected once more, adjacent to the excision biopsy site, on the day of the surgery. This should be done about 1 hour before surgery to maximize the chance that the tracer has migrated to the sentinel lymph node and to minimize movement of the tracer to second-tier nodes that, although mildly radiolabeled, should not be removed as part of the biopsy procedure.

The handheld gamma probe is used to transcutaneously confirm the location of the sentinel lymph node as marked at lymphoscintigraphy—whether in standard regional nodal basins, or ectopic and in-transit sites between the primary melanoma and the regional nodal basin—immediately prior to the planned surgical procedure, either in the surgical holding area and/or upon arrival in the operating room.

Most patients prefer general anesthesia for this procedure, since significant mobilization of tissue is often required to achieve primary closure of the melanoma site following wide excision, and extensive dissection is occasionally needed at the sentinel lymph node biopsy sites, especially in obese patients. In some cases, however, monitored sedation with adequate local anesthesia may be used. Once adequate anesthesia is obtained, approximately 2 to 3 mL of vital blue dye are administered intradermally, similar to the way the radiocolloid is administered. The injection sites are massaged for approximately 2 to 3 minutes to encourage uptake by the cutaneous lymphatics. This injection is usually performed using 1 mL syringes and 25- or 27-gauge needles. The surgeon should ensure that a true intradermal injection is performed, since subcutaneous injection (sometimes noticeable by minimal resistance to injection and the lack of blue-colored blush and wheal of the adjacent skin), may result in inadequate uptake of the dye by the cutaneous afferent lymphatic channels and lack of uptake by the sentinel nodes.

Following injection of the vital blue dye, the patient is properly positioned for surgery and appropriately prepped and draped. Whenever possible, intraoperative lymphatic mapping and sentinel lymphadenectomy is

TABLE 10-5. Locations of sentinel nodes from primary melanomas in various body sites.

| Melanoma Site | Area | n* | %* |
|---|---|---|---|
| Posterior trunk (n = 1057) | | | |
| | Axilla | 913 | 86 |
| | Groin | 105 | 10 |
| | Triangular intermuscular space | 134 | 13 |
| | Cervical—Level II | 1 | |
| | —Level III | 4 | 0.5 |
| | —Level IV | 15 | 1.5 |
| | —Level V | 108 | 11 |
| | Supraclavicular | 139 | 13 |
| | Postauricular | 1 | |
| | Occipital | 4 | 0.5 |
| | Paravertebral or paraaortic | 22 | 2 |
| | Retroperitoneal | 9 | 1 |
| | Interval node | 130 | 12 |
| Anterior trunk (n = 211) | | | |
| | Axilla | 184 | 87 |
| | Groin | 31 | 15 |
| | Cervical—Level II | 1 | 0.5 |
| | —Level III | 3 | 1.5 |
| | —Level IV | 3 | 1.5 |
| | —Level V | 6 | 3 |
| | Supraclavicular | 27 | 14 |
| | Costal margin | 6 | 3 |
| | Internal mammary | 2 | 1 |
| | Interval node | 18 | 8.5 |
| Head and Neck (n = 508) | | | |
| | Parotid | 178 | 35 |
| | Cervical—Level I | 103 | 20 |
| | —Level II | 321 | 63 |
| | —Level III | 79 | 16 |
| | —Level IV | 56 | 11 |
| | —Level V | 113 | 22 |
| | Supraclavicular | 53 | 10 |
| | Occipital | 62 | 12 |
| | Postauricular | 88 | 17 |
| | Axillary | 9 | 2 |
| | Interval node | 25 | 5 |
| Upper limb (n = 571) | | | |
| | Axilla | 563 | 99 |
| | Epitrochlear | 36 | 6 |
| | Cervical—Level V | 3 | 0.5 |
| | Supraclavicular | 36 | 6 |
| | Triangular intermuscular space | 3 | 0.5 |
| | Interpectoral | 2 | 0.3 |
| | Infraclavicular | 1 | 0.2 |
| | Interval node | 23 | 4 |
| Lower limb (n = 712) | | | |
| | Groin | 712 | 100 |
| | Popliteal | 38 | 5 |
| | Interval | 4 | 0.5 |

Legend:
*n—number, and % = percentage of patients with drainage to the site indicated.
*Source:* Uren RF, Howman-Giles R, Thompson JF. Patterns of lymphatic drainage from the skin in patients with melanoma. J Nucl Med. 2003;44(4):570–582. Adapted by permission of the Society of Nuclear Medicine.

performed prior to the wide local excision. With the patient prepped and draped, areas of increased focal radiotracer uptake in the first basin are confirmed with the handheld gamma probe. A small, usually approximately 3-cm, incision is then made overlying the area of increased focal radiotracer uptake activity. Before making this incision, usually the nodal basin is marked as if a formal lymph node dissection were being performed; this ensures that the incision can be incorporated into a completion lymph node dissection incision, including the biopsy site and cavity, if the sentinel node contains pathological evidence of metastatic melanoma. Once the areolar tissue of the nodal basin is entered, often immediate rescanning of the biopsy site with the gamma probe can direct further dissection. The sentinel node can then be identified by blunt dissection toward the area of increasing radiotracer uptake. Subtle manipulation of the angle of the gamma probe helps to precisely locate the direction of the required dissection; this is particularly helpful in patients who are obese, in whom the sentinel node is likely several centimeters below the surface of the skin. Repeating this maneuvering ensures that the dissection proceeds in as directed a fashion as possible. In addition, blue-stained lymphatic channels can be traced to a draining lymph node, while in many cases, gamma probe-directed dissection results in the immediate identification of a blue-stained sentinel node, since co-localization of blue dye and radiotracer uptake is common (3,72). Once identified, this node is secured with a suture and gently elevated. Surrounding fatty tissue is dissected with electrocautery, and vascular and lymphatic structures are identified and ligated with ties to minimize bleeding and seroma formation. In this fashion, the lymph node is harvested, and ex-vivo radiotracer counts are obtained with the handheld gamma probe and documented in the patient's chart, the operative record, and the pathology sheet.

Although some surgeons may question the need for the blue dye, we strongly believe that it provides an invaluable adjunct and remains a critical component of the lymphatic mapping technique. The dye provides a visual aid that not only confirms that the node is a sentinel lymph node, but also facilitates localization of sentinel nodes when transcutaneous localization of the colloid is unsuccessful; it also helps to minimize dissection when gamma probe localization is achieved.

The sentinel node is visually inspected for evidence of gross metastatic disease. If it has none—the most common scenario—no frozen section analysis of the lymph node is performed. For a lymph node that appears grossly suspicious (e.g., obvious melanin pigment and/or tumor), a frozen section examination may be performed to confirm the diagnosis, if concomitant completion lymph node dissection is being considered and has been discussed with the patient in advance. At M.D. Anderson, frozen section analysis is reserved for highly suspicious nodes only, since many sentinel lymph nodes that appear "abnormal" often simply represent reaction to the initial biopsy procedure. If frozen section analysis were routinely performed, subsequent additional examination of these nodes might be hampered and may not provide optimal tissue for careful permanent section analysis using serial section and immunohistochemistry (108).

After removal of the sentinel lymph node, the basin is rescanned using the gamma probe. If an area of increased focal radiotracer activity is again identified, the above-outlined procedure is repeated. Any additional sentinel lymph nodes are harvested, and their uptake of blue dye and ex-vivo counts documented. They are numbered sequentially within a nodal basin and submitted for permanent section pathological analysis. Background radiotracer activity in the nodal basin signifies that all sentinel lymph nodes have been removed. Copious irrigation and verification of hemostasis of the sentinel node biopsy cavity is subsequently performed. In general, these incisions are closed in 2 layers using absorbable interrupted dermal sutures followed by a running subcuticular stitch. Drains are rarely required for sentinel node biopsy sites, since in most cases use of the handheld gamma probe permits limited dissection of the nodal basin (and therefore little disruption of the lymphatics).

Careful attention to patient positioning in the operating room is necessary to ensure that all components of lymphatic mapping and sentinel lymph node biopsy are achievable. Positioning must take into account not only the location of the primary melanoma and the regional nodal basins as well as in-transit or ectopic sites at risk for metastatic disease, but also potential donor sites for skin grafting. Careful study of the preoperative lymphoscintigram provides most of the information necessary to develop an operative positioning strategy, especially when multiple nodal basins or in-transit or ectopic sites are anticipated or identified.

## General Principles of Operating Room Positioning Strategies

Several concepts should be considered when developing the operating room positioning strategy for lymphatic mapping and sentinel lymphadenectomy (125). The positioning strategy should:

1. Minimize the number of patient position changes required to achieve and complete the planned surgery without compromising the surgeon's ability to approach regional nodal basins.
2. Provide easy access to the regional nodal basin(s).
3. Enable the surgeon to approach the regional lymph node basin(s) with predominant drainage first.

4. Provide adequate exposure of in-transit and ectopic lymphatic sites to permit scanning with a handheld gamma probe.

5. Permit rescanning of the regional nodal basin(s) following wide local excision of the primary melanoma.

6. Minimize shine-through from the primary site, which may obscure identification of sentinel lymph nodes in adjacent regional nodal basins.

7. Take into consideration the potential need to approach 1 or more regional nodal basins after the wide local excision.

8. Provide adequate exposure of the wide local excision site (primary melanoma) and maximize the potential for proper closure of this site.

9. Provide adequate access to a potential split-thickness or full-thickness skin graft donor site (if necessary for closure of the primary excision site) or rotational flap reconstruction sites (in special circumstances).

## Approach to Patients with Irregular Lymphatic Drainage Patterns

Patterns of lymphatic drainage from the skin are highly variable from patient to patient, and drainage to "unexpected" nodal basins and multiple nodal basins is not uncommon (see Table 10-5). Sentinel lymph nodes may be identified in interval and, less commonly, in ectopic sites. Interval nodes are located along the course of a lymphatic channel between a primary melanoma and a standard nodal basin; these nodes can be found in any area of the body, but are most common with cutaneous melanomas of the trunk and distal limbs. A not uncommon presentation is a patient with a distal extremity primary lesion with lymphatic drainage to a sentinel node in the epitrochlear or popliteal basin. The incidence of sentinel lymph nodes appearing in interval locations is 1% to 7% (127,137,138). Occasionally they are found in ectopic locations, most commonly in patients with truncal primary melanomas. In patients undergoing lymphoscintigraphy as part of the diagnostic workup and treatment of truncal melanoma, sentinel nodes have been identified in the triangular intermuscular space in 13% of patients, and through the posterior body wall in the para-aortic, paravertebral, and retroperitoneal areas in 3% of patients with back melanomas (128,129). Melanomas on the back also drain over the shoulders to sentinel lymph nodes in the neck in 20% of patients (128). In addition, it is not uncommon to see truncal and head and neck melanomas drain to contralateral nodal sites (127). Contralateral groin metastasis from lower extremity melanoma is extremely rare but has been reported (139). In the head and neck, unexpected lymphatic drainage is seen in about 30% of patients (133,140). This involves drainage to post-auricular nodes, contralateral drainage, drainage up to the neck, drainage to interval nodes, and drainage from the scalp down to nodes at the neck base bypassing the upper cervical nodes, parotid, post-auricular and occipital nodes.

Although the number of reported cases is small, it appears that sentinel lymph nodes of either the interval or ectopic type can harbor metastatic melanoma. The incidence of ectopic sentinel node positivity can be as high as 14% (127,129,137,138), and that of positive interval as well as ectopic sentinel lymph nodes is high enough to warrant preoperative lymphoscintigraphy, careful intraoperative gamma probe search for ectopic and interval nodes, and excisional biopsy when identified. If this biopsy reveals metastatic melanoma, the patient is at risk for involvement of more proximal regional nodes; therefore, a positive ectopic sentinel node biopsy indicates the need for treatment of the next draining basin with surgical lymphadenectomy or radiotherapy. For example, positive sentinel lymph node biopsy in the epitrochlear area should prompt ipsilateral axillary node dissection.

Management of the interval or ectopic area is controversial. With few data to guide treatment decisions, the previous recommendation was to reexplore and exenterate the lymphatic tissue around the area of a positive ectopic or interval node. Recent data, however, questions this practice in patients with disease identified by sentinel lymph node biopsy, based on the finding that, at reexploration, much less additional metastatic disease is usually identified (141).

In summary, the sentinel node is not always found in the nearest node field, and is best defined as any lymph node receiving direct lymphatic drainage from a primary tumor site. Interval nodes, which lie along the course of a lymphatic vessel between a lesion site and a recognized node field, may be found in a patient with melanoma, especially on the distal extremity and trunk. Drainage to the epitrochlear region from the hand and arm, and to the popliteal region from the foot and leg is more common than was previously thought. Drainage across the midline of the body and to ectopic sites is frequent with axially located primary melanomas. Micrometastatic disease can be present in any sentinel node, regardless of location, and for the sentinel lymph node biopsy technique to be accurate, all true sentinel nodes must be biopsied in every patient (130,135).

## Approach to Patients with Previous Wide Local Excisions

Some patients will present for consideration of lymphatic mapping and sentinel lymphadenectomy following previous wide local excision of the primary melanoma. Although this is technically feasible, there is at least theoretical concern that the procedure may be less accurate than in a case with an intact primary lesion. Lymphatic drainage of the skin surrounding the wide local excision site may be different from that of the original lesion, and disruption of the afferent lymphatics from the original site could alter or obstruct lymphatic flow to the sentinel node. In general, we advocate a selective approach to this subgroup, and carefully detail the potential limitations to all patients in whom sentinel lymphadenectomy following wide excision is planned. Our initial experience with 105 patients who had a previous wide local excision in the absence of significant rotational flap suggests that the approach is reasonable, since the sentinel node positivity rate was similar to that for more than 1,400 patients mapped during the same time period (with a similar overall pattern of clinicopathologic risk factors) for whom wide local excision had not been performed (142). Others have shown that sentinel node biopsies can successfully identify clinically occult nodal metastases in patients who have had previous wide local excision of a melanoma, and caution that the false-negative rate in patients with rotation flap closures should be taken into consideration (143,144).

## Desmoplastic Histology

Desmoplastic melanoma is characterized by an admixture of spindled melanocytes and desmoplastic stroma. It tends to occur in the head and neck region, and can be locally infiltrative, especially along neural and vascular structures. At least 1 report has suggested that desmoplastic melanoma has a higher rate of local recurrence and a poorer overall prognosis than other cutaneous melanoma histologic types (145), but recent reports from large melanoma treatment centers indicate that it is not associated with a worse prognosis. In 1998, the Sydney Melanoma Unit reported on 280 patients with either desmoplastic melanoma (n = 190) or neurotropic desmoplastic melanoma (n = 90). The 5-year overall survival of the patients in this study was 75%, and was related to several well-known prognostic factors, including tumor thickness and mitotic activity (146).

Regional nodal spread appears to occur less frequently with desmoplastic melanoma than with other histologic types. In the experience reported from Memorial Sloan-Kettering Cancer Center in New York, there were few nodal metastases at diagnosis or during follow-up, and no patients with desmoplastic melanoma had a positive sentinel lymph node (147). In contrast, however, Su and colleagues (148) reported that in a series of 33 patients with desmoplastic neurotropic melanoma undergoing sentinel lymphadenectomy, 4 (12%) were found to harbor micrometastases in the sentinel lymph node; none had any additional nonsentinel lymph node metastases at completion lymph node dissection. A recent review of the experience at the University of Texas M.D. Anderson Cancer Center, which included 1,850 patients undergoing sentinel lymphadenectomy, found a low incidence of sentinel node metastasis (2%) in a group of 47 patients with pure desmoplastic melanoma, despite their having thicker primary tumors at presentation (149,150). Interestingly, patients with "mixed" desmoplastic melanoma (N = 19)—defined as less than 90% of the invasive component of the melanoma having desmoplastic features— or nondesmoplastic melanoma (N = 1785) had a similar incidence of a positive sentinel lymph nodes (15.8% and 17.5%, respectively). Given these results, the role of sentinel lymphadenectomy in patients with desmoplastic melanoma is not yet well defined.

## Summary

Over the past 3 decades, there has been considerable evolution in the approach to the patient with clinically negative regional lymph node basins. Initially, elective lymph node dissection for patients with intermediate and thick primary melanoma was advocated. Support for this more aggressive approach came from large clinical trials, which showed a survival benefit for certain subsets of patients undergoing elective nodal dissection. This approach, however, exposes patients, the majority of whom do not harbor microscopic disease, to the potential morbidity of a lymph node dissection.

Subsequently, the technique of sentinel lymphadenectomy was introduced. Its ability to identify patients with microscopic lymph node involvement using a minimally invasive approach has obvious advantages over a treatment algorithm that includes routine elective lymph node dissection. Overall, the technique of sentinel lymphadenectomy has been shown to reliably identify those patients who are most likely to benefit from completion lymphadenectomy, while sparing those with negative nodes the morbidity of an additional surgical procedure. The prognostic power and ultimate success of this procedure is dependent on excellent communication and coordination among the surgeon, nuclear medicine physician, radiologist, and pathologist.

The advent of the sentinel lymph node technique has ushered in a new era of molecular pathological analysis of the lymph node. Rather than traditional routine histologic examination, the sentinel lymph node is now subjected to more extensive pathological examination with step sectioning, immunohistochemistry, and more recently, RT-PCR. In the future, cDNA microarray technology will make possible a genomic approach to melanoma classification, potentially allowing the identification of genetic markers or expression profiles that might be important for diagnosis, prognosis, and even therapy

(151–153). The particular combination of sentinel lymph node pathological and molecular examinations that maximize both sensitivity and specificity (i.e., overall clinical accuracy of metastasis detection) remains a topic of active investigation.

Recent reports suggest that not only is the extent of microscopic tumor burden in the sentinel lymph nodes a strong predictor of clinical outcome, it may be a key determinant of likely involvement of additional nodes in the same basin as well (62,63,89,92,154). Indeed, in a setting of truly submicroscopic disease, the sentinel lymph node biopsy procedure may prove to be both therapeutic and diagnostic, but this requires further study. Long-term results of the MSLT will address and hopefully answer many of these questions.

Other frontiers in the treatment of early-stage melanoma include defining the role of sentinel lymphadenectomy in patients with T1 primary tumors and determining which patients receive the most/least benefit from a completion lymphadenectomy following positive sentinel lymphadenectomy. These are a few of the many questions that remain unanswered in this complex disease.

# References

1. Morton DL, Wen DR, Wong JH, et al. Technical details of intraoperative lymphatic mapping for early stage melanoma. *Arch Surg*. 1992;127:392–399.
2. Albertini JJ, Cruse CW, Rapaport D, et al. Intraoperative radio-lymphoscintigraphy improves sentinel lymph node identification for patients with melanoma. *Ann Surg*. 1996;223:217–224.
3. Gershenwald JE, Tseng CH, Thompson W, et al. Improved sentinel lymph node localization in patients with primary melanoma with the use of radiolabeled colloid. *Surgery*. 1998;124:203–210.
4. Krag DN, Meijer SJ, Weaver DL, et al. Minimal-access surgery for staging of malignant melanoma. *Arch Surg*. 1995;130:654–658.
5. Gershenwald JE, Thompson W, Mansfield PF, et al. Multi-institutional melanoma lymphatic mapping experience: the prognostic value of sentinel lymph node status in 612 stage I or II melanoma patients. *J Clin Oncol*. 1999;17:976–983.
6. Reintgen D, Balch C, Kirkwood J, et al. Recent advances in the care of the patient with malignant melanoma. *Ann Surg*. 1997;225:1–14.
7. Reintgen D, Cruse CW, Wells K, et al. The orderly progression of melanoma nodal metastases. *Ann Surg*. 1994;220:759–767.
8. Uren RF, Howman-Giles R, Thompson JF, et al. Lymphoscintigraphy to identify sentinel lymph nodes in patients with melanoma. *Melanoma Res*. 1994;4:395–399.
9. Gershenwald JE, Colome MI, Lee JE, et al. Patterns of recurrence following a negative sentinel lymph node biopsy in 243 patients with stage I or II melanoma. *J Clin Oncol*. 1998;16:2253–2260.
10. Robert ME, Wen DR, Cochran AJ. Pathological evaluation of the regional lymph nodes in malignant melanoma. *Semin Diagn Pathol*. 1993;10:102–115.
11. Lane N, Lattes R, Malm J. Clinicopathological correlations in a series of 117 malignant melanomas of the skin of adults. *Cancer*. 1958;11:1025–1043.
12. Gupta TK. Results of treatment of 269 patients with primary cutaneous melanoma: a 5-year prospective study. *Ann Surg*. 1977;186:201–209.
13. Cochran AJ, Wen DR, Morton DL. Occult tumor cells in the lymph nodes of patients with pathological stage I malignant melanoma. An immunohistological study. *Am J Surg Pathol*. 1988;12:612–618.
14. Wang X, Heller R, VanVoorhis N, et al. Detection of submicroscopic lymph node metastases with polymerase chain reaction in patients with malignant melanoma. *Ann Surg*. 1994;220:768–774.
15. Reintgen D, Albertini J, Berman C, et al. Accurate nodal staging of malignant melanoma. *Cancer Control*. 1995;2:405–414.
16. Goydos JS, Ravikumar TS, Germino FJ, et al. Minimally invasive staging of patients with melanoma: sentinel lymphadenectomy and detection of the melanoma-specific proteins MART-1 and tyrosinase by reverse transcriptase polymerase chain reaction. *J Am Coll Surg*. 1998;187:182–188.
17. Goydos JS, Patel KN, Shih WJ, et al. Patterns of recurrence in patients with melanoma and histologically negative but RT-PCR-positive sentinel lymph nodes. *J Am Coll Surg*. 2003;196:196–204.
18. Shivers SC, Wang X, Li W, et al. Molecular staging of malignant melanoma: correlation with clinical outcome. *JAMA*. 1998;280:1410–1415.
19. Ribuffo D, Gradilone A, Vonella M, et al. Prognostic significance of reverse transcriptase-polymerase chain reaction-negative sentinel nodes in malignant melanoma. *Ann Surg Oncol*. 2003;10:396–402.
20. Balch CM, Soong SJ, Murad TM, et al. A multifactorial analysis of melanoma: III. Prognostic factors in melanoma patients with lymph node metastases (stage II). *Ann Surg*. 1981;193:377–388.
21. Reintgen D, Cox E, McCarty K, et al. Efficacy of elective lymph node dissection in patients with intermediate thickness primary melanoma. *Ann Surg*. 1983;198:379–385.
22. McCarthy W, Shaw H, Milton G. Efficacy of elective lymph node dissection in 2347 patients with clinical stage I malignant melanoma. *Surg Gynecol Obstet*. 1985;161:575–580.
23. Morton DL, Wanek L, Nizze JA, et al. Improved long-term survival after lymphadenectomy of melanoma metastatic to regional nodes. Analysis of prognostic factors in 1134 patients from the John Wayne Cancer Clinic. *Ann Surg*. 1991;214:491–499.
24. Balch CM, Milton GW, Cascinelli N, et al. Elective lymph node dissection: pros and cons. In: Balch CM, Houghton AN, Milton S, eds. *Cutaneous Melanoma*. Philadelphia: Lippincott; 1992.

25. Balch CM, Soong SJ, Bartolucci AA, et al. Efficacy of an elective regional lymph node dissection of 1 to 4 mm thick melanomas for patients 60 years of age and younger. *Ann Surg.* 1996;224:255–266.

26. Cascinelli N, Morabito A, Santinami M, et al. Immediate or delayed dissection of regional nodes in patients with melanoma of the trunk: a randomized trial. WHO Melanoma Programme. *Lancet.* 1998;351:793–796.

27. Balch CM, Buzaid AC, Atkins MB, et al. A new American Joint Committee on Cancer staging system for cutaneous melanoma. *Cancer.* 2000;88:1484–1491.

28. Ross M, Reintgen D, Balch C. Selective lymphadenectomy: emerging role for lymphatic mapping and sentinel lymph node biopsy in the management of early stage melanoma. *Semin Surg Oncol.* 1993;9:219–223.

29. Pawlik TM, Ross MI, Gershenwald JE. Lymphatic mapping in the molecular era. *Ann Surg Oncol.* 2004;11:362–374.

30. Rousseau DL Jr, Ross MI, Johnson MM, et al. Revised American Joint Committee on Cancer staging criteria accurately predict sentinel lymph node positivity in clinically node-negative melanoma patients. *Ann Surg Oncol.* 2003;10:569–574.

31. Thompson JF, Scolyer RA, Kefford RF: Cutaneous melanoma. Lancet 2005;365:687–701.

32. Thompson J: The Sydney Melanoma Unit experience of sentinel lymphadenectomy for melanoma. *Ann Surg Oncol.* 2001;8:44S-47S.

33. Kammula US, Ghossein R, Bhattacharya S, et al. Serial follow-up and the prognostic significance of reverse transcriptase-polymerase chain reaction—staged sentinel lymph nodes from melanoma patients. *J Clin Oncol.* 2004;22:3989–3996.

34. Romanini A, Manca G, Pellegrino D, et al. Molecular staging of the sentinel lymph node in melanoma patients: correlation with clinical outcome. *Ann Oncol.* 2005;16:1832–1840.

35. Thompson JF, McCarthy WH, Bosch CM, et al. Sentinel lymph node status as an indicator of the presence of metastatic melanoma in regional lymph nodes. *Melanoma Res.* 1995;5:255–260.

36. Gogel BM, Kuhn JA, Ferry KM, et al. Sentinel lymph node biopsy for melanoma. *Am J Surg.* 1998;176:544–547.

37. Morton DL, Thompson JF, Essner R, et al. Validation of the accuracy of intraoperative lymphatic mapping and sentinel lymphadenectomy for early-stage melanoma. *Ann Surg.* 1999;230:453–465.

38. Jansen L, Nieweg OE, Peterse JL, et al. Reliability of sentinel lymph node biopsy for staging melanoma. *Br J Surg.* 2000;87:484–489.

39. Carcoforo P, Soliani G, Bergossi L, et al. Reliability and accuracy of sentinel node biopsy in cutaneous malignant melanoma. *Tumori.* 2002;88:S14–S16.

40. Ross MI. The case for elective lymphadenectomy. *Surg Oncol Clin North Am.* 1992;1:205.

41. Godellas CV, Berman CG, Lyman G, et al. The identification and mapping of melanoma regional nodal metastases: minimally invasive surgery for the diagnosis of nodal metastases. *Am Surg.* 1995;61:97–101.

42. Rayatt SS, Hettiaratchy SP, Key A, et al. Psychosocial benefits of sentinel lymph node biopsy in the management of cutaneous malignant melanoma. *Br J Plast Surg.* 2002;55:95–99.

43. Wrightson WR, Wong SL, Edwards MJ, et al. Complications associated with sentinel lymph node biopsy for melanoma. *Ann Surg Oncol.* 2003;10:676–680.

44. Blumenthal R, Banic A, Brand C, et al. Morbidity and outcome after sentinel lymph node dissection in patients with early-stage malignant cutaneous melanoma. *Swiss Surg.* 2002;8:209–214.

45. Schijven MP, Vingerhoets AJ, Rutten HJ, et al. Comparison of morbidity between axillary lymph node dissection and sentinel node biopsy. *Eur J Surg Oncol.* 2003;29:341–350.

46. Golshan M, Martin W, Dowlatshahi K. Sentinel lymph node biopsy lowers the rate of lymphedema when compared with standard axillary lymph node dissection. *Am Surg.* 2003;69:209–211.

47. Thomas JM, Clark MA. Selective lymphadenectomy in sentinel node-positive patients may increase the risk of local/in-transit recurrence in malignant melanoma. *Eur J Surg Oncol.* 2004;30:686–691.

48. Estourgie SH, Nieweg OE, Kroon BB. High incidence of in-transit metastases after sentinel node biopsy in patients with melanoma. *Br J Surg.* 2004;91:1370–1371.

49. van Poll D, Thompson JF, Colman MH, et al. A sentinel node biopsy does not increase the incidence of in-transit metastasis in patients with primary cutaneous melanoma. *Ann Surg Oncol.* 2005;12:597–608.

50. Pawlik TM, Ross MI, Thompson JF, et al. The risk of in-transit melanoma metastasis depends on tumor biology and not the surgical approach to regional lymph nodes. *J Clin Oncol.* 2005;23:4588–4590.

51. Pawlik TM, Ross MI, Johnson MM, et al. Predictors and natural history of in-transit melanoma after sentinel lymphadenectomy. *Ann Surg Oncol.* 2005;12:587–596.

52. Kang JC, Wanek LA, Essner R, et al. Sentinel lymphadenectomy does not increase the incidence of in-transit metastases in primary melanoma. *J Clin Oncol.* 2005;23:4764–4770.

53. Balch CM, Soong SJ, Gershenwald JE, et al. Prognostic factors analysis of 17,600 melanoma patients: validation of the American Joint Committee on Cancer melanoma staging system. *J Clin Oncol.* 2001;19:3622–3634.

54. Ferrone CR, Panageas KS, Busam K, et al. Multivariate prognostic model for patients with thick cutaneous melanoma: importance of sentinel lymph node status. *Ann Surg Oncol.* 2002;9:637–645.

55. McMasters KM, Sondak V, Lotze M, et al. Recent advances in melanoma staging and therapy. *Ann Surg Oncol.* 1999;6:467–475.

56. Zettersten E, Shaikh L, Ramirez R, et al. Prognostic factors in primary cutaneous melanoma. *Surg Clin North Am.* 2003;83:61–75.

57. Gershenwald JE, Mansfield P, Lee J, et al. Role for lymphatic mapping and sentinel lymph node biopsy in patients with thick (> or =4 mm) primary melanoma. *Ann Surg Oncol.* 2000;7:160–165.

58. Thompson JF, Shaw H. The prognosis of patients with thick primary melanomas: is regional lymph node status

relevant and does removing positive regional nodes influence outcome? *Ann Surg Oncol.* 2002;9:719–722.

59. Balch CM, Buzaid AC, Soong SJ, et al. Final version of the American Joint Committee on Cancer staging system for cutaneous melanoma. *J Clin Oncol.* 2001;19:3635–3648.

60. Gershenwald JE, Prieto VG, Colome-Grimmer MI, et al. The prognostic significance of microscopic tumor burden in 945 melanoma patients undergoing sentinel lymph node biopsy. *Proc Am Soc Clin Oncol.* New Orleans, LA; 2000:51a.

61. Andtbacka RH, Gershenwald JE, Prieto VG, et al. Microscopic tumor burden in sentinel lymph nodes best predicts nonsentinel lymph node involvement in patients with melanoma. *J Clin Oncol.* 2006;24(suppl): 8004.

62. Gershenwald JE, Prieto V, Johnson M. AJCC stage III (nodal) criteria accurately predict survival in sentinel node-positive melanoma patients. 3rd International Sentinel Node Congress. Yokohama, Japan; 2002.

63. Gershenwald JE, Berman RS, Porter G, et al. Regional nodal basin control is not compromised by previous sentinel lymph node biopsy in patients with melanoma. *Ann Surg Oncol.* 2000;7:226–231.

64. Carlson GW, Murray DR, Lyles RH, et al. The amount of metastatic melanoma in a sentinel lymph node: does it have prognostic significance? *Ann Surg Oncol.* 2003;10: 575–581.

65. Gershenwald JE, Buzaid AC, Ross MI. Classification and staging of melanoma. *Hematol Oncol Clin North Am.* 1998;12:737–765.

66. Porter GA, Ross MI, Berman RS, et al. Significance of multiple nodal basin drainage in truncal melanoma patients undergoing sentinel lymph node biopsy. *Ann Surg Oncol.* 2000;7:256–261.

67. McMasters KM, Wong SL, Edwards MJ, et al. Factors that predict the presence of sentinel lymph node metastasis in patients with melanoma. *Surgery.* 2001;130:151–156.

68. Wagner JD, Gordon MS, Chuang TY, et al. Predicting sentinel and residual lymph node basin disease after sentinel lymph node biopsy for melanoma. *Cancer.* 2000;89: 453–462.

69. Sondak VK, Taylor JM, Sabel MS, et al. Mitotic rate and younger age are predictors of sentinel lymph node positivity: lessons learned from the generation of a probabalistic model. *Ann Surg Oncol.* 2004;11:247–258.

70. Azzola MF, Shaw HM, Thompson JF, et al. Tumor mitotic rate is a more powerful prognostic indicator than ulceration in patients with primary cutaneous melanoma: an analysis of 3661 patients from a single center. *Cancer.* 2003;97:1488–1498.

71. Francken AB, Shaw HM, Thompson JF, et al. The prognostic importance of tumor mitotic rate confirmed in 1317 patients with primary cutaneous melanoma and long follow-up. *Ann Surg Oncol.* 2004;11:426–433.

72. Thompson JF, Shaw HM. Should tumor mitotic rate and patient age, as well as tumor thickness, be used to select melanoma patients for sentinel node biopsy? *Ann Surg Oncol.* 2004;11:233–235.

73. Salman S, Rogers G. Prognostic factors in thin cutaneous malignant melanoma. *J Dermatol Surg Oncol.* 1990;16: 413–418.

74. Leon P, Daly JM, Synnestvedt M, et al. The prognostic implications of microscopic satellites in patients with clinical stage I melanoma. *Arch Surg.* 1991;126:1461–1468.

75. Kesmodel SB, Karakousis GC, Botbyl JD, et al. Mitotic rate as a predictor of sentinel lymph node positivity in patients with thin melanomas. *Ann Surg Oncol.* 2005;12: 449–458.

76. Clark WH Jr, Elder DE, Guerry D, et al. Model predicting survival in stage I melanoma based on tumor progression. *J Natl Cancer Inst.* 1989;81:1893–1904.

77. Bedrosian I, Faries MB, Guerry D, et al. Incidence of sentinel node metastasis in patients with thin primary melanoma (<1 mm) with vertical growth phase. *Ann Surg Oncol.* 2000;7:262–267.

78. Lee RJ, Gibbs JF, Proulx GM, et al. Nodal basin recurrence following lymph node dissection for melanoma: implications for adjuvant radiotherapy. *Int J Radiat Oncol Biol Phys.* 2000;46:467–474.

79. Pidhorecky I, Lee RJ, Proulx G, et al. Risk factors for nodal recurrence after lymphadenectomy for melanoma. *Ann Surg Oncol.* 2001;8:109–115.

80. Ballo MT, Strom E, Zagars G, et al. Adjuvant irradiation for axillary metastases from malignant melanoma. *Int J Radiat Oncol Biol Phys.* 2002;52:964–972.

81. Calabro A, Singletary S, Balch C. Patterns of relapse in 1001 consecutive patients with melanoma nodal metastases. *Arch Surg.* 1989;124:1051–1055.

82. Slingluff CL Jr, Stidham K, Ricci W, et al. Surgical management of regional lymph nodes in patients with melanoma: experience with 4682 patients. *Ann Surg.* 1994;219: 120–130.

83. Sabel MS, Griffith K, Sondak VK, et al. Predictors of nonsentinel lymph node positivity in patients with a positive sentinel node for melanoma. *J Am Coll Surg.* 2005; 201:37–47.

84. Lee JH, Essner R, Torisu-Itakura H, et al. Factors predictive of tumor-positive nonsentinel lymph nodes after tumor-positive sentinel lymph node dissection for melanoma. *J Clin Oncol.* 2004;22:3677–3684.

85. Bilchik AJ, Giuliano A, Essner R, et al. Universal application of intraoperative lymphatic mapping and sentinel lymphadenectomy in solid neoplasms. *Cancer J Sci Am.* 1998;4:351–358.

86. Cascinelli N, Belli F, Santinami M, et al. Sentinel lymph node biopsy in cutaneous melanoma: the WHO Melanoma Program experience. *Ann Surg Oncol.* 2000;7:469–474.

87. Starz H, Balda BR, Kramer KU, et al. A micromorphometry-based concept for routine classification of sentinel lymph node metastases and its clinical relevance for patients with melanoma. *Cancer.* 2001;91:2110–2211.

88. Reeves ME, Delgado R, Busam KJ, et al. Prediction of nonsentinel lymph node status in melanoma. *Ann Surg Oncol.* 2003;10:27–31.

89. Scolyer RA, Li LX, McCarthy SW, et al. Micromorphometric features of positive sentinel lymph nodes predict involvement of nonsentinel nodes in patients with melanoma. *Am J Clin Pathol.* 2004;122:532–539.

90. McMasters KM, Chao C, Wong SL, et al. Interval sentinel lymph nodes in melanoma. *Arch Surg.* 2002;137:543–547.

91. Shaw HM, Thompson JF. Frequency of nonsentinel lymph node metastasis in melanoma. *Ann Surg Oncol.* 2002;9:934; author reply 934–935.

92. Dewar DJ, Newell B, Green MA, et al. The microanatomic location of metastatic melanoma in sentinel lymph nodes predicts nonsentinel lymph node involvement. *J Clin Oncol.* 2004;22:3345–3349.

93. McMasters KM, Wong SL, Edwards MJ, et al. Frequency of nonsentinel lymph node metastasis in melanoma. *Ann Surg Oncol.* 2002;9:137–141.

94. Cochran AJ, Wen DR, Huang RR, et al. Prediction of metastatic melanoma in nonsentinel nodes and clinical outcome based on the primary melanoma and the sentinel node. *Mod Pathol.* 2004;17:747–755.

95. Scolyer RA, Thompson JF, McCarthy SW. Sentinel lymph nodes in malignant melanoma: extended histopathologic evaluation improves diagnostic precision. *Cancer.* 2004;101:2141–2142; author reply 2142–2143.

96. Dessureault S, Soong SJ, Ross MI, et al. Improved staging of node-negative patients with intermediate to thick melanomas (>1 mm) with the use of lymphatic mapping and sentinel lymph node biopsy. *Ann Surg Oncol.* 2001;8:766–770.

97. Morton DL, Thompson JF, Cochran AJ, et al. Interim results of the multicenter selective lymphadenectomy trial (MSLT-I) in clinical stage I melanoma. 2005 ASCO Annual Meeting. Orlando, FL, 2005:7500.

98. Cochran AJ. The pathologist's role in sentinel lymph node evaluation. *Semin Nucl Med.* 2000;30:11–17.

99. Prieto VG, Clark S. Processing of sentinel lymph nodes for detection of metastatic melanoma. *Ann Diagn Pathol.* 2002;6:257–264.

100. Cook MG, Green MA, Anderson B, et al. The development of optimal pathological assessment of sentinel lymph nodes for melanoma. *J Pathol.* 2003;200:314–319.

101. Koopal SA, Tiebosch AT, Albertus Piers D, et al. Frozen section analysis of sentinel lymph nodes in melanoma patients. *Cancer.* 2000;89:1720–1725.

102. Gibbs JF, Huang P, Zhang P, et al. Accuracy of pathologic techniques for the diagnosis of metastatic melanoma in sentinel lymph nodes. *Ann Surg Oncol.* 1999;6:699–704.

103. Clary BM, Lewis J, Brady M, et al. Should frozen section analysis of the sentinel node be performed in patients with melanoma? *Eur J Nucl Med.* 1999;26:S68.

104. Tanis PJ, Boom RP, Koops HS, et al. Frozen section investigation of the sentinel node in malignant melanoma and breast cancer. *Ann Surg Oncol.* 2001;8:222–226.

105. Stojadinovic A, Allen PJ, Clary BM, et al. Value of frozen-section analysis of sentinel lymph nodes for primary cutaneous malignant melanoma. *Ann Surg.* 2002;235:92–98.

106. Cochran AJ, RR H, J G, et al. Current practice and future directions in pathology and laboratory evaluation of the sentinel node. *Ann Surg Oncol.* 2001;8:13–17.

107. Morton LM: Minimally invasive staging of melanoma: invited commentary. *J Am Coll Surg.* 1998;187:188–190.

108. Scolyer RA, Thompson JF, Gershenwald JE, et al. Intraoperative frozen section evaluation of sentinel nodes may reduce the accuracy of pathologic assessment. *J Am Coll Surg.* 2005;201(5):821–823.

109. Creager AJ, Shiver S, Shen P, et al. Intraoperative evaluation of sentinel lymph nodes for metastatic melanoma by imprint cytology. *Cancer.* 2002;94:3016–3022.

110. Bachter D, Balda B, Vogt H, et al. Primary therapy of malignant melanomas: sentinel lymphadenectomy. *Int J Dermatol.* 1998;37:278–282.

111. Blaheta HJ, Schittek B, Breuninger H, et al. Lymph node micrometastases of cutaneous melanoma: increased sensitivity of molecular diagnosis in comparison to immunohistochemistry. *Int J Cancer.* 1998;79:318–323.

112. Fisher ER, Swamidoss S, Lee C, et al. Detection and significance of occult axillary node metastases in patients with invasive breast cancer. *Cancer.* 1978;42:2025–2031.

113. Wells CA, Heryet A, Brochier J, et al. The immunocytochemical detection of axillary micrometastases in breast cancer. *Br J Cancer.* 1984;50:193–197.

114. Reintgen DS, Einstein A. The role of research in cost containment. *Cancer Control.* 1995;2:425–431.

115. Yu LL, Flotte TJ, Tanabe KK, et al. Detection of microscopic melanoma metastases in sentinel lymph nodes. *Cancer.* 1999;86:617–627.

116. Messina JL, Glass LF, Cruse CW, et al. Pathologic examination of the sentinel lymph node in malignant melanoma. *Am J Surg Pathol.* 1999;23:686–690.

117. Baisden BL, Askin F, Lange J, et al. HMB-45 immunohistochemical staining of sentinel lymph nodes: a specific method for enhancing detection of micrometastases in patients with melanoma. *Am J Surg Pathol.* 2000;24:1140–1146.

118. Sarantou T, Chi DD, Garrison DA, et al. Melanoma-associated antigens as messenger RNA detection markers for melanoma. *Cancer Res.* 1997;57:1371–1376.

119. Mocellin S, Hoon DSB, Pilati P, et al. Sentinel lymph node ultrastaging in patients with melanoma: a systematic review and meta-analysis of prognosis. *J Clin Oncol.* 2007;25:1588–1595.

120. Wrightson WR, Wong SL, Edwards MJ, et al. Reverse transcriptase-polymerase chain reaction (RT-PCR) analysis of nonsentinel nodes following completion lymphadenectomy for melanoma. *J Surg Res.* 2001;98:47–51.

121. Bieligk SC, Ghossein R, Bhattacharya S, et al. Detection of tyrosinase mRNA by reverse transcription-polymerase chain reaction in melanoma sentinel nodes. *Ann Surg Oncol.* 1999;6:232–240.

122. Blaheta HJ, Schittek B, Breuninger H, et al. Detection of melanoma micrometastasis in sentinel nodes by reverse transcription-polymerase chain reaction correlates with tumor thickness and is predictive of micrometastatic disease in the lymph node basin. *Am J Surg Pathol.* 1999;23:822–828.

123. Bostick PJ, Morton DL, Turner RR, et al. Prognostic significance of occult metastases detected by sentinel lymphadenectomy and reverse transcriptase-polymerase chain reaction in early-stage melanoma patients. *J Clin Oncol.* 1999;17:3238–3244.

124. Li W, Stall A, Shivers SC, et al. Clinical relevance of molecular staging for melanoma: a comparison of RT-PCR and immunohistochemistry staining in sentinel lymph nodes of patients with melanoma. *Ann Surg.* 2000;231:795–803.

125. Aloia TA, Gershenwald JE. Management of early-stage cutaneous melanoma. *Curr Probl Surg.* 2005;42:460–534.

126. Gershenwald J, Sumner W, Porter G. Role of sentinel lymph node biopsy in patients with thin (<1 mm) cutaneous melanoma. 53rd Annual Meeting of the Society of Surgical Oncology. New Orleans, LA; 2000.

127. Thompson JF, Uren RF. Anomalous lymphatic drainage patterns in patients with cutaneous melanoma. *Tumori.* 2001;87:S54–S56.

128. Uren RF, Howman-Giles R, Thompson JF. Lymphatic drainage from the skin of the back to retroperitoneal and paravertebral lymph nodes in melanoma patients. *Ann Surg Oncol.* 1998;5:384–387.

129. Uren RF, Howman-Giles R, Thompson JF, et al. Lymphatic drainage to triangular intermuscular space lymph nodes in melanoma on the back. *J Nucl Med.* 1996;37:964–966.

130. Uren RF, Thompson J, Howman-Giles R. Sentinel nodes, interval nodes, lymphatic lakes, and accurate sentinel node identification. *Clin Nucl Med.* 2000;25:234–236.

131. Mariani G, Erba P, Manca G, et al. Radioguided sentinel lymph node biopsy in patients with malignant cutaneous melanoma: the nuclear medicine contribution. *J Surg Oncol.* 2004;85:141–151.

132. Mariani G, Gipponi M, Moresco L, et al. Radioguided sentinel lymph node biopsy in malignant cutaneous melanoma. *J Nucl Med.* 2002;43:811–827.

133. de Wilt JH, Thompson JF, Uren RF, et al. Correlation between preoperative lymphoscintigraphy and metastatic nodal disease sites in 362 patients with cutaneous melanomas of the head and neck. *Ann Surg.* 2004;239:544–552.

134. Uren RF. Lymphatic drainage of the skin. *Ann Surg Oncol.* 2004;11:179S-185S.

135. Uren RF, Howman-Giles R, Thompson JF. Patterns of lymphatic drainage from the skin in patients with melanoma. *J Nucl Med.* 2003;44:570–582.

136. Thompson JF, Uren RF: Lymphatic mapping and sentinel node biopsy for melanoma. *Expert Rev Anticancer Ther.* 2001;1:446–452.

137. Uren RF, Howman-Giles R, Thompson JF, et al. Interval nodes: the forgotten sentinel nodes in patients with melanoma. *Arch Surg.* 2000;135:1168–1172.

138. Sumner WE, Ross MI, Mansfield PF, et al. Implications of lymphatic drainage to unusual sentinel lymph node sites in patients with primary cutaneous melanoma. *Cancer.* 2002;95:354–360.

139. Thompson JF, Saw RP, Colman MH, et al. Contra-lateral groin node metastasis from lower limb melanoma. *Eur J Cancer.* 1997;33:976–977.

140. O'Brien CJ, Uren RF, et al. Prediction of potential metastatic sites in cutaneous head and neck melanoma using lymphoscintigraphy. *Am J Surg.* 1995;170:461–466.

141. Delman K, Cormier J, Ross M, et al. Surgical management of melanoma patients with epitrochlear or popliteal lymph node metastases. 57th Annual Meeting of the Society of Surgical Oncology. New York; 2004.

142. Gannon CJ, Rousseau DL Jr, Ross MI, et al. Sentinel lymph node biopsy after previous wide local excision accurately reflects the status of the regional nodal basin in patients with primary melanoma. 4th Annual International Sentinel Node Conference. Los Angeles; 2004.

143. Leong WL, Ghazarian DM, McCready DR. Previous wide local excision of primary melanoma is not a contra-indication for sentinel lymph node biopsy of the trunk and extremity. *J Surg Oncol.* 2003;82:143–146.

144. McCready DR, Ghazarian DM, Hershkop MS, et al. Sentinel lymph-node biopsy after previous wide local excision for melanoma. *Can J Surg.* 2001;44:432–434.

145. Carlson JA, Dickersin GR, Sober AJ, et al. Desmoplastic neurotropic melanoma: a clinicopathologic analysis of 28 cases. *Cancer.* 1995;75:478–494.

146. Quinn MJ, Crotty KA, Thompson JF, et al. Desmoplastic and desmoplastic neurotropic melanoma: experience with 280 patients. *Cancer.* 1998;83:1128–1135.

147. Gyorki DE, Busam K, Panageas K, et al. Sentinel lymph node biopsy for patients with cutaneous desmoplastic melanoma. *Ann Surg Oncol.* 2003;10:403–407.

148. Su LD, Fullen DR, Lowe L, et al. Desmoplastic and neurotropic melanoma. *Cancer.* 2004;100:598–604.

149. Pawlik T, Ross M, Johnson M, et al. The use of sentinel lymph node biopsy for primary cutaneous desmoplastic melanoma, 4th Annual International Sentinel Node Conference. Los Angeles, CA; 2004.

150. Pawlik TM, Ross MI, Prieto VG, et al. Assessment of the role of sentinel lymph node biopsy for primary cutaneous desmoplastic melanoma. *Cancer.* 2006;106:900–906.

151. Bittner M, Meltzer P, Chen Y, et al. Molecular classification of cutaneous malignant melanoma by gene expression profiling. *Nature.* 2000;406:536–540.

152. Baldi A, Santini D, De Luca A, et al. cDNA array technology in melanoma: an overview. *J Cell Physiol.* 2003;196:219–223.

153. Gershenwald JE, Bar-Eli M. Gene expression profiling of human cutaneous melanoma: are we there yet? *Cancer Biol Ther.* 2004;3:121–123.

154. Cochran AJ, Lana A, Wen D. Histomorphometry in the assessment of prognosis in stage II malignant melanoma. *Am J Surg Pathol.* 1989;13:600–604.

# 11
# Dynamic Sentinel Lymph Node Biopsy in Penile Carcinoma

Simon Horenblas, Bin K. Kroon, Renato A. Valdés Olmos, and Omgo E. Nieweg

Squamous cell carcinoma accounts for more than 95% of malignant penile neoplasms. The pattern of dissemination is predominantly lymphogenic to the inguinal nodes. Treatment of patients with penile carcinoma and proven inguinal metastases is straightforward, and consists of treatment of the primary lesion and regional lymph node dissection. For individuals with impalpable nodes, however, treatment has been a subject of debate for many years. Routine elective inguinal lymph node dissection leads to overtreatment in the majority of patients because of the low incidence of occult lymph node metastases. On the other hand, a wait-and-see policy harbors the risk of patients presenting with metastasis at a stage when cure is no longer possible (1). Unfortunately, primary tumor characteristics are rather unreliable in predicting occult metastases (2,3). In addition, staging with computerized tomography and magnetic resonance imaging has so far not been shown to improve the accuracy of detecting occult metastases (4). Staging with ultrasound along with fine-needle aspiration biopsy is more accurate, but still has a relatively low sensitivity (5). The challenge is to accurately detect the patient who requires a lymph node dissection. For this purpose, sentinel lymph node biopsy may be an option.

## History

Removal of the primary tumor and its associated lymph nodes has been the hallmark of surgical oncology since the pioneering work of Halstead on breast cancer. The primary drainage of penile carcinoma is to the inguinal region, and secondary drainage is to the lymph nodes in the pelvis. It was not until the late 1800s that bilateral inguinal lymphadenectomy was recommended for the treatment of documented inguinal metastases (6). In 1907, Young (8) published a paper on "a radical operation for the cure of cancer of the penis" recommending simultaneous penectomy and bilateral lymphadenectomy. While oncologically sound, these early reports enumerated a long list of complications, tempering enthusiasm for this surgical procedure. Improved anatomic knowledge based on 450 cadaver dissections by Daseler and associates led to more precise surgery of the inguinal lymphatic basin (9). A further refinement, described by Baronofsky in 1948, was the technique of covering the femoral vessels by rotating the sartorius muscle (7). Despite these improvements, inguinal lymphadenectomy for penis cancer remained a procedure fraught with postoperative sequelae, especially debilitating lymph edema of the lower limbs and genital region. While this was inevitable in patients with lymphatic invasion, it was a high price to pay for those without histologic evidence of lymph node metastasis, which was more often than not the case.

In 1977, Cabañas proposed an approach for treatment of penile carcinoma based on the concept that the lymphatic system of the penis drains to 1 node or a group of lymph nodes—the "sentinel node(s)"—that appeared to be the primary site of metastases from penile carcinoma (10). The sentinel lymph node was considered the guardian of the lymphatic basin, obviating a lymph node dissection if it proved to be tumor-negative. This concept was based on a study using lymphangiograms made via the dorsal lymph vessels of the penis in conjunction with anatomic dissections. The identification and removal of such a node was founded on static anatomic landmarks, but did not take into account the individual variation in lymphatic drainage patterns. Despite the revolutionary nature of this concept, it failed to gain international acceptance. It was not accurate enough in daily clinical practice, and after the publication of several false-

Portions of this chapter are reprinted from Kroon BK, Horenblas S, Nieweg OE. Contemporary management of penile squamous cell carcinoma. J Surg Oncol 2005;89:43–50. Reprinted with permission of Wiley-Liss, Inc. a subsidiary of John Wiley & Sons, Inc.

negative case reports, the procedure was considered too unreliable for staging.

Efforts concentrated on surgical methods to diminish postoperative morbidity. One of these was the modified lymphadenectomy proposed by Catalona (11); by restricting the boundaries of dissection and preserving the saphenous vein, morbidity was decreased without presumed loss of accuracy. However, this procedure is still associated with significant morbidity (12,13), and its accuracy was called into question after publication of false-negative procedures (14,15). And so the controversy over lymphadenectomy continued, with some proposing early lymphadenectomy at the time of treatment of the primary tumor, versus proponents of a "therapeutic lymphadenectomy" at the time of proven lymph node metastases.

The wider acceptance of the sentinel lymph node concept in melanoma and breast cancer and the reliability of lymphatic mapping pioneered by Morton and associates (16) led to a revival of interest in the procedure for penile carcinoma. In 2000, the first results were published by Horenblas et al. (17). The procedure, described as dynamic sentinel node biopsy, was based on individual mapping with the aid of dynamic lymphoscintigraphy and blue dye.

## Epidemiology and Etiology of Penile Carcinoma

Penile carcinoma is a rare tumor type in Western countries and accounts for less than 1% of male cancers in these regions (18,19). On the other hand, in developing countries this percentage can be as high as 10% (20,21). Although the disease mostly affects men older than 50 years, it is not unusual in younger persons; it is primarily seen in uncircumcised men. Phimosis is present in most of the patients and seems to be a risk factor (22). Other risk factors are chronic infection and tobacco use (22,23). Penile carcinoma also is associated with high-risk human papilloma virus, a sexually transmittable virus, which can be detected in approximately 30% of the tumors (24,25).

## Clinical Presentation, Natural Course, Diagnosis, and Staging

Almost all penile cancers (>90%) arise at the glans and prepuce, and only a small minority at the shaft. Clinical presentation ranges from an induration to an ulcer or a warty lesion. Neglect will result in corpora involvement.

This carcinoma has a strong tendency for lymphatic spread, with hematogenic dissemination only in cases with advanced nodal metastasis. Without treatment, most patients develop metastases and usually die within 2 years after diagnosis of the primary lesion. In general, patients die because of locoregional progression or from distant metastases (26–28).

The inguinal lymph nodes are the first site of metastasis, followed by the pelvic nodes and sometimes the retroperitoneal nodes. In rare cases, the liver, lungs, and bones are involved (29). The accuracy of palpation is not sufficient to select patients in whom inguinal lymphadenectomy is necessary. Palpable inguinal lymphadenopathy is present at diagnosis in 30% to 60% of the patients (30); in about half of these persons, this is caused by metastatic invasion, and in the other half by inflammatory reactions (31).

The easiest way to confirm lymph node metastases in patients with palpable lymph nodes is by fine-needle aspiration cytology. Obviously, the result is only reliable if positive; false-negative rates are reported up to 29% (4,32). If negative, another fine-needle aspiration is recommended with a brief delay; if negative again, and in the presence of clinical suspicion, an excisional biopsy should follow (33). Occult nodal metastasis is present in approximately 20% of patients presenting with impalpable lymph nodes (31). The most commonly used staging system in penile carcinoma is the 2002 American Joint Committee on Cancer TNM classification (Table 11-1).

TABLE 11-1. American Joint Committee on Cancer TNM classification for penile carcinoma.

| | |
|---|---|
| TX | Primary tumor cannot be assessed |
| T0 | No evidence of primary tumor |
| Tis | Carcinoma in situ |
| Ta | Noninvasive verrucous carcinoma |
| T1 | Tumor invades subepithelial connective tissue |
| T2 | Tumor invades corpus spongiosum or cavernosum |
| T3 | Tumor invades urethra or prostate |
| T4 | Tumor invades other adjacent structures |
| NX | Regional lymph nodes cannot be assessed |
| N0 | No regional lymph node metastasis |
| N1 | Metastasis in a single superficial inguinal lymph node |
| N2 | Metastasis in multiple or bilateral superficial inguinal lymph nodes |
| N3 | Metastasis in deep inguinal or pelvic lymph node(s), unilateral or bilateral |
| MX | Distant metastasis cannot be assessed |
| M0 | No distant metastasis |
| M1 | Distant metastasis |

*Source:* Used with the permission of the American Joint Committee on Cancer (AJCC), Chicago, Illinois. The original source for this material is Greene FL et al., AJCC Cancer Staging Manual, Sixth Edition (2002) published by Springer-New York, www.springeronline.com.

## Primary Tumor Prognosticators for Lymph Node Metastasis

The depth of invasion (T-stage) and the grade (G) of the primary tumor are the most important indicators for lymphatic spread. Grading for squamous cell carcinoma—as well-differentiated (G1), intermediately differentiated (G2), and poorly differentiated (G3)—is based on the work of Broders (34). Several series showed a relation between poorly differentiated tumors and the presence of lymph node metastases. Deeply infiltrating tumors (>T1) also have a high propensity for nodal spread (3,12,35–37). In contrast, low-grade tumors (G1-2) and superficial tumors (Tis-1) have a limited tendency to metastasize. By combining these factors, risk profiles for occult lymph node metastases have been identified (38,39). Patients with a superficial, low-grade tumor (Tis-1, G1) rarely have occult lymph node metastasis, and it has been well established that a careful wait-and-see policy is justified in these persons. In all other tumor types, the risk of occult nodal metastasis is higher, and various experts recommend elective lymph node dissection in these cases (21,40,41).

## Lymphatic Drainage of the Penis

The regional lymph nodes of the penis are located in the groin, and their anatomy has been described by various authors (6,42,43). It is customary to divide the inguinal nodes into 2 groups, superficial and deep. The superficial nodes are located beneath the Scarpa's fascia and above the fascia lata covering the muscles of the thigh; 8 to 25 nodes are present. The deep inguinal lymph nodes, which number 3 to 5, are situated around the fossa ovalis, the opening in the fascia lata where the saphenous vein drains into the femoral vein. The deep inguinal nodes connect the superficial inguinal nodes to upper-tier regional lymph nodes, that is, the pelvic nodes. In addition to receiving afferent lymphatic vessels from the superficial nodes, the deep inguinal nodes also receive lymphatic vessels draining directly from the deeper penile structures. The distinction of superficial and deep inguinal lymph nodes is only relevant from an academic point of view, because clinically the 2 sets of lymph nodes cannot be distinguished by physical examination (palpation). (72) The so-called Cloquet lymph node is the most constant and usually the largest inguinal node, located just underneath the inguinal ligament and medially to the femoral vein. A horizontal line and a vertical line drawn through the point where the saphenous vein merges with the femoral vein divide the inguinal region into 4 sections; with some individual variation, penile carcinoma metastasizes most frequently to lymph nodes located in the craniomedial section, and lymphoscintigraphic studies have shown that in most cases such metastatic involvement is bilateral (44,45,72). Pelvic lymph nodes number approximately 12 to 20 on each side and are located in the obturator fossa around the iliac vessels. Inguinal lymphadenectomy consists of removal of all regional nodes in the groin, and pelvic lymphadenectomy comprises removal of all pelvic nodes.

## Lymphadenectomy and Identification of Occult Lymph Node Metastases

Lymphadenectomy is curative in up to 80% of the patients who present with 1 or 2 invaded lymph nodes. Even in those with pelvic node involvement, cure by surgery alone can still be obtained (1,46). The extent and timing of lymphadenectomy have been debated at length. A scientifically sound answer to these questions can be given only after prospective randomized trials, but the rarity of penile carcinoma precludes this type of clinical effort. To date, the answers can only be obtained from large single-institution experiences.

Patients with proven lymphatic metastasis must undergo lymphadenectomy, but how extensive the surgery should be is debatable. In general, 30% of patients with positive inguinal lymph nodes have involved pelvic nodes as well. In this regard, the proportion of patients with metastatic involvement of pelvic lymph nodes increases with the increasing number of metastatic lymph nodes found during inguinal lymphadenectomy (1,47). Patients with 1 positive inguinal node and no involvement of the highest lymph node in the dissection specimen have a low likelihood of pelvic involvement. Additional unilateral pelvic node dissection of the affected site is recommended in all others with inguinal node involvement. The probability of bilateral involvement is also related to the number of involved lymph nodes in the resected specimen; with 2 or more metastases, the probability of occult contralateral involvement is approximately 30% and warrants elective contralateral inguinal lymph node dissection (1).

## Wait-and-See versus Early Lymph Node Dissection

For many years, the timing of lymph node dissection in patients without clinical signs of nodal metastatic disease has been controversial. Some support early lymph node dissection, defined as that carried out in a patient with nonpalpable regional lymph nodes, while others favor therapeutic lymph node dissection, carried out at the first sign of palpable lymph node involvement (1,21,40,48,49). At the heart of the matter is the unreliability of primary tumor characteristics and clinical methods to detect occult metastases.

Early lymphadenectomy seems unwarranted, since it is unnecessary in up to 80% of the patients because of the low incidence of occult lymph node metastases (31,51). Furthermore, inguinal lymph node dissection is associated with major morbidity such as lymph edema, wound infection, skin necrosis, and seroma. Contemporary series report complication rates up to 80% (12,13,50,52). On the other hand, a wait-and-see policy may decrease survival. In recent years, several retrospective single-institution studies have shown survival benefit from immediate resection of occult lymph node metastases (48,49).

## Modified Inguinal Lymph Node Dissection

Since the report by Catalona et al. (11), modified inguinal lymph node dissection has been advocated as an alternative to standard node dissection. In this procedure, the saphenous vein is spared and thick skin flaps are preserved. A much smaller amount of lymphatic tissue is removed, compared to that in standard inguinal node dissection. As expected, the rate of complications of the modified procedure is lower than that of the standard procedure (12–14,52–54). On the other hand, modified dissection is unnecessary in the majority of patients, as no tumor will be found in the resected specimen. Moreover, the reliability of this approach has been questioned (14,15).

# Dynamic Sentinel Lymph Node Biopsy

Sentinel lymph node biopsy might be a good option for select patients who will benefit from dissection. At the Netherlands Cancer Institute in Amsterdam, 140 patients underwent this procedure between 1994 and 2004 (51); few other investigators have published their initial experiences with sentinel node biopsy in penile carcinoma, but they describe small series or case reports (55–59). The largest other study to date was reported by Perdona et al. and concerned 17 patients (60).

## Lymphoscintigraphy

To localize the sentinel node preoperatively, lymphoscintigraphy is usually performed after intradermal, peritumoral injections of colloid particles labeled with $^{99m}$Tc. The tracer is transported through the lymphatic channels to the first draining nodes in the groin and made visible on the lymphoscintigram as "hot spots." Lymph node uptake is based on the ingestion of the colloid particles by the macrophages, and this receptor-mediated phagocytosis may be improved by the activation of an increased number of receptors. Lymphoscintigraphy is usually performed the day before surgery. The reasons for using lymphoscintigraphy in the sentinel node procedure are various, and include the following: (1) to point out the draining lymph node field at risk for metastatic disease; (2) to indicate the number of sentinel nodes; (3) to help distinguish first-tier lymph nodes from second-tier nodes; (4) to identify lymph nodes in unpredictable locations; and (5) to mark the location of a sentinel lymph node on the skin. In European countries, the most commonly used tracer is $^{99m}$Tc nanocolloid with a particle size of less than 80 nm; typically, a dose of about 80 MBq is administered. Application of a spray containing lidocaine (Xylocaine 10%) at the injection site 30 minutes before tracer administration is recommended, to ensure that subsequent tracer injections are well tolerated and relatively easy to perform. A volume of 0.3 mL tracer fluid is subsequently administered intradermally around the tumor in 3 depots of 0.1 mL, and each depot injected raises a wheal. The tracer is injected proximally from the tumor. For large tumors not restricted to the glans, the tracer can be administered in the prepuce. Injection margins within 1 cm from the primary tumor are recommended. In patients who have undergone a previous excision, the injections may be administered around the scar using similar margins, although it is unclear whether lymphatic drainage is altered by removal of the tumor. Images are produced using a gamma camera with a low-energy, high-resolution collimator.

Sentinel node lymphoscintigraphy must be sequential, with images obtained at various time intervals. It should accommodate the sentinel lymph node concept, visualizing the lymphatic channels and identifying the lymph nodes receiving direct drainage from the tumor. To detect these sentinel nodes, gamma camera acquisition consists of 2 parts: dynamic and static. After tracer injection, dynamic acquisition is begun for a period of 20 minutes to study the lymphatic flow. Subsequently, anterior and lateral static views are obtained using a flood source to facilitate orientation; static images will be repeated after 30 minutes, and 2 hours. Guided by the imaging, the location of the sentinel lymph node is marked on the skin to enable intraoperative localization using a handheld gamma ray probe, usually the following day (45).

At the Netherlands Cancer Institute in Amsterdam, lymphatic drainage to both groins was seen in 79% of the patients (Figure 11-1), unilateral drainage in 19% (Figure 11-2), and no drainage in 2%. A mean number of 1.3 sentinel lymph nodes per groin were visualized. One study showed nonvisualization of sentinel nodes in 11% of the mapped groins (44). Visualization appears to depend on the administered tracer dose, so for optimal results, the administered dose of activity should be sufficient. The tumor load in the lymph nodes also may play

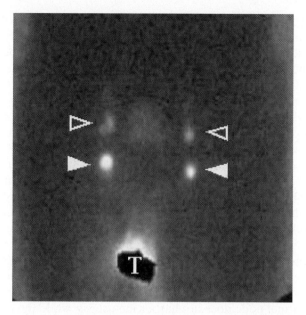

FIGURE 11-1. Preoperative anterior lymphoscintigraphic image after intradermal injection of $^{99m}$Tc-nanocolloid around the primary tumor (T), showing drainage to both groins, with visualization of 1 sentinel lymph node in both groins (solid arrows) and further drainage to the second-echelon nodes (open arrows).

a role in nonvisualization. Blocking of afferent lymph vessels by tumor cells precludes tracer uptake in these nodes, possibly leading to a false-negative procedure (61).

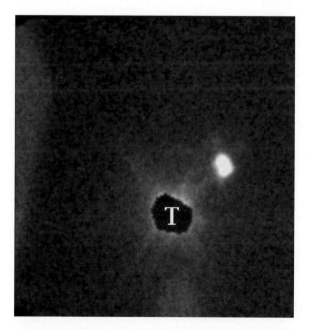

FIGURE 11-2. Preoperative anterior lymphoscintigraphic image after intradermal injection of $^{99m}$Tc-nanocolloid around the primary tumor (T), showing unilateral drainage to 1 inguinal sentinel lymph node in the right groin.

## Patent Blue

Intraoperatively, patent blue dye can visualize lymphatic vessels and helps to differentiate sentinel lymph nodes from second-echelon nodes. However, the use of blue dye alone seems insufficient to reliably detect sentinel nodes. Differences between lymphatic mapping with radiolabeled colloid and with blue dye occur fairly often (17,51,62). Almost all harvested sentinel nodes in our series were "hot," whereas only about 70% were blue as well. The 2 lymphatic mapping techniques are complementary; if we had used only blue dye, we would have missed almost 30% of the sentinel lymph nodes. This may be caused by differences in the characteristics of the 2 tracers or the site of injection, or a difference in the injected volume. In general, separate physicians administer the radiolabeled colloid and blue dye, which may result in differences in injection technique and injection sites. Finally, the injected volume of blue dye is often greater than the volume of the radiopharmaceutical, which also may cause a different outcome.

## First Results of Dynamic Sentinel Lymph Node Biopsy: and Modifications Based on First Results

Between 2000 and 2002, the early results of dynamic sentinel lymph node biopsy in penile carcinoma were published (17,45,62). Most sentinel nodes could be surgically identified with the aid of the tracer and the dye. Approximately 25% of the patients had a tumor-positive sentinel node, and only these patients underwent additional inguinal lymph node dissection. The morbidity was limited, but the reliability of the procedure was not satisfactory, as a false-negative rate of 22% was reported initially.

Since the success of this novel procedure is determined by the false-negative rate, our 6 false-negative cases were analyzed (61). In 1 patient, 1 groin was not explored for blue dye because lymphoscintigraphy did not identify a sentinel node on that side. In a second patient, additional serial sectioning and immunohistochemical staining of the sentinel node revealed metastasis. In 3 patients, blockage of inflow and rerouting of lymph due to gross tumor involvement of the sentinel lymph node might have caused failure; the true sentinel node was probably bypassed and the tracers diverted to another one that was falsely labeled sentinel. In the sixth patient, the wrong node was taken out due to a low radioactivity level in the sentinel lymph node during surgery.

Based on the failures, adaptations have been made to the technique. Nonvisualization of a sentinel node on 1 side may be caused by a metastasis blocking the lymph flow, and exploration of the groin after blue dye injection may still reveal a blue vessel leading to a nonradioactive sentinel node. Therefore, exploration for blue vessels was introduced as a standard procedure in our sentinel lymph node biopsy practice in the case of nonvisualization on the scintigram. We also adjusted routine pathological analysis, because of the pathological sampling error. Serial sectioning was introduced as well, and immunohistochemistry was added to standard staining. Finally, high-resolution ultrasonography with fine-needle aspiration cytology (ultrasonography-guided FNAC) became a routine examination for patients before a scheduled dynamic sentinel lymph node biopsy, in an effort to avoid false-negative cases caused by gross involvement of the sentinel node and tumor blocking; these nodes in particular might be picked up by ultrasound. With the introduction of ultrasonography, there have been no further false-negative sentinel node biopsy results at our institute. The sensitivity of ultrasonography-guided FNAC in detecting clinically occult lymph node metastases was 39%, with 100% specificity (5), and this has proved to be a useful tool for preoperative screening of clinically node-negative groins in patients with penile cancer scheduled to undergo sentinel lymph node biopsy. By detecting occult metastases, patients could immediately be scheduled for complete inguinal lymphadenectomy, avoiding unnecessary sentinel node procedures in groins with a positive node confirmed on ultrasonography-guided FNAC.

## Reliability of Lymphoscintigraphy

A variable lymphatic drainage pattern could be another cause of the false-negative sentinel lymph node procedures. To examine this, we evaluated the reproducibility of lymphoscintigraphy in 20 patients with penile carcinoma in whom imaging was performed twice. The results of this study were a 100% concordance of the 2 lymphoscintigrams for the depiction of nodal basins, number of sentinel lymph nodes, and node location. Moreover, all sentinel lymph nodes that were visualized during the first lymphoscintigram showed increased radioactivity after repeat injection of the radiolabeled colloid, and the correlation for the count rates at the first and the second scintigraphic examinations was statistically significant.

Thus, lymphoscintigraphy in patients with penile carcinoma had 100% reproducibility in the assessment of inguinal drainage in all 20 patients studied. These data suggest that lymphoscintigraphy is safe and that intra-individual variability in lymphatic drainage is an unlikely explanation for false-negative sentinel lymph node procedures.

## Overall Results of Dynamic Sentinel Lymph Node Biopsy (1994–2004)

Based on the experience of 140 procedures performed over more than 10 years, there are several benefits of dynamic sentinel lymph node biopsy in patients with penile carcinoma (51). First, the procedure prevents a relevant number of unnecessary lymph node dissections, and therefore decreases morbidity of staging these patients. Second, the procedure results in markedly improved staging, as histopathologic analysis focuses on only 1 lymph node (or a few at most) rather than on several nodes, as is harvested during conventional lymphadenectomy. The lymph node(s)—the sentinel node(s), i.e. those most likely to harbor metastasis—can therefore be extensively analyzed by serial sectioning and immunohistochemical staining. Third, the high prognostic value of the sentinel lymph node status has now been well proven (51): prognosis of patients whose sentinel lymph node is metastatic is poorer than that of patients whose sentinel node is nonmetastatic. In particular, disease-free survival of patients whose sentinel lymph node is metastatic is 26% shorter than in patients whose sentinel node does not harbor metastasis, while the corresponding reduction in 5-year overall survival is 30%. Moreover, multivariate analysis identified tumor status of the sentinel lymph node as the only significant prognostic factor (51). Thus, tumor status of the sentinel lymph node might in the future be incorporated in the TNM classification system for penile carcinoma, which has already occurred for patients with melanoma or with breast cancer (see chapters 8, 9, and 10).

## The Role of Dynamic Sentinel Lymph Node Biopsy in Unilateral Clinically Node-Positive Patients

Since lymphatic drainage of penile carcinoma is most frequently bilateral, it might be inferred that patients with clinically positive inguinal lymph nodes on 1 side should undergo mandatory bilateral lymphadenectomy, even if the contralateral side is clinically negative. Clinical evidence of even unilateral involvement of inguinal lymph nodes is a contraindication to lymphoscintigraphy and sentinel lymph node biopsy. Nevertheless, our experience shows that lymphatic mapping is helpful in this condition as well, to select those patients who only need unilateral lymphadenectomy on the clinically positive side. In 12 out of 17 patients with unilateral clinically positive inguinal nodes, the sentinel lymph node on the contralateral side was negative for tumor metastasis. Thus these 12 patients only underwent unilateral rather than bilateral lymphadenectomy (51).

## Micrometastasis versus Macrometastasis

No additional tumor-positive lymph node was found in approximately 80% of the patients when completion groin dissection was performed after an involved sentinel node had been removed (51). Thus, in retrospect most sentinel node-positive patients underwent an unnecessary additional lymph node dissection. Prognostic factors may identify sentinel node-positive patients who can be spared the additional surgery and its accompanying morbidity. To characterize this subgroup, we compared patients with and those without additional positive lymph nodes in the dissection specimen. The size of the sentinel node metastases seems to predict the presence of additional positive lymph nodes. In other tumor types, efforts are also being taken to predict nonsentinel node involvement. In breast cancer, for instance, it has been shown that a combination of the primary tumor size and the size of the sentinel node metastasis is predictive of the chance of nonsentinel node involvement. Based on these criteria, it has been proposed that axillary clearance be omitted in patients with a low risk of additional lymph node involvement (63). In melanoma, Lee et al. found that a thicker primary tumor and a larger sentinel lymph node metastasis are factors correlating with the incidence of tumor-positive nonsentinel nodes (64). According to Starz et al. the risk of additional involvement was determined by the number of melanoma deposits in the sentinel node, their location, and their morphology (65).

# Future Developments

## Completing Dissection

Although patients with micrometastasis in their sentinel nodes never had additional lymph node involvement, our series of patients is small and, in retrospect, 1 of our false-negative cases had only a micrometastasis in the sentinel lymph node (61). Therefore, more data from other groups are needed before completing lymph node dissection can be omitted in such patients.

## Imaging Alternatives for Dynamic Sentinel Lymph Node Biopsy

Magnetic resonance lymphography is a promising technique to detect occult lymph node metastases. A recently developed lymph node-specific contrast agent allows identification of clinically occult metastasis. This contrast agent, known as ultra-small particles of iron oxide (USPIO), is injected intravenously and taken up primarily by macrophages in the lymph nodes. The presence of USPIO in the node results in signal intensity loss (darkening) on T2-weighted sequences. Metastatic tissue displaces the macrophages filled with USPIO, and the metastatic part of the node continues to remain high in signal intensity (whitening) (66,67). Thus, metastasis within the lymph node shows as white filling defect.

Metastases as small as 1 mm have been detected using this technique. In a mouse model, even as few as 1000 tumor cells were depicted (68). Preliminary results in penile carcinoma are promising (69), and improvement of this technique could mean that sentinel lymph node biopsy is (partly) replaced in the future.

## Microarray

New molecular technological advances may help unravel the biologic behavior of neoplastic diseases. Important prognostic information obtained by these advanced technologies provides may be useful in detecting patients at high risk of occult lymph node metastases in penile carcinoma. Genome-wide profiling may make it possible to determine the biology of the disease based on the primary lesion; the recently developed DNA microarray gene-expression might fulfill this promise (68,70). Experience with this novel technique in head and neck squamous cell carcinoma shows potential (71). In the near future it may be possible to predict occult metastases by means of this technique with high specificity and sensitivity.

# Conclusions

Penile carcinoma predominantly spreads to the inguinal lymph nodes. Current primary tumor characteristics cannot predict lymph node involvement accurately, clinical methods to detect occult metastases are inadequate, and the morbidity of inguinal lymph node dissection is substantial. Therefore, sentinel lymph node biopsy is attractive in patients with clinically node-negative penile carcinoma.

Preoperative lymphoscintigraphy is mandatory to identify the sentinel nodes. Results of lymphoscintigraphy proved to be highly reproducible. In our experience, sentinel node biopsy in penile carcinoma is of important diagnostic and prognostic value at the cost of only minor morbidity. Based on the false-negative results during the first years, adaptations in the technique were made. Preoperative ultrasonography with fine-needle aspiration cytology was added, and the pathological analysis was expanded with serial sectioning and immunohistochemical staining. Exploration of groins with no visualization on scintigram and intraoperative palpation of the wound were introduced. No more false-negative results occurred after these changes were made. To further decrease morbidity, one should focus on finding prognostic factors for additional lymph node involvement and thus identify sentinel node-positive patients in whom additional complementary dissection can be avoided.

In conclusion, sentinel node lymph biopsy is a promising technique for staging patients with clinically node-negative penile carcinoma. The reliability has to be investigated further by others before it can be recommended as standard procedure.

## References

1. Horenblas S, van Tinteren H, Delemarre JF, et al. Squamous cell carcinoma of the penis. III. Treatment of regional lymph nodes. *J Urol.* 1993;149:492–497.
2. Lopes A, Hidalgo GS, Kowalski LP, et al. Prognostic factors in carcinoma of the penis: multivariate analysis of 145 patients treated with amputation and lymphadenectomy. *J Urol.* 1996;156:1637–1642.
3. Slaton JW, Morgenstern N, Levy DA, et al. Tumor stage, vascular invasion and the percentage of poorly differentiated cancer: independent prognosticators for inguinal lymph node metastasis in penile squamous cancer. *J Urol.* 2001;165:1138–1142.
4. Horenblas S, van Tinteren H, Delemarre JF, et al. Squamous cell carcinoma of the penis: accuracy of tumor, nodes and metastasis classification system, and role of lymphangiography, computerized tomography scan and fine needle aspiration cytology. *J Urol.* 1991;146:1279–1283.
5. Kroon BK, Horenblas S, Deurloo EE, et al. Ultrasonography-guided fine-needle aspiration cytology before sentinel node biopsy in patients with penile carcinoma. *BJU Int.* 2005;95:517–521.
6. Crawford ED, Daneshgari F. Management of regional lymphatic drainage in carcinoma of the penis. *Urol Clin North Am.* 1992;19:305–317.
7. Baronofsky ID. Technique for inguinal node dissection. *Surgery.* 1948;24:555–567.
8. Young HH. A radical operation for the cure of cancer of the penis. *J Urol.* 1931;26:285.
9. Daseler EH, Anson BJ, Reimann AF. Radical excision of the inguinal and iliac lymph glands: a study based upon 450 anatomical dissections and upon supportive clinical observations. *Surg Gynecol Obstet.* 1948;87:679–694.
10. Cabanas RM. An approach for the treatment of penile carcinoma. *Cancer.* 1977;39:456–466.
11. Catalona WJ. Modified inguinal lymphadenectomy for carcinoma of the penis with preservation of saphenous veins: technique and preliminary results. *J Urol.* 1988;140:306–310.
12. Bevan-Thomas R, Slaton JW, Pettaway CA. Contemporary morbidity from lymphadenectomy for penile squamous cell carcinoma: the M.D. Anderson Cancer Center Experience. *J Urol.* 2002;167:1638–1642.
13. Kroon BK, Lont AP, Valdes Olmos RA, et al. Morbidity of dynamic sentinel node biopsy in penile carcinoma. *J Urol.* 2005;173:813–815.
14. Lopes A, Rossi BM, Fonseca FP, et al. Unreliability of modified inguinal lymphadenectomy for clinical staging of penile carcinoma. *Cancer.* 1996;77:2099–2102.
15. d'Ancona CA, de Lucena RG, Querne FA, et al. Long-term follow-up of penile carcinoma treated with penectomy and bilateral modified inguinal lymphadenectomy. *J Urol.* 2004;172:498–501.
16. Morton DL, Wen DR, Wong JH, et al. Technical details of intraoperative lymphatic mapping for early stage melanoma. *Arch Surg.* 1992;127:392–399.
17. Horenblas S, Jansen L, Meinhardt W, et al. Detection of occult metastasis in squamous cell carcinoma of the penis using a dynamic sentinel node procedure. *J Urol.* 2000;163:100–104.
18. Landis SH, Murray T, Bolden S, et al. Cancer statistics, 1999. *CA Cancer J Clin.* 1999;49:8–31.
19. Frisch M, Friis S, Kjaer SK, et al. Falling incidence of penis cancer in an uncircumcised population (Denmark 1943–90). *BMJ.* 1995;311:1471.
20. Persky L. Epidemiology of cancer of the penis. Recent results. *Cancer Res.* 1977;60:97–109.
21. Ornellas AA, Seixas AL, Marota A, et al. Surgical treatment of invasive squamous cell carcinoma of the penis: retrospective analysis of 350 cases. *J Urol.* 1994;151:1244–1249.
22. Dillner J, Meijer CJ, von Krogh G, et al. Epidemiology of human papillomavirus infection. *Scand J Urol Nephrol Suppl.* 2000;205:194–200.
23. Harish K, Ravi R. The role of tobacco in penile carcinoma. *Br J Urol.* 1995;75:375–377.
24. Ferreux E, Lont AP, Horenblas S, et al. Evidence for at least 3 alternative mechanisms targeting the p16INK4A/cyclin D/Rb pathway in penile carcinoma, one of which is mediated by high-risk human papillomavirus. *J Pathol.* 2003;201:109–118.
25. Griffiths M. Detection of human papilloma virus DNA in semen from patients with intrameatal penile warts. *Genitourin Med.* 1990;66:229–230.
26. Burgers JK, Badalament RA, Drago JR. Penile cancer. Clinical presentation, diagnosis, and staging. *Urol Clin North Am.* 1992;19:247–256.
27. Misra S, Chaturvedi A, Misra NC. Penile carcinoma: a challenge for the developing world. *Lancet Oncol.* 2004;5:240–247.
28. Kroon BK, Horenblas S, Nieweg OE. Contemporary management of penile squamous cell carcinoma. *J Surg Oncol.* 2005;89:43–50.
29. Culkin DJ, Beer TM. Advanced penile carcinoma. *J Urol.* 2003;170:359–365.
30. Horenblas S, van Tinteren H, Delemarre JF, et al. Squamous cell carcinoma of the penis. II. Treatment of the primary tumor. *J Urol.* 1992;147:1533–1538.
31. Abi-Aad AS, deKernion JB. Controversies in ilioinguinal lymphadenectomy for cancer of the penis. *Urol Clin N Am.* 1992;19:319–324.
32. Senthil Kumar MP, Ananthakrishnan N, Prema V. Predicting regional lymph node metastasis in carcinoma of the penis: a comparison between fine-needle aspiration cytology, sentinel lymph node biopsy and medial inguinal lymph node biopsy. *Br J Urol.* 1998;81:453–457.
33. Horenblas S. Lymphadenectomy for squamous cell carcinoma of the penis. Part 2: the role and technique of lymph node dissection. *BJU Int.* 2001;88:473–483.
34. Broders AC. Carcinoma: grading and practical applications. *Arch Pathol Lab Med.* 1926;2:376–381.
35. Villavicencio H, Rubio-Briones J, Regalado R, et al. Grade, local stage and growth pattern as prognostic factors in carcinoma of the penis. *Eur Urol.* 1997;32:442–447.
36. Solsona E, Iborra I, Ricos JV, et al. Corpus cavernosum invasion and tumor grade in the prediction of lymph node condition in penile carcinoma. *Eur Urol.* 1992;22:115–118.

37. Demkow T. The treatment of penile carcinoma: experience in 64 cases. *Int Urol Nephrol*. 1999;31:525–531.

38. McDougal WS. Carcinoma of the penis: improved survival by early regional lymphadenectomy based on the histological grade and depth of invasion of the primary lesion. *J Urol*. 1995;154:1364–1366.

39. Solsona E, Iborra I, Rubio J, et al. Prospective validation of the association of local tumor stage and grade as a predictive factor for occult lymph node micrometastasis in patients with penile carcinoma and clinically negative inguinal lymph nodes. *J Urol*. 2001;165:1506–1509.

40. Theodorescu D, Russo P, Zhang ZF, et al. Outcomes of initial surveillance of invasive squamous cell carcinoma of the penis and negative nodes. *J Urol*. 1996;155:1626–1631.

41. Koch MO, McDougal WS. Penile carcinoma: the case for primary lymphadenectomy. *Cancer Treat Res*, 1989;46:55.

42. Cabanas RM. Anatomy and biopsy of sentinel lymph nodes. *Urol Clin North Am*. 1992;19:267–276.

43. Dewire D, Lepor H. Anatomic considerations of the penis and its lymphatic drainage. *Urol Clin North Am*. 1992;19:211–219.

44. Kroon BK, Valdes Olmos R, Nieweg OE, et al. Nonvisualization of sentinel lymph nodes in penile carcinoma. *Eur J Nucl Med Mol Imaging*. 2005;32:1096–1099.

45. Valdes Olmos RA, Tanis PJ, Hoefnagel CA, et al. Penile lymphoscintigraphy for sentinel node identification. *Eur J Nucl Med*. 2001;28:581–585.

46. Lopes A, Bezerra AL, Serrano SV, Hidalgo GS. Iliac nodal metastases from carcinoma of the penis treated surgically. *BJU Int*. 2000;86:690–693.

47. Srinivas V, Morse MJ, Herr HW, et al. Penile cancer: relation of extent of nodal metastasis to survival. *J Urol*. 1987;137:880–882.

48. McDougal WS, Kirchner FK Jr, Edwards RH, Killion LT. Treatment of carcinoma of the penis: the case for primary lymphadenectomy. *J Urol*. 1986;136:38–41.

49. Johnson DE, Lo RK. Management of regional lymph nodes in penile carcinoma. Five-year results following therapeutic groin dissections. *Urology*. 1984;24:308–311.

50. Ravi R. Morbidity following groin dissection for penile carcinoma. *Br J Urol*. 1993;72:941–945.

51. Kroon BK, Horenblas S, Meinhardt W, et al. Dynamic sentinel node biopsy in penile carcinoma: evaluation of 10 years experience. *Eur Urol*. 2005;47:601–606.

52. Bouchot O, Rigaud J, Maillet F, et al. Morbidity of inguinal lymphadenectomy for invasive penile carcinoma. *Eur Urol*. 2004;45:761–765.

53. Colberg JW, Andriole GL, Catalona WJ. Long-term follow-up of men undergoing modified inguinal lymphadenectomy for carcinoma of the penis. *Br J Urol*. 1997;79:54–57.

54. Parra RO. Accurate staging of carcinoma of the penis in men with nonpalpable inguinal lymph nodes by modified inguinal lymphadenectomy. *J Urol*. 1996;155:560–563.

55. Wawroschek F, Vogt H, Bachter D, et al. First experience with gamma probe guided sentinel lymph node surgery in penile cancer. *Urol Res*. 2000;28:246–249.

56. Han KR, Brogle BN, Goydos J, et al. Lymphatic mapping and intraoperative lymphoscintigraphy for identifying the sentinel node in penile tumors. *Urology*. 2000;55:582–585.

57. Akduman B, Fleshner NE, Ehrlich L, et al. Early experience in intermediate-risk penile cancer with sentinel node identification using the gamma probe. *Urology*. 2001;58:65–68.

58. Steinbecker KM, Muruve NA. Lymphoscintigraphy for penile cancer. *J Urol*. 2000;163:1251–1252.

59. Izawa J, Kedar D, Wong F, et al. Sentinel lymph node biopsy in penile cancer: evolution and insights. *Can J Urol*. 2005;12(suppl 1):24–29.

60. Perdona S, Gallo L, Claudio L, et al. Role of crural inguinal lymphadenectomy and dynamic sentinel lymph node biopsy in lymph node staging in squamous-cell carcinoma of the penis. Our experience. *Tumori*. 2003;89:276–279.

61. Kroon BK, Horenblas S, Estourgie SH, et al. How to avoid false-negative dynamic sentinel node procedures in penile carcinoma. *J Urol*. 2004;171:2191–2194.

62. Tanis PJ, Lont AP, Meinhardt W, et al. Dynamic sentinel node biopsy for penile cancer: reliability of a staging technique. *J Urol*. 2002;168:76–80.

63. Hwang RF, Krishnamurthy S, Hunt KK, et al. Clinicopathologic factors predicting involvement of nonsentinel axillary nodes in women with breast cancer. *Ann Surg Oncol*. 2003;10:248–254.

64. Lee JH, Essner R, Torisu-Itakura H, et al. Factors predictive of tumor-positive nonsentinel lymph nodes after tumor-positive sentinel lymph node dissection for melanoma. *J Clin Oncol*. 2004;22:3677–3684.

65. Starz H, Balda BR, Kramer KU, et al. A micromorphometry-based concept for routine classification of sentinel lymph node metastases and its clinical relevance for patients with melanoma. *Cancer*. 2001;91:2110–2121.

66. Harisinghani MG, Barentsz J, Hahn PF, et al. Noninvasive detection of clinically occult lymph-node metastases in prostate cancer. *N Engl J Med*. 2003;348:2491–2499. Erratum in *N Engl J Med*. 2003;349:1010.

67. Rockall AG, Sohaib SA, Harisinghani MG, et al. Diagnostic performance of nanoparticle-enhanced magnetic resonance imaging in the diagnosis of lymph node metastases in patients with endometrial and cervical cancer. *J Clin Oncol*. 2005;23:2813–2821. Erratum in *J Clin Oncol*. 2005;23:4808.

68. Wunderbaldinger P, Josephson L, Bremer C, et al. Detection of lymph node metastases by contrast-enhanced MRI in an experimental model. *Magn Reson Med*. 2002;47:292–297.

69. McDougal WS. Preemptive lymphadenectomy markedly improves survival in patients with cancer of the penis who harbor occult metastases. *J Urol*. 2005;173:681.

70. van de Vijver MJ, He YD, van't Veer LJ, et al. A gene-expression signature as a predictor of survival in breast cancer. *N Engl J Med*. 2002;347:1999–2009.

71. Roepman P, Wessels LF, Kettelarij N, et al. An expression profile for diagnosis of lymph node metastases from primary head and neck squamous cell carcinomas. *Nat Genet*. 2005;37:182–186.

72. Horenblas S. Lymphadenectomy for squamous cell carcinoma of the penis. Part 1: diagnosis of the lymph node metastasis. *BJU Int*. 2001;88:467–472.

# 12
# Sentinel Lymph Node Biopsy in Cancer of the Head and Neck

Luca Calabrese, David Soutar, Jochen Werner, Roberto Bruschini, Concetta De Cicco, and Fausto Chiesa

## The History of Neck Metastasis in Head and Neck Squamous Cell Carcinoma

Squamous cell carcinoma of the upper aerodigestive tract represents 90% of all malignant neoplasms developing in the head and neck. The main risk factors are alcohol and tobacco, and their effects are multiplicative (1). The age-standardized incidence rate of head and neck cancer (around 1990) in males exceeds 30/100,000 in regions of France, Hong Kong, the Indian subcontinent, Central and Eastern Europe, Spain, Italy, Brazil, and among US blacks. In women, high rates (>10/100,000) are found in the Indian subcontinent, Hong Kong, and the Philippines. The tongue is the most common site in the oral cavity, followed by the floor of the mouth, lip, gingival and retromolar trigone (1).

Prognosis depends on the stage, with mortality ranging from 10% for stage I tumors to 70% for stage IV. The neck is a critical point in the management of head and neck squamous cell carcinoma. The 5-year survival rate of tongue squamous cell carcinoma, whatever the pathology (pT) stage, is 73% for pN0 cases, 40% when nodes are positive without extracapsular spread (pN+ECS-), and 29% when nodes are positive with extracapsular spread (pN+ECS+: $p < 0.00001$) (2).

The risk of neck metastasis depends on the site, size, grading, and depth of infiltration of the tumors. The oropharynx and hypopharynx are at most risk. The tonsil, hypopharynx, base of the tongue, and supraglottic portion of the larynx show 73%, 70%, 65%, and 55% rates of nodal metastases, respectively, when the primary lesion is diagnosed, and often neck nodes are the first sign of disease. Metastatic neck nodes can be diagnosed preoperatively in up to 95% of cases by palpation in combination with either ultrasonography, computed tomography (CT), magnetic resonance (MR), or fine-needle aspiration cytology (FNAC). Positron emission tomography (PET) shows promise, but is expensive and needs further investigation. However, the main problem is detecting micrometastases (cN0 pN1), which are found in up to 50% of patients with cN0 tongue squamous cell lesions who undergo neck dissection (1,3). At present, no clinical staging modalities or biological markers reveal the presence of nodal micrometastases; for this reason, the treatment of N0 neck in early tongue squamous cell tumors is debated (4,5).

Because of the morbidity associated with neck dissection (such as hemorrhage, nerve injury, pain, or lymphedema [6,7]), several studies have compared a wait-and-see policy in patients with clinically N0 tumors with elective neck dissection, and the results showed a worse prognosis in cases that later develop cN+ and undergo delayed neck dissection (8–16). However, improved survival was observed in cN0 that was revealed to be pN1 after elective neck dissection (3,8,17–20).

Treatment modality of the neck is based on that of the primary lesion: neck dissection, in the case of surgical removal of the tumor; or radiotherapy on the primary lesion and the neck. When the neck is treated by surgery, 3 modalities are available: en-bloc neck dissection; contemporary noncontinuous neck dissection; and delayed neck dissection. En-bloc dissection is indicated when surgical removal of the primary lesion or the reconstructive technique requires an approach through the neck. Delayed dissection is preferred when the primary lesion has been treated by interstitial radiotherapy, or when surgical removal of the primary lesion does not require approach through the neck. Neck dissection of ipsilateral I–V levels (modified radical neck dissection) is the standard therapy for metastases from a lateralized primary tumor. In these cases, treatment of the contralateral neck is still under debate.

The decision to perform bilateral neck dissection is based on the site and/or stage of the primary lesion; cancers on the anterior floor of the mouth, the base of the tongue, and all those crossing the midline are treated with this procedure. If contralateral metastases are preoperatively suspected, bilateral neck dissection is mandatory, regardless of the stage and site of the primary tumor. Positive nodes are often located at levels II and III. Several studies have shown that selective neck dissection, which implies removal of the lymph nodes in levels with a higher probability of being metastatic, has the same survival rate as that for radical modified neck dissection (18).

## Rationale of the Sentinel Node Biopsy in Head and Neck Tumors

The sentinel node is the first node reached by the lymphatic stream, assuming an orderly and sequential drainage from the tumor site, and it should be predictive of the nodal stage. In clinical practice, it is tested to avoid morbidity from unnecessary lymph node dissection. This technique is routinely used in breast cancer and malignant melanoma surgery, due to the high morbidity of axillary and groin dissection; in these patients, the sentinel node has a main role in staging and in selecting those for adjuvant treatments. Instead, in head and neck cancer neck dissection is a key part of the treatment, and the presence of metastatic lymph nodes in the neck have more than a mere prognostic value.

Unlike with breast cancer and melanoma, head and neck cancers present several problems that can complicate the routine use of sentinel node biopsy. These include:

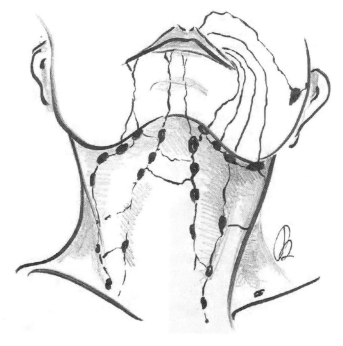

FIGURE 12-1. Complexity of the lymphatic network in the neck.

- the complex functional anatomy of the lymphatic tree (see Figure 12-1);
- broad intra-individual variation in the distribution of metastatic nodes from the same primary lesion site;
- the presence of 5% to 8% of contralateral metastatic nodes in lateralized primary lesions.

Sentinel lymph node biopsy in the head and neck is used in many centers, but strictly within clinical trials, mainly to guide the decision making on the neck management modality in cN0 cases treated with a transoral approach (4,21–25); for those cases that require an approach through the neck, a lymphatic mapping technique is under study that aims to preoperatively identify all the levels reached by the lymphatic stream from the primary site.

## Topographic and Functional Anatomy of Lymphatic Drainage of the Upper Aerodigestive Tract

There are about 800 lymphatic nodes in the human body, and approximately 300 of them are located in the head and neck area. The lymphatic network of the mucosa of the aerodigestive tract consists of narrow-meshed superficial and wide-meshed deep vessels. Beside lymphatic capillaries, precollectors are rarely found in the superficial network. Into the deeper layer, lymphatic valves are observed more frequently than in the superficial lymphatic plexus. Generally, the thickness of the walls of the precollector vessels increases from the subepithelial to the submucous layer, due to an efficacious muscle layer that allows the lymphatic stream to progress. The most relevant aspects of the complex lymphatic network of the upper aerodigestive tract have been reviewed (26,27). See also Chapter 7 of this book.

## Oral Cavity

The mucosa of the oral cavity is pervaded by a continuous tangled superficial and deep lymphatic network. About 8 to 10 collectors drain the lymph from the lip and buccal mucosa across the buccinator muscle and along the facial vessels to the submandibular fossa.

The lymphatic density of the mouth floor is higher than that of the upper and lower lip, gingiva, and buccal mucosa. The main lymphatic drainage here occurs alongside the mandibular axis to the collectors draining to the submandibular fossa. Single collectors drain from the anterior mouth floor to the submental area, and from the posterior part alongside the medial surface of the angle of mandible to the oropharynx.

The tongue is pervaded by a dense lymphatic network, and lymphatic density of the mucosa is higher than that of the muscles. Lingual lymphatic flow reveals regional differences. From the ventral undersurface of the tongue, lymphatic transport occurs mainly in a medial direction, and from there in a dorsal direction via at least 2 main collectors. Together with the lymph fluid of the mouth floor, a small part of the lymph flows to the submandibular region. Lymph fluid from the mucosa of the tongue dorsum is drained mainly in a lateral direction, and from there to the submandibular region via marginal collectors, and in the area of the tongue floor in a craniojugular direction. Lymph fluid of the mucosa around the median line flows in a vertical direction, in the area of the middle third of the tongue, via 5 to 7 collectors situated between the genioglossal muscles. From the posterior portion of the tongue, lymph is drained via collectors drawing through the pharyngeal wall together with the dorsal lingual veins; most of these collectors run to the cranio-jugular area. Collectors of the left and right part of the tongue communicate via precollectors that cross the midline. Crossings of the midline can be observed from the lingual surface to the mylohyoid muscle (28).

## Oropharynx

Lymphatic drainage of the palatine gingiva of the upper jaw occurs via the lymphatic system of the hard and soft palate. Here the mucosa is pervaded by a dense superficial and deeply situated lymphatic network. Few crossing lymph vessels are located in the midline of the hard palate; significant crossing of the midline can only be detected in the deep part of the soft palate, including the uvula. At the anterior and posterior palatine arch, lymph collectors are directed alongside the palatoglossal muscle and the palatopharyngeal muscle.

The palatine tonsils reveal the highest lymphatic density below the squamous epithelium and in lateral areas adjacent to the tonsillar fossa. Septal lymph vessels can also be detected, as well as lymph vessels in the interfollicular and subreticular lymphatic tissue. Penetration of lymph vessels can only be observed in the area of penetration of blood vessels in the capsule formed by fascia of the upper pharyngeal constrictor muscle (26).

## Larynx

The laryngeal mucosa contain 2 communicating lymphatic networks: one narrow-meshed and superficial, the other wide-meshed and deeply situated. Both are connected with those of the pharynx and trachea. Lymphatic network of the larynx is characterized by regional differences in density, and no barrier divides the network into a superior or inferior part, or into a left and a right part. In the superficial lymphatic network, numerous vessels

crossing the midline can be observed. The submucous network, however, rarely crosses to the contralateral side. The lymphatic density of the larynx is highest in the supraglottic area. Exceptions to this are the mucosa in the area of the epiglottic petiole and the tissue around the thyroepiglottic ligament. The lymph fluid of the supraglottic space drains in a mediolateral direction via 3 to 6 collectors through the lateral part of the thyrohyoid membrane; that of the laryngeal surface of the epiglottis drains to the lingual surface of the epiglottis. The main drainage occurs via the free epiglottic edge, but a small part of the lymph fluid flows through porus-like holes localized in the epiglottic cartilage.

In the vocal cords, the mucosa contains few precollectors, and no lymph collectors. The vocalis muscle has significantly more precollectors than the mucosa, and the muscle tissue holds 2 to 3 collectors. In the vocal ligament, lymph vessels are observed sporadically. The connective tissue of the vocal cord tendon contains few initial lymphatic sinuses and infrequent precollectors.

The highest density of lymph collectors can be observed in the supraglottic region in the triangle formed by the epiglottis, ventricular fold, and aryepiglottic fold. About 2 cm below the glottic level, regular, mainly horizontally directed lymph collectors can be observed in the mucosa (29).

## Hypopharynx

Together with the lymph fluid of the glottic and supraglottic areas, lymph of the cranial hypopharyngeal area flows mainly in a dorsoventral direction, and from the retrolaryngeal mucosa in a mediolateral direction to collectors in the lateral part of the thyrohyoid area adjacent to the superior laryngeal artery. Lymph of the caudal hypopharyngeal area is drained via collectors in the cricothyroid membrane. Another drainage pathway occurs in a cranio-caudal direction at the hypopharynx's posterior wall, along a midline that is crossed by numerous lymph vessels (27,28).

## Direction of Lymphatic Drainage

### Oral cavity

The lymphatic stream goes from the anterior oral cavity to the level I nodes; from the upper lip to the intraparotid nodes, and from the lateral tongue and posterior floor of the mouth to level II nodes.

### Oropharynx

The lymphatic drainage from the palatine tonsil and the base of the tongue goes to the level II nodes. Occasionally, collectors drain to the retropharyngeal lymph nodes and level III nodes (28).

## Larynx

The lymphatic fluid drains from the supraglottic and glottic areas and the cranial part of the hypopharynx to level II and III nodes. Lymph from the subglottic area goes to the conus elasticus and through the cricotracheal ligament to level III and VI nodes (30–34).

## Hypopharynx

The lymphatic stream goes to level II, III, and IV nodes; from the posterior wall of the pharynx, it flows to the retropharyngeal nodes and from there to level II and III nodes.

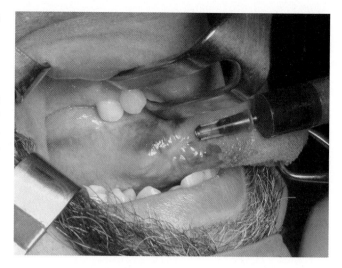

FIGURE 12-2. Peritumoral injection of blue dye and $^{99m}$Tc-albumin nanocolloids in the tongue. (Dr. Franco Ionna, G. Pascale National Cancer Institute of Naples, Italy.)

## The History of Sentinel Lymph Node Biopsy in Head and Neck Squamous Cell Carcinoma

In head and neck squamous cell carcinoma, the first successful sentinel node biopsy was performed in 1996 by Alex and Krag on a patient with a supraglottic carcinoma (35). Two years later, Bilchik et al. included 5 patients with head and neck cancer in a report on sentinel node biopsy in a variety of neoplasms (36). The techniques for identification of sentinel node in head and neck cancer were widely debated. Pitman et al., injecting blue dye alone (Figure 12-2), were unable to find any sentinel nodes in the neck in 16 patients (11). Koch et al. using a radiocolloid and intraoperative gamma probe, were only able to identify sentinel nodes in 2 out of 5 patients with oral and oral pharyngeal squamous cell carcinoma (37). In 1999, Shoaib et al. suggested a method of sentinel node biopsy for squamous cell carcinoma of the head and neck that was largely based on Morton's experience in melanoma. They suggested a triple diagnostic approach of preoperative lymphoscintigraphy, intraoperative blue dye (Figure 12-3, see Color Plate), and gamma probe localization (Figure 12-4) (38).

Several centers throughout the world began using sentinel lymph node biopsy within a research protocol. In June 2001, the first international conference in sentinel node biopsy in mucosal head and neck cancer was held in Glasgow, bringing together 22 centers. Examination of pooled data from these centers demonstrated a learning curve for the technique, with significantly improved results in centers that had performed more than 10 cases. Overall, sentinel node identification was 98%, and the sensitivity of the procedure was 90% (39). Two years later, at the second international conference in Zurich, results from more than 20 centers were accumulated.

Pooled data on 397 N0 patients were available for study. The identification rate was 97%, and many centers were reporting 100% identification rates using preoperative lymphoscintigraphy and a handheld gamma probe for lymphatic mapping as minimal requirements (40). The importance of examining the sentinel nodes in considerable pathological detail became clear.

The majority of published reports have been validation studies to demonstrate the reliability and reproducibility of this technique. Such studies have included a neck dissection to identify whether the sentinel nodes

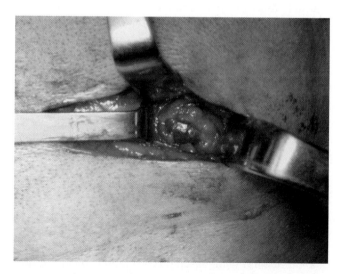

FIGURE 12-3. Intraoperative identification of the sentinel node (colored by blue dye). (Dr. Franco Ionna, G. Pascale National Cancer Institute of Naples, Italy.) (See Color Plate.)

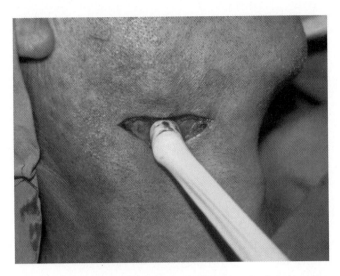

FIGURE 12-4. Intraoperative search of the sentinel node, using a handheld gamma probe. (Dr. Franco Ionna, G. Pascale National Cancer Institute of Naples, Italy.)

are a true reflection of the presence or absence of metastatic disease in the neck nodes (24,38–42).

To improve the accuracy of the technique, additional pathology was required, including step sectioning and immunohistochemistry. The technique was not useful in the N+ neck, likely because of changes in hydrostatic pressure within the involved lymph nodes. Its main function was in staging the cN0 neck in T1 and T2 tumors that could be treated intra-orally.

The 20 centers that presented their results at the second international conference in Zurich in 2003 show remarkable similarity. In reporting on this conference and reviewing the available literature, Stoeckli et al. demonstrated an identification rate of 97% (range 90–100%), and a negative predictive value of a negative sentinel node for the remainder of the neck of 96% (range 88–100%) (40). This overview established the high reliability and accuracy of the sentinel node biopsy. In his series of 90 patients with squamous cell carcinoma, Werner showed a sensitivity of 96.7%, confirming the role of serial sectioning and also the requirement that all radioactive sentinel nodes be removed (41). The majority of series have demonstrated that the technique does not isolate 1 node, but usually 2 to 3 sentinel nodes, which require detailed pathological investigation. In 2003, the American College of Surgeons Oncology Group opened a validation study for patients with T1 and T2 clinically and radiologically N0 squamous cell carcinoma of the oral cavity. This trial is expected to accrue sufficient numbers by the end of 2006.

Ross et al. recently published the preliminary results of a multicenter trial, based on the Canniesburn sentinel node biopsy protocol (43). The 6 centers enrolled in this study accrued 134 clinically N0 cases with T1/T2 tumors

of the oral cavity and oropharynx. Seventy-nine cases underwent sentinel node biopsy alone to stage the neck, and in 55 cases sentinel node biopsy was performed in combination with an elective neck dissection. The identification rate was 93%; out of these 125 cases, 42 (34%) were upstaged demonstrating metastasis, 32 using hematoxylin and eosin (H&E) stain (26%) and 10 (11%) requiring additional pathology with step serial sectioning and immunohistochemistry. The overall sensitivity of the technique was 93%. Problems were encountered with tumors on the floor of the mouth, where identification of the sentinel node was 86% compared to 97% for other sites, and sensitivity was only 80% compared to 100% for the other sites. The close proximity of the floor of mouth to the draining nodal basin provides difficulties in identifying and harvesting the sentinel node, because of close proximity with the injection site, even when using software masking techniques and lead shields. This multicenter study is due to be updated in 2006 and is the only one to date where comparisons have been made between sentinel node biopsy alone and sentinel node biopsy with elective neck dissection.

## Morbidity of the Sentinel Node Biopsy

A discussion of the morbidity of the sentinel node biopsy requires defining the morbidity of the standard surgical approach for the cN0 neck. In the Western world, the surgical treatment provides selective neck dissection. With respect of valid data, few reports focus on morbidity rates in patients who underwent selective neck dissection for cN0 neck tumors.

A recent study by Cappiello et al. compares the results of clinical and electrophysiologic investigations of shoulder function in patients affected by head and neck carcinoma who were treated with concomitant surgery on the primary lesion and the neck, with different selective neck dissections (44). Two groups of 20 patients each matched for gender and age were selected according to the type of neck dissection received: those in group A had selective neck dissection involving clearance of levels II to IV, and those in group B had clearance of levels II to V. At least 1 year following surgery, patients underwent evaluation of shoulder function by means of a questionnaire, clinical inspection, strength and motion tests, electromyography of the upper trapezius and sternocleidomastoid muscles, and electroneurography of the spinal accessory nerve. A slight strength impairment of the upper limb, a slight motor deficit of the shoulder, and shoulder pain were observed in 0%, 5%, and 15% of patients in group A, and in 20%, 15%, and 15% of patients in group B, respectively. On inspection, in group B shoulder droop, shoulder protraction, and scapular flaring were present in 30%, 15%, and 5% of patients, respectively. One patient (5%) in group A showed shoulder droop as the only significant finding. In group B, muscle strength and arm movement impairment were found in 25% of patients, 25% showed limited shoulder flexion, and 50% had abnormalities of shoulder abduction with contralateral head rotation. In contrast, only 1 patient (5%) in group A presented slight arm abduction impairment. Electromyographic abnormalities were less frequently found in group A than in group B (40% versus 85% [P = 0.003]), and the distribution of abnormalities recorded in the upper trapezius muscle and sternocleidomastoid muscle was quite different: 20% and 40% in group A, versus 85% and 45% in group B, respectively. Only 1 case of total upper trapezius muscle denervation was observed in group B. In both groups, electroneurographic data from the treated side of the neck showed a statistically significant increase in latency (P = 0.001) and decrease in amplitude (P = 0.008) compared with the contralateral side. There was no significant difference in electroneurographic data from the side with and the side without dissection in either group. Although a high number of abnormalities was found on electrophysiological testing, only a limited number of patients, mostly in group B, displayed shoulder function disability affecting daily activities. The study data confirmed that clearance of the posterior triangle of the neck increases shoulder morbidity. However, subclinical nerve impairment can be observed even after selective neck dissection (levels II–IV) if the submuscular recess is routinely dissected.

In 2004, Laverick et al. published a prospective study to compare health-related quality of life in patients having no neck dissection and in those having selective dissection, with particular reference to shoulder dysfunction (45). A total of 270 patients undergoing primary lesion surgery for previously untreated oral and oropharyngeal squamous cell carcinoma were studied using the Washington Quality of Life questionnaire, administered on the day before surgery and at 6 months, 12 months, and more than 18 months after surgery. In the group, no neck dissection was performed in 58 of the patients (21%), while a unilateral dissection was performed in 181 (65%) and a bilateral dissection in 39 (14%). Patients with no neck dissection and those with unilateral level III or IV dissections had similar mean scores for shoulder dysfunction, whereas patients with unilateral level V and bilateral level III and IV dissections recorded much worse scores on average. The results confirm the clinical impression that there is little subjective morbidity associated with shoulder dysfunction after a unilateral level III or IV neck dissection, compared with patients undergoing primary lesion surgery without a neck dissection. More extensive surgery in the neck, whether bilaterally removing levels I to III or IV, or extending posteriorly to include level V, is associated with statistically significantly worse shoulder dysfunction.

Today, no prospective data have been published comparing the rate of shoulder dysfunction or subjective morbidity between patients who underwent sentinel node biopsy and those in whom selective neck dissection has been performed. The first critical issue to be discussed is the extent of skin incision. Some authors postulate a 1- to 2-cm skin incision as a safe standard procedure for sentinel node biopsy, but this should be strongly rejected. Such small skin incisions are unsuitable to identify deeply located cervical lymph nodes in levels IIA, IIB, and III, and accidental damage to neighboring nerval, vascular, or lymphatic structures (e.g., chylus fistula) seems more likely. With the several suture techniques available, a larger incision should be favored, which does not unnecessarily compromise the patients' safety, quality of life, and postoperative shoulder function. Sufficient overview and identification of anatomical landmarks are required to prevent damage to the accessory nerve, which the authors have seen occur repeatedly in undersized skin incision. At this time, no valid data exist supporting a reduction of subjective or functional morbidity in sentinel lymph node biopsy, when compared to selective neck dissection (43–45).

## From the Sentinel Lymph Node Biopsy to Lymphatic Mapping Dissection

The majority of head and neck squamous cell carcinomas require combined resection through the neck or flap reconstruction due to locally advanced tumors; if surgical procedures on the neck are performed for a cancer, a lymphatic dissection is always required, as in case of cN0.

Moreover, surgical management of patients following sentinel node biopsy remains controversial, especially regarding the type of elective lymphadenectomy to be performed in the case of metastatic involvement of the sentinel lymph node. A further obstacle to the application of sentinel node biopsy in head and neck cancers is that the technique does not resolve the problem of in-transit metastases due to tumor emboli within the lymphatic collectors between the tumor site and the sentinel lymph node.

To solve these issues, studies are looking at whether lymphoscintigraphy can supply a complete mapping of the lymphatic drainage before surgery, both to plan the type of intervention and to guide lymphadenectomy selecting the laterocervical levels to be dissected. Results of a recent study (46) suggest that it is possible to plan in advance a "super-selective" neck dissection tailored to each patient through preoperative mapping.

For a dynamic evaluation, a low-weight tracer (colloidal sulphide particle size <50 nm) was used (46). Each patient received a maximum total activity of 40 MBq in

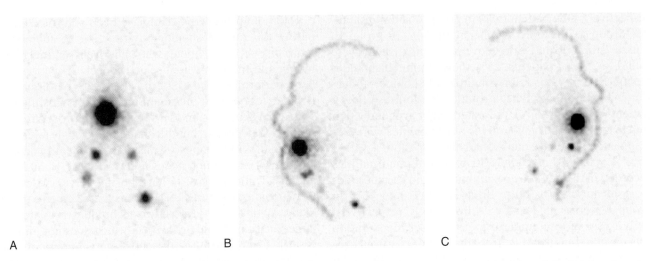

A                                          B                                          C

Figure 12-5. Static lymphoscintigraphy in the anterior (A), left lateral (B), and right lateral (C) views of the head and neck.

3 injections around the primary lesion, with an injected volume of 0.1 mL for each aliquot. After injection, patients were instructed to rinse their mouths thoroughly with tap water, to remove any residual radiocolloid.

A dynamic acquisition started after administration of radiocolloid for 15 minutes in anterior view (30 seconds/frame). Static images of the head and neck in anterior and lateral views were acquired 30 minutes and 2 hours after injection (see Figure 12-5), with the patient lying in a supine position and the head extended, collecting 100 Kcts. A $^{57}$Co point source was used to place an ink marker on the cutaneous projection of the "hot spots" (the main steps of the procedure are shown in Figure 12-6). Moreover, to correctly determine the anatomical position of the lymph node draining the injection area, single photon emission tomography-computed tomography (SPECT-CT) scan was performed, employing a hybrid system in which CT and SPECT systems are combined. The system allows the simultaneous acquisition of anatomical and functional information (see Figure 12-7, see

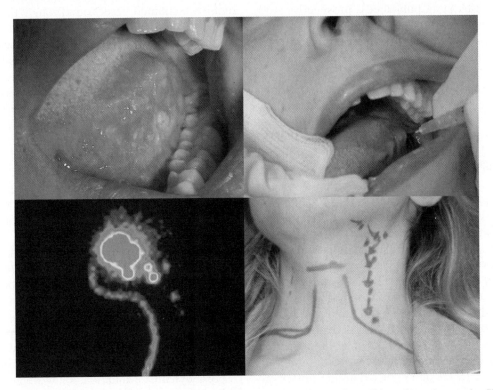

Figure 12-6. Example of lymphoscintigraphic mapping, showing multiple homolateral lymph nodes at the IIA, III, and IV levels (according to Robbins classification).

FIGURE 12-7. Lymphoscintigraphic images obtained using a SPECT/CT gamma camera for better anatomic localization of the sentinel node. (See Color Plate.)

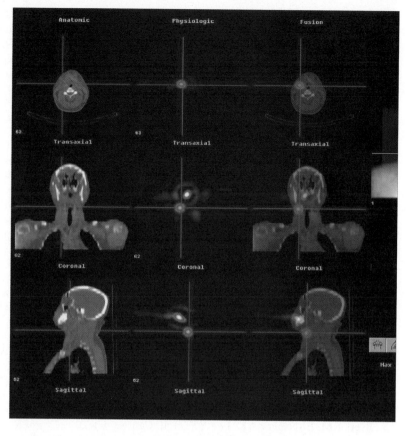

Color Plate). Functional anatomical fusion is used to generate and review the slices created from co-registered functional and anatomical imaging data. Planar images of the specimen were gathered immediately after the surgical operation, to mark each lymph node that picked up radiocolloids and order them according to level (Figure 12-8). These images were compared with preoperative lymphoscintigraphy and with pathological findings.

The preliminary results on a small selected group of patients suggest that lymphoscintigraphy aimed at lymphatic mapping determination may optimize the extent of neck surgery, both reducing related morbidity and assuring oncological radicality, due to the selection of neck levels potentially at risk to harbor cancer.

## Conclusion

Prognosis of head and neck squamous cell carcinoma gets worse as nodal involvement increases; in cN+ cases, neck dissection is potentially curative with a low morbidity. Management of the cN0 neck in patients remains controversial. Sentinel node biopsy is a reliable technique in selected cN0 cases, but the procedure is still experimental and should not be performed outside validation trials, as the second international conference on sentinel node biopsy in mucosal head and neck cancer suggested (40). Successful application of sentinel node biopsy in the head and neck region requires experience and technical adaptation, including preoperative lymphoscintigraphy.

These technical restrictions may limit the practical application of lymphatic mapping and sentinel node biopsy in mucosal malignancies of the head and neck. Stoeckli (40) gives the following indications for sentinel node biopsy, within clinical trials:

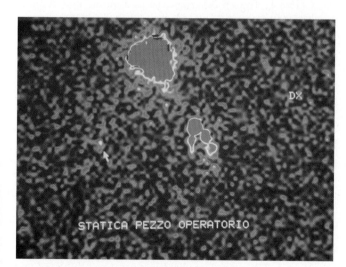

FIGURE 12-8. Ex-vivo scintigraphy of a surgical specimen (the arrow points to a contralateral labeled lymph node).

1. Staging of the ipsilateral neck in unilateral T1, T2, and N0 tumors.
2. Staging of the ipsilateral and contralateral neck in midline tumors or tumors crossing the midline, T1, T2, and N0.
3. Staging of the contralateral neck in midline tumors or tumors crossing the midline, T1, T2, N2A.

Moreover, lymphoscintigraphy aims at lymphatic drainage determination and could allow planning an individual neck dissection, thus reducing the related morbidity and assuring the oncological radicality.

## References

1. Shah JP, Johnson NW, Batsakis JG. *Oral Cancer.* Ed. London: Martin Dunitz, Taylor and Francis Group, 2003.
2. Myers JN, Greemberg JS, Mo V, et al. Extracapsular spread. A significant predictor of treatment failure in patients with squamous cell carcinoma of the tongue. *Cancer.* 2001;92:2364–2373.
3. Haddadin KJ, Soutar DS, Oliver RJ, et al. Improved survival for patients with clinically T1/T2, N0 tongue tumors undergoing a prophylactic neck dissection. *Head Neck.* 1999;21:517–525.
4. Ionna F, Chiesa F, Longo F, et al. Prognostic value of sentinel node in oral cancer. *Tumori.* 2002;88:S18–S19.
5. Byers RM, El-Naggar AK, Lee YY, et al. Can we detect or predict the presence of occult nodal metastases in patients with squamous carcinoma of the oral tongue? *Head Neck.* 1998;20:138–144.
6. Taylor JC, Terrell JE, Ronis DL, et al. University of Michigan Head and Neck Cancer Team. Disability in patients with head and neck cancer. *Arch Otolaryngol Head Neck Surg.* 2004;130:764–769.
7. Genden EM, Ferlito A, Shaha AR, et al. Complications of neck dissection. *Acta Otolaryngol.* 2003;123:795–801.
8. Vandenbrouck C, Sancho-Garnier H, Chassagne D, et al. Elective versus therapeutic radical neck dissection in epidermoid carcinoma of the oral cavity: results of a randomized clinical trial. *Cancer.* 1980;46:386–390.
9. Nieuwenhuis EJ, Castelijns JA, Pijpers R, et al. Wait-and-see policy for the N0 neck in early-stage oral and oropharyngeal squamous cell carcinoma using ultrasonography-guided cytology: is there a role for identification of the sentinel node? *Head Neck.* 2002;24:282–289.
10. Yuen AP, Wei WI, Wong YM, et al. Elective neck dissection versus observation in the treatment of early oral tongue carcinoma. *Head Neck.* 1997;19:583–588.
11. Pitman KT, Johnson JT, Edington H, et al. Lymphatic mapping with isosulfan blue dye in squamous cell carcinoma of the head and neck. *Arch Otolaryngol Head Neck Surg.* 1998;124:790–793.
12. Weiss MH, Harrison LB, Isaacs RS. Use of decision analysis in planning a management strategy for the stage N0 neck. *Arch Otolaryngol Head Neck Surg.* 1994;120:699–702.
13. Steiner W, Hommerich CP. Diagnosis and treatment of the N0 neck of carcinomas of the upper aerodigestive tract. Report of an international symposium, Gottingen, Germany, 1992. *Eur Arch Otorhinolaryngol.* 1993;250:450–456.
14. Eschwege F, Bridier A, Luboinski B. Principles and techniques of irradiation for the N0 neck. *Eur Arch Otorhinolaryngol.* 1993;250:439–441.
15. Jones AS, Phillips DE, Helliwell TR, et al. Occult node metastases in head and neck squamous carcinoma. *Eur Arch Otorhinolaryngol.* 1993;250(8):446–449.
16. Bataini JP. Radiotherapy in N0 head and neck cancer patients. *Eur Arch Otorhinolaryngol.* 1993;250:442–445.
17. Yii NW, Patel SG, Rhys-Evans PH, et al. Management of the N0 neck in early cancer of the oral tongue. *Clin Otolaryngol.* 1999;24:75–79.
18. Brazilian Head and Neck Cancer Study Group. Results of a prospective trial on elective modified radical classical versus supraomohyoid neck dissection in the management of oral squamous carcinoma. *Am J Surg.* 1998;176:422–427.
19. Kowalski LP, Medina JE. Nodal metastases: predictive factors. *Otolaryngol Clin North Am.* 1998;31:621–637.
20. Jones AS, Phillips DE, Helliwell TR, et al. Occult node metastases in head and neck squamous carcinoma. *Eur Arch Otorhinolaryngol.* 1993;250:446–449.
21. Kohno N, Ohno Y, Kihara K, et al. Feasibility of sentinel lymph node radiolocalization in neck node-negative oral squamous cell carcinoma patients. *ORL J Otorhinolaryngol Relat Spec.* 2003;65:66–70.
22. Thompson JF, Uren RF, Shaw HM. Location of sentinel lymph nodes in patients with cutaneous melanoma: new insights into lymphatic anatomy. *J Am Coll Surg.* 1999;189:195–204.
23. Shoaib T, Soutar DS, MacDonald DG, et al. The accuracy of head and neck carcinoma sentinel lymph node biopsy in the clinically N0 neck. *Cancer.* 2001;91:2077–2083.
24. Mozzillo N, Chiesa F, Botti G, et al. Sentinel node biopsy in head and neck cancer. *Ann Surg Oncol.* 2001;8(suppl):103S–105S.
25. Chiesa F, Tradati N, Calabrese L. Sentinel node biopsy, lymphatic pattern and selective neck dissection in oral cancer. *Oral Dis.* 2001;7:317–318.
26. Werner JA, Dünne AA, Myers JN. Functional anatomy of the lymphatic drainage system of the upper aerodigestive tract and its role in metastasis of squamous cell carcinoma. *Head Neck.* 2003;25:322–332.
27. Werner JA, Davis RK. *Metastases in Head and Neck Cancer.* New York: Springer; 2004.
28. Werner JA. Untersuchungen zum Lymphgefässsystem von Mundhöhle und Rachen. *Laryngorhinootologie.* 1995;74:622–628.
29. Werner JA, Schunke M, Lippert BM. The laryngeal lymph vessel system of the human. A morphologic and lymphography study with clinical viewpoints. *HNO.* 1995;43:525–531.
30. Most A. Über die Lymphgefässe und Lymphdrüsen des Kehlkopfes. *Anat Anz.* 1899;15:387–393.
31. Most A. Über den Lymphgefässapparat von Kehlkopf und Trachea und seine Beziehungen zur Verbreitung krankhafter Prozesse. *Dtsch Z Chir.* 1900; 57:199–230.

32. Most A. Über den Lymphapparat von Nase und Rachen. *Arch Anat Physiol*. 1901;75–94.

33. Werner JA, Dünne AA, Ramaswamy A, et al. Sentinel node detection in N0 cancer of the pharynx and larynx. *Br J Cancer*. 2002;87:711–715.

34. Werner JA, Dunne AA, Ramaswamy A, et al. Number and location of radiolabeled, intraoperatively identified sentinel nodes in 48 head and neck cancer patients with clinically staged N0 and N1 neck. *Eur Arch Otorhinolaryngol*. 2002;259:91–96.

35. Alex JC, Krag DN. The gamma-probe-guided resection of radiolabeled primary lymph nodes *Surg Oncol Clin N Am*. 1996;5:33–41.

36. Bilchik AJ, Giulino A, Essner R, et al. Universal application of intraoperative lymphatic mapping and sentinel lymphadenectomy in solid neoplasms. *Cancer J Sci Am*. 1998;4:351–358.

37. Koch WM, Choti MA, Civelek AC, et al. Gamma probe directed biopsy of the sentinel node in oral squamous cell carcinoma. *Arch Autolaryngol Head Neck Surg*. 1998;124:455–459.

38. Shoaib T, Soutar DS, Prosser JE, et al. A suggested method for sentinel node biopsy in squamous cell carcinoma of the head and neck. *Head Neck*. 1999;21:728–753.

39. Ross GL, Shoaib T, Soutar DS, et al. The first international conference on sentinel node biopsy in mucosal head and neck cancer and adoption of a multicenter trial protocol. *Ann Surg Oncol*. 2002;9:406–410.

40. Stoeckli SJ, Pfaltz M, Ross G, et al. The second international conference on sentinel node biopsy in mucosal head and neck cancer. *Ann Surg Oncol*. 2005;12:919–924.

41. Werner BA, Dunne AA, Ramaswany A, et al. The sentinel node concept in head and neck cancer: solution for the controversies in the N0 neck. *Head Neck*. 2004;26:603–611.

42. Barzan L, Sulfaro S, Albertio F, et al. Gamma probe accuracy in detecting the sentinel lymph node in clinically $N_O$ squamous cell carcinoma of the head and neck. *Ann Otol Rhinol Laryngol*. 2002;111:794–798.

43. Ross GL, Soutar DS, MacDonald G, et al. Sentinel node biopsy in head and neck cancer: preliminary results of a multi-center trial. *Ann Surg Oncol*. 2004;11:690–696.

44. Cappiello J, Piazza C, Giudice M, et al. Shoulder disability after different selective neck dissections (levels II-IV versus levels II-V): a comparative study. *Laryngoscope*. 2005;115:259–263.

45. Laverick S, Lowe D, Brown JS, et al. The impact of neck dissection on health-related quality of life. *Arch Otolaryngol Head Neck Surg*. 2004;130:149–154.

46. De Cicco C, Trifirò G, Calabrese L, et al. Lymphatic mapping to tailor selective lymphadenectomy in tongue carcinoma cN0: beyond the sentinel node concept. *Eur J Nucl Med Mol Imaging*. 2006;33:900–905.

# 13
# Sentinel Lymph Node Biopsy in Gynecologic Malignancies

Emilio Bombardieri, Marco Maccauro, Rosanna Fontanelli, Francesco Raspagliesi, and Giovanni Paganelli

## Background

Lymph node status is one of the most relevant factors for prognostic and therapeutic strategies for every cancer. It is a powerful predictor of survival in patients with early malignant tumors of the vulva, cervix, and uterus (1). For most cancers, the standard therapeutic approach consists of radical resection of the primary tumor with extensive lymphadenectomy. Malignant diseases require appropriate staging to ensure that the surgery does not exceed the minimum required (2). However, preoperative evaluation of lymph node status to establish the optimal extent of surgical dissection is difficult. It is well known that incorrect staging can affect short- and long-term morbidity and mortality.

In vulvar cancer, which drains preferentially to the inguinofemoral nodes, lymph node status can be evaluated by physical examination; but the clinical assessment may be inaccurate, because metastases may be present in normal nodes and cancer-free nodes may be enlarged by inflammatory conditions. In cervical and endometrial cancers, lymphatic drainage involves mainly the pelvic lymph nodes, which are difficult to evaluate clinically (3). Several imaging modalities are used for the visualization of lymph nodal invasion; but morphologic imaging (ultrasonography, magnetic resonance, computed tomography) lacks diagnostic specificity, and the new nuclear medicine imaging ($^{18}$F-fluorodeoxyglucose-positron emission tomography, FDG-PET) lacks sensitivity (4,5). With morphologic imaging, enlarged or suspicious lymph nodes are commonly detected, but the correlation with histologic findings is not high. In addition, normal nodes not depicted by diagnostic imaging sometimes may contain microscopic foci of metastases.

The sentinel node concept provides a valid alternative to systematic lymphadenectomy. The method is minimally invasive, offers accurate preoperative staging of the node status, and can reduce morbidity related to the lymph node dissection. Initial studies were carried out with vital blue dye as a tracer; the use of radiocolloid has led to the rediscovery of lymphoscintigraphy, which shows tumoral lymphatic drainage and preoperative sentinel lymph node localization (6,7). The intraoperative detection of sentinel nodes is accomplished with a gamma detector. Thus, sentinel nodes can be identified by injecting either blue dye or radiocolloid, or both tracers in combination. The concept has been accepted worldwide for many malignancies, such as melanoma and breast cancer.

However, use of the sentinel lymph node procedure in gynecologic malignancies is still open to debate. The procedure's feasibility has been demonstrated, and much evidence in the literature shows that this approach can provide an accurate preoperative lymph node staging. However, standardization of the different methods (tracers, modalities of injection, protocols of detection, staining, interpretation of pathological positivity, macro- or micrometastases, etc.) is yet to be determined, mainly for endometrial cancer. At present, prospective studies are insufficient to support the clinical usefulness of this procedure in early gynecologic cancers. This chapter summarizes the most important clinical experience.

## Vulvar Cancer

Vulvar cancer is a rare disease that accounts for approximately 4% of gynecologic cancers. The median age of patients with invasive vulvar cancer is approximately 65 to 70 years. Epidemiologic, histopathologic, and viral data suggest that patients with invasive squamous cell carcinoma of the vulva can be divided in 2 groups with different etiologies: 1 associated with human papillomavirus (HPV) infection, and 1 not associated with it. The lymphatic system that drains the vulva frequently crosses the midline, and even minimally invasive tumors may spread to regional lymph nodes (8). In most cases, the initial locoregional metastasis is located in superficial inguinal nodes. Cancer may metastasize to the deep femoral lymph nodes, and then to the pelvic lymph nodes. However, metastases have been reported to the deep femoral lymph nodes without involvement of the superficial inguinal nodes, especially from carcinoma of the clitoris. Metastasis of vulvar carcinoma to contralateral nodes is uncommon in patients with lateralized lesions.

Prognosis is strongly correlated with the presence and number of inguinal node metastases. Homesley et al. reported 5-year survival rates of 91% for patients with negative inguinal lymph nodes, and 75%, 36%, and 24%, respectively, for patients with 1 to 2, 3 to 4, or 5 to 6 positive nodes. Patients with bilateral nodes had a survival rate of 25% compared with 71% for patients with unilateral involvement (8,9). Patients with pelvic node metastases show a particularly poor survival rate.

The traditional operative approach consists of radical resection of the vulva and bilateral inguinofemoral lymphadenectomy, which leads to an overall 5-year survival rate of approximately 90% in patients with stage I disease. In principle, radiotherapy was thought to have little role in the treatment of vulvar cancer. This radical surgery is often associated with significant physical and psychological complications, while at the same time patients with multiple positive nodes continue to have a poor prognosis. In recent years, less aggressive surgery for the early stages of disease have been proposed by several surgeons and oncologists, including separate vulvar and groin incisions, partial vulvectomy with or without inguinofemoral lymphadenectomy, or radiotherapy alone. This also considers that a limited number of patients (from 10% to 25%) with isolated vulvar involvement show inguinal lymph node metastases, and thus inguinal dissection does not have clinical value in the remaining majority of

this group of women. The morbidity of inguinofemoral lymphadenectomy is well known and includes leg edema (30% to 35%), wound breakdown and infections (25% to 30%), and a consequent poor quality of life.

The first publication on the identification of the sentinel node in patients with vulvar cancer appeared in 1994. Levenback et al. studied a series of 9 patients using perilesional intradermal injection of isosulfan blue during surgery, and they were able to identify the sentinel lymph nodes intraoperatively (10). The sentinel lymph nodes were depicted in 7 of 12 basins, and the procedure correctly described the lymph node status: there were no false-negative sentinel lymph nodes or positive nonsentinel nodes. In 1995 and 2001, the same authors published 2 other contributions using blue dye, for a series of 21 and 52 patients, respectively (11,12) (see Table 13-1). They obtained sentinel node identification rates of 66% and 88%, respectively, and no false-negative results. The reliability of the colorimetric method was discussed by Ansink et al. who used isosulfan blue in a multicentric study in a series of 51 patients (13). The detection rate was 56%, and on the basis of these data, the authors concluded that the sentinel node procedure with blue dye alone was not feasible in vulvar carcinoma because of its low negative predictive value. They recommended that the dissection be performed extensively, without considering the information provided by the sentinel node procedure. The poor predictive value of the colorimetric method is evident as well in other studies based on dual labeling with blue dye and radiocolloid. In 10 patients with early stage vulvar cancer, De Hullu et al. obtained an identification rate of 100%, but the intraoperative blue dye injection confirmed the sentinel nodes identified by radiocolloid uptake in only 56% of nodes

TABLE 13-1. Relevant clinical experiences with sentinel node procedures in vulvar cancer.

| Author, year, reference | Number of patients | Technique | Detection rate (%) | Positive sentinel nodes (%) | False-negative rate (%) |
|---|---|---|---|---|---|
| Levenback et al. 1995 (11) | 21 | C | 66 | 33 | 0 |
| Decesare et al. 1997 (15) | 10 | R | 100 | 30 | 0 |
| Ansink et al. 1999 (13) | 51 | C | 56 | 17 | 18 |
| Sideri et al. 2000 (16) | 44 | R | 100 | 29 | 0 |
| De Cicco et al. 2000 (17) | 37 | R | 100 | 21 | 0 |
| De Hullu et al. 2000 (21) | 59 | C and R | 100 | 32* | 0 |
| Terada et al. 2000 (20) | 9 | C and R | 100 | 30* | 0 |
| Levenback et al. 2001 (12) | 52 | C | 88 | 19* | 0 |
| Molpus et al. 2001 (18) | 11 | C and R | 91 | 27* | 0 |
| Tavares et al. 2001 (19) | 15 | C and R | 100 | 20 | 0 |
| Sliutz et al. 2002 (22) | 26 | R | 100 | 35* | 0 |
| Zambo et al. 2002 (23) | 10 | R | 100 | 30* | 0 |
| Piug-Tintore et al. 2003 (24) | 26 | C and R | 96 | 31* | 0 |
| Moore et al. 2003 (25) | 29 | C and R | 100 | 34* | 0 |
| Merisio et al. 2005 (26) | 20 | R | 100 | | 1 |

Legend:
C—colorimetric method
R—radioactive method
*Step sectioning and immunohistochemical staining in lymph nodes negative at Hematoxylin and Eosin (HE) staining

detected (14). The low identification rate achieved by blue dye alone may be explained by the small volume of patent blue injected (0.5–1 mL), a parameter that could affect detection. However, in our opinion radioisotopic tracer is far better for the diagnosis of lymphatic involvement due to its ability to detect and provide complete topographic information.

The first report on the use of radiolabeling of sentinel lymph nodes in vulvar cancer was published by Decesare et al. in 1997 (15). They injected 14.8 MBq of $^{99m}$Tc-sulphur colloid at the site of primary vulvar carcinoma in 10 patients, obtaining an identification rate of 100%. Patients underwent bilateral inguinal and femoral lymphadenectomy. A total of 4 groins (3 patients) were positive for metastases. In 1 patient, only the sentinel lymph node was positive for disease. In a second patient, 2 unilateral nodes were positive for disease and both were identified with the gamma probe as sentinel nodes. In a third patient, a single sentinel node was positive for malignancy in each groin, and multiple nonsentinel nodes were positive. In no case was the sentinel node negative when other nonsentinel nodes were positive. The advantage of the injection of a radioactive tracer is that the sentinel node can be located transcutaneously, and this can aid the surgeon in planning the incision and identifying the sentinel node.

Sideri et al. confirmed the feasibility of surgical identification of inguinal sentinel lymph nodes using lymphoscintigraphy and a gamma probe in patients with early vulvar cancer (16). $^{99m}$Tc-labeled colloid human albumin was administered perilesionally in 44 patients (20 patients with T1 vulvar cancer, 23 with T2, and 1 patient with a lower-third vaginal cancer). All patients had complete inguinofemoral node dissection, and the nodes underwent separate pathologic evaluation. A total of 77 groins were dissected in 44 patients. Sentinel nodes were identified in all the studied groins. Thirteen cases had positive nodes, with the sentinel lymph nodes positive in all of them. In 10 cases, the sentinel node was the only positive one. The remaining 31 patients showed negative sentinel lymph nodes, all of them negative for lymph node metastases.

Many authors have reported on dual labeling in the sentinel node procedure (17–20). De Hullu et al. published the results of a prospective study on 59 patients with primary vulvar carcinoma (21). All the patients underwent sentinel node detection with the combined technique: preoperative lymphoscintigraphy with $^{99m}$Tc-labelled nanocolloid and intraoperative blue dye. Radical excision of primary tumor with unilateral or bilateral inguinofemoral lymphadenectomy was subsequently performed. Sentinel nodes and lymphadenectomy specimens were sent for separate histopathologic examinations. The day before surgery, the investigators injected 60 MBq of $^{99m}$Tc-colloid intrader-

mally around the tumor. The following day, at the start of surgery, 2 mL of patent blue was injected at the same sites. In 59 patients, 107 inguinofemoral lymphadenectomies were performed, 11 unilateral and 48 bilateral. All sentinel nodes as observed on preoperative scintigraphy were identified intraoperatively; the identification rate was 100%. Routine histopathologic examination detected lymph node metastases in 27 groins, all of which were detected by the sentinel node procedure. The negative predictive value for a negative sentinel node was 100%.

Since then, pathologic evaluation of the sentinel lymph node has evolved from routine evaluation with bisection of the node to ultrastaging with serial sections stained with hematoxylin and eosin (H&E). Some authors have added immunohistochemical staining. Ultrastaging and immunohistochemistry demonstrated 4 additional metastases in 102 sentinel nodes with negative results at the first routine pathologic test. It was concluded that the sentinel node procedure with the combined technique is highly accurate in predicting inguinofemoral node status in patients with early stage vulvar cancer. In addition, step sectioning and immunohistochemistry could increase the diagnostic sensitivity in showing metastases.

Various authors have confirmed that combining ultrastaging with serial sectioning and immunohistochemical staining can increase the detection of micrometastases in sentinel nodes that were negative by H&E staining, and this can reduce the risk of recurrence (22,23). Puig-Tintore et al. studied this procedure in 26 patients with squamous cell carcinoma of the vulva (24). The day before surgery, 2 or 3 doses of 27.7 to 37 MBq of $^{99m}$Tc-colloid were injected intradermally around the lesion. Immediately before surgery, peritumoral injections of blue dye were given at the same sites. Dissection of the sentinel nodes was followed by standard lymphadenectomy and vulvar exeresis. Pathological ultrastaging was carried out by evaluating at least 4 histopathological sections of every lymph node (400 micron thickness) using H&E and immunostaining against cytokeratin. Sentinel nodes were identified in 96% of patients; the nodes were unilateral in 19 patients (76%), and bilateral in 6 (24%). A total of 46 sentinel nodes were isolated. Metastases were localized in 3 sentinel nodes from 8 patients (30.8%); of these, 38% presented micrometastasis detected only in ultrastaging. No metastatic spread was diagnosed in nonsentinel lymph nodes, when sentinel nodes were negative in patients without clinically suspicious adenopathy. No inguinal recurrences were observed during follow-up of 15 patients in whom groin dissection was unilateral. The authors concluded that inguinofemoral dissection can be confidently avoided when sentinel node metastases are excluded by histologic ultrastaging.

There is no consensus on the usefulness of the addition of immunohistochemical staining to H&E staining in the pathological evaluation of sentinel nodes. A recent study by Moore et al. demonstrated that the combination with immunohistochemical staining does not increase the detection of micrometastases (25). The author evaluated the value of immunohistochemical staining in inguinal sentinel lymph nodes found to be negative for metastatic disease by H&E staining. Twenty-nine patients with squamous cell carcinoma of the vulva underwent an inguinal sentinel lymph node dissection: 19 patients had inguinal dissection negative for metastatic involvement, 2 patients had bilateral inguinal metastases, and 8 patients had unilateral inguinal metastasis. Forty-two groin dissections with sentinel lymph node biopsies were carried out; 12 groins were positive for metastatic disease and 30 were negative on the basis of ultrastaging with H&E staining. A total of 107 sentinel lymph nodes were obtained, of which 18 nodes with metastatic invasion were identified by ultrastaging and staining with H&E. Two sentinel nodes showed metastasis less than 0.3 mm, and 16 had metastasis greater than 2 mm. Eighty-nine sentinel lymph nodes found to be negative for metastasis by H&E staining were also negative for micrometastasis on evaluation with an anti-pancytokeratin antibody. In conclusion, Moore et al. said that with the use of detailed serial sectioning or ultrastaging, all metastases and micrometastases should be detected.

Merisio et al. (26) confirmed the diagnostic accuracy of sentinel lymph node detection by preoperative lymphoscintigraphy with $^{99m}$Tc-labeled nanocolloid (see Figure 13-1), followed by radioguided intraoperative detection. Twenty patients were studied, with 9 with T1 stage tumors and 11 with T2 N0 M0. Sentinel node detection was 100%. Thirty inguinofemoral lymphadenectomies were performed, and pathological examination revealed 17 true negative nodes, 2 true positive, and 1 false negative. The overall accuracy of detection was 95%. Our group, however, published a case report in which, using $^{99m}$Tc-nanocolloid alone, we found a false negative sentinel node in a woman with vulvar cancer (27).

Plante et al. (28) carried out a general evaluation of 353 cases from 12 studies to summarize the clinical reliability of the sentinel lymph node procedure in vulvar cancer. The sentinel node detection rate was 92%. Only 3 groin recurrences have been documented so far (<1%). The critical review of the literature seems to suggest that the combined approach with blue dye and lymphoscintigraphy is superior to blue dye alone for sentinel node detection. Complications with this procedure are rare and usually not severe, except for the possibility of an anaphylactic reaction to the blue dye (around 1%). Based on these data, the authors suggest that the sentinel lymph node mapping technique is feasible in vulvar cancer

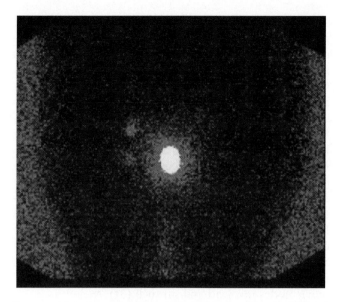

Figure 13-1. Late lymphoscintigraphy (static acquisitions) obtained in a patient with vulvar cancer, showing visualization of 2 sentinel lymph nodes located in the right inguinal region. Transmission images obtained with a flood source placed beneath the patient help to identify anatomic structures.

and may become a valuable alternative to the traditional groin and pelvic lymphadenectomy. However, results have not been controlled for in large multicentric trials, and the technique should still be validated in prospective clinical trials.

## Cervical Cancer

For women aged 20 to 40, cervical cancer is the second leading cause of cancer death after breast cancer, and represents 18% of deaths from gynecologic cancer. Biological and epidemiologic studies have demonstrated a strong relationship between human papillomavirus (HPV), cervical intraepithelial neoplasia, and invasive carcinoma of the cervix. This tumor may extend to the lower uterine segment, to the vagina, or into the paracervical regions. Invasive cancer can spread to the bladder or the rectum and may become fixed to the pelvic wall. The cervix has a rich network of lymphatics, distributed in 3 anastomotic plexuses draining the mucosal, muscularis, and serosal layers. The most important lymphatic trunks exit from the uterine isthmus in 3 branches (29). The upper branch follows the uterine artery and terminates in the hypogastric nodes. The middle branch drains to obturator and external lymph nodes. The lower branch joins a posterior course with gluteal, common iliac, presacral, and subaortic nodes. Additional posterior lymphatic channels drain to the rectal lymph nodes or continue to subaortic nodes. The incidence of pelvic and paraaortic node involvement depends mainly on the stage. The frequency of pelvic node invasion is 1% to 20% for stage IB tumors; 20% to 35% for stage IIA; 35% to 45% for stage IIB; and 40% to 55% for stage II. In paraaortic node invasion, the frequency is 2% to 10% for stage IB tumors; 10% to 15% for stage IIA; 16% to 20% for stage IIB; and 26% to 35% for stage III. The most important prognostic factors are related to FIGO (International Federation of Gynecology and Obstetrics) stage and a number of tumor characteristics included in the staging system. Lymph node metastases are an important predictor of prognosis. Patients treated with radical hysterectomy for stage IIIB tumors show a survival rate of approximately 90% in cases of negative nodes, and 50% for patients with positive nodes (30). Several authors have reported a strict correlation between the number of pelvic nodes involved and survival (31).

The traditional treatment of early cervical cancer consists of surgery (radical hysterectomy and pelvic lymphadenectomy) and/or radiotherapy (32–34). As described previously, the main problem is that pelvic lymph node invasion is present only in 1% to 20% of women with stage IB cervical cancer. This means that for approximately 80% of these patients, pelvic lymphadenectomy does not provide any major clinical benefit; on the contrary, the procedure sometimes causes vessel and nerve damage. In many cases, postoperative radiotherapy is required, and consequently edema of the legs and lymphocele are other possible adverse effects. This is why the presence or absence of metastatic disease in pelvic lymph nodes has a strategic value in cervical cancer.

The evolution of surgery in recent years has led to less aggressive surgical treatment of early cervical cancer, with more attention paid to the quality of life without compromising survival. In series of selected patients with invasive tumors, trachelotomy is used to preserve fertility. The sentinel lymph node procedure appears to have several advantages. First, sentinel lymph node biopsy provides reliable information, so the complications of pelvic lymphadenectomy can be avoided, especially in those patients with stage I cervical cancer that is free from pelvic lymph space involvement. Second, the detection rate of lymph node metastases seems to be increased by the use of multiple sectioning and immunohistochemical staining. This procedure was shown to be able to detect occult micrometastases that are responsible of pelvic recurrences in patients with negative standard histologic findings.

Echt et al. published the first study on sentinel lymph node biopsy in cervical cancer using a blue dye (35). This tracer was injected into the cervix of 13 women, and the following laparotomy correctly identified the sentinel node in only 15% of cases. Since this unsuccessful attempt, the detection rate of sentinel lymph nodes described in the literature ranges between 60% and 100% independently by the surgical route, the colorimetric method, or the radioactive tracer and the detection protocol (Table 13-2). Medl et al. and O'Boyle et al. published the first reports of lymphatic mapping with isosulfan blue and sentinel node biopsy (36,37). Dargent et al. studied the largest series of patients injecting the patent blue violet alone (38). The blue violet was injected around the tumor in 35 patients, then laparoscopy was

TABLE 13-2. Relevant clinical experiences with sentinel node procedures in cervical cancer.

| Author, year, reference | Number of patients | Technique | Sentinel node detection rate (%) | Positive sentinel node (patients number) | False-negative rate (%) |
|---|---|---|---|---|---|
| Echt et al. 1999 (35) | 13 | C | 15 | 2 | 0 |
| Medl et al. 2000 (36) | 3 | C | 100 | 3 | 0 |
| O'Boyle et al. 2000 (37) | 20 | C | 60 | 3 | 0 |
| Dargent et al. 2000 (38) | 35 | C | 100 | 11 | 0 |
| Kamprath et al. 2000 (39) | 18 | R* | 89 | 1 | 0 |
| Verheijn et al. 2000 (41) | 10 | C and R | 80 | 1* | 0 |
| Lantzsch et al. 2001 (40) | 14 | R | 93 | 1* | 0 |
| Malur et al. 2001 (42) | 50 | C and R | 78 | 5 | 17 |
| Levenback et al. 2002 (43) | 39 | C and R | 100 | 8* | 11 |
| Barranger et al. 2003 (44) | 13 | C and R | 92 | 2 | 0 |
| Chung et al. 2003 (45) | 26 | C and R | 100 | 1 | 0 |
| Martinez-Palones et al. 2004 (46) | 25 | C and R | 92 | 3* | 0 |
| Pijpers et al. 2004 (47) | 34 | C and R | 97 | 12 | 0 |
| Niikura et al. 2004 (48) | 20 | C and R | 90 | 3* | 0 |
| Marchiole et al. 2004 (51) | 29 | C and R | 100 | 3* | 12,5 |
| Angioli et al. 2005 (49) | 37 | R | 89 | 6 | 0 |

Legend:
C—colorimetric method
R—radioactive method
*Step sectioning and immunohistochemical staining in lymph nodes negative at Hematoxylin and Eosin (HE) staining.

performed and the positive lymph nodes sought. Positive sentinel nodes were removed and systematic dissection was performed on 69 pelvic sidewalls; dissection was not performed in the second side when the assessment of the first side suggested surgery should not be performed. One or more sentinel nodes were found in 59 of 69 dissections. An important result of this investigation is the demonstrated correlation between the rate of failure and the amount of blue dye injected: 50% for 1.5 mL, 17% for 2 mL, and 10% after injection of 4 mL. In 4 cases, 2 sentinel lymph nodes were identified; therefore, the overall number of sentinel lymph nodes detected reached 63. In 11 pelvic wall dissections performed in 8 patients, 1 or more metastatic lymph nodes were found. The node that was positive by blue dye was the sentinel lymph node, or 1 of them, in all cases. The laparoscopic procedure with patent blue alone identified sentinel nodes in 100% of the patients. Kamprath et al. and Lantzsch et al. first used the radioisotopic method, injecting $^{99m}$Tc-labeled nanocolloid preoperatively in patients with early cervical cancer (39,40). They had no false-negative results and concluded that this method was feasible for determining the extent of the disease. Other authors have obtained good results using the same injection technique for sentinel node detection combined with blue dye for visual detection (41–49).

Malur et al. compared patent blue alone, radiocolloid alone, and a combination of the 2 reagents (42). They studied 50 patients with cervical cancer: 32 with FIGO stage I tumors, 16 with stage II, and 2 with stage IV. The patients underwent sentinel lymph node detection during the primary operation (radical laparoscopic vaginal or abdominal hysterectomy). The day before surgery, 50 MBq of $^{99m}$Tc-labeled albures colloid was injected into the cervix; blue dye injection was performed during surgery at the same locations. The detection rate was 78%. Lymph node metastases were diagnosed in 10 patients, and the sentinel node detection rates were 55% with blue alone, 76% with radiocolloid alone, and 90% with the combination. Recently, in a series of 39 patients Levenback et al. obtained a 100% identification rate with dual labeling and a laparotomy procedure (43).

Barranger et al. looked at the feasibility of the laparoscopic sentinel lymph node procedure with combined radioisotopic and patent blue labeling (44). Sentinel lymph nodes were identified in 12 of 13 patients (tumor stage I-IIa), and a median of 10.5 pelvic lymph nodes per patient (range 4–17) were removed. No lymph node involvement was detected in sentinel lymph nodes with H&E staining, while immunohistochemical studies found 4 metastatic sentinel nodes in 2 patients, with micrometastases in 2 sentinel nodes from the first patient and isolated tumor cells in 2 sentinel nodes from the second. No false-negative sentinel node results were obtained.

Chung et al. carried out a prospective study on 26 patients with FIGO stage I-IIa cervical cancer. The author stressed the importance of the correct use of the intraoperative gamma probe (45). Sentinel lymph nodes were successfully localized using a combination of lymphoscintigraphy and an intraoperative gamma probe in all 26 cases. However, in 2 cases, sentinel nodes were localized using the gamma probe. Martinez-Palones et al. examined 25 patients with stage I-II tumors using $^{99m}$Tc-labeled human serum albumin and isosulfan blue dye injection (46). Complete pelvic or paraaortic lymphadenectomy was carried out in all cases by laparoscopy or surgery. A total of 51 sentinel nodes were identified in 23 patients by lymphoscintigraphy; 61 sentinel lymph nodes were detected intraoperatively, with a mean of 2.5 nodes per patient by a gamma probe, and a mean of 1.9 nodes per patient after a blue dye injection. Microscopic nodal metastases (4 lymph nodes) were confirmed in 12% of the cases previously detected as sentinel lymph nodes. The remaining 419 nodes after pelvic lymphadenectomy (nonsentinel nodes) were histologically negative (100% negative predictive value). Pijpers et al. evaluated the sentinel node procedure in 34 patients after peritumoral injection of 140 MBq of $^{99m}$Tc-colloidal albumin and single blue dye injection before the laparoscopy (47). Lymphoscintigraphy revealed 70 sentinel lymph nodes in 50 basins during dynamic imaging, and 83 sentinel nodes in 63 basins at late imaging. Sentinel lymph nodes were found in 97% of the patients. Among the radioactive lymph nodes resected, 74 were considered sentinel nodes, of them 53 were blue as well. All the resected nodes were examined pathologically at frozen section. In 17 basins of 12 patients, tumor-positive lymph nodes were depicted. Based on sentinel node histology, the authors reported that the treatment has been changed in 9 patients (26%). Data published by Niikura et al. with the combined use of the $^{99m}$Tc-labelled colloid and blue dye on 20 consecutive patients, indicated 46 sentinel lymph nodes were detected (48)—11 sentinel lymph nodes (24%) were detected only through radioactivity, and 2 (4%) were detected only through blue dye. The sensitivity, specificity, and negative predictive value for sentinel lymph node detection were 100%. Angioli et al. obtained favorable results as well by using the radioisotopic tracer alone (49). Thirty-seven patients with stage IB1 tumors were enrolled in this study, and sentinel nodes were identified with preoperative lymphoscintigraphy in 89% of the patients. The intraoperative detection rate was 70%. During surgery, the sentinel lymph node was revealed bilaterally in 31% of the patients; in 15%, 2 sentinel lymph nodes on the same site of the lymphatic vessels were detected. Metastatic sentinel nodes were found in 23% of the patients. There was no case with a positive nonsentinel lymph node in the presence of a negative sentinel node.

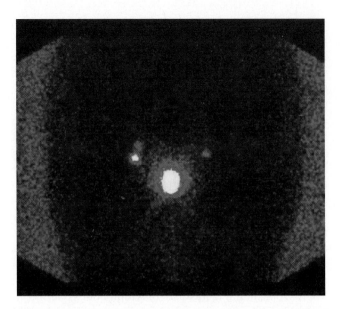

FIGURE 13-2. Late lymphoscintigraphy (static acquisitions) obtained in a patient with cervical cancer, showing visualization of sentinel lymph nodes located in the right (2 nodes) and left (1 node) external iliac regions. Transmission images obtained with a flood source placed beneath the patient help to identify anatomic structures.

The sentinel lymph node procedure in early cervical cancer has confirmed that the main lymphatic drainage from the cervix goes to the external iliac nodes (Figure 13-2); this happens in 60% to 85% of the cases. It is quite rare to find sentinel nodes in the common iliac region (0% to 17%). A limited number of sentinel lymph nodes are reported in the paraaortic region and the inguinal area (43,50). In general, the authors believe the sentinel node procedure is a reliable method to assess the lymph nodal status in early cervical cancer. Niikura analyzed 9 large studies involving 295 patients, and the summarized detection rate was 85% (48). The overall sensitivity, specificity, and negative predictive value were 99%, 100%, and 99%, respectively. These rates are encouraging, in spite of the presence of some isolated cases of false-negative results. Obviously, the false-negative rate is important, since it may influence the frequency of recurrences and patient survival. However, while the number of false-negative findings described worldwide in the clinical experience seems to be low (42,43), Marchiole et al. have reported a considerable number of false-negative findings on 29 consecutive patients treated with pelvic laparoscopy, lymphadenectomy, and radical surgery (51). The incidence of micrometastases was evaluated by multilevel node sectioning and immunohistochemical staining, and the rate of false-negative results was 12%. In addition, some cases have had micrometastases in nonsentinel nodes, even when sentinel nodes were found to be negative for cancer in biopsy. This issue

needs further investigation, specifically in regard to: 1) better standardization of the sentinel lymph node procedure; 2) larger perspective studies; and 3) better definitions of the most correct indications. Thus, while sentinel lymph node biopsy in patients with early stage cervical cancer is feasible and predicts accurately the nodal involvement, currently there is not sufficient evidence that the sentinel lymph node procedure alone can replace pelvic lymphadenectomy.

## Endometrial Cancer

Neoplasia of the uterus is the most common group of gynecologic malignancies. The majority of these diseases consist of epithelial tumors. Endometrial carcinoma is a typical disease of postmenopausal women. The tumor grows in the uterine cavity, and may spread to the endometrial surface and then to the lower uterine segment and cervix. Aggressive cancer invades myometrium and lymphatic vessels. Lymphatic channels draining the fundus join the paraaortic lymph nodes in the upper abdomen, while those from the middle and lower uterus go to the pelvic nodes. A few lymphatic vessels follow the round ligaments to the superficial inguinal nodes (52). This complex network explains how nodal metastases can occur everywhere, and with any combination (both in the pelvic and paraaortic regions). A tumor crossing the serosa may invade the bladder, colon, or adnexa and tumor cell may esfoliate in the peritoneal cavity. The staging of endometrial cancer is performed with surgery. The main prognostic factors are histologic grade, depth of myometrial invasion, tumor spread to adnexal organs, lymph node status, and distant metastases (53).

The management of endometrial cancer at early stages consists of peritoneal cytology, hysterectomy with salpingo-oophorectomy, and lymph node sampling (54). The strategies to evaluate lymph node involvement differ by groups: pelvic lymphadenectomy is recommended by FIGO, while the Gynecological Oncology Group advocates systematic pelvic and paraaortic lymphadenectomy (55). To date, in many centers pelvic lymph node dissection is performed on a routine basis, and paraaortic lymphadenectomy is not systematically carried out (56,57). However, these procedures cannot be applied without risk to patients, considering the high frequency of the side effects, and the characteristics of these patients who are often affected by diabetes or obesity. In addition, in early stage endometrial cancer, the frequency of lymph node metastasis is low and the surgical morbidity is not negligible (58,59).

For these reasons, the feasibility of lymphoscintigraphy and sentinel lymph node biopsy has been assessed in several studies looking for an alternative diagnostic

TABLE 13-3. Relevant clinical experiences with sentinel node procedures in endometrial cancer.

| Author, year, reference | Number of patients | Site of injection | Technique | Sentinel node detection rate (%) | Iliac location of sentinel node (number) | Paraaortic location of sentinel node (number) | False-negative rate (%) |
|---|---|---|---|---|---|---|---|
| Burke et al. 1996 (60) | 15 | SSM | C | 67 | 19 | 12 | 0 |
| Echt et al. 1999 (35) | 8 | SSM | C | 0 | — | — | — |
| Holub et al. 2002 (61) | 13 | SSM | C | 62 | 8 | 0 | |
| | 12 | PC | | 83 | 10 | 0 | |
| Pelosi et al. 2003 (62) | 16 | PC | C and R | 100 | 24 | 0 | 0 |
| Niikura et al. 2004 (63) | 28 | PT | R | 100 | 41 | 30 | 0 |
| Barranger et al. 2003 (64) | 17 | PC | C and R | 100 | 42 | 0 | 0 |
| Raspagliesi et al. 2004 (65) | 18 | PT | C and R | 100 | 41 | 12 | 0 |
| Maccauro et al. 2005 (66) | 26 | PT | C and R | 100 | 48 | 14 | 0 |

Legend:
C—colorimetric method
PC—pericervical injection
PT—peritumoral
R—radioactive method
SSM—subserosal myometrial injection

option to lymphadenectomy and to minimize invasive procedures. Table 13-3 lists the most relevant results obtained by the different authors (60–66).

Burke et al. and Echt et al. used the colorimetric technique with subserosal myometrium injection (60,35). The aim was to determine the feasibility of intraperitoneal lymphatic mapping of the uterine cancer as a tool for identifying target sites for lymph node biopsy during staging laparotomy. Using isosulfan blue dye injected into the subserosal myometrium at 3 sites, Burke et al. were successful in visualizing the sentinel nodes, even if the rate of detection was not elevated. Deposition of dye into identifiable lymph nodes was seen in 10 out of 15 cases (67%), in a total of 31 nodes. The locations of lymph nodes were 12 paraaortic, 6 common iliac, and 13 pelvic sites. Microscopic nodal metastases to sentinel lymph nodes were detected in 2 of 4 women with proven metastatic invasion. Holub et al. used the blue dye, injecting the tracer in subserosal myometrium in 13 patients, and in both subserosal myometrium and pericervical regions in 12 patients (61). The resulting detection rate was better when the injection was performed via the pericervical region.

In the studies of Pelosi et al. and Barranger et al. $^{99m}$Tc-labeled nanocolloid and blue dye were injected in the pericervical regions (62,64). The detection rate was high in these investigations (100%). Pelosi et al. observed 16 consecutive patients with FIGO cancer stage Ib; lymphoscintigraphy and laparoscopically assisted intraoperative sentinel lymph node procedures were performed. In 15 of 16 patients, 24 sentinel lymph nodes were detected at lymphoscintigraphy. The location was only in the internal iliac region, with 6 lymph nodes monolateral and 9 bilateral. In histologic analysis, 3 of the 24 were positive for micrometastases, whereas the remaining 21 were negative. No other surgically dissected lymph nodes revealed metastases. Barranger examined 16 patients with endometrial cancer stage I and 1 patient with stage II who underwent a laparoscopic sentinel node procedure based on combined radiocolloid and patent blue, injected pericervically. The patients had pelvic lymphadenectomy and hysterectomy after the sentinel node procedure. Sentinel lymph nodes were identified in 16 of 17 patients (94.1%). Macrometastases were depicted in 3 sentinel nodes from 2 patients by H&E staining. In 3 other patients, immunohistochemical analysis identified 6 micrometastases in nodes and 1 node with clusters of tumor cells. No false-negative findings were described, and no paraaortic locations were found.

An interesting approach was introduced by Niikura et al. who injected the $^{99m}$Tc-colloid hysteroscopically (63). The authors examined 28 patients with endometrial cancer who underwent total hysterectomy, bilateral salpingo-oophorectomy, or total pelvic lymphadenectomy. Preoperative lymphoscintigraphy was carried out by injecting $^{99m}$Tc-labeled phytate into the endometrium during hysteroscopy. The radiopharmaceutical was dissolved in patent blue and injected the day before surgery into the peritumoral endometrium. The blue dye was not used to detect sentinel nodes, but to check the penetration of the tracer in the subendometrial layer without leakage. This procedure allowed detection of at least 1 sentinel node (82%) in 23 of the 28 patients. Sentinel nodes were identified in 21 of 22 patients (95%) whose tumor did not penetrate more than 50% of the myometrium wall. Radioactive lymph nodes were described in the paraaortic area in 18 patients. The

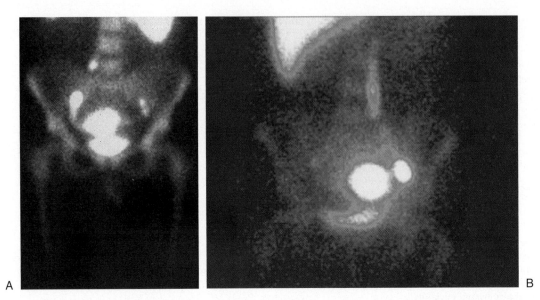

FIGURE 13-3. Late lymphoscintigraphy (static acquisitions) obtained in 2 patients with endometrial cancer. Rich blood vascularity of the endometrium results in early systemic passage of an important fraction of the radiocolloid injected interstitially, with ensuing visualization of the overall reticulo-endothelial system (bone marrow, liver, and spleen). Although this relatively high radioactivity background can interfere with intraoperative gamma counting for sentinel lymph node localization, the outline of the body structures helps to identify the location of the nodes in preoperative imaging. (A) Visualization of sentinel lymph nodes in the right and left internal iliac regions and in the right paraaortic region. (B) Visualization of sentinel lymph nodes in the right and left external iliac regions and in the left paraaortic region.

overall accuracy in detecting lymph node metastases was 100%. In 2 consecutive studies, our group at the National Tumor Institute (Istituto Nazionale Tumori) in Milan demonstrated the feasibility of the sentinel lymph node technique by peritumoral tracer injection (65,66). Maccauro et al. observed 26 women who had hysteroscopic injection of 111 MBq of $^{99m}$Tc-labeled nanocolloid and blue dye administered subendometrially around the tumor. On the same day, each patient underwent lymphoscintigraphy (Figure 13-3), followed 3 to 4 hours later by a hysterectomy with bilateral salpingo-oophorectomy and pelvic lymphadenectomy. Paraaortic lymphadenectomy was also performed in cases of papillary carcinoma (7 of 26 patients). All sentinel lymph nodes were removed and examined with H&E and immunohistochemical techniques. The sensitivity of this technique was 100%: lymph node metastases were found in 4 out of the 26 patients (15%)—bilaterally in the external iliac region (1 patient), unilaterally in the external iliac region (1 patient), unilaterally in the common iliac region (1 patient), and unilaterally in the paraaortic region (1 patient). In all 4 cases, metastases were located within sentinel nodes detected by lymphoscintigraphy. Only 10 of the 26 patients had significant blue dye staining. All blue-stained lymph nodes were radioactive. This experience shows that in patients with endometrial cancer, lymphatic mapping and sentinel lymph node biopsy can define the topographic distribution of the lymphatic network and also accurately detect lombo-aortic and pelvic metastasis within sentinel nodes. These findings suggest that this procedure is feasible and can be useful in choosing the best management strategy of endometrial cancer.

## Conclusions

Examining the data published in the literature and considering our institutional experience, we conclude that the sentinel lymph node procedure allows the selective targeting of the first draining node, in which the initial metastasis will arise. A negative sentinel lymph node indicates a high probability of an absence of metastases in the regional lymph nodes. There is no doubt that this procedure is useful for sentinel node sampling, and the combined use of lymphoscintigraphy with a gamma probe, whether or not associated with blue dye, is one of the most interesting staging procedures available in surgical oncology. The main unresolved issue is whether this procedure can substitute for surgery in preoperative staging, thus avoiding lymph node dissection in early gynecological cancer. Our opinion is that this concept is close to being introduced into clinical practice for vulvar cancer; however, further study is required to evaluate the validity of the technique for cervical and endometrial cancers.

# References

1. Levenback C. Intraoperative lymphatic mapping and sentinel node identification: gynaecologic applications. *Recent Results Cancer Res.* 2000;157:150–158.

2. Zambo K, Koppan M, Paal A, Schmidt E, Tinneberg HR, Bodis J. Sentinel lymph nodes in gynaecological malignancies: frontline between TNM and clinical staging system? *Eur J Nucl Med Mol Imaging.* 2003;30:1684–1688.

3. Barranger E, Darai E. Lymphatic mapping for gynaecologic malignancies. *Semin Oncol.* 2004;31:392–402.

4. Scheidler J, Hricak H, Yu KK, Subak L, Segal MR. Radiological evaluation of lymph node metastases in patients with cervical cancer. A meta-analysis. *JAMA.* 1997;278:1096–1101.

5. Grahek D, Barranger E, Darai E, Uzan S, Talbot JN. Role of [$^{18}$F]-fluorodeoxyglucose positron emission tomography for the initial detection, staging, search for recurrences and restaging of gynecological and breast cancers. *Gynecol Obstet Fertil.* 2005;33:371–381.

6. Paganelli G, De Cicco C, Chinol M. Sentinel node localization by lymphoscintigraphy: a reliable technique with widespread applications. *Recent Results Cancer Res.* 2000;157:121–129.

7. Morton DL, Wen DR, Wong JH, et al. Technical details of intraoperative lymphatic mapping for early stage melanoma. *Arch Surg.* 1992;127:392–399.

8. Binder SW, Huang I, Fu YS, Hacker NF, Berek JS. Risk factors for the development of lymph node metastasis in vulvar squamous cell carcinoma. *Gynecol Oncol.* 1990;37:9–16.

9. Homesley HD, Bundy BN, Sedlis A, et al. Assessment of current International Federation of Gynecology and Obstetrics staging of vulvar carcinoma relative to prognostic factors for survival (a Gynecologic Oncology Group study). *Am J Obstet Gynecol.* 1991;164:997–1003; discussion 1003–1004.

10. Levenback C, Burke TW, Gershenson DM, Morris M, Malpica A, Ross MI. Intraoperative lymphatic mapping for vulvar cancer. *Obstet Gynecol.* 1994;84:163–167.

11. Levenback C, Burke TW, Morris M, Malpica A, Lucas KR, Gershenson DM. Potential applications of intraoperative lymphatic mapping in vulvar cancer. *Gynecol Oncol* 1995;59:216–220.

12. Levenback C, Coleman RL, Burke TW, Bodurka-Bevers D, Wolf JK, Gershenson DM. Intraoperative lymphatic mapping and sentinel node identification with blue dye in patients with vulvar cancer. *Gynecol Oncol.* 2001;83:276–281.

13. Ansink AC, Sie-Go DM, van der Velden J, et al. Identification of sentinel lymph nodes in vulvar carcinoma patients with the aid of a patent blue V injection: a multicenter study. *Cancer.* 1999;86:652–656.

14. De Hullu JA, Doting E, Piers DA, et al. Sentinel lymph node identification with technetium-99m-labeled nanocolloid in squamous cell cancer of the vulva. *J Nucl Med.* 1998;39:1381–1385.

15. Decesare SL, Fiorica JV, Roberts WS, et al. A pilot study utilizing intraoperative lymphoscintigraphy for identifica-

tion of the sentinel lymph nodes in vulvar cancer. *Gynecol Oncol.* 1997;66:425–428.

16. Sideri M, De Cicco C, Maggioni A, et al. Detection of sentinel nodes by lymphoscintigraphy and gamma probe guided surgery in vulvar neoplasia. *Tumori.* 2000;86:359–363.

17. De Cicco C, Sideri M, Bartolomei M, et al. Sentinel node biopsy in early vulvar cancer. *Br J Cancer.* 2000;82:295–299.

187. Molpus KL, Kelley MC, Johnson JE, Martin WH, Jones HW 3rd. Sentinel lymph node detection and microstaging in vulvar carcinoma. *J Reprod Med.* 2001;46:863–869.

19. Tavares MG, Sapienza MT, Galeb NA Jr, et al. The use of $^{99m}$Tc-phytate for sentinel node mapping in melanoma, breast cancer and vulvar cancer: a study of 100 cases. *Eur J Nucl Med.* 2001;28:1597–1604.

20. Terada KY, Shimizu DM, Wong JH. Sentinel node dissection and ultrastaging in squamous cell cancer of the vulva. *Gynecol Oncol.* 2000;76:40–44.

21. De Hullu JA, Hollema H, Piers DA, et al. Sentinel lymph node procedure is highly accurate in squamous cell carcinoma of the vulva. *J Clin Oncol.* 2000;18:2811–2816.

22. Sliutz G, Reinthaller A, Lantzsch T, et al. Lymphatic mapping of sentinel nodes in early vulvar cancer. *Gynecol Oncol.* 2002;84:449–452.

23. Zambo K, Schmidt E, Hartmann T, et al. Preliminary experiences with sentinel lymph node detection in cases of vulvar malignancy. *Eur J Nucl Med Mol Imaging.* 2002;29:1198–1200.

24. Puig-Tintore LM, Ordi J, Vidal-Sicart S, et al. Further data on the usefulness of sentinel lymph node identification and ultrastaging in vulvar squamous cell carcinoma. *Gynecol Oncol.* 2003;88:29–34.

25. Moore RG, Granai CO, Gajewski W, Gordinier M, Steinhoff MM. Pathologic evaluation of inguinal sentinel lymph nodes in vulvar cancer patients: a comparison of immunohistochemical staining versus ultrastaging with hematoxylin and eosin staining. *Gynecol Oncol.* 2003;91:378–382.

26. Merisio C, Berretta R, Gualdi M, et al. Radioguided sentinel lymph node detection in vulvar cancer. *Int J Gynecol Cancer.* 2005;15:493–497.

27. Raspagliesi F, Ditto A, Fontanelli R, et al. False-negative sentinel node in patients with vulvar cancer: a case study. *Int J Gynecol Cancer.* 2003;13:361–363.

28. Plante M, Renaud MC, Roy M. Sentinel node evaluation in gynecologic cancer. *Oncology (Williston Park, N. Y.).* 2004;18:75–87.

29. Plentl AA, Friedman EA. Lymphatics of the cervix. In: *Lymphatic System of the Female Genitalia.* Philadelphia: WB Saunders; 1971:75.

30. Averette HE, Nguyen HN, Donato DM, et al. Radical hysterectomy for invasive cervical cancer. A 25-year prospective experience with the Miami technique. *Cancer.* 1993;71:1422–1437.

31. Inoue T, Chihara T, Morita K. The prognostic significance of the size of the largest nodes in metastatic carcinoma from the uterine cervix. *Gynecol Oncol.* 1984;19:187–193.

32. Landoni F, Maneo A, Colombo A, et al. Randomized study of radical surgery versus radiotherapy for stage Ib-IIa cervical cancer. *Lancet.* 1997;350:535–540.

33. Sakuragi N, Satoh C, Takeda N, et al. Incidence and distribution pattern of pelvic and para-aortic lymph node metastasis in patients with Stages IB, IIA, and IIB cervical carcinoma treated with radical hysterectomy. *Cancer.* 1999;85:1547–1554.

34. Lecuru F, Taurelle R. Transperitoneal laparoscopic pelvic lymphadenectomy for gynecologic malignancies (I). Technique and results. *Surg Endosc.* 1998;12:1–6.

35. Echt ML, Finan MA, Hoffman MS, Kline RC, Roberts WS, Fiorica JV. Detection of sentinel lymph nodes with Lymphazurin in cervical, uterine, and vulvar malignancies. *South Med J.* 1999;92:204–208.

36. Medl M, Peters-Engl C, Schutz P, Vesely M, Sevelda P. First report of lymphatic mapping with isosulfan blue dye and sentinel node biopsy in cervical cancer. *Anticancer Res.* 2000;20:1133–1134.

37. O'Boyle JD, Coleman RL, Bernstein SG, Lifshitz S, Muller CY, Miller DS. Intraoperative lymphatic mapping in cervix cancer patients undergoing radical hysterectomy: a pilot study. *Gynecol Oncol.* 2000;79:238–243.

38. Dargent D, Martin X, Mathevet P. Laparoscopic assessment of the sentinel lymph node in early stage cervical cancer. *Gynecol Oncol.* 2000;79:411–415.

39. Kamprath S, Possover M, Schneider A. Laparoscopic sentinel lymph node detection in patients with cervical cancer. *Am J Obstet Gynecol.* 2000;182:1648.

40. Lantzsch T, Wolters M, Grimm J, et al. Sentinel node procedure in Ib cervical cancer: a preliminary series. *Br J Cancer.* 2001;14:791–794.

41. Verheijen RH, Pijpers R, van Diest PJ, Burger CW, Buist MR, Kenemans P. Sentinel node detection in cervical cancer. *Obstet Gynecol.* 2000;96:135–138.

42. Malur S, Krause N, Kohler C, Schneider A. Sentinel lymph node detection in patients with cervical cancer. *Gynecol Oncol.* 2001;80:254–257.

43. Levenback C, Coleman RL, Burke TW, et al. Lymphatic mapping and sentinel node identification in patients with cervix cancer undergoing radical hysterectomy and pelvic lymphadenectomy. *J Clin Oncol.* 2002;20:688–693.

44. Barranger E, Grahek D, Cortez A, Talbot JN, Uzan S, Darai E. Laparoscopic sentinel lymph node procedure using a combination of patent blue and radioisotope in women with cervical carcinoma. *Cancer.* 2003;97:3003–3009.

45. Chung YA, Kim SH, Sohn HS, Chung SK, Rhim CC, Namkoong SE. Usefulness of lymphoscintigraphy and intraoperative gamma probe detection in the identification of sentinel nodes in cervical cancer. *Eur J Nucl Med Mol Imaging.* 2003;30:1014–1017.

46. Martinez-Palones JM, Gil-Moreno A, Perez-Benavente MA, Roca I, Xercavins J. Intraoperative sentinel node identification in early stage cervical cancer using a combination of radiolabeled albumin injection and isosulfan blue dye injection. *Gynecol Oncol.* 2004;92:845–850.

47. Pijpers R, Buist MR, van Lingen A, et al. The sentinel node in cervical cancer: scintigraphy and laparoscopic gamma probe-guided biopsy. *Eur J Nucl Med Mol Imaging.* 2004;31:1479–1486.

48. Niikura H, Okamura C, Akahira J, et al. Sentinel lymph node detection in early cervical cancer with combination 99mTc phytate and patent blue. *Gynecol Oncol.* 2004;94:528–532.

49. Angioli R, Palaia I, Cipriani C, et al. Role of sentinel lymph node biopsy procedure in cervical cancer: a critical point of view. *Gynecol Oncol.* 2005;96:504–509.

50. Hauspy J, Verkinderen L, De Pooter C, Dirix LY, van Dam PA. Sentinel node metastasis in the groin detected by technetium-labeled nanocolloid in a patient with cervical cancer. *Gynecol Oncol.* 2002; 86:358–360.

51. Marchiole P, Buenerd A, Scoazec JY, Dargent D, Mathevet P. Sentinel lymph node biopsy is not accurate in predicting lymph node status for patients with cervical carcinoma. *Cancer.* 2004;100:2154–2159.

52. Larson DM, Johnson K, Olson KA. Pelvic and para-aortic lymphadenectomy for surgical staging of endometrial cancer: morbidity and mortality. *Obstet Gynecol.* 1992;79: 998–1001.

53. DiSaia PJ, Creasman WT, Boronow RC, Blessing JA. Risk factors and recurrent patterns in Stage I endometrial cancer. *Am J Obstet Gynecol.* 1985;151:1009–1015.

54. Annual report on the results of treatment in gynecologic cancer. *Int J Gynecol Obstet.* 1989;28:189–190.

55. American Joint Committee on Cancer. In: *Manual for Staging of Cancer.* Philadelphia: Lippincott; 1992:155–157.

56. Belinson Jl, Lee KR, Badger GJ, Pretorius RG, Jarrell MA. Clinical stage I adenocarcinoma of the endometrium—analysis of recurrences and the potential benefit of staging lymphadenectomy. *Gynecol Oncol.* 1992; 44:17–23.

57. Benedetti Panici Pl, Scambia G, Baiocchi G, Greggi S, Mancuso S. Technique and feasibility of radical para-aortic and pelvic lymphadenectomy for gynecologic malignancies: a prospective study. *Int Gynecol Cancer.* 1991;1: 133–140.

58. Corn BW, Lanciano RM, Greven KM, et al. Impact of improved irradiation technique, age, and lymph node sampling on the severe complication rate of surgically staged endometrial cancer patients: a multivariate analysis. *J Clin Oncol.* 1994;12:510–515.

59. Arduino S, Leo L, Febo G, Tessarolo M, Wierdis T, Lanza A. Complications of pelvic and para-aortic lymphadenectomy in patients with endometrial cancer. *Eur J Gynecol Oncol.* 1997;18:208–210.

60. Burke TW, Levenback C, Tornos C, Morris M, Wharton JT, Gershenson DM. Intra-abdominal lymphatic mapping to direct selective pelvic and para-aortic lymphadenectomy in women with high-risk endometrial cancer: results of a pilot study. *Gynecol Oncol.* 1996;62:169–173.

61. Holub Z, Jabor A, Kliment L. Comparison of 2 procedures for sentinel lymph node detection in patients with endometrial cancer: a pilot study. *Eur J Gynaecol Oncol.* 2002;23:53–57.

62. Pelosi E, Arena V, Baudino B, et al. Pre-operative lymphatic mapping and intra-operative sentinel lymph node detection in early stage endometrial cancer. *Nucl Med Commun.* 2003;24:971–975.

63. Niikura H, Okamura C, Utsunomiya H, et al. Sentinel lymph node detection in patients with endometrial cancer. *Gynecol Oncol.* 2004;92:669–674.

64. Barranger E, Grahek D, Cortez A, Talbot JN, Uzan S, Darai E. Laparoscopic sentinel lymph node procedure using a combination of patent blue and radioisotope in women with cervical carcinoma. *Cancer.* 2003;97:3003–3009.

65. Raspagliesi F, Ditto A, Kusamura S, et al. Hysteroscopic injection of tracers in sentinel node detection of endometrial cancer: a feasibility study. *Am J Obstet Gynecol.* 2004;191:435–439.

66. Maccauro M, Lucignani G, Aliberti G. Sentinel lymph node detection following the hysteroscopic peritumoral injection of [99m]Tc-labelled albumin nanocolloids in endometrial cancer. *Eur J Nucl Med Mol Imaging.* 2005;32:569–74.

# 14
# Sentinel Lymph Node Biopsy in Cancers of the Gastrointestinal Tract

Yuko Kitagawa, Sukamal Saha, and Masaki Kitajima

Despite the significant clinical contribution of the sentinel lymph node concept to the effective treatment in melanoma and breast cancer (1,2), most surgeons have reserved judgment on its applicability to upper gastrointestinal (GI) malignancies (3,4), mainly due to multidirectional lymphatic flow from the gastrointestinal tract and the widespread and random patterns of lymph node metastasis in GI malignancies. Anatomic skip metastases were found in 50% to 60% of esophageal cancers and 20% to 30% of gastric cancers in a retrospective analysis of the location of solitary metastases (5,6). Sano et al. reported that the perigastric nodal area close to the primary tumor is the first site of metastasis in only 62% of gastric cancers, based on a retrospective analysis of cases of solitary metastasis (7). In cases of lower rectal cancer, a relatively high incidence of lateral lymph node metastasis, including skip metastasis, has been reported (8). Based on these clinical observations, extended radical procedures such as esophagectomy with 3-field lymph node dissection, gastrectomy with D2 lymphadenectomy, and extended lymphadenectomy with lateral node dissection for rectal cancer have become standard surgical treatment in Japan, even for clinically node negative cases (9–11). However, randomized trials (12,13) have demonstrated a significant increase in morbidity and mortality with such aggressive procedures. To minimize the morbidity and mortality of the surgery, it may be possible to use information from sentinel lymph node biopsy to modify the surgical procedure.

Lymph node involvement is one of the most important prognostic factors in gastrointestinal cancers and assists in the planning of multimodality treatment. The clinical significance of the sentinel lymph node as a reliable diagnostic indicator in colorectal cancer has been reported previously (14,15).

The utility of sentinel lymph node mapping in GI cancers is related to: (1) the incidence of metastasis in relatively early-stage (cT1-T2) disease; (2) the anatomic distribution of sentinel lymph nodes and the target organs; and (3) the feasibility of function-preserving surgery. This chapter presents the technical aspects, current status, and clinical applications of sentinel lymph node mapping in gastrointestinal cancer.

## Sentinel Lymph Node Mapping for Gastric Cancer

In the past 5 years, several single institutional studies have described the value of the sentinel lymph node concept in patients with gastric cancer (Table 14-1) (16). Unexpected skip metastases might be accounted for by aberrant drainage from the primary lesion. In cases of gastric cancer, 5% to 10% of sentinel lymph nodes are located in the second compartment and not in the perigastric nodes, i.e., the first compartment. In our experience, sentinel lymph node mapping identifies these cases. Lymphatic drainage routes from the lower stomach are relatively complicated; the distribution of sentinel lymph nodes is unique to each patient and is not predictable without actual lymphatic mapping.

As with sentinel lymph node mapping of other organs, the reliability of the procedure must be confirmed by multicenter prospective clinical trials. Two major well-designed large-scale clinical trials of sentinel node mapping for gastric cancer for open surgery have been initiated in Japan. The Gastric Cancer Surgical Study Group of the Japan Clinical Oncology Group (JCOG) has organized a multicenter prospective study of sentinel lymph node mapping with the dye-guided method, using subserosal injection of indocyanine green. The Japan Society of Sentinel Node Navigation Surgery (SNNS) is also conducting a multicenter prospective trial of sentinel lymph node mapping, using both blue dye and radioactive colloid. The results of these clinical trials should provide information on the value of this procedure for gastric cancer. If the JCOG study reveals favorable results in terms of false-negative rates, the dye-guided

TABLE 14-1. Single institutional results of sentinel lymph node mapping for gastric cancer.

| Author | Year and Publication | Method | Total | Detection rate | Sensitivity |
|---|---|---|---|---|---|
| Kitagawa et al. | 2000, *Surg Clin N Am* | RI | 36 | 97% | 100% |
| Hiratsuka et al. | 2001, *Surgery* | Dye | 77 | 99% | 90% |
| Yasuda et al. | 2001, *Tokai J Exp Clin Med* | RI | 26 | 100% | 82% |
| Ichikura et al. | 2002, *World J Surg* | Dye | 62 | 100% | 85% |
| Kitagawa et al. | 2002, *Br J Surg* | RI | 145 | 95% | 92% |
| Carlini et al. | 2002, *J Exp Clin Cancer Res* | Dye | 40 | 100% | 87% |
| Hayashi et al. | 2003, *J Am Coll Surg* | RI + Dye | 31 | 100% | 100% |
| Miwa et al. | 2003, *Br J Surg* | Dye | 211 | 96.2% | 89% |
| Gretschel et al. | 2003, *Chirurg* | RI | 15 | 93% | 89% |
| Yasuda et al. | 2003, *Jpn J Clin Oncol* | RI | 21 | 100% | 100% |
| Tonouchi et al. | 2003, *Dig Surg* | RI + Dye | 17 | 100% | 100% |
| Simsa et al. | 2003, *Acta Chir Belg* | Dye | 22 | 100% | 56% |
| Ryu et al. | 2003, *Eur J Surg Oncol* | Dye | 71 | 92% | 100% |
| Kim et al. | 2003, *Hepatogastroenterology* | RI | 22 | 91% | 82.2% |
| Song et al. | 2004, *Am J Surg* | Dye | 27 | 96% | 100% |
| Nimura et al. | 2004, *Br J Surg* | Dye | 84 | 99% | 100% |
| Karube et al. | 2004, *J Surg Oncol* | RI + Dye | 41 | 100% | 92% |
| Kim et al. | 2004, *Ann Surg* | RI | 46 | 93.5% | 84.6% |
| Osaka et al. | 2004, *Clin Cancer Res* | Dye | 57 | 100% | 100% |

Legend:

RI—radioisotopic.

*Source:* Kitagawa et al., 2005 (16), by permission.

method will become routine practice for open surgery in a wide range of institutions. If not, introduction of the radioguided method may be considered, or further technical improvements may be added, even for open surgery. If the SNNS study demonstrates acceptable detection rates and low false-negative rates, the next step would be to conduct a feasibility study of laparoscopic sentinel lymph node mapping for gastric cancer. Since there are several remaining technical issues, we are in a transitional phase to the clinical applications.

As with other solid tumors, the dual tracer method using radioactive colloid and dye is recommended for detection of sentinel lymph nodes in gastric cancer. The type of dye, the injection routes (submucosal or subserosal), the tracer volume, and the observation timing (17) are issues that need to be standardized. The current protocol of sentinel lymph node mapping for gastric cancer using the dual tracer method in Keio University Hospital is presented in Table 14-2 (17).

## Indication

Cases with clinically apparent lymph node metastasis should be excluded, because the purpose of this technique is to identify clinically undetectable lymph node involvement. Clinical T3 and T4 tumors, in which original lymphatic drainage routes might be obstructed and altered, are also excluded. Clinical T1 or T2 tumors with primary lesion diameter of <4 cm would be suitable, for which modified resection could be applicable in cases of negative sentinel lymph node status. Further exclusion criteria, such as histologic types, require analysis based on prospective multicenter trials.

## Injection of Radioactive Tracer

In initial pilot studies, we chose to inject $^{99m}$Tc-tin colloid, which has a relatively large particle size. In our experience, tin colloid migrates into the sentinel lymph nodes within 2 hours and remains there for more than 20 hours

TABLE 14-2. Current protocol for sentinel lymph node mapping for gastric cancer using the dual-tracer method (Keio University Hospital).

***Indication:***
cT1 N0 M0 (single lesion, no previous treatments)
Diameter of primary lesion < 4 cm
***Radioguided method***
Tracer: $^{99m}$Tc-tin colloid (0.3 mCi at the time of surgery)
Administration of tracer: endoscopic submucosal injection 0.5 mL × 4 points
Timing of administration: day before surgery
Sentinel lymph node detection: Gamma probing (Navigator, Tyco Health Care, Japan)
***Dye-guided method***
Tracer: 1% isosulfan blue (Lymphazurin, Tyco Health Care, Japan)
Administration of tracer: endoscopic submucosal injection 0.5 mL × 4 points
Timing of administration: intraoperative
Sentinel lymph node detection: blue node identification within 15 minutes

*Source:* Kitagawa et al., 2005 (17), modified by permission of Wiley-Liss, Inc. a subsidiary of John Wiley & Sons, Inc.

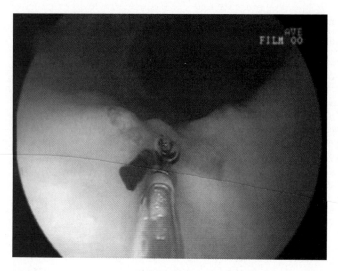

FIGURE 14-1. Endoscopic injection of the radioactive tracer into the submucosal layer of the lesion in a case of early gastric cancer.

through phagocytosis by macrophages. The day before surgery, $^{99m}$Tc-tin colloid solution in a volume of 2 mL (150 MBq) is injected in 4 quadrants into the submucosal layer of the primary lesion, using an endoscopic puncture needle (Figure 14-1). Endoscopic injection enables us to perform accurate injection of the tracer.

## Intraoperative Detection of the Sentinel Lymph Node

For intraoperative detection, the gastrocolic ligament should be divided to visualize all possible directions of lymphatic flow from the stomach. Blue dye (1% isosulfan blue) is injected using intraoperative endoscopy, in exactly the same manner used for the preoperative injection of the radioactive tracer. For cT1 N0 gastric cancer, the primary lesion is not always palpable from the serosal side, and accurate injection of tracer particles is not easy with the subserosal approach. Within 15 minutes, blue lymphatic vessels and nodes can be detected. Although there are limitations to the dye-directed method, such as the fast transit of the dye and blind sites in dense fat, blue dye is useful for visualizing the lymphatic vessels. At the same time, a handheld gamma probe is used to locate the radioactive sentinel lymph node. Intraoperative gamma probing is also feasible in thoracoscopic or laparoscopic surgery, using a special gamma detector introducible from a trocar port. Technical errors that appear using a single agent approach are reduced by adding a second approach for lymphatic mapping. The radioguided method allows confirmation of the complete harvest of sentinel lymph nodes by gamma probe, while the blue dye procedure permits real-time observation of the visu-

alized lymphatic vessels. Thus, we recommend a combination of visible tracer and radioguided methods for systematic lymphatic mapping of gastric cancer.

## Sentinel Lymph Node Sampling

Generally, 2 types of sentinel lymph node sampling procedures for gastric cancer have been described. The pickup method is a well-established, simple method already used for breast cancer and melanoma (18). Sentinel lymphatic basin dissection is a focused lymph node dissection of hot and blue nodes (Figure 14-2). Prior reports have demonstrated that sentinel lymphatic basins contained truly positive nodes, even in cases with false-negative sentinel node biopsy results (19).

## Clinical Applications

Clinically, T1 N0 gastric cancer is a good place to start to try to modify the therapeutic approach. From the data reported in the literature, micrometastases tend to be limited within the sentinel lymph basins for this cancer, so the basins are good targets for selective lymphadenectomy for patients with potential risk of micrometastasis. As indicated in Figure 14-3 (17), patients with positive sentinel lymph nodes after selective dissection of sentinel basins can be treated with conventional radical surgery. Furthermore, laparoscopic local resection is theoretically feasible for curative treatment of sentinel lymph node-negative early gastric cancer (20). In Japan, clinical applications of this novel, minimally invasive approach could have a great impact on patient care for gastric cancer, because 60% to 70% of gastric cancer cases treated in major institutions belong to this category.

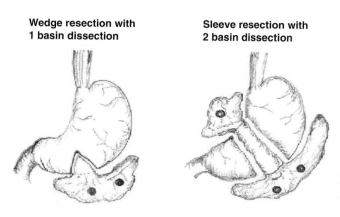

**Wedge resection with 1 basin dissection**

**Sleeve resection with 2 basin dissection**

FIGURE 14-2. Function-preserving surgery for gastric cancer using sentinel lymph node basin dissection. (Reprinted from Kitagawa et al., 2005 [17], with permission from Wiley-Liss, Inc. a subsidiary of John Wiley & Sons, Inc.)

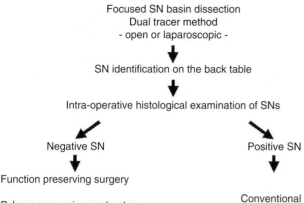

FIGURE 14-3. An individualized surgical approach for early gastric cancer based on sentinel node biopsy (SN = sentinel lymph node). (From Kitagawa Y, et al. Recent advances in sentinel node navigation for gastric cancer: a paradigm shift of surgical management. J Surg Oncol 2005;90:147–52. Reprinted with permission from Wiley-Liss, Inc. a subsidiary of John Wiley & Sons, Inc. [17].)

## Sentinel Lymph Node Mapping for Esophageal Cancer

Sentinel lymph node mapping for esophageal cancer is relatively more complicated than that for gastric cancer. Often, the dye-guided method is not feasible here, because frequently regional lymph nodes of the thoracic esophagus are pigmented by anthracosis, and it is difficult to identify the blue nodes. In organs such as the esophagus and rectum, real-time observation of the lymphatic route using dye is impossible without operative mobilization of the primary site; however, the mobilization destroys the active lymphatic flow from the primary lesion. For these reasons, the radioguided method has been preferred for sentinel node mapping in esophageal cancer.

Only a few studies have demonstrated the feasibility and validity of the sentinel lymph node concept in esophageal cancer (21,22); in Western countries, the number of early-stage esophageal cancers is limited, so it is difficult to perform clinical studies. In esophageal cancer, sentinel lymph nodes are multiple and widely spread, from the cervical to abdominal areas. In more than 80% of the cases, at least 1 sentinel lymph node is located in the second or third compartment of regional lymph nodes (21). This characteristic distribution of sentinel nodes is attributed to the multidirectional lymphatic drainage routes from the esophagus. It is essential that multicentric validation studies for sentinel lymph node mapping for esophageal cancer be planned and conducted.

## Injection of Radioactive Tracer

The procedure for preoperative endoscopic injection of radioactive tracer is basically the same as that described for gastric cancer. The day before surgery, $^{99m}$Tc-tin colloid solution in a volume of 2 mL (150 MBq) is injected in 4 quadrants in the submucosal layer of the primary lesion, using an endoscopic puncture needle.

## Lymphoscintigraphy

Preoperative lymphoscintigraphy, taken 3 hours after tracer injection, is useful in detecting sentinel lymph nodes in unexpected sites distant from the primary esophageal cancer lesion (Figure 14-4). The distribution of sentinel lymph nodes in esophageal cancer is wide, ranging from the cervical to the abdominal areas, and preoperative lymphoscintigraphy is essential for sentinel lymph node sampling.

## Intraoperative Sentinel Lymph Node Sampling

Sentinel lymph nodes located in the cervical area can be identified through percutaneous gamma probing. These nodes can be resected by a less invasive procedure. As in gastric cancers, laparoscopic detection and sampling of abdominal sentinel lymph nodes is feasible. However, sampling of mediastinal sentinel lymph nodes is complicated and invasive, because mobilization of the thoracic esophagus is required. In addition, shine-through from the primary lesion is also an obstacle for gamma probing here.

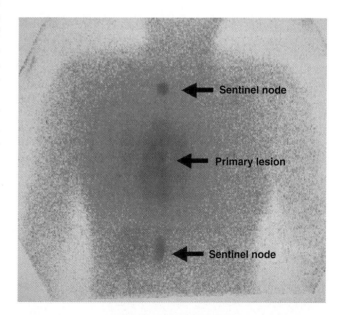

FIGURE 14-4. Preoperative lymphoscintigram of patient with thoracic esophageal cancer.

## Clinical Applications

Metastatic status of regional lymph nodes is an important prognostic factor in patients with esophageal cancer. Ando et al. reported a randomized trial of postoperative adjuvant chemotherapy with cisplatin and fluorouracil (5FU) versus surgery alone (23); there was a reduction in relapse rates in esophageal carcinoma patients who underwent adjuvant chemotherapy compared to surgery alone, particularly in those with lymph node metastasis. Therefore, detection of micrometastasis in lymph nodes is clinically important for patients with esophageal cancer.

Although a number of studies report underestimation of micrometastasis in regional lymph nodes using conventional staging procedures, the application of intensive examinations, such as step sectioning, immunohistochemistry, and reverse transcription-polymerase chain reaction (RT-PCR), for all resected lymph nodes is not practical. A focused examination of sentinel lymph nodes may help resolve this issue.

## Selective Lymphadenectomy Based on Sentinel Lymph Node Status

Transthoracic extended esophagectomy with 3-field radical lymph node dissection has been a standard procedure in Japan for thoracic esophageal cancer because of its widely spread and unpredictable metastatic patterns (9). The indications of upper mediastinal lymph node dissection for cervical esophageal cancer and of lower mediastinal lymph node dissection for abdominal esophageal cancer are controversial. Sentinel lymph node mapping would provide significant information for an individualized selective lymphadenectomy, based on node status.

Unlike that in breast cancer, complete sampling of multiple and widespread sentinel lymph nodes in esophageal cancer is not minimally invasive. At present, local resection of the primary lesion of esophageal cancer with negative sentinel lymph node is not practical. However, selective and modified lymphadenectomy targeted on sentinel basins for clinically N0 esophageal cancer should become feasible and clinically useful; in our experience, clinically undetectable micrometastases in cT1 N0 esophageal cancer tend to be limited within sentinel basins. Although 3-field lymph node dissection is recognized as an extensive and curative procedure for thoracic esophageal cancer, its prognostic significance is still controversial, and uniform application of this highly invasive procedure could increase the morbidity and reduce quality of life after surgery. Therefore, individualized selective lymphadenectomy for cN0 esophageal cancer patients based on sentinel lymph node status seems to be a reasonable surgical approach (24). The incidence of carcinoma of the esophagogastric junction, including Barrett carcinoma, has been on the rise in Western countries and more recently in Japan, and several surgical approaches exist for it (25). Individualized resection and lymph node dissection for Barrett carcinoma based on lymphatic mapping will become an important topic in surgical oncology for the upper GI tract, as shown in Figure 14-5 (26).

## Nonsurgical Approaches

Recently, chemoradiotherapy has attracted attention as a multidisciplinary curative treatment for cT1 N0 esophageal cancer. Although an acceptable effect on local control has been reported in this approach, distant lymph node recurrence in the area outside of the irradiation field is a serious problem in long-term observations. In

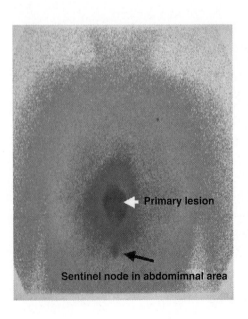

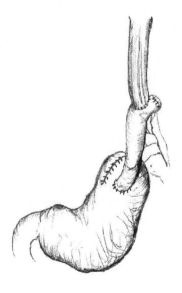

FIGURE 14-5. Modified surgery for adenocarcinoma of esophagogastic junction based on the sentinel lymph node concept. Limited proximal gastrectomy with jejunal interposition can be applied in the case of negative abdominal sentinel node. (Reprinted with permission from Kitagawa Y, et al. Sentinel lymph node mapping in esophogeal and gastric cancer. Cancer treatment research, selective sentinel lymphadenectomy for human solid cancer. Leong S, Kitagawa M, eds. Springer Science, NY, USA 123-139, 2005.)

FIGURE 14-6. Individualized irradiation field for patients with cT1 N0 esophageal cancer based on the distribution of sentinel lymph nodes.

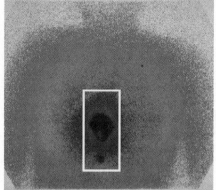
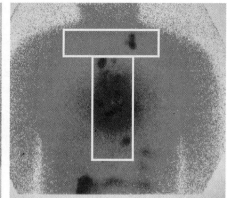

this approach, control of micrometastases is essential. Lymphoscintigrams revealing the distribution of sentinel nodes are useful in designing the field of irradiation in each individual case. Currently, we are performing curative chemoradiotherapy for cT1 N0 esophageal cancer patients with an individualized irradiation field, instead of long T-type uniform irradiation fields (Figure 14-6).

## Sentinel Lymph Node Mapping for Colon Cancer

Since the first reported feasibility study in 1997, there have been numerous publications validating sentinel lymph node mapping as a highly accurate and powerful upstaging technique for colorectal cancers (27–32). Studies have also evaluated the usefulness of various tracers, such as Fluorescein and $^{99m}$Tc-sulphur colloid, used either in combination or individually, and explored new techniques such as laparoscopic, ex-vivo, and minimally invasive approaches to sentinel lymph node mapping for colorectal tumors.

Recently, a poorly designed multicenter prospective trial for sentinel lymph node staging in colorectal cancer was published with disappointing results (33) (a false-negative rate of 54%). Inappropriate criteria that included patients with advanced tumors and technical errors in the initial learning phase among participating institutes with limited experience may have contributed to this discouraging result. At present, an international prospective clinical trial is ongoing, including leading institutions from all over the world.

### Dye-Guided Method

The dye-guided method using intraoperative subserosal injection is popular as a procedure for detecting sentinel lymph nodes in colon cancer. At the time of laparotomy, the location of the tumor is identified either manually by palpation, or visually by recognizing the endoscopic tat-

tooing in patients who underwent polypectomy during colonoscopy. The tumor-bearing portion of the colon is mobilized by dividing the lateral peritoneal attachments and any adhesions present. Precautions must be taken to avoid cutting through the peritoneum covering the mesentery, to prevent any disruption of the mesenteric lymphatic pathways that lead to the lymph nodes.

Once the tumor-bearing area is isolated, 1 to 2 mL of Lymphazurin 1% is injected using a tuberculin syringe and a 30-gauge needle. The dye is injected subserosally, in a circumferential manner around the primary tumor. Care should be taken to avoid spillage of the dye onto the surface of the mesentery or injection into the bowel lumen. Intraluminal injection of the dye can lead to its absorption away from the primary tumor and may highlight lymph nodes that are not the "true" sentinel nodes. This in turn can lead to higher false-negative rates and lower accuracy, as seen in the study by Joosten et al. (34).

Usually within 5 to 10 minutes of the injection, the blue dye travels via the lymphatics to the nearby mesenteric lymph nodes, which turn pale to deep blue. The first through fourth blue nodes with the most direct drainage from the primary tumor are marked with suture as "sentinel lymph node(s)." The sentinel nodes are most often seen on the retroperitoneal surface and marked accordingly for future identification by the pathologist. Because the blue dye often travels quickly through the lymphatics and lymph nodes, the "true" sentinel nodes may soon lose their blue color; thus, by the time the specimen reaches the pathologist, the dye may be found in lymph nodes further down the lymphatic chain, while the "true" sentinel node may not be blue at all. This underscores the importance of the initial tagging of the nodes with suture at the time of their identification intraoperatively. In the event that in-vivo identification of 1 or more sentinel lymph nodes is not accomplished during the operation, an additional 1 to 2 mL of Lymphazurin 1% can be injected ex vivo. This might allow the pathologist to identify a sentinel node during pathologic dissection of the mesentery. Once the sentinel lymph nodes are identified, a standard oncologic resection is performed that includes adequate proximal and distal margins, along with the regional lymph nodes in the attached mesentery. Occasionally, a blue node may be identified outside of the usual lymphatic area; it should be considered a sentinel node and included within the margins of the resection. In patients with unusually thick or fatty mesentery, limited surgical dissection of the mesenteric fat may be required to identify the blue-stained lymph nodes.

## Clinical Applications

As with most other solid malignancies, the tumor stage at the time of initial diagnosis remains the most important prognostic factor for predicting survival in colorectal cancer. Although surgery alone is considered curative for patients in which the disease is confined within the bowel wall (American Joint Committee on Cancer [AJCC] stages I and II), survival decreases dramatically by about 25% to 35% once the disease has spread beyond the bowel wall and into the draining lymph nodes (AJCC stage III). The addition of adjuvant chemotherapy following surgical resection has been shown to be curative in more than one-third of patients with nodal metastasis (35,36). Therefore, diagnostic accuracy of nodal metastasis remains critical for the proper prediction of survival and appropriate therapeutic planning. The sentinel lymph node mapping technique provides an ideal avenue for highly accurate staging of patients with colon cancer.

As for minimally invasive and modified surgery, sentinel lymph node mapping for colon cancer has a relatively small impact in comparison with other GI cancers, because of the anatomical and functional factors associated with the colon. However, identification of aberrant mesenteric lymphatic drainage patterns is useful to confirm the need to extend planned resection margins.

# Sentinel Lymph Node Mapping for Rectal Cancer

## Radioguided Method

Lymphatic mapping with the dye-guided method is not practical for rectal cancer, because of the same anatomical situation as in esophageal cancer (37)—in organs such as the esophagus and rectum, real-time observation of the lymphatic route using dye is difficult without operative mobilization of the primary site, but the mobilization itself destroys the active lymphatic flow from the primary lesion. For these reasons, the radioguided method or dual tracer method has been preferred for sentinel lymph node mapping in rectal

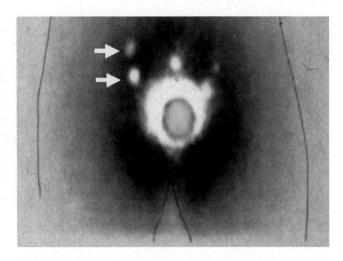

Figure 14-7. Sentinel lymph nodes in rectal cancer located in the lateral area detected by preoperative lymphoscintigraphy. (Reprinted from Kitagawa Y, et al. The role of sentinal lymph nodes in gastrointestinal cancer. Surgical Clinics of North America, 2000;80(6):1799–1809, with permission from Elsevier.)

cancer. Radioactive colloid is injected into the lesion's submucosal layer the day before surgery, using an endoscopic puncture needle. Preoperative lymphoscintigraphy, taken 3 hours after the tracer injection, aids in detecting sentinel lymph nodes in the lateral area draining the primary lesion of lower rectal cancer (Figure 14-7). A gamma probe is useful to locate sentinel lymph nodes near the pelvic wall.

## Clinical Applications

Successful sentinel lymph node detection has great potential in surgical treatment for rectal cancer. As with colon cancer, accurate staging targeted to sentinel nodes would help determine the indications for adjuvant treatment. More intensive examination of sentinel nodes, including immunohistochemistry with step sectioning or detection of specific markers by RT-PCR, would then be feasible.

With cases of lower rectal cancer, a relatively high incidence of lateral lymph node metastasis, including skip metastasis, has been reported (8). However, extended lymphadenectomy with lateral node dissection frequently affects quality of life for the patient after surgery, due to the destruction of autonomic nervous tissue. Thus, the clinical benefits of extensive lateral lymphadenectomy are regarded as limited. Where there is no metastasis in pararectal sentinel lymph nodes and no distribution of sentinel nodes in the lateral area, lateral lymphadenectomy would be unnecessary. In 10% of the cases with lower rectal cancer in our series, distribution of sentinel nodes in lateral lymph nodes was observed (37); those in the lateral area would be the functional first compartment of the lymphatic drainage routes, and a selective and partial lateral lymph node sampling, including the sentinel node, would be beneficial for accurate staging and effective lymphadenectomy.

## Conclusions

Based on recent single institutional reports and multicenter studies of sentinel lymph node mapping, the concept seems valid for gastrointestinal cancer. Although further accumulation of evidence based on large-scale multicenter clinical trials using standard protocols is required, this technique would be a great tool for performing individualized surgical and nonsurgical treatment for patients with gastrointestinal cancer (38).

## References

1. Reintgen D, Cruse CW, Wells K, et al. The orderly progression of melanoma nodal metastases. *Ann Surg.* 1994; 220:759–767.
2. Cox CE, Pendas S, Cox JM, et al. Guidelines for sentinel node biopsy and lymphatic mapping of patients with breast cancer. *Ann Surg.* 1998;227:645–653.
3. Maruyama K, Sasako M, Kinoshita T, et al. Can sentinel node biopsy indicate rational extent of lymphadenectomy in gastric cancer surgery? *Langenbecks Arch Surg.* 1999;384:149–157.
4. Siewert JR, Sendler A. Potential and futility of sentinel node detection for gastric cancer. *Recent Result Cancer Res.* 2000;157:259–269.
5. Kosaka T, Ueshima N, Sugaya J, et al. Lymphatic route of the stomach demonstrated by gastric carcinomas with solitary lymph node metastasis. *Surg Today.* 1999;29:695–700.
6. Matsubara T, Ueda M, Kaisaki S, et al. Localization of initial lymph node metastasis from carcinoma of the thoracic esophagus. *Cancer.* 2000;89:1869–1873.
7. Sano T, Katai H, Sasako M, et al. Gastric lymphadenectomy and detection of sentinel nodes. *Recent Results Cancer Res.* 2000;157:253–258.
8. Moriya Y, Sugihara K, Akatsu T, Fujita S. Importance of extended lymphadenectomy with lateral node dissection for advanced rectal cancer. *World J Surg.* 1997;21:728–732.
9. Akiyama H, Tsurumaru M, Udagawa H, et al. Radical lymph node dissection for cancer of the thoracic esophagus. *Ann Surg.* 1994;220:364–373.
10. Maruyama K, Gunven P, Okabayashi K, et al. Lymph node metastases of gastric cancer. General pattern in 1931 patients. *Ann Surg.* 1989;210:596–602.
11. Mori T, Takahashi K, Yasuno M. Radical resection with autonomic nerve preservation and lymph node dissection techniques in lower rectal cancer and its results: the impact of lateral lymph node dissection. *Langenbecks Arch Surg.* 1998;383:409–415.
12. Bonenkamp JJ, Hermans J, Sasako M, et al. Extended lymph-node dissection for gastric cancer. Dutch Gastric Cancer Group. *N Engl J Med.* 1999;340:908–914.
13. Hulsher JBF, van Sandick JW, de Boer AGEM, et al. Extended transthoracic resection compared with limited transhiatal resection for adenocarcinoma of the esophagus. *N Engl J Med.* 2002;347:1662–1669.
14. Saha S, Wiese D, Badin J, et al. Technical details of sentinel lymph node mapping in colorectal cancer and its impact on staging. *Ann Surg Oncol.* 2000;7:120–124.
15. Bilchik AJ, Saha S, Wiese D, et al. Molecular staging of early colon cancer on the basis of sentinel node analysis: a multicenter phase II trial. *J Clin Oncol.* 2001;19:1128–1136.
16. Kitagawa Y, Kitano S, Kubota T, et al. Minimally invasive surgery for gastric cancer—a confluence of two major streams. *Gastric Cancer.* 2005;8:103–110.
17. Kitagawa Y, Fujii H, Kumai K, et al. Recent advances in sentinel node navigation for gastric cancer: a paradigm shift of surgical management. *J Surg Oncol.* 2005;90: 147–151.
18. Hiratsuka M, Miyashiro I, Ishikawa O, et al. Application of sentinel node biopsy to gastric cancer surgery. *Surgery.* 2001;129:335–340.
19. Miwa K, Kinami S, Taniguchi K, et al. Mapping sentinel nodes in patients with early-stage gastric carcinoma. *Br J Surg.* 2003;90:178–182.
20. Kitagawa Y, Ohgami M, Fujii H, et al. Laparoscopic detection of sentinel lymph nodes in gastrointestinal cancer: a novel and minimally invasive approach. *Ann Surg Oncol.* 2001;8(9S):86–89.
21. Kitagawa Y, Fujii H, Mukai M, et al. The role of sentinel lymph node in gastrointestinal cancer. *Surg Clin N Am.* 2000;80:1799–1809.
22. Yasuda S, Shimada H, Chino O, et al. Sentinel lymph node detection with Tc-99m tin colloids in patients with esophagogastric cancer. *Jpn J Clin Oncol.* 2003;33:68–72.
23. Ando N, Iizuka T, Ide H et al. Surgery plus chemotherapy compared with surgery alone for localized squamous cell carcinoma of the thoracic esophagus: a Japan Clinical Oncology Group Study—JCOG9204. *J Clin Oncol.* 2003; 21:4592–4596.
24. Kitajima M, Kitagawa Y. Surgical treatment of esophageal cancer—the advent of the era of individualization. *N Engl J Med.* 2002;21:1705–1709.
25. Vizcaino AP, Moreno V, Lambert R, et al. Time trends incidence of both major histologic types of esophageal carcinomas in selected countries, 1973–1995. *Int J Cancer.* 2002;99:860–868.
26. Stein HJ, Sendler A, Siewert JR. Site-dependent resection techniques for gastric cancer. *Surg Oncol Clin N Am.* 2002;11:405–414.
27. Saha S, Dan AG, Viehl CT, Zuber M, Wiese. Sentinel lymph node mapping in colon and rectal cancer—its impact on staging, limitations, and pitfalls. In: Leong S, Kitajima M, Kitagawa Y, eds. *Selective Sentinel Lymphadenectomy for Human Solid Cancer.* New York: Springer Science; 2005.

28. Saha S, Bilchik A, Wiese D, et al. Ultrastaging of colorectal cancer by sentinel lymph node mapping technique—a multicenter trial. *Ann Surg Oncol.* 2001;8:94–98.

29. Paramo J, Summerall J, Poppiti R, et al. Validation of sentinel node mapping in patients with colon cancer. *Ann Surg Oncol.* 2002;9:550–554.

30. Bendavid Y, Latulippe J, Younan R, et al. Phase I study on sentinel lymph node mapping in colon cancer: a preliminary report. *J Surg Oncol.* 2002;79:81–84.

31. Bilchik A, Saha S, Tsioulias G, et al. Aberrant drainage of missed micrometastases: the value of lymphatic mapping and focused analysis of sentinel lymph nodes in gastrointestinal neoplasms. *Ann Surg Oncol.* 2001;8:82–85.

32. Fitzgerald T, Khalifa M, Zahrani M, et al. Ex vivo sentinel lymph node biopsy in colorectal cancer: a feasibility study. *J Surg Oncol.* 2002;80:27–32.

33. Bertagnolli M, Miedema B, Redston M, et al. Sentinel node staging of resectable colon cancer. Results of a multicenter study. *Ann Surg.* 2004;240:624–628.

34. Joosten J, Strobbe L, Wauters C, et al. Intraoperative lymphatic mapping and the sentinel node concept in colorectal carcinoma. *Br J Surg.* 1999;86:482–486.

35. Cohen AM, Kelsen D, Saltz L, et al. Adjuvant therapy for colorectal cancer. *Curr Prob Cancer.* 1998;22:5–65.

36. Wolmark N, Rockette H, Fisher B, et al. The benefit of leucovorin-modulated fluorouracil as postoperative adjuvant therapy for primary colon cancer: Results from National Surgical Adjuvant Breast and Bowel protocol C-03. *J Clin Oncol.* 1993;11:1879–1887.

37. Kitagawa Y, Watanabe M, Hasegawa H, et al. Sentinel node mapping for colorectal cancer with radioactive tracer. *Dis Colon Rectum.* 2002;45:1476–1480.

38. Kitagawa Y, Fujii H, Mukai M, Kubo A, Kitajima M. Sentinel lymph node mapping in esophageal and gastric cancer—impact on individualized minimally invasive surgery. In: Leong S, Kitajima M, Kitagawa Y, eds. *Selective Sentinel Lymphadenectomy for Human Solid Cancer.* New York: Springer Science; 2005:123–139.

# 15
# Sentinel Lymph Node Biopsy in Prostatic Cancer

Alexander Winter, Harry Vogt, Dorothea Weckermann, Rolf Harzmann, and Friedhelm Wawroschek

The identification of lymph drainage has significant clinical importance for tumor spread in prostatic cancer. Pelvic lymph node metastases indicate a poor prognosis for patients with clinically localized prostate cancer. The prognosis depends on nodal cancer volume (1), extracapsular extension (2), and the number of prostatic nodes affected (3). It is not clear whether the more valuable prognostic factor is the diameter of the largest metastases, or the total number of positive lymph nodes (4).

In addition to being of prognostic value, lymph node status in prostate cancer is also of tremendous therapeutic relevance, since common standards still include renunciation of local curative therapy (e.g., radical prostatectomy, radiotherapy) with positive lymph node findings, and hormonal withdrawal therapy may be performed (5). A few studies have demonstrated the potential therapeutic benefit of pelvic lymphadenectomy (3,6–8).

## Prediction and Detection of Lymph Node Metastases in Prostate Cancer

Techniques for identifying metastases must have high sensitivity (to avoid unnecessary and stressful treatment) and high specificity (not to deprive a patient of promising/curative treatment). Statements regarding lymph node status in prostate cancer are based on radiologic imaging, predictive nomograms, and different surgical techniques of pelvic lymphadenectomy (9), including different histopathologic techniques of lymph node examination.

## Radiologic Imaging

Often lymph node metastases are revealed at the time of surgery. None of the currently available means of radiologic imaging provides sufficient identification of affected lymph nodes with a metastatic diameter of up to 5 mm. Computed tomography (CT) scans and magnetic resonance imaging (MRI) are routinely performed for the primary diagnostics of lymph node metastases in prostate cancer. Radioimmunoscintigraphy, positron emission tomography (PET) scans, and PET-CT are limited to investigative studies. Lymphangiography, which was performed frequently in the 1970s (10), proved to be useless for the identification of micrometastases.

CT scans and MRI are not able to identify lymph node metastases in the absence of nodal enlargement. Since pelvic lymph nodes are frequently enlarged without bearing metastases, the size of the nodes does not accurately reveal whether it is benign or malignant. In 1999, Tigueret et al. (11) showed that on average, positive lymph nodes were smaller than negative nodes in patients with clinically localized prostate cancer (axial size >1 cm in 76% and >5 mm in 26% of positive nodes). Subsequently, they concluded that lymph node size should not be used as a predictor of the presence of node metastases.

In 1995, Wolf et al. (12) reviewed a total of 25 studies (1,354 patients) on pelvic lymph node staging in clinically localized prostate cancer. They were unable to find any difference in the accuracy of CT and MRI (sensitivity 36%, specificity 97%). Both Wolf's review and another meta-analysis from Scheidler et al. (13) imply that positive imaging results are inconclusive and merely demonstrate the need for further investigation if a treatment decision rests on nodal status. Van Poppel et al. (14) reached an extraordinarily high sensitivity of 77% by combining CT and fine-needle aspiration cytology. With the inclusion of diagnostic cytology, the specificity was 100%. Negative biopsy results were verified by means of a distinctive form of pelvic lymphadenectomy (the average number of removed lymph nodes was 12.9). This technique has not yet become general practice. The diagnostic value of lymph node size as a criterion for differentiation between malignant and benign remains controversial and is discussed in these special collectives (11). Advances in MRI technology, such as dynamic contrast-enhanced MRI (15), or the development of a lymph node-specific contrast agent (16) may improve the diagnostic value of preoperative imaging. These techniques seem most feasible for reducing the number of false positive examinations. Ultra-small, superparamagnetic iron oxide particles have not yet been approved for diagnostics.

Disappointingly, immunoscintigraphy using an indium-labelled antibody against a prostate-specific membrane antigen (ProstaScint, Cytogen, US) does not yield distinctly better results than CT or MRI. The sensitivity of this method was between 44% and 75%, with a specificity of 80% to 86% (17–19). At present, immunoscintigraphy should be limited to investigative studies, since a predictive value of only 66.7% was achieved in a group of patients at high risk for lymph node metastases (19).

Similarly, PET using 2-fluoro-2-deoxy-d-glucose (FDG-PET) or $^{11}$C-acetate results in a great number of small lymph node metastases going undetected. Sensitivity of 30% to 75% and specificity of 72% to 100% have been described (20–26). Studies with fluorocholine PET-CT and $^{11}$C-Choline-PET-CT did not show higher sensitivity (27,28).

## Predictive Nomograms

Nomograms have attempted to predict the probability of nodal involvement for an individual patient, based on preclinical data and multivariate analyses (29–31). The probability of lymph node metastases increases with the level of prostate-specific antigen (PSA), biopsy grade (Gleason score), and clinical T stage (Figure 15-1).

These nomograms are based on the results of large surgical series of pelvic lymphadenectomy and radical prostatectomy. The largest published series is that of Partin et al. (33), who analyzed the results of more than 4000 patients in 3 institutions, and subsequently more than 5000 patients in the nomogram update (34). In the update of the Partin tables, the likelihood of lymph node metastases was 0% to 2% in men with PSA < 10, biopsy Gleason score < 6, and clinical stage < T2b (cancer in 1 lobe). Patients with clinical stage T2c and identical PSA and biopsy Gleason scores had a 0% to 3% risk of lymphatic spread (34).

Cangiannos and colleagues (35) showed that besides the clinical stage, Gleason score, and PSA, a fourth variable incorporating institution-specific prevalence of

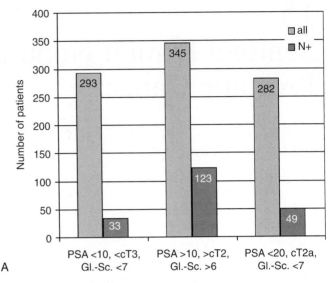

A

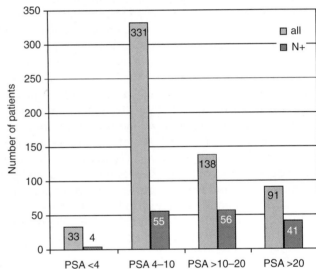

B

FIGURE 15-1. The number of lymph node-positive patients depending on the preoperative PSA-level (A) and preoperative parameters (B) n = 638 patients. (Wawroschek et al. 2005 [32]. Reprinted with permission.)

lymph node invasion also represented a statistically significant predictor of nodal metastases. They used multi-institutional data from 7,014 patients treated at 6 centers on 3 continents, and found that institution-specific prevalence of positive lymph nodes ranged from 1.5% to 7%. Possible reasons for these discrepancies are institution-specific population differences and variations relating to the extent of lymphadenectomy and/or the pathological evaluation of the lymphadenectomy specimen.

Further information on the probability of lymph node metastasis is gained through the extent and grade of tumor involvement in prostate sextant biopsies, and the tumor involvement of the seminal vesicles, in biopsies and through positive basal prostate biopsies (36,37). Conrad et al. (38,39) stated the number of biopsies containing Gleason grade 4 or 5, and the presence of predominantly Gleason grade 4 and 5 disease in any biopsy was the best predictor of lymph node metastases. They identified 3 risk groups, dependent on the number of biopsies harboring prostate cancer with Gleason score > 7: 1) 4 to 6 biopsies with Gleason score > 7 (45%); 2) 1 to 3 biopsies with Gleason score > 7 (19%); no biopsy with Gleason score > 7 (2%).

In another analysis, the number of biopsies involved with Gleason grade 4–5 and a preoperative PSA serum level >15 ng/ml was demonstrated as a significant predictor for positive lymph nodes (40).

Unfortunately, the use of predictive nomograms to forecast lymph node status does not offer a sufficient degree of reliability for the majority of patients. Nomograms are partly based on results from studies with large patient populations, and the performance of distinctively limited forms of pelvic lymphadenectomy creates additional uncertainty. The percentage of N+-stages varies depending on the treated patient population and the extent and technique of lymphadenectomy (41–43).

However, based on the results of the numerous published nomograms, in many centers pelvic staging lymphadenectomy is no longer performed in patients with relatively favorable initial tumor data (PSA < 10 ng/mL, Gleason score < 7, and clinical stage < T2). However, we identified positive lymph nodes by radioguided surgery in patients with PSA < 10 ng/mL and biopsy Gleason score < 6 in 6.8% (positive biopsies in 1 lobe) and 10.7% (positive biopsies in both lobes) of patients (44).

## Staging Lymphadenectomy

Pelvic lymphadenectomy remains the gold standard for identification of lymph node metastases. Staging is expected to safely detect metastatic spread. In addition, a staging lymphadenectomy should not prove too morbid, since it may not be a curative therapy. On the other hand, data published by Catalona (45) suggest that lymphadenectomy has therapeutic value, based on an intermediate follow-up without biochemical relapse in about 20% of patients with lymph node metastases. The prognostic relevance of lymph node status is unanimously regarded as high: Kapadia and colleagues demonstrated that the number of positive

nodes was the only independent predictor of survival (46).

Surgical standards for pelvic lymphadenectomy in prostate cancer do not exist in the current literature. The least invasive variation—mostly carried out by means of laparoscopic pelvic lymphadenectomy—removes only the lymphatic tissue of the obturator fossa, which is confined to the external iliac vein and to the obturator nerve (47,48). In 1996, Weingärtner et al. (49) concluded that about 20 lymph nodes must be dissected by means of the widespread standard of modified pelvic lymphadenectomy, from lymphatic tissue surrounding the external iliac artery and vein, the obturator fossa, and the obturator nerve. In contrast, Schuessler et al. (50) regard as the surgical standard the resection of lymphatic tissue surrounding the common iliac artery, the external iliac artery and vein, the genitofemoral nerve, the obturator fossa, and the region medial to the internal iliac artery surrounding its anterior arterial branches. They describe this dissection, minus the lymphatic tissue of the common iliac artery and lateral to the external iliac artery, as the limited or modified dissection. In Germany, the most current variant of these recommendations is published in the guidelines of the German Urologic Association and merely includes the lymphatic tissue of the obturator fossa and surrounding the internal iliac artery (51).

Extended pelvic lymphadenectomy has been shown to be associated with an increased risk of complications such as lymphocele, venous thrombosis, lower extremity edema, and ureteral injury (52). Due to high morbidity related to extended dissection and the operative time of about 2.5 hours (53), the dissection area has been reduced in most centers. Stone et al. (54) were able to prove the obvious interdependency between the complication rate and the number of dissected lymph nodes: 2.1% in cases averaging 9.3 lymph nodes, versus 35.9% in cases averaging 17.8 lymph nodes. Our own investigations (55) also showed a significant increase in the complication rate—especially lymphatic complications—dependent on the number of resected lymph nodes: 1 to 5 lymph nodes, 10.5%; 6 to 10 lymph nodes, 12.4%; 11 to 15 lymph nodes, 15.1%; 16 to 20 lymph nodes, 24.3%; more than 21, 26.6%.

In most cases, studies with a low complication rate of pelvic dissection only have about 10 dissected lymph nodes in their specimens (47,56), or do not specify the number of dissected lymph nodes (57). The latter in particular makes evaluation of surgical treatment more difficult (see Table 15-1).

Several studies of complete pelvic lymphadenectomy in prostate cancer patients revealed that reduction of the dissection area decreased the sensitivity of detection of metastases (37,42,50,54,59,60). McDowell

TABLE 15-1. Complication rate of pelvic lymphadenectomy, type of lymphadenectomy, and number of resected lymph nodes.

| Author, year, reference | Number of patients | Complications (%) | Type of lymphadenectomy | Number of lymph nodes |
|---|---|---|---|---|
| Paul et al. 1983 (58) | 150 | 51 | extended open | — |
| McDowell et al. 1990 (59) | 217 | 22 | extended open | — |
| Schuessler et al. 1993 (50) | 147 | 31 | extended laparoscopic | 45 |
| Lezin et al. 1997 (57) | 22 | 9.1 | minilaparotomie | — |
| | 22 | 31.8 | modified laparoscopic | — |
| Fahlenkamp et al. 1997 (47) | 200 | 12.5 | modified laparoscopic | 11 |
| Herrell et al. 1997 (56) | 38 | 20 | modified open | 9 |
| Winter et al. 2005 (55) | 163 | 23.3 | SLNE + extended open | 22 |
| | 117 | 24.8 | SLNE + modified open | 21 |
| | 216 | 15.3 | SLNE | 12 |

Legend:
SLNE—sentinel lymphadenectomy
*Source:* Wawroschek F, Hamm M, et al: Urol Int 2003;71:129–135. (43). Adapted with permission from S. Karger AG, Basel, Switzerland.

et al. (59) found isolated lymphatic spread in the presacral region and the tissue surrounding the branches of the internal iliac artery (superior and inferior vesical arteries, internal pudendal artery, hypogastric region) in 29% of patients with lymph node metastases. Limiting the dissection area to the obturator fossa results in missing about 50% to 60% of the N+ patients (43,50,61–63).

## History of Prostate Lymphoscintigraphy

After the first report of the selective uptake of interstitially injected radiocolloid by regional lymph nodes in 1953 by Shermann and Ter Pogossian (64) using $^{198}$Au, lymphatic drainage of most organs was subsequently investigated scintigraphically.

The first prostate lymphoscintigraphies in the late 1970s aimed to examine the intraprostatic lymph system and visualize the regional lymphatic drainage of the prostate. Clinicians had assumed that lack of lymph node visualization might indicate the presence of metastases. Menon et al. (65) first verified the debated existence of intraprostatic lymphatic pathways by intraprostatic injection of a tracer in a canine model. The injection was carried out through a transvesical access in 9 dogs and revealed a scintigraphical depiction of lymph nodes from different lymphatic drainage areas in each case. Experiments by Kaplan et al. (66) with 9 dogs rendered comparable results. Between 1 and 4 lymph nodes were depicted each time. In 1 dog, a digitally guided, transrectal intraprostatic injection with subsequent successful lymphoscintigraphy was performed for the first time.

Gardiner et al. (67,68) were the first to demonstrate lymphatic pathways by transrectal injection with a $^{99m}$Tc-labeled tracer (particle size 4–12 nm) into the human prostate capsule. Transperineal injections into the parenchyma, open, and periprostatic injections had not been successful. A uni- or bilateral lymph drainage was shown in all 40 patients with injections close to the capsule. In 1990, using a comparable technique Zuckier et al. (69) demonstrated a partly contralateral pelvic lymphatic drainage in 8 out of 9 patients with prostate cancer; the remaining patient underwent a repeat injection under similar conditions to show identical lymphatic drainage. Whether it was possible to depict the whole lymphatic drainage pathways of the prostate remained uncertain, since the only possible means of verifying the results with certainty—operative and histologic examination in lymph node-positive patients with prostate cancer—was carried out later. The chronology of prostate lymphoscintigraphy is shown in Table 15-2.

## Implementation of the Sentinel Lymph Node Concept in Prostate Cancer

These scintigraphic studies of the prostate's lymphatic drainage formed the basis for the introduction of the sentinel lymph node concept for prostate carcinoma. In 1998, scintigraphy combined with intraoperative detection via a gamma probe was applied for the first time to identify a sentinel node (72). More than 630 patients have now been evaluated (32,44,73), and the sentinel lymph node concept has been established in prostate cancer by many groups (62,63,74,75).

TABLE 15-2. Chronology of prostate lymphoscintigraphy in canines and patients.

| Author, year, reference | Group | Injection technique | Radiotracer | Results |
|---|---|---|---|---|
| Menon et al. 1977 (65) | 9 dogs | Open procedure; transvesical, intraprostatic | $^{198}$Au colloid | Positive scintigraphy in all dogs |
| Gardiner, et al. 1979 (67) | 25 patients | Transrectal into the prostate capsule, transurethral, transabdominal | $^{99m}$Tc-antimony sulphide colloid 0.05 mL | Transrectal successful in every case (n = 7), intraprostatic injection: negative scintigraphy |
| Gardiner et al. 1979 (68) | 33 patients | Transrectal | $^{99m}$Tc-antimony sulphide colloid | Positive scintigraphy in every case |
| Stone et al. 1979 (70) | 30 patients | Transurethral, transperineal, superficial perineal | $^{99m}$Tc-phytate and $^{99m}$Tc-antimony sulphide colloid | Most successful: the perineal injection into the posterior prostatic capsule with antimony sulphide colloid |
| Kaplan et al. 1980 (66) | 9 dogs, 1 patient with pc | dogs: transvesical intraprostatic; patient: transrectal | $^{99m}$Tc-antimony sulphide colloid 0.1 mL | Positive scintigraphy in every dog and 1 patient |
| Zuckier et al. 1990 (69) | 10 patients with pc | Transrectal, including unilateral | $^{99m}$Tc-antimony sulphide colloid 0.2 mL | Contralateral lymphatic drainage in case of unilateral inj. |
| Horenblas et al. 1992 (71) | 11 patients with pc | perineal into the ischiorectal fossa | $^{99m}$Tc-antimony sulphide colloid 0.2 mL | negative lymphoscintigraphy had no predictive value (specificity 13%) |

Legend:
pc—prostate cancer

## Clinical Evaluation of Sentinel Lymph Node Excision in Prostate Cancer

For sentinel lymph node detection, $^{99m}$Tc-nanocolloid (62,73,76,77), $^{99m}$Tc-rhenium sulphur colloid (63), or $^{99m}$Tc-phytate (74) are used. The injected volumes and the interval between injection and surgery have varied. In the first clinical examinations (72), $^{99m}$Tc-nanocolloid (Nanocoll, Nycomed Amersham Sorin, Italy) was injected transrectally into the prostate the day before lymphadenectomy under ultrasound guidance. In most cases, the 18 to 22-hour interval between injection and surgery was determined by the 6-hour half-life of the radiocolloid. Prior to injection, patients were administered a broad-spectrum antibiotic (e.g., Ciprobay), which was continued until postoperative day 2. In early studies, a single central injection was given to each prostate lobe; 100 MBq per lobe in a total injected volume of about 2 mL were given. Based on the results of canine studies, a minimum of 2 injections into each prostate lobe are now given, in a reduced injection volume of 0.6 mL for each side (78). Figure 15-2 shows a sono-guided transrectal injection.

Takashima and colleagues (74) injected $^{99m}$Tc-phytate into the peripheral zone of each prostate lobe (40 MBq/ 0.1 mL per side; 80 MBq/0.2 mL in total) under transrectal ultrasonographic guidance 5 to 6 hours before surgery. Other injection procedures are listed in Table 15-3.

## Strategies of Tracer Injection and the Influence on Lymphoscintigraphy in Human and Animal Studies

The identification of sentinel lymph nodes in prostate cancer is different than the technique used with other tumors. In breast cancer (79), penis cancer (80,81), and malignant melanoma (82,83), in most centers a well-directed peritumoral injection is placed only to observe the lymphatic drainage of the tumor. In prostate cancer, however, it is not known from which part of the organ the metastatic spread originates. Therefore, the aim of prostate lymphoscintigraphy must be the imaging of all primarily draining lymph nodes of the prostate. Inevitably, 1 or more sentinel nodes will be present among them.

The quality of prostate lymphoscintigraphy has to be evaluated not only by the sentinel node detection rate, but also by the proportion of low-isotope accumulating sentinel nodes. These can be missed intraoperatively, and so sentinel lymph nodes of lesser radioactivity are a major problem in prostate lymphoscintigraphy. Single lymph nodes with a high uptake actually increase the value of average sentinel lymph node uptake, but are not

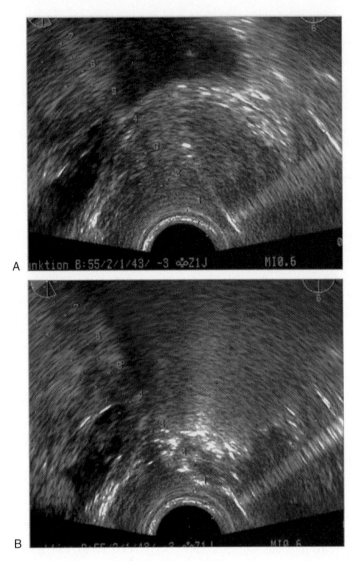

FIGURE 15-2. Transrectal application of sentinel tracer into the prostate under ultrasound guidance: (A) before injection, (B) after injection with intraprostatic diffusion of fluid.

TABLE 15-3. Sentinel tracer injection in patients with prostate cancer.

| Author, year, reference | Patients | Injection technique | Radiotracer | Results |
|---|---|---|---|---|
| Wawroschek et al. 2001 2003 2005 (73,44,32) | 638 | Transrectal bilateral; 100 MBq per lobe, total volume 2 mL; single central application; in later studies: 100 MBq per lobe, volume 0.6 mL each side; minimally 2 injections into each lobe | [99m]Tc-nanocolloid | Positive scintigraphy in 92.6% of patients, intraoperative SLN-detection 96.9%, average 6.3 SLN |
| Rudoni et al. 2002 (62) | 48 | Transrectal | [99m]Tc-nanocolloid technetium Tc | Intraoperative, average 0.9 SLN |
| Takashima et al. 2004 (74) | 24 | Transrectal 80 MBq/0.2 mL in total; bilateral, peripheral zone | [99m]Tc-labeled phytate | Positive scintigraphy in 70.8% of patients, intraoperative average 4.1 SLN |
| Bastide et al. 2004 (63) | 34 | Transrectal bilateral; 60 MBq/0.6 mL in total; peripheral zone | [99m]Tc-rhenium sulphur colloid | Positive scintigraphy in 85.3% of patients, intraoperative SLN-detection 67.7% |

Legend:
SLN—sentinel lymph node

necessary for intraoperative identification. The aim has to be an even sentinel lymph node uptake and a reduction of the number of sentinel nodes with low activity. The latter can be missed in the 2-day protocol.

Studies with surgically removed prostates show a highly inhomogeneous tracer distribution, with concentration at the injection sites (84). Animal experiments were conducted to clarify the influence of different injection techniques on tracer distribution, and individual reproducibility tested via repeated tracer injections. These studies also examined whether individual factors or injection technique was responsible for the observed strong variations in lymph node activity. To transfer results from animal studies to human, the anatomy of the prostate lymph drainage and the injection requirements had to be comparable. There is evidence from the anatomy of prostatic lymph drainage in humans and in dogs that different areas of the prostate have a variable drainage region (85); different lymphatic drainage from the periurethral and peripheral zone is the only difference between the human and canine prostate (86).

The canine studies showed that the number of sentinel nodes of the same dog was increased after central injection (1 per lobe), compared to peripheral injection (2 times per lobe). Some sentinel lymph nodes show a higher uptake after peripheral injection, and others after the central one. The representation of sentinel lymph nodes was reproducible in 5 out of 6 dogs with central injection. The different injection techniques are demonstrated in Figure 15-3.

Lymphatic flow is initialized by an increase in the interstitial pressure triggered by a certain volume of fluid that causes distention of the endothelial cells mediated by anchoring filaments. Therefore, the volume for initializing lymphatic flow depends on tissue density. For subdermal application in malignant melanoma or penile cancer, small volumes (0.1 to 0.2 mL) seem appropriate, whereas larger volumes of 3 to 8 mL are needed for peritumoral application in breast cancer (87). Apparently, this does not reflect the physiological condition, and individual reports have demonstrated good results with much smaller volumes (88). In prostate lymphoscintigraphy of canines, as a reduction of the prostate volume from 10% to 1% demonstrated reproducible results in sentinel lymph node uptake (84), this should be preferred as the physiological way of administration. Furthermore, the varying activities in sentinel nodes in repeated tests with identical injection technique and injection volumes clearly demonstrate that the amount of isotope uptake is not an appropriate criterion for sentinel lymph node identification (78,84,89).

Compared with previous prostate lymphoscintigraphies in canines (66,65), in our study (78) the number of identified lymph nodes was increased and locations were detected that until now could not be demonstrated with

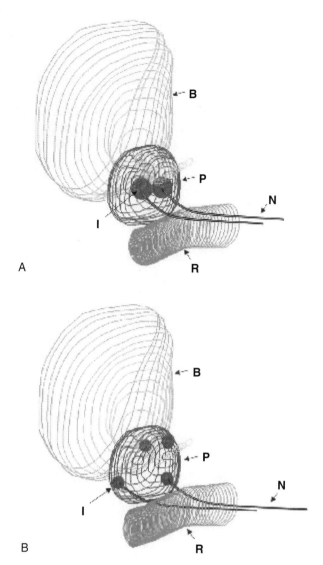

FIGURE 15-3. Scheme of the: (A) intraprostatic central and (B) peripheral injection technique (B = bladder, P = prostate, N = needle, R = rectum, I and dark grey points = injection sites). (From Wawroschek F, Wengenmair H, Senekowitsch-Schmidtke R, et al. Prostate lymphoscintigraphy for sentinel lymph node identification in canines: reproducibility, uptake, and biokinetics depending on different injection strategies. Urol Res 2003;31:152–158. Reprinted with permission from Springer.)

dyes or lymphoscintigraphy. One reason for this might be the different experimental methods (e.g., the amount of radioactivity, the radiopharmaceutical agent, the injection volume, and the injection technique) from the previous investigations.

However, as a consequence of the animal investigations, we are convinced that a combination of central and peripheral injections and a reduced volume lead to a more homogenous intraprostatic tracer distribution and optimal prostate lymphoscintigraphy.

## The Technique of Prostate Lymphoscintigraphy

Lymphoscintigraphy has been performed at different intervals following injection. Bastide et al. and Brenot-Rossi et al. (63,90) carried out scintigraphy 2 hours after injection. In our practice, approximately 15 minutes to a few hours after injection, scintigraphies were executed in anterior and posterior view using a low-energy all-purpose (LEAP) collimator at 100,000 counts/view or 10 minutes time for acquisition (Figure 15-4). Alternatively, single photon emission computed tomography (SPECT) or an image fusion system consisting of a gamma camera with integrated x-ray tube could be used (76,77).

Takashima et al. (74) used planar imaging 15 minutes and 3 hours after RI injection, along with a SPECT scan 3 hours after injection, to identify sentinel nodes. In their first patient, the radioactive tracer was injected the day before surgery. However, because the sentinel node identified at 3 hours after injection could not be identified 24 hours after, SPECT was performed for the remaining patients 3 hours after injection.

## Intraoperative Detection of Sentinel Lymph Nodes

The intraoperative detection of sentinel lymph nodes requires highly sensitive probes (for low sentinel lymph node activity) with good shielding properties (sentinel nodes may be localized very closely to the prostate, and high background activity may be present), high local resolution (for discrimination of neighboring lymph nodes), and low detector size (because of limited room in operative cavity). For these reasons, only semiconductor or scintillation detectors are appropriate. The gamma probes must be collimated and optimized for the different tracers. Probes are available in different forms for open and laparoscopic detection (e.g., C-TRAK system, Care Wise, US; Szintiprobe MR-100, Pol.Hi.Tech., Italy; Navigator GPS, AutoSuture, Japan).

## The Operative Procedure

Depending upon the intended therapy for the prostate cancer (e.g., radiotherapy, or perineal or retropubic prostatectomy), pelvic lymphadenectomy can be carried out via different surgical accesses: laparotomy, minilaparotomy, or laparoscopy.

Initially, to evaluate the sensitivity of the sentinel-guided pelvic lymphadenectomy, an extended lymph node dissection was performed (common iliac, external iliac, obturator, internal iliac, and presacral regions) (74,75,91). Alternatively, a standard lymphadenectomy (obturator fossa and external iliac regions) (64) was executed in addition to dissection of the sentinel nodes. The above is in contrast to conventional procedures with limited lymphadenectomy. At the beginning of our studies, all patients received sentinel lymphadenectomy plus dissection of the lymph nodes from the obturator fossa and the external iliac (a so-called modified lymphadenectomy). Analysis after 121 patients (91,92) showed that sentinel lymphadenectomy in comparison to modified lymphadenectomy has a sensitivity of about 96%. This result was significantly better ($p < 0.05$) than resection of the obturator lymph nodes only. We subsequently modified our study protocol, and the extent of pelvic lymphadenectomy varied depending on the preoperative risk factors between sentinel lymphadenectomy only (PSA < 10 ng/mL, Gleason score < 7 in biopsy, and clinical stage < T3) and sentinel lymphadenectomy with additional extended pelvic lymphadenectomy (PSA > 10 ng/mL, Gleason > 6 in biopsy, or clinical stage > T2) (see Figure 15-1).

## Histopathologic Examination and the Influence on Lymph Node Status

Different studies demonstrate that the extent of pelvic lymphadenectomy not only has a significant influence on lymph node status, but also on the nature of the histo-

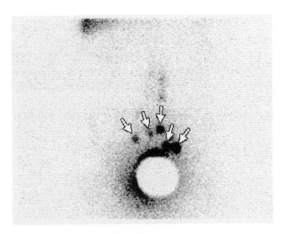

RVL 100'PI

FIGURE 15-4. Representative scintigraphy shows 5 sentinel lymph nodes (arrows). Sites were detected intraprostatively by probe as the right external iliac vein, dorsal right umbilical artery, left presacral region, left internal iliac artery, and left obturator fossa.

TABLE 15-4. Number (%) of node-positive patients who would have been detected provided only lymph nodes from different regions were investigated based on different histopathological techniques.[†]

| Technique of histopathology | Step sections | Serial sections | Immunohistochemistry in serial |
|---|---|---|---|
| SLNE, obturator fossa, external iliac and other regions | 86.7 (69.3–96.2) | 96.7 (82.8–99.9) | 100 (88.4–100) |
| SLNE, obturator fossa, external iliac and other regions | 86.7 (69.3–96.2) | 96.7 (82.8–99.9) | 100 (88.4–100) |
| SLNE, obturator fossa, external iliac region | 83.3 (65.3–94.4) | 87.5 (71–96.5) | 96.7 (82.8–99.9) |
| SLNE (all regions possible) | 79.3 (60.3–92) | 89.7 (72.7–97.8) | 93.1 (77.2–99.2) |
| Obturator fossa, external iliac region | 73.3* (54.1–87.7) | 73.3* (54.1–87.7) | 73.3* (54.1–87.7) |
| Obturator fossa | 46.7** (28.3–65.7) | 46.7** (28.3–65.7) | 46.7** (28.3–65.7) |

[†]The sensitivity of sentinel lymphadenectomy (SLNE) is related to 29 patients, because identifying sentinel lymph nodes in 1 node-positive patient was impossible. The so-called other regions included those nonsentinel nodes outside the standard dissection area, which had been dissected during sentinel lymphadenectomy (95% confidence interval).
*Significant, $p < 0.05$
**Significant, $p < 0.01$
*Source:* Reprinted from Wawroschek et al., 2003 (94), with permission from Elsevier.

pathologic examination (serial section, immunohistochemistry, and RT-PCR) (93–96).

In one study (95), 194 patients with prostate cancer were examined: 36 received sentinel lymphadenectomy plus extended pelvic lymphadenectomy; 112 received sentinel lymphadenectomy plus modified pelvic lymphadenectomy; 37 had only sentinel lymphadenectomy; 8 had modified pelvic lymphadenectomy; and 1 received pick-up pelvic lymphadenectomy. The sentinel lymph nodes were completely embedded and examined by step sections (2 mm). Serial sections (5 systematically distributed sections of 4 μm between each step section) and immunohistochemical staining (pancytokeratin antibody) of 1 serial section followed in a later preparation if metastases were not present in the step sections. All nonsentinel nodes had at least 1 section at the largest diameter. Larger lymph nodes were examined with further step sections in concordance with the Association of Directors of Anatomic and Surgical Pathology (ADASP) recommendation (96). Additionally, in the first 100 patients nonsentinel nodes were examined like sentinel nodes. The results are shown in Table 15-4. A diagnostic improvement of about 14% has been reached through extended histopathologic techniques. For example, using conventional histologic technique, lymph node metastases were found in 5% of patients with preoperative PSA < 10 ng/mL, clinical T2 stage, and Gleason score in biopsy < 7. By adding serial sections, metastases were found in 11.3%.

The PSA-specific RT-PCR combined with (immuno)-histology is a new revealing supplementary technique for the detection of tumor cells in sentinel nodes of prostate cancer patients. Haas et al. (95) showed that 4 of 12 patients with biochemical relapse, but without immunohistologically detectable tumor cells, were RT-PCR-positive for PSA.

## Results of Sentinel Lymph Node Identification

Sentinel lymph nodes were detectable with lymphoscintigraphy in 71% to 93% of patients with prostate cancer (61,63,74). Prostate lymphoscintigraphy seemed only to be influenced by neoadjuvant hormonal therapy, provided it was the selected treatment over a longer period of time (>3 months). This might be the cause for a low number of sentinel nodes in Takashima's investigation (70.8%), in which 75% of the patients were treated with hormonal deprivation. Also, a previous transurethral resection or transvesical surgery of the prostate leads to postoperative alterations in lymphatic drainage.

Wengenmair et al. (97) demonstrated a high interindividual variance of uptake. In 10 randomly selected patients, the determination of radionuclide distribution and its time course were made via "regions of interest" over prostate, bladder, liver, spleen, and the sentinel nodes (Figure 15-5 and Table 15-5). Depiction of the lymphatic pathways was only possible in 11% of the cases. The essential sentinel lymph node criteria were the persistent accumulation of activity and the anatomical localization.

## Intraoperative Sentinel Lymph Node Detection

The authors (32) dissected an average of 6.3 sentinel lymph nodes. Sentinel nodes were detected intraoperatively in 618 of 638 patients (96.9%). An earlier study (73) showed that 78.9% of 350 patients with at least 1 sentinel lymph node had between 2 and 8 sentinel lymph nodes. There was no significant relationship between the

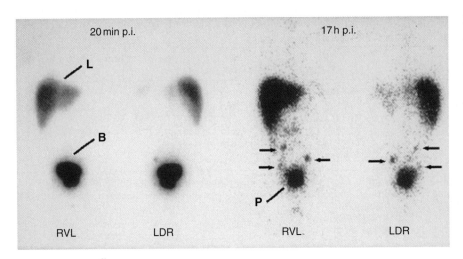

20 min p.i.                    17 h p.i.

RVL          LDR              RVL.           LDR

FIGURE 15-5. Whole-body scan with distribution of radioactivity into the liver (L), bladder (B), prostate (P), and sentinel lymph nodes (black arrows).

number of sentinel nodes, tumor stage, and the number of sentinel nodes in node-positive and -negative patients (5.8 versus 5.5, respectively). Radioactive lymph nodes that could not clearly be identified as a subordinated lymph node on the basis of the anatomical localization and knowledge of the lymphoscintigraphy were classed as sentinel nodes. In 78.6%, the number of intraoperatively identified sentinel lymph nodes exceeded that determined by scintigraphy. In 16.4% of the cases, dissection of all sentinel lymph nodes was impossible. This was the case mainly in laparoscopy (6 out of 7) or minilaparotomy (16 out of 69 cases). Non-resectable or reidentifiable sentinel lymph nodes were mostly located in areas that were difficult to access surgically (internal iliac region, pararectal, presacral). Sentinel nodes could be located anywhere in the minor pelvis, but the most frequently occurring location was the internal iliac nodes (32%). The location of sentinel nodes is shown in Figure 15-6.

In 10 patients, it was not possible to identify at least 1 sentinel lymph node (2.9%) intraoperatively: 1 patient received neoadjuvant hormonal therapy for 3 years, 2 had laparoscopic surgery, and 3 had previously undergone transurethral or transvesical prostate surgery for benign enlargement. In 4 cases, no reason was obvious for failed sentinel lymph node identification. In an additional 5 patients, the intraoperative measuring was not applied (e.g., macrometastases). Of 23 patients who had a previous transurethral resection or transvesical prostatectomy, 4 showed no sentinel lymph nodes. This limitation was significant ($\alpha < 0.005$, $\chi 2$ test).

The investigations by Brenot-Rossi et al. (90) and Bastide et al. (63) also showed the majority of sentinel nodes located in the internal iliac region (77.8% and 58.4%, respectively).

Takashima et al. (74) identified sentinel lymph nodes in 17 out of 24 patients (70.8%) by lymphoscintigraphy,

TABLE 15-5. Average uptake of different organs in prostate lymphoscintigraphy.

| Organ | Average uptake % (range) |
|---|---|
| Prostate | 15.8 (7.7–28) |
| bladder | 24.5 (4.3–47) |
| Liver | 25 (12.2–47.2) |
| Spleen | 2.1 (0.7–3.6) |
| Bone marrow | 32 (21.9–54.2) |
| Sentinel lymph nodes | 0.12 (0.007–0.63) |

*Source:* Data from Wengenmair et al., 2002 (97).

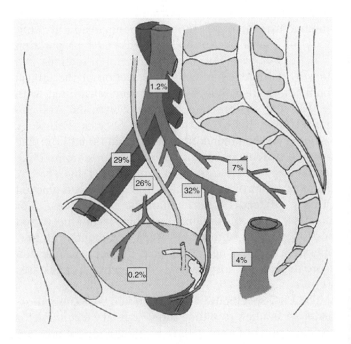

FIGURE 15-6. Distribution of sentinel lymph nodes based on intraoperative findings (n = 638 patients): external iliac region 29%, obturator fossa 26%, presacral 7%, internal iliac region 32%, paravesical 0.2%, pararectal 7%, and common iliac region 1.2%. (Data from Wawroschek et al. 2005 [32].)

in 21 out of 24 patients (87.5%) by in-vivo examination, and in 23 out of 24 (95.8%) patients by ex-vivo measuring. They identified a maximum of 1 to 10 sentinel nodes, with a mean of 4.2 (with scintillation counter). Bastide (63) detected sentinel lymph nodes in only 67.7% of the patients.

## Detection of Lymph Node Metastases

Evaluation of 638 patients resulted in 24.5% lymph node-positive cases. The incidence of node-positive patients depends on preoperative prostate-specific antigen (PSA) and tumor classification of prostatectomy specimens (see Figure 15-1). Further analysis of 333 patients with sentinel lymphadenectomy and extended pelvic lymphadenectomy showed 109 node positive and 3 false-negative patients. Thus, sensitivity was 97.4%. By using immunohistochemistry and serial section examinations of all dissected lymph nodes in 100 patients, sensitivity decreased to 93.1%. If only the sentinel lymph node with the highest radioactivity had been resected, there would have been a further decrease to 74.2%; whereas sensitivity increased to 85% by resection of the most radioactive lymph node of both sides.

In contrast, we demonstrated a sensitivity of 79.2% (44) for the modified pelvic lymphadenectomy. In the same study, in 16 of 24 assessable patients only the sentinel lymph node was positive. Metastases were often exclusively located in the hypogastric region, a region that is normally not included in different forms of modified pelvic (standard) lymphadenectomies. More than half of the node-positive patients would have been falsely classified as pN0-stage if the lymph nodes of the obturator fossa only had been resected.

In cases with comparatively favorable preoperative prognostic factors (PSA < 10 ng/mL, clinical stage < T3, and Gleason score < 7 in prostate biopsy), we found lymph node metastases in 11.8%, although staging lymphadenectomy is not the standard for these patients (44).

Rudoni et al. (62) detected 43 sentinel lymph nodes in 48 patients; 20 were located outside the usual lymphadenectomy area. Metastases were found in 5 sentinel nodes, and 2 of these were also located outside the usual lymphadenectomy area. No metastases were found in nonsentinel nodes.

Brenot-Rossi et al. (90) found lymph node metastases in 4 out of 27 patients only in sentinel lymph nodes. Two were in the hypogastric area, and 2 in the obturator fossa.

The work by Bastide et al. (63) identified lymph node metastases in 4 patients (11.7%). In 3 of these cases they were located in a sentinel lymph node, and in 2 cases, the metastasis was in a sentinel node outside of the pelvic chain.

Takashima et al. (74) detected lymph node metastases in 3 out of 43 patients by manifestation of the hot nodes themselves and in the vicinity of neighboring nodes. False-negative cases with metastases in nodes other than the hot nodes were not encountered. Seven out of 9 metastases were located in the internal iliac region.

In Egawa's investigation (75), 1 patient with extensive lymph node metastasis showed a false-negative lymph node. The sensitivity was 90% in this series.

## Conclusions

There are no universally accepted surgical standards of pelvic staging lymphadenectomy for prostate cancer. Because of high morbidity from extended pelvic lymphadenectomy and the lengthy operating time, the extent of dissection has been decreased at most centers. Published data of extended pelvic lymphadenectomy in prostate cancer point out that any limitation of the dissection area results in a reduced detection rate of metastases. The widespread limitation of the dissection area to the so-called obturator fossa lymph nodes results in missing about 50% of node-positive patients.

Radioguided lymph node dissection offers a reduced time of resection and lower morbidity compared to the extended forms of pelvic lymphadenectomy, without having to expect a significantly reduced detection of metastases.

In contrast to the clinical algorithms, which provide statistical probabilities for populations of patients with similar clinical variables, the pelvic lymphadenectomy renders a precise lymph node staging and a potential benefit for the individual patient. It has been clearly demonstrated that more patients than previously believed are bearing micrometastasis in particular, especially in the case of clinically localized prostate cancer.

As a consequence, lymph node surgery including the primary draining prostate lymph nodes is essential for most patients treated with curative intent (radiotherapy and prostatectomy). This might not "only" be of prognostic relevance for the patient, but also may have a therapeutic significance. Recent data from centers (e.g., Bern, Augsburg) which perform extended pelvic surgery in cases of radical prostatectomy demonstrate that patients with singular lymph node metastasis may be free of PSA recurrence in long-term follow-ups.

Because of the considerable individual variance of prostatic lymph drainage and the inadequacy of alternative non-operative techniques for the identification of lymph node metastases, the sentinel lymphadenectomy in prostate cancer seems to offer a major improvement in clinical practice.

# References

1. Cheng L, Pisansky TM, Ramnani DM, et al. Extranodal extension in lymph node-positive prostate cancer. *Mod Pathol*. 2000;13:113–118.

2. Griebling TL, Ozkutlu D, See WA, et al. Prognostic implications of extracapsular extension of lymph node metastases in prostate cancer. *Mod Pathol*. 1997;10:804–809.

3. Cheng L, Zincke H, Blute ML, et al. Risk of prostate carcinoma death in patients with lymph node metastasis. *Cancer*. 2001;91:66–73.

4. Cheng L, Bergstralh EJ, Cheville JC, et al. Cancer volume of lymph node metastasis predicts progression in prostate cancer. *Am J Surg Pathol*. 1998;22:1491–1500.

5. Aus G, Abbou CC, Pacik D, et al. EAU guidelines on prostate cancer. *Eur Urol*. 2001;40:97–101.

6. Bader P, Burkhard FC, Markwalder R, et al. Disease progression and survival of patients with positive lymph nodes after radical prostatectomy. Is there a chance of cure? *J Urol*. 2003;169:849–854.

7. Heidenreich A, Ohlmann CH, Polyakov S. Anatomical extent of pelvic lymphadenectomy in bladder and prostate cancer. *Eur Urol*. 2005;4(suppl):15–24.

8. Messing EM, Manola J, Sarosdy M, et al. Immediate hormonal therapy versus observation after radical prostatectomy and pelvic lymphadenectomy for node positive prostate cancer: at 10 years results of EST3886. *J Clin Oncol*. 2004;22:abstract 4570.

9. Parker CC, Husband J, Dearnaley DP. Lymph node staging in clinically localized prostate cancer. *Prostate Cancer Prostatic Dis*. 1999;2:191–199.

10. Harzmann R, Bichler KH. Stellenwert der Lymphangiographie bei Tumoren der ableitenden Harnwege und des männlichen Genitale. *Med Klin*. 1977;72:183–197.

11. Tigueret R, Gheiler EL, Tefilli MV, et al. Lymph node size does not correlate with the presence of prostate cancer metastases. *Urology*. 1999;53:367–371.

12. Wolf J, Cher M, Dall´Era M, et al. The use and accuracy of cross-sectional imaging and fine needle aspiration cytology for detection of pelvic lymph node metastases before radical prostatectomy. *J Urol*. 1995;153:993–999.

13. Scheidler J, Hricak H, Yu KY, et al. Radiological evaluation of lymph node metastases in patients with cervical cancer: a meta-analysis. *JAMA*. 1997;278:1096–1101.

14. Van Poppel H, Ameye F, Oyen R, et al. Accuracy of combined computerized tomography and fine needle aspiration cytology in lymph node staging of localized prostatic carcinoma. *J Urol*. 1994;151:1310–1314.

15. Barentsz JO, Jager GJ, van Vierzen PB, et al. Staging urinary bladder cancer after transurethral biopsy: value of fast dynamic contrast-enhanced MR imaging. *Radiology*. 1996;201:185–193.

16. Harisinghani MG, Saini S, Slater GJ, et al. MR imaging of pelvic lymph nodes in primary pelvic carcinoma with ultrasmall superparamagnetic iron oxide (Combidex): preliminary observations. *J Magn Reson Imaging*. 1997;7:161–167.

17. Babaian RJ, Sayer J, Podoleff DA, et al. Radioimmunoscintigraphy of pelvic lymph nodes with 111-indium-labeled monoclonal anti-body CYT-356. *J Urol*. 1994;152:1952–1955.

18. Hinkle GH, Burgers JK, Neal CE, et al. Multicenter radioimmunoscintigraphic evaluation of patients with prostate carcinoma using indium-111 capromab pendetide. *Cancer*. 1998;83:739–747.

19. Polascik TJ, Manyak MJ, Haseman MK, et al. Comparison of clinical staging algorithms and 111indium-capromab pendetide immunoscintigraphy in prediction of lymph node involvement in high-risk prostate carcinoma patients. *Cancer*. 1999;85:1586–1592.

20. Rigo P, Paulus BJ, Kaschten BJ, et al. Oncological applications of positron emission tomography with fluorine-18 fluorodeoxyglucose. *Eur J Nucl Med*. 1996;23:1641–1674.

21. Shreve PD, Grossmann HB, Gross MD, et al. Metastatic prostate cancer: initial findings of PET with 2-desoxy-2-(F-18)fluoro-*D*-glucose. *Radiology*. 1996;199:751–756.

22. Heicapell R, Müller-Mattheis V, Reinhardt M. Staging of pelvic lymph nodes in neoplasm of the bladder and prostate by positron emission tomography with 2-($^{18}$F)-2-deoxy-D-glucose. *Eur Urol*. 1999;40:481–487.

23. Fricke E, Machtens S, Hofmann M, et al. Positron emission tomography with $^{11}$C-acetate and $^{18}$F-FDG in prostate cancer patients. *Eur J Nucl Med Mol Imag*. 2003;30:607–611.

24. Sanz G, Robles JE, Gimenez M, et al. Positron emission tomography with 18fluorine-labeled deoxyglucose: utility in localized and advanced prostate cancer. *Br J Urol*. 1998;84:1028–1031.

25. Seltzer MA, Barbaric Z, Belldegrun A, et al. Comparison of helical computerized tomography, positron emission tomography and monoclonal antibody scans for evaluation of lymph node metastases in patients with prostate specific antigen relapse after treatment for localized prostate cancer. *J Urol*. 1999;162:1322–1328.

26. Sung J, Espiritu Jl, Segall GM, et al. Fluorodeoxyglucose positron emission tomography studies in the diagnostic and staging of clinically advanced prostate cancer. *BJU Int*. 2003;92:24–27.

27. Janetschek G, Langsteger W, Leeb K, et al. Detection of lymph node metastases in patients with clinically localized prostate cancer: comparison of 18 fluor cholin PET-CT with laparoscopic sentinel lymph node dissection and extended lymph node dissection. *Eur Urol*. 2005;3(suppl 4):68.

28. Bartsch Jun. G, Gottfried HW, Rinnab L, et al. Lymph node staging in prostate cancer by the use of 11C-choline-PET/CT scan imaging. *Eur Urol*. 2005;3(suppl 4):67.

29. Ackermann DA, Barry JU, Wicklund RA, et al. Analysis of risk factors associated with prostate cancer extension to the surgical margin and pelvic node metastasis at radical prostatectomy. *J Urol*. 1993;150:1845–1850.

30. Bluestein DL, Bostwick DG, Bergstrahl EJ, et al. Eliminating the need for bilateral pelvic lymphadenectomy in selected patients with prostate cancer. *J Urol*. 1994;151:1315–1320.

31. Dunzinger M, Sega W, Madersbacher S, et al. Predictive value of the anatomical location of ultrasound-guided systematic sextant prostate biopsies for the nodal status of

patients with localized prostate cancer. *Eur Urol.* 1997;31: 317–322.

32. Wawroschek F, Harzmann R, Weckermann D. Wertigkeit der Sentinel-Lymphknotenbiopsie bei urologischen Tumoren. *Urologe (A).* 2005;44:630–634.

33. Partin AW, Kattan MW, Subong ENP, et al. Combination of prostate-specific antigen, clinical stage, and Gleason score to predict pathological stage of localized prostate cancer. *JAMA.* 1997;277:1445–1451.

34. Partin AW, Mangold LA, Lamm DM, et al. Contemporary update of prostate cancer staging nomograms (Partin tables) for the new millennium. *Urology.* 2001;58:843–848.

35. Cangiannos I, Karakiewicz P, Eastham JA, et al. A preoperative nomogram identifying decreased risk of positive pelvic lymph nodes in patients with prostate cancer. *J Urol.* 2003;170:1798–1803.

36. Stock RG, Stone NN, Ianuzzi C. Seminal vesicle biopsy and laparoscopic pelvic lymph node dissection: implications for patient selection in the radiotherapeutic management of prostate cancer. *Int J Oncol Biol Phys.* 1995;33: 815–821.

37. Stone NN, Stock RG, Unger P. Indications for seminal vesicle biopsy and laparoscopic pelvic lymph node dissection in men with localized carcinoma of the prostate. *J Urol.* 1995;154:1392–1396.

38. Conrad S, Graefen M, Pichlmeier U, et al. Systematic sextant biopsies improve preoperative prediction of pelvic lymph node metastases in patients with clinically localized prostatic carcinoma. *J Urol.* 1998;159:2023–2029.

39. Conrad S, Graefen M, Pichlmaer U, et al. Prospective validation of an algorithm with systematic sextant biopsy to predict lymph node metastasis in patients with clinically localized prostate cancer. *J Urol.* 2002;167:521.

40. Naya Y, Babaian RJ. The predictors of pelvic lymph node metastasis at radical retropubic prostatectomy. *J Urol.* 2003;170:2306–2310.

41. Heidenreich A, Varga Z, Knobloch von R. Extended pelvic lymphadenectomy in patients undergoing radical prostatectomy: high incidence of lymph node metastasis. *J Urol.* 2002;167:1681–1686.

42. Bader P, Burkhard FC, Markwalder R, et al. Is a limited lymph node dissection an adequate staging procedure for prostate cancer? *J Urol.* 2002;168:514–518.

43. Wawroschek F, Hamm M, Weckermann D, et al. Lymph node staging in clinically localized prostate cancer. *Urol Int.* 2003;71:129–135.

44. Weckermann D, Wawroschek F, Harzmann R. Is there a need for pelvic lymph node dissection in low-risk prostate cancer patients prior to definitive local therapy? *Eur Urol.* 2005;47:45–51.

45. Catalona WJ, Smith DS. Cancer recurrence and survival rates after anatomic radical retropubic prostatectomy for prostate cancer: intermediate-term results. *J Urol.* 1998; 160:2428–2434.

46. Kapadia K, Bochner B, Groshen S, et al. Lymph node positive disease in radical prostatectomy patients: preoperative predictors and subsequent outcome. *J Urol.* 1999;161(suppl):1147.

47. Fahlenkamp D, Müller W, Schönberger B, et al. Laparoskopische pelvine Lymphadenektomie (LPLA) in der Diagnostik des lokoregionären Prostatakarzinoms. *Akt Urol.* 1997;28:35–42.

48. Winfield HN, Donovan JF, See WA, et al. Urological laparoscopic surgery. *J Urol.* 1991;146:941–948.

49. Weingärtner K, Ramaswamy A, Bittinger A, et al. Anatomical basic for pelvic lymphadenectomy in prostate cancer: results of an autopsy study and implications for the clinic. *J Urol.* 1969;156:1969–1971.

50. Schuessler WW, Pharand D, Vancaille TG. Laparosopic standard pelvic node dissection for carcinoma of the prostate: is it accurate? *J Urol.* 1993;150:898–901.

51. Leitlinien zur Diagnostik von Prostatakarzinomen. Mitteilungen der DGU und des BDU. *Urologe A.* 1999;38: 388–401.

52. Clark T, Parekh DJ, Cookson MS, et al. Randomized prospective evaluation of extended versus limited lymph node dissection in patients with clinically localized prostate cancer. *J Urol.* 2003;169:145–148.

53. Paul DB, Loening SA, Narayana AS, et al. Morbidity from pelvic lymphadenectomy in staging carcinoma of the prostate. *J Urol.* 1983;129:1141–1144.

54. Stone NN, Stock RG, Unger P. Laparoscopic pelvic lymph node dissection for prostate cancer: comparison of the extended and modified techniques. *J Urol.* 1997;158:1891–1894.

55. Winter A, Vogt C, Weckermann D, et al. Komplikationsraten verschiedener LA-Techniken beim Klinisch lokalisierten prostatakarzinom im vergleich. *Der Urologe.* 2005;44(Suppl 1):79.

56. Herrell SD, Trachtenberg J, Theodorescu D. Staging pelvic lymphadenectomy for localized carcinoma of the prostate: a comparison of 3 surgical techniques. *J Urol.* 1997;157: 1337–1339.

57. Lezin MS, Cherrie R, Cattolica E. Comparison of laparoscopic and mini-laparotomy pelvic lymphadenectomy for prostate cancer staging in a community practise. *Urology.* 1997;49:60–64.

58. Paul DB, Loening SA, Narayana AS, et al. Morbidity from pelvic lymphadenectomy in staging carcinoma of the prostate. *J Urol.* 1983;129:1141–1144.

59. McDowell GC, Johnson JW, Tenney DM, et al. Pelvic lymphadenectomy for staging clinically localized prostate cancer: indications, complications, and results in 217 cases. *Urology.* 1990;35:476–482.

60. Golimbu M, Morales P, Al Askari S, et al. Extended pelvic lymphadenectomy for prostatic cancer. *J Urol.* 1979;121: 617–620.

61. Wawroschek F, Vogt H, Wengenmair H, et al. Prostate lymphoscintigraphy and radioguided surgery for sentinel lymph node identification in prostate cancer. *Urol Int.* 2003;70:303–310.

62. Rudoni M, Sacchetti GM, Leva L, et al. Recent applications of the sentinel lymph node concept: preliminary experience in prostate cancer. *Tumori.* 2002;88: 16–17.

63. Bastide C, Brenot-Rossi I, Garcia S, et al. Feasibility and value of the isotope sentinel node mapping technique in prostate cancer. *Prog Urol.* 2004;14:501–506.

64. Sherman AI, Ter Pogossian M. Lymph node concentrative colloidal gold following interstitial injection. *Cancer.* 1953;6:1238–1244.

65. Menon M, Menon S, Strauss HW, et al. Demonstration of the existence of canine prostatic lymphatics by radioisotope technique. *J Urol.* 1977;118:274–277.

66. Kaplan WD, Whitmore WF, Gittes RF. Visualization of canine and human prostatic lymph nodes following intraprostatic injection of technetium 99m antimony sulfide colloid. *Invest Radiol.* 1980;15:34–38.

67. Gardiner RA, Fitzpatrick JM, Constable AR, et al. Human prostatic lymphoscintigraphy: a preliminary report. *Br J Urol.* 1979;51:300–303.

68. Gardiner RA, Fitzpatrick JM, Constable AR, et al. Improved techniques in radionuclide imaging of prostatic lymph nodes. *Br J Urol.* 1979;51:561–564.

69. Zuckier LS, Finkelstein M, Kreutzer ER, et al. Technetium-99m antimony sulphide colloid lymphoscintigraphy of the prostate by direct transrectal injection. *Nucl Med Commun.* 1990;11:589–596.

70. Stone AR, Merrick MV, Chisholm GD. Prostatic lymphoscintigraphy. *Br J Urol.* 1979;51:556–560.

71. Horenblas S, Nuyten MJ, Hoefnagel CA, et al. Detection of lymph node invasion in prostatic carcinoma with iliopelvic lympho-scintigraphy. *Br J Urol.* 1992;69:180–182.

72. Wawroschek F, Vogt H, Weckermann D, et al. Radioisotope-guided pelvic lymph node dissection for prostate cancer. *J Urol.* 2001;166:1715–1719.

73. Wawroschek F, Vogt H, Wengenmair H, et al. Prostate lymphoscintigraphy and radioguided surgery for sentinel lymph node identification in prostate cancer: technique and results of the first 350 cases. *Urol Int.* 2003;70:303–310.

74. Takashima H, Egawa M, Imao T, et al. Validity of sentinel lymph node concept for patients with prostate cancer. *J Urol.* 2004;171:2268–2271.

75. Egawa M, Fukuda M, Takashima H, et al. Application of sentinel node navigation surgery to prostate cancer. *Gan To Kagaku Ryoho.* 2005;32:117–120.

76. Wurm T, Eichhorn K, Corvin S, et al. Anatomic-functional image fusion allows intraoperative sentinel node detection in prostate cancer patients. *Eur Urol.* 2004;3(suppl 2):140.

77. Corvin S, Eichhorn K, Wurm T, et al. Radioisotope guided laparoscopic pelvic lymph node dissection—a novel technique for prostate cancer staging. *Eur Urol.* 2004;3(suppl 2):140.

78. Wawroschek F, Wengenmair H, Senekowitzsch-Schmidtke R, et al. Prostate lymphoscintigraphy for sentinel lymph node identification in canines: reproducibility, uptake, and biokinetics depending on different injection strategies. *Urol Res.* 2003;31:152–158.

79. Miltenburg DM, Miller C, Karamlou TB, et al. Meta-analysis of sentinel lymph node biopsy in breast cancer. *J Surg Res.* 1999;84:138–142.

80. Horenblas S, Jansen L, Meinhardt W, et al. Detection of occult metastasis in squamous cell carcinoma of the penis using a dynamic sentinel node procedure. *J Urol.* 2000;163:100–104.

81. Wawroschek F, Vogt H, Bachter D, et al. R. First experience of gamma probe-guided sentinel lymph node surgery in penile cancer. *Urol Res.* 2000;28:246–249.

82. Morton DL, Wen DR, Wong JH, et al. Technical details of intraoperative lymphatic mapping for early stage melanoma. *Arch Surg.* 1992;127:392–399.

83. Morton DL, Wen DR, Cochran AJ. Management of early stage melanoma by intraoperative lymphatic mapping and selective lymphadenectomy. An alternative to routine elective lymphadenectomy or watch and wait. *Surg Oncol Clin N Am.* 1990;1:247.

84. Wengenmair HE. *Biokinetische und messtechnische Grundlagen zum szintigraphischen und intraoperativen Nachweis von Wächterlymphknoten der Prostata mit $^{99m}$Tc-Nanokolloid.* Aachen: Shaker Verlag, 2005.

85. Suzuki T, Kurokawa K, Yamanaka H, et al. Lymphatic drainage of the prostate gland in canines. *Prostate.* 1992;21:279.

86. Aumüller G. Morphologie der normalen Prostata und experimentelle Modelle der Prostataforschung. In: Helpap B, Senge T, Vahlensieck W, editors. *Die Prostata.* Frankfurt: pmi; 1983:15.

87. Gallowitsch HJ. Lymphoscintigraphy and dosimetry. In: Munz DL, ed. *The Sentinel Lymph Node Concept in Oncology. Facts and Fiction.* Munich: W. Zuckschwerdt; 2001:57.

88. Uren RF, Howman-Giles RB, Thompson JF, et al. Mammary lymphoscintigraphy in breast cancer. *J Nucl Med.* 1995;36:1775.

89. McMasters KM, Reintgen DS, Ross MI, et al. Sentinel lymph node biopsy for melanoma: how many radioactive nodes should be removed? *Ann Surg Oncol.* 2001;8:192.

90. Brenot-Rossi I, Bastide C, Garcia S, et al. Limited pelvic lymphadenectomy using the sentinel lymph node procedure in patients with localized prostate carcinoma: a pilot study. *Eur J Nucl Med Mol Imaging.* 2005;32:635–640.

91. Wawroschek F, Vogt H, Weckermann D, et al. The sentinel lymph node concept in prostate cancer—first results of gamma probe-guided sentinel lymph node identification. *Eur Urol.* 1999;36:595–600.

92. Moul JW, Lewis DJ, Ross AA, et al. Immunohistologic detection of prostate cancer pelvic lymph node micrometastases: correlation to preoperative serum prostate-specific antigen. *Urology.* 1994;43:68–73.

93. Gomella LG, White JL, Mccue PA, et al. Screening for occult nodal metastasis in localized carcinoma of the prostate. *J Urol.* 1993;149:776–778.

94. Wawroschek F, Wagner Th, Hamm M, et al. The influence of serial sections, immunohistochemistry, and extension of pelvic lymph node dissection on the lymph node status in clinically localized prostate cancer. *Eur Urol.* 2003;43:132–137.

95. Haas J, Wagner T, Wawroschek F, et al. Combined application of RT-PCR and immunohistochemistry on paraffin embedded sentinel lymph nodes of prostate cancer patients. *Pathol Res Pract.* 2005;200:763–770.

96. Lawrence WD. ADASP recommendations for processing and reporting of lymph node specimens submitted for evaluation of metastatic disease. *Virchows Arch*. 2001;439: 601–603.

97. Wengenmair H, Kopp J, Vogt H, et al. Sentinel lymph node diagnostic in prostate carcinoma. II. Biokinetics and dosimetry of $^{99m}$Tc-nanocolloid after intraprostatic injection. *Nucl Med*. 2002;412:102–107.

# 16
# Radioguided Biopsy of the Sentinel Lymph Node in Patients with Non-Small Cell Lung Cancer

Giuseppe Boni, Gianpiero Manca, Franca M.A. Melfi, Marco Lucchi, Alfredo Mussi, and Giuliano Mariani

## The Clinical Problem

Lung cancer is one of the most common malignancies in the Western world, accounting for more cancer deaths than the next 4 most frequent cancers combined. In the year 2000, the worldwide incidence of non-small cell lung cancer was close to 1,000,000 cases; in 2004, there were approximately 174,000 cases of lung cancer in the United States alone, resulting in more than 160,000 deaths (1). The overall low 5-year survival rate for patients diagnosed with lung cancer (15%) is especially discouraging. Such poor long-term survival is probably related to the fact that early-stage disease is asymptomatic, and thus the onset of symptoms marks the presence of advanced, mostly incurable disease.

Once a diagnosis of non-small cell lung cancer is confirmed, patients should be staged as accurately as possible on the basis of clinical, radiologic, and pathological information. Staging based on the TNM (tumor, nodes, and metastases) classification, as recommended by the American Joint Committee for Cancer (AJCC) (2), is the primary determinant of survival for these patients (3,4). The main goals of staging are to assist in determining appropriate treatment options (surgery versus nonsurgical therapies) and in predicting prognosis.

Traditional staging modalities include history and physical exams, laboratory tests, and noninvasive staging techniques such as conventional chest x-ray, computed tomography (CT), bone scan, magnetic resonance imaging, and positron emission tomography. If these tests do not demonstrate the presence of metastatic disease or unresectable local disease, then further invasive staging procedures may be necessary, including bronchoscopy, mediastinoscopy, and video-assisted thoracoscopic surgery.

Additional invasive modalities for defining the N stage, such as complete thoracic lymphadenectomy or nodal sampling (both performed during surgical resection of the primary tumor), may help to further stratify patients into appropriate therapeutic and prognostic categories. In this regard, mediastinal lymph node dissection can result in the implementation of effective therapeutic strategies when it helps discover nodal metastatic non-small cell lung cancer, as lymph node status is an important prognostic indicator (5,6). However, this procedure is not therapeutic per se, and may even be harmful for patients with lymph node metastasis.

Thus, the role of complete mediastinal lymph node dissection versus sampling at the time of thoracotomy remains controversial. Advocates of complete lymphadenectomy assert that without complete resection of nodal tissue, residual cancer may remain, leading to poorer prognosis due to locoregional recurrence and understaging of disease (7,8). Proponents of lymph node sampling argue that it does not impair local immune factors, which may reduce the potential for local recurrence, and is not associated with increased morbidity, such as increased perioperative blood loss, recurrent nerve injury, chylothorax, or bronchopleural fistula (9). To date, no survival advantage has clearly been demonstrated using either technique.

To further investigate this issue, the American College of Surgeons Oncology Group (ACOSOG) is conducting a large prospective randomized trial of more than 1000 patients, comparing complete mediastinal lymph node dissection to standard lymph node sampling only (10). The study's primary objective is to evaluate any effect on survival, and secondary objectives include evaluation of disease-free survival, postoperative complications, and potential for identification of occult metastatic disease in the dissected lymph nodes. Although it will be years before the survival objective is answered, preliminary results on the impact of mediastinal lymph node dissection seem to indicate no increase in morbidity or mortality rates associated with this surgical procedure.

Thus, while there is no dispute over the prognostic impact of lymph node pathological status, whether to perform a complete dissection or only lymph node sampling at the time of lung cancer resection remains a controversial issue. This is a crucial issue in patients with operable lung cancers, since the presence of lymph node involvement may decrease their 5-year survival rate by nearly 50%, as compared to that of similar patients without nodal metastases (11).

Since prognosis for patients with non-small cell lung cancer does not seem to be affected by complete mediastinal lymph node dissection (even if performed with alleged therapeutic intent), it can be speculated that morbidity of selective mediastinal lymph node sampling and pathologic staging of lung cancer can be improved with sentinel lymph node mapping. Sentinel node mapping and biopsy would enable surgeons to accurately stage the mediastinum in patients with non-small cell lung cancer, while avoiding more or less extensive lymph node dissection and its associated complications.

## The Sentinel Lymph Node Concept

Although several studies on lymphatic mapping in patients with non-small cell lung cancer have been published, all proving that sentinel lymph nodes exist in this type of tumor (12–18), sentinel node biopsy cannot yet be considered as part of the clinical practice for this disease.

Although lung resection for non-small cell lung cancer combined with mediastinal lymph node dissection lead to greater production of postoperative exudates than with resection alone, the morbidity of mediastinal lymph node dissection is not particularly relevant (10). In this regard, the main advantage of sentinel node mapping and biopsy lies in directing extensive histopathologic examination selectively to the first node receiving lymph draining from the non-small cell lung tumor. Exquisitely sensitive analysis techniques—such as serial sectioning of virtually the entire lymph node for conventional hematoxylin and eosin (H&E) staining or immunohistochemistry, and reverse transcription-polymerase chain reaction (RT-PCR) analysis—can be applied, increasing the chance of detecting occult micrometastatic nodal disease (13,18). In fact, more careful pathologic evaluation (immunohistochemistry versus H&E staining) of lymph nodes that were previously reported negative for metastatic involvement in resected lung cancer patients has revealed micrometastatic disease in over 20% of such patients classified as pN0, thus determining upstage of the disease for a sizable fraction (19,20).

Both such "ultrastaging" (made possible by restricting pathological analysis to the sentinel node) and the recognition of the most frequent patterns of mediastinal distribution of lymph draining from the locations of non-small cell lung cancer may have a profound effect on the future modality of lung cancer staging. If confirmed by large-scale studies, these results might lead to a revision of the TNM staging system for non-small cell lung cancer, so as to include information on the number of involved nodes and the degree of nodal invasion.

## Non-Radionuclide Methods for Sentinel Lymph Node Mapping

Several techniques have been described for using non-radionuclide tracers to map the sentinel lymph node in patients with non-small cell lung cancer (12,21,22). In 1999, Little et al. first reported on intraoperative lymphatic mapping of the sentinel node in these patients using the vital dye isosulfan blue (12). However, it was often difficult to visually detect the pattern of distribution of the blue dye reaching anthracotic lymph nodes in the thoracic cavity, so the resulting identification rate of the sentinel node (46%) was too low to be clinically useful. An even lower identification rate (6.3%) was reported by Sugi et al. using indocyanine green as the vital dye (21). In addition, it should be noted that, although rare, anaphylactic reactions to these dyes have been reported (22).

A more novel approach has been based on magnetic recognition (23), whereby colloidal ferumoxides (superparamagnetic iron) are injected at the periphery of the tumor during thoracotomy. A highly sensitive, handheld magnetometer is then used to detect ex-vivo the magnetic force of the ferumoxides within the lymph nodes excised during mediastinal dissection, thus helping to identify the sentinel node(s). Although the preliminary results indicate that this approach is feasible and safe, so far it is not suitable for effective in-vivo sentinel node mapping.

## Radionuclide Methods for Sentinel Lymph Node Mapping

In 2000, Liptay et al. were the first to describe the surgical technique of radioguided localization of sentinel lymph nodes in patients with non-small cell lung cancer (13). Their approach involved peritumoral injection of the radiocolloid at the time of thoracotomy (74 MBq of $^{99m}$Tc-sulfur colloid, filtered through a 0.22 μm filter, subdivided into 4 aliquots injected equatorially), as soon as the tumor could be exposed. The surgery then proceeded normally, paying particular care to avoid direct handling of the peribronchial lymphatics until the last portion of the resection. After performing radioactive counting of both the primary tumor and visible lymph node stations with a handheld gamma counter, anatomic resection with a full mediastinal node dissection was performed, followed by histopathology of all the resected nodes. Sentinel lymph nodes were defined as any nodal station with in-vivo radioactivity readings 3 times greater than background measurements in the chest cavity. By adopting this criterion, multiple sentinel node stations were identified in approximately 15% of the cases. Radioactive nodes identified as sentinel nodes were examined using both conventional H&E staining and immunohistochemistry employing an anticytokeratin monoclonal antibody.

The mean migration time of the radiocolloid through the lymphatics was 63 minutes (range: 23–170 min) and did not prolong the operation. Radioguided localization was not associated with increased morbidity.

The success rate in sentinel node identification was 82%, and the false-negative rate (i.e., finding metastasis in a nonsentinel node) was about 5%. Metastatic disease was found in the sentinel nodes of 12 out of 37 patients (32%). In 3 patients, immunohistochemistry and complete serial section analysis identified micrometastasis in sentinel nodes that had turned negative at conventional H&E staining, thus upstaging these patients from N0 to N1. Although most sentinel nodes identified by intraoperative gamma counting were located in the proximal lobar and hilar stations (N1), 22% were in the mediastinal space (N2), either in addition to those in the more proximal lobar/hilar stations, or only found in the mediastinum (thus with a "skip pattern" of nodal drainage).

The authors concluded that the intraoperative technique was feasible and safe. However, they reported that the technique did not ensure useful radioactivity counting rates from the upper mediastinal lymph nodes intraoperatively, due to a somewhat high interfering background caused by radiocolloid that had migrated from the lung parenchyma (the injection site) into the trachea. Identification of mediastinal sentinel nodes had

to be based on ex-vivo counting following mediastinal lymph node dissection. Obviously, this is an important limitation in the perspective of adopting mediastinal lymph node sampling directed specifically to sentinel lymph nodes.

To overcome this drawback, Liptay et al. modified the original technique by simply decreasing the amount of radioactivity injected into the tumor from the original total dose of 74 MBq to about 9 MBq. This dose adjustment allowed a relevant reduction in background radiation from the injection site, enhancing the ability to identify sentinel node stations by in-vivo gamma probe counting (18).

An alternative approach was described in 2002 by Nomori et al. (14,15), based on CT-guided injection of 220 to 300 MBq of $^{99m}$Tc-tin colloid, administered as a single peritumoral bolus the day before surgery. Lymphoscintigraphic imaging was performed only in a pilot phase of the study, to monitor progression of lymphatic drainage (Figure 16-1). On the following day, intraoperative gamma-probe counting was used to search for sentinel nodes. These authors reported an 87% success rate in sentinel node identification, with about 85% of such nodes being lobar/hilar and 15% located in the mediastinum. Interestingly, no false-negative sentinel nodes were reported (14). Subsequently, other groups (16,21) have adopted a similar approach (CT-guided preoperative radiocolloid injection), reporting a sentinel node identification rate (67%–87%) similar to that obtained with the intraoperative injection procedure originally described by Liptay et al.

The most important advantage of the preoperative injection technique is that it enables intraoperative gamma counting for the upper mediastinal lymph node as well, since any radioactivity that may have migrated from the injection site into the trachea is cleared during

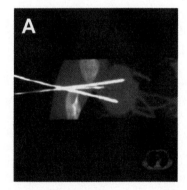 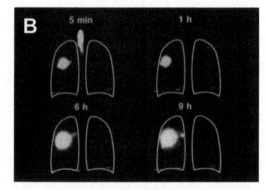

FIGURE 16-1. (A) Transthoracic computed tomographic (CT)-guided injection of a radiocolloid in non-small cell lung cancer (3 different positions of the 23-gauge needle utilized for injection within the tumor mass). (B) Sequential lymphoscintigraphy showing time-course progression of $^{99m}$Tc-tin colloid administered by CT-guided injection in a patient with non-small cell lung cancer. After some intraparenchymal diffusion of the injected radiocolloid (migrating in part also to the trachea, as observed in the early imaging time), hilar lymph nodes are clearly depicted at the 6-hour imaging, when tracheal radioactivity has completely cleared away. (Panel (A) Reprinted from Melfi et al. [16], with permission from Elsevier; (B) Reprinted from Nomori et al. [14], with permission from American Association for Thoracic Surgery.)

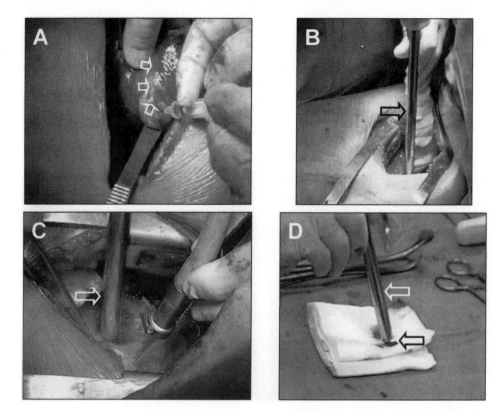

FIGURE 16-2. Sequential phases of radioguided biopsy of the sentinel lymph node in a patient with non-small cell lung cancer, according to the intraoperative radiocolloid injection procedure. (A) Injection of $^{99m}$Tc-albumin nanocolloid at the periphery of the tumor (indicated by white open arrows) immediately after exposing the lung during thoracotomy. (B) The search for the sentinel lymph node(s) using a handheld intraoperative gamma probe (indicated by a black open arrow) at the lobar/hilar level. (C) The search for sentinel lymph node(s) using the gamma probe (indicated by a white open arrow) in the mediastinum. (D) Ex-vivo counting of a sentinel lymph node (indicated by a black open arrow) using the gamma probe (indicated by a white open arrow).

the intervening period between the injection and surgery (24 hours apart).

Lardinois et al. described an interesting alternative to CT-guided injection, using instead preoperative transbronchoscopic injection of the radiocolloid (80 Mbq of $^{99m}$Tc-albumin nanocolloid). With this technique (which was not associated with any complication), the authors reported a 95% success rate in the identification of sentinel nodes; 21% were located in the mediastinum, while more than 1 sentinel node was found in 63% of patients. Metastatic involvement was discovered in 47% of the patients; in 2 patients, immunohistochemistry and extensive serial sectioning revealed micrometastasis that had gone undetected with conventional H&E staining (17).

Based on these reports indicating the feasibility of both pre- and intraoperative modalities of radiocolloid injection for identifying the first sites of potential nodal metastases of non-small cell lung cancer, Melfi et al. (from Pisa) explored both mapping procedures: for 19 patients, using CT-guided preoperative injection of 37 MBq of $^{99m}$Tc-albumin nanocolloid; and for 10 patients, using intraoperative injection (see Figure 16-2). As a slight modification to Nomori's approach, the CT-guided radiocolloid injection was performed 1 to 2 hours rather than 24 hours before surgery. The cumulative success rate in sentinel lymph node identification was 96%, and no false-negative results were observed (i.e., metastatic involvement of nonsentinel nodes). The only failure in sentinel node identification (poor migration of the radiocolloid) was observed in 1 patient with a large tumor (6.5 cm). Similar to other reports, 2 different sentinel nodes were found in 28% of patients, and about 20% of the sentinel nodes were located in the mediastinum (with a skip pattern of lymph drainage in 2 patients). Furthermore, in 2 patients immunohistochemistry revealed micrometastasis that had gone undetected with conventional H&E staining. No complications were observed during the mapping procedure; in particular, no pneumothorax or bleeding was observed during the intratumoral injection under CT guidance (the needle used for radiocolloid injection is 23-gauge) (16). The above pattern of results obtained by the Pisa group has subsequently been confirmed in a group of more than 60 patients in an ongoing clinical trial (unpublished results).

## Conclusion

Although several studies and ongoing trials have demonstrated the feasibility and safety of radioguided biopsy of the sentinel lymph node in patients with non-small cell lung cancer, a standard technique has not yet been established (24).

While lymphatic mapping and radioguided biopsy of the sentinel node in non-small cell lung cancer may allow a more accurate characterization of unique patterns of lymphatic drainage from the tumor, the potential role of sentinel node evaluation for limiting mediastinal node dissection (especially in patients with small tumors and clinically negative lymph nodes) remains to be determined. In this regard, possible patterns of skip lymphatic drainage are a cause of special concern. However, sentinel lymph node identification may direct accurate histopathologic evaluation, especially with extensive serial sectioning and immunohistochemistry analysis. If obtained intraoperatively, such staging information may assist the surgeon in adopting the adequate level of nodal dissection for individual patients.

Further experience and large-scale multicenter trials of sentinel lymph node mapping in non-small cell lung cancer are necessary before this surgical procedure is widely accepted for treating this type of cancer and avoiding complete mediastinal lymphadenectomy in patients with early-stage tumors.

## References

1. Jemal RC, Tiwari T, Murray, et al. Cancer statistics, 2004. *CA Cancer J Clin.* 2004;54:8–29.
2. Greene FL, Page DL, Fleming ID, et al. *AJCC Cancer Staging Handbook.* 6th edition. New York: Springer; 2002.
3. Nesbitt JC, Putnam JB, Walsh GL, Roth JA, Mountain CF. Survival in early-stage non-small cell lung cancer. *Ann Thorac Surg.* 1995;60:466–472.
4. Mountain CF. Revisions in the international system for staging lung cancer. *Chest.* 1997;111:1710–1717.
5. Keller SM, Adak S, Wagner H, Johnson DH. Mediastinal lymph node dissection improves survival in patients with stages II and IIIa non-small cell lung cancer. Eastern Cooperative Oncology Group. *Ann Thorac Surg.* 2000;70:358–365 (discussion 365–366).
6. Naruke T, Goya T, Tsuchiya R, Suemasu K. The importance of surgery to non-small cell carcinoma of lung with mediastinal lymph node metastasis. *Ann Thorac Surg.* 1988;46:603–610.
7. Passlick B, Kubuschock B, Sienel W, et al. Mediastinal lymphadenectomy in non-small cell lung cancer: effectiveness in patients with or without nodal micrometastases—results of a preliminary study. *Eur J Cardiothoacr Surg.* 2002;21:520–526.
8. Naruke T, Tsuchiya R, Kondo H, Nakayama H, Asamura H. Lymph node sampling in lung cancer: how should it be done? *Eur J Cardiothorac Surg.* 1999;16:17–24.
9. Izbicki JR, Thetter O, Habekost M, et al. Radical systematic mediastinal lymphadenectomy in non-small cell lung cancer: a randomized controlled trial. *Brit J Surg.* 1994; 81:229–235.
10. Allen MS, Darling G, Pechet T, et al. Morbidity and mortality of major pulmonary resections in patients with early-stage lung cancer: initial results of the randomized, prospective ACOSOG Z0030 Trial. *Ann Thorac Surg.* 2006;81:1013–1019.
11. Mountain CF, Dresler CM. Regional lymph node classification for lung cancer staging. *Chest.* 1997;111:1718–1723.
12. Little AG, DeHoyos A, Kirgan DM, et al. Intraoperative lymphatic mapping for non-small cell lung cancer: the sentinel node technique. *J Thorac Cardiovasc Surg.* 1999;117:220–234.
13. Liptay MJ, Masters GA, Winchester DJ, et al. Intraoperative radioisotope sentinel lymph node mapping in non-small cell lung cancer. *Ann Thorac Surg.* 2000;70:384–389.
14. Nomori H, Horio H, Naruke T, Orikasa H, Yamazaki K, Suemasu K. Use of technetium-99m tin colloid for sentinel lymph node identification in non-small cell lung cancer. *J Thorac Cardiovasc Surg.* 2002;1243:486–492.
15. Nomori H, Watanabe K, Ohtsuka T, Naruke T, Suemasu K. In vivo identification of sentinel lymph nodes for clinical stage I non-small cell lung cancer for abbreviation of mediastinal lymph node dissection. *Lung Cancer.* 2004; 46:49–55.
16. Melfi FM, Chella A, Menconi GF, et al. Intraoperative radioguided lymph node biopsy in non-small cell lung cancer. *Eur J Cardiothorac Surg.* 2003;23:214–220.
17. Lardinois D, Brack T, Gaspert A, et al. Bronchoscopic radioisotope injection for sentinel lymph-node mapping in potentially resectable non-small-cell lung cancer. *Eur J Cardiothorac Surg.* 2003;23:824–827.
18. Liptay MJ, Grondin SC, Fry WA, et al. Intraoperative sentinel lymph node mapping in non-small-cell lung cancer improves detection of micrometastases. *J Clin Oncol.* 2002; 20:1984–1988.
19. Kubuschock B, Passlick B, Izbicki JR, et al. Disseminated tumor cells in lymph nodes as a determinant for survival in surgically resected non-small cell lung cancer. *J Clin Oncol.* 1999;17:19–24.
20. Riquet M, Manac'h D, Pimpec-Barthes F, et al. Prognostic significance of surgical-pathologic N1 disease in non-small cell carcinoma of the lung. *Ann Thorac Surg.* 1999;67:1572–1576.
21. Sugi K, Fukuda M, Nakamura H, Kaneda Y. Comparison of 3 tracers for detecting sentinel lymph nodes in patients with clinical N0 lung cancer. *Lung Cancer.* 2003;39:37–40.

22. Albo D, Wayne JD, Hunt KK, et al. Anaphylactic reactions to isosulfan blue dye during sentinel lymph node biopsy for breast cancer. *Am J Surg.* 2001;182:393–398.

23. Nakagawa T, Minamiya Y, Katayose Y, et al. A novel method for sentinel lymph node mapping using magnetite in patients with non-small cell lung cancer. *J Thorac Cardiovasc Surg.* 2003;126:563–567.

24. Minamiya Y, Ogawa J-I. The current status of sentinel lymph node mapping in non-small cell lung cancer. *Ann Thorac Cardiovasc Surg.* 2005;11:67–72.

# 17
# Sentinel Lymph Node Biopsy in Thyroid Cancer

Massimo Salvatori, Domenico Rubello, Michael J. O'Doherty, Maria Rosa Pelizzo, and Giuliano Mariani

Intraoperative lymphatic mapping and sentinel lymph node dissection are based on the concept that tumor status of the sentinel lymph node—the first node in the regional nodal basin that drains a primary tumor—reflects the tumor status of that basin's remaining lymph nodes (1). This technique has been extensively validated in patients with melanoma and breast cancer and has been investigated in other solid tumors, such as thyroid carcinoma (2–4). However, differentiated thyroid carcinoma (DTC) is perhaps the only tumor in the human body where the presence of locoregional nodal metastasis has no bearing on the patient's long-term survival, and therefore the role of the lymph node surgery is debatable and controversial (5).

In this context, the utility of sentinel lymph node dissection in the surgical management of patients with DTC remains to be fully defined, and the technique has been restricted to formal clinical research (6). However, preliminary reports indicate that sentinel lymph node dissection may be applicable easily and successfully in thyroid cancer, with an acceptable diagnostic accuracy (7,8).

## Lymphatic Drainage and Lymph Node Compartments in the Neck

Surgical management of patients with DTC requires an understanding of the lymphatic drainage of the thyroid.

The lymphatic drainage of the thyroid is extensive. In general, the lymphatics accompany the veins, but in contrast to the veins, their direction of flow is not always predictable. Collecting lymph channels draining the intraglandular capillaries are found beneath the thyroid capsule, and these channels in turn drain into the lymph vessels associated with the capsule and may cross-communicate with the isthmus and the opposite lobe. The lymphatic system of the neck is contained in the cellulo-adipose tissue delineated by the aponeurosis enveloping the muscles, vessels, and nerves (9). It consists of the following:

- The superior lymph vessels drain the isthmus and the medial superior portion of the thyroid lobes, ascend in front of the larynx, and terminate in the subdigastric lymph nodes of the internal jugular chain.
- The median inferior lymph vessels descend with the inferior vein to the pretracheal nodes.
- The lateral collecting group drains superiorly to the anterior and superior nodes of the jugular chain, and inferiorly to the lateral and inferior nodes of the internal jugular vein.

Numerous classifications have been proposed to describe the location and the anatomic boundaries of lymph node groups in the neck, using either surgical landmarks, physical assessment criteria, or computed tomography and magnetic resonance imaging (10). The most commonly used have been defined by the American Joint Committee on Cancer (AJCC) and the American Academy of Otolaryngology-Head and Neck Surgery (AAO-HNS) (11,12). These classifications use a levels system (Figure 17-1), in which certain lymph node groups are located within each level of the neck (Table 17-1) (9,13). The levels' boundaries are defined by surgically visible bones, muscles, blood vessels, and nerves, with successive refinements suggested using radiological landmarks; further definition of sublevels has been proposed (Figure 17-2) (9).

This level-based system, originally described by head and neck surgeons at Memorial Sloan-Kettering Hospital in New York, divides the neck into 5 regions on each side, with a sixth region used to classify the lymph nodes in the anterior neck (12). The region defined as level Ia is a unique median region that contains the submental nodes, while level Ib contains the submandibular nodes. These nodes are not at risk for har-

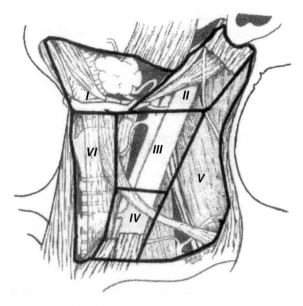

FIGURE 17-1. The level system most widely used to describe the location of lymph nodes in the neck. (Robbins et al. [14], by permission from Elsevier.)

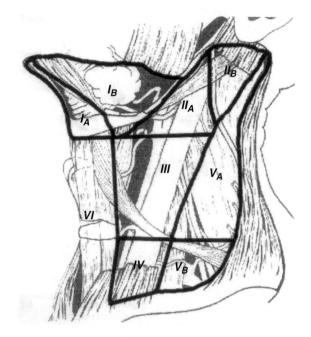

FIGURE 17-2. Division of neck levels I, II, and V into sublevels. (Robbins et al. [14], by permission from Elsevier.)

boring metastases from DTC, but may contain metastatic disease when the primary site involved is the lip, buccal mucosa, anterior nasal cavity, or soft tissue of the cheek (12,14).

Level II extends from the base of the skull to the carotid bifurcation or the caudal border of the body of the hyoid bone. It contains the upper jugular lymph nodes located around the upper one-third of the internal jugular vein and the upper spinal accessory nerve (level IIa), and posteriorly to the spinal accessory nerve (level IIb). These nodes are at greatest risk of harboring metastases from cancers of the nasal cavity, oral cavity, nasopharynx, oropharynx, hypopharynx, larynx, and the major salivary glands (12).

Level III is the caudal extension of level II and contains the middle jugular lymph node group, including the jugulo-omohyoid nodes, located around the middle third

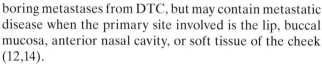

TABLE 17-1. Lymph nodes groups located within each level of the neck.

| Level | Lymph Node Group |
|---|---|
| Ia | Submental nodes |
| Ib | Submandibular nodes |
| Iia | Upper jugular nodes, anterior to spinal accessory nerve |
| Iib | Upper jugular nodes, posterior to spinal accessory nerve |
| III | Middle jugular nodes |
| IV | Lower jugular nodes |
| Va | Posterior triangle nodes (spinal accessory group) |
| Vb | Posterior triangle nodes (supraclavicular group) |
| VI | Central compartment lymph nodes |

*Source:* Robbins et al. (12), by permission from Elsevier.

of the internal jugular vein. The highly variable lymph nodes at this level have the greatest risk of harboring metastases from cancers of the oral cavity, nasopharynx, oropharynx, hypopharynx, and larynx (12).

Level IV extends from the caudal limit of level III to the clavicle and includes the lower jugular lymph nodes surrounding the lower third of the internal jugular vein. It has a variable number of nodes , which receive afferent lymphatics primarily from levels III and V, and collecting lymphatics from the hypopharynx, larynx, and thyroid gland. Level IV nodes are at high risk of harboring metastases from cancers of the hypopharynx, larynx, and cervical esophagus (12).

Levels Va and Vb include all the lymph nodes contained within the posterior triangle, collectively referred to as the posterior triangle group. This group is composed predominantly of the nodes located along the spinal accessory nerve, the transverse cervical artery, and the supraclavicular nodes that are not involved in the drainage of head and neck cancers except skin tumors (9).

Level VI, also called the anterior (central) neck compartment, contains the pretracheal and paratracheal nodes, the precricoid (Delphian) node, and the perithyroidal nodes, including the lymph nodes along the recurrent laryngeal nerves (14). These nodes and their connecting lymphatic channels are often pathways for the spread of papillary thyroid carcinoma, and it is recommended that they be removed during surgery for thyroid cancer (15).

# Incidence and Pattern of Lymph Node Metastases

The majority of patients with papillary thyroid carcinoma with lymph node metastases have these metastases at the time of initial presentation; less frequently, metastatic lesions in lymph nodes are found at follow-up, indicating either an incomplete initial treatment or the presence of an aggressive tumor (16). Shaha et al. (17) reported a 56% incidence of clinically apparent nodal metastasis at the time of initial presentation, and only 5% subsequent development of nodal metastasis (61% cumulative incidence).

The reported incidence of nodal metastasis in DTC depends on the size of the involved nodes, the histological variety, the age of the patient, the extent of lymphnode surgery, and the number of sections examined by the pathologist. Macroscopic or clinically apparent nodal involvement ranges between 15% and 50% (5); microscopic metastases have been found in up to 80% of adult patients with papillary thyroid carcinoma (5).

The highest incidence of nodal metastasis is noted in young individuals (up to 80% of children), who, however, have excellent prognosis, demonstrating that the age at initial diagnosis is one of the most important prognostic factors in multivariate analysis (16).

The central compartment (level VI) is involved in approximately 90% of node-positive (N+) patients (18). It was not involved in 15.3%, 8.9%, and 10% of the series of N+ patients reported by Mirallie et al. (18), Ozaki et al. (19), and Frankenthaler et al. (20), respectively.

There is also a high frequency of lateral node involvement among patients with positive nodes, ranging from 51% to 100% of the reported series (18,20,21), with the caudal portions of the cervicolateral compartments (level III, IV) involved more frequently than the cranial portions (22). Supraclavicular node involvement is the third site involved, with a reported 10% to 52% rate among N+ patients (18,20).

Contralateral node involvement in the presence of a uni-nodular thyroid tumor has been reported in 18.4% of patients (18,21). Mediastinal node involvement is infrequent, and in most cases is localized in the anterosuperior mediastinum. In the absence of systematic dissection, their frequency—which has been reported to range between 1.9% and 15% (18,20,23)—cannot be reliably evaluated.

The distribution of cervical metastatic involvement is not related to the tumor's site in the thyroid lobe (18). However, when the tumor is located in the upper third of the thyroid, subdigastric lymph nodes are often involved (18), and tumors arising in the isthmus may cause bilateral cervical metastases (24) or increased nodal recurrence on the contralateral side in patients with initial unilateral lymph node metastases (25).

The size of the primary cancer has been linked to the site of lymph node metastases, with carcinomas of less than 10 mm shown to have nodal metastases to the paratracheal area, and rarely to the jugular nodes (26).

# Prognostic Significance of Lymph Node Metastases

In general, locoregional lymph node metastasis of most malignant tumors is considered to worsen prognosis, and extensive resection can improve the outcome for these patients (27). However, nodal involvement has little influence on the long-term survival of patients with papillary thyroid carcinoma, and an extensive literature review shows that lymph node metastases at presentation of the initial tumor are not associated with a decrease in patient survival rate (16). In particular, large-scale studies were not able to attribute the status of independent prognostic factors to subclinical nodal involvement (28). These results are reflected in the commonly used thyroid cancer patient risk assessment systems (AMES, AGES, MACIS, etc.), in that neck nodal metastases are not used to predict overall patient survival.

However, cervical lymph node metastases have been associated with an increased incidence of locoregional recurrence (16), and extracapsular invasion of lymph node metastases has been reported to be an indicator of distant metastases and of poor prognosis in patients with thyroid papillary carcinoma (29). The TNM scoring system requires assessment of nodal involvement in the staging of patients older than age 45 yr (30). In patients with follicular carcinoma, the impact of nodal disease on survival is controversial.

Finally, some authors have evaluated the hypothesis that distant metastasis can occur via an indirect pathway involving lymph node dissemination (22,31). Although less important than extrathyroidal growth, lymph node metastasis may represent an alternative mechanism of distant metastasis in papillary thyroid cancer. A direct pathway of disease extension from neck to lung has been suggested, because [131]I scans can show tracts of uptake between the thyroid bed and the lungs, especially behind the sternoclavicular joints (31).

# Neck Dissection in the Management of Thyroid Cancer

The surgical management of lymph node metastases, in particular during the first operation, for patients with DTC has been an ongoing source of debate, because the benefit of node dissection on recurrence and survival is controversial (5). Appropriate application and extension of lymph node dissection is based mainly on histologic type, the stage of the primary tumor, and the extent of nodal involvement, but often depends more on the attitudes of the surgeon than on the clinical characteristics (14).

In cases with gross clinical or ultrasound evidence of lymph node involvement, there is no debate about the need and prognostic benefit of a neck dissection in addition to a total thyroidectomy (15). The management of apparently normal lymph nodes, however, is much more conservative. To date, there is no evidence proving a general benefit of routine prophylactic neck dissection for papillary thyroid cancer. As a result, most surgeons currently do not perform neck dissection in patients with apparently normal nodes.

Nevertheless, Japanese surgeons use prophylactic node dissection in patients with proven papillary thyroid cancer even in the absence of clinically suspicious nodal involvement (cN0). This decision is based on the high rate of occult lymph node metastasis and the favorable clinical results. Noguchi et al. found metastatic nodal involvement on histologic examination in 82% of patients with clinically negative nodal disease (32), and Hamming et al. (33) reported 70% of patients who were clinically node negative as having metastatic nodal disease after prophylactic modified neck dissection. Hamming et al. (33) did find more locoregional recurrences in the group of patients that did not have a prophylactic modified neck dissections, and others (34–36) have reported that compartment-oriented nodal dissections decrease locoregional recurrence and improve survival.

Other surgical strategies in the presence of apparently normal cervical lymph nodes include node picking, prophylactic routine neck dissection of the ipsilateral central and jugular compartments, or prophylactic lymphadenectomy of the ipsilateral central compartments (12).

A nonsurgical therapeutic alternative uses 100 to 150 mCi of $^{131}$I to destroy occult micrometastases in clinically negative nodes, but the efficacy of this approach remains to be proven.

Based on the definition of the neck levels, the Committee for Head and Neck Surgery and Oncology of the AAO-HNS proposed the following definitions of the various lymph node dissection procedures:

- Radical neck dissection is the standard basic procedure for cervical lymphadenectomy, where levels I to V are removed with the internal jugular vein, the sternocleidomastoid muscle, and the spinal accessory nerve.
- When modification of the radical neck dissection involves preservation of 1 or more non-lymphatic structures, the procedure is termed modified radical neck dissection.
- When the modification of the radical neck dissection involves preservation of 1 or more lymph node groups, the procedure is termed selective neck dissection.
- When the modification involves removal of additional lymph node groups or non-lymphatic structures relative to the radical neck dissection, the procedure is termed an extended radical neck dissection.

In patients with DTC, en-bloc dissection of regional nodes either through modified radical neck dissection or, more likely, selective neck dissection of the indicated nodal levels represents appropriate treatment in 2 categories of patients. These include patients with clinically positive preoperative regional nodal disease, and those with metastatic disease demonstrated at thyroidectomy in the central neck compartment (level VI) or the mid/lower jugular nodes (levels III, IV) (14).

It is inappropriate: 1) to perform prophylactic modified radical neck dissection or selective neck dissection of the lateral regional nodal levels in clinically N0 patients; 2) to perform local excision of individual nodes or nodal aggregates ("berry picking") in N+ patients; or 3) to perform radical neck dissection that sacrifices uninvolved cervical structures in patients with regional thyroid malignancy (14). However, an aggressive surgical approach is indicated in patients with medullary thyroid carcinoma, because of this tumor's predilection to metastasize through nodal and extranodal tissues and its lack of response to adjuvant therapy (14).

Appropriate applications for lymph node dissection include: 1) standard central neck dissection of all patients, to include the superior mediastinal tissues; 2) ipsilateral elective modified radical neck dissection in patients with positive central neck nodes or large primary tumors, especially with familial-type medullary thyroid carcinoma; 3) bilateral elective modified radical neck dissection in patients with histologically proven bilateral lymph nodes metastases; and 4) ipsilateral or bilateral lymphadenectomy in previously thyroidectomized N0 patients with rising or persistently elevated serum levels of the specific tumor marker (thyroglobulin or calcitonin) (14).

## Techniques for Sentinel Lymph Node Biopsy in DTC

Only patients with lymph node metastases may benefit from lymph node treatment. Therefore, before neck dissection is carried out, the status of the lymph nodes should be identified before selecting the therapeutic strategy. Sentinel node dissection in patients with DTC may help identify which nodes harbor occult metastases and can be used to decide on selective lymph node dissection, radioiodine treatment, or both. During thyroidectomy, a sentinel node dissection can be performed using the vital dye technique, lymphoscintigraphy, and gamma probe, or using a combined technique.

## Vital Dye Technique

In Japan in 1982, Ozaki et al. (19) first used thyroid chromo-lymphography by chlorophyll and iodinated oil for diagnosis of cervical lymph node metastases in thyroid cancer patients. Metastasis was more often found in the colored nodes, with metastasis-positive rates in colored nodes and non-colored nodes of 46.4% and 22.7%, respectively. They supposed that the flow of dye predicted the lymphatic flow of the cancer cells from the tumor, thus supporting the sentinel lymph node concept for thyroid cancer patients.

To date, 10 studies have described the use of a vital dye technique for identifying the sentinel node in thyroid cancer patients (1,37–45) (Table 17-2). The first description of sentinel lymph node dissection applied to DTC by a vital dye was reported by Kelemen et al. (37) from the John Wayne Cancer Institute in Santa Monica, California. Haigh and Giuliano from the same institute reported an update of the technique (1). In this institute, at the time of initial thyroid surgery, after exposure of the thyroid by a standard transverse low-collar skin incision and lateral retraction of the strap muscles, 0.5 to 1 mL of 1% isosulfan blue dye (Lymphazurin) is injected into the thyroid nodule using a tuberculin syringe. The thyroid gland is not extensively mobilized before injection, so that lymphatic drainage remains intact. Usually within seconds, but sometimes up to 1 to 2 minutes, the blue dye is seen to pass through lymphatic channels toward the sentinel node. Once identified, all blue-stained nodes are removed. Extreme caution must be exercised (especially during a total thyroidectomy) that parathyroid glands are not removed with sentinel node dissection; when in doubt, a small incisional biopsy of the blue-stained structure can confirm it is a lymph node. The excised sentinel nodes are submitted for frozen section, and after the node is halved along its long axis, it is examined with Diff-Quik stain. Permanent sections are evaluated by pathologic examination with hematoxylin and eosin staining, and if negative at 2 levels, immunohistochemistry using anticytocheratin antibodies is performed on an additional 2 sections (1).

Johnson et al. (38) explored the sentinel lymph node biopsy technique for 3 out of 11 patients with Hürthle cell tumors, injecting isosulfan blue directly into the tumor or the portions of the lobe affected by it once the thyroid was exposed. Great care was taken to minimize dissection and any disruption of the lymphatics until 20 minutes after the dye injection. The thyroid surgical resection was performed after the sentinel lymph node biopsy, and in all cases parathyroid glands not stained by vital dye were easily identified.

After exposure of the thyroid, Dixon et al. (39) injected isosulfan blue vital dye into the tumor in increments of 0.1 mL until a blue-stained lymphatic was seen, or until no lymphatics could be identified after multiple injections (up to 0.7 mL, using a tuberculin syringe). Following each injection, the thyroid gland was replaced into its normal anatomic position for 1 to 2 minutes before proceeding with lymphatic mapping.

Pelizzo et al. (41) used patent blue V dye at a concentration of 0.5% and a dose of 0.25 mL/cm of the neoplasm's greatest diameter. To avoid spillage, the stain was injected slowly, applying little pressure and blotting the site with a wad of cotton wool when the needle was withdrawn.

Similar techniques were used by Arch-Ferrer et al. (43) Tsugawa et al. (40) Nakano et al. (42) and Takami

TABLE 17-2. Review of literature on vital dye technique for sentinel lymph node dissection in thyroid cancer.

| Author | Year | Vital dye | Volume | Injection site |
|---|---|---|---|---|
| Kelemen (37) | 1998 | Isosulfan blue | — | Intra |
| Johnson (38) | 1999 | Isosulfan blue | — | Peri |
| Dixon (39) | 2000 | Isosulfan blue | ~0.7 mL | |
| Haigh (1) | 2000 | Isosulfan blue | 0.5–1.0 mL | Intra |
| Tsugawa (40) | 2000 | Patent blue V | 0.2 mL | Intra |
| Pelizzo (41) | 2001 | Patent blue V | 0.25 mL/cm | Intra |
| Nakano (42) | 2004 | Isosulfan blue | 0.2 mL × 2 | Peri |
| Arch-Ferrer (43) | 2001 | Isosulfan blue | 0.5 mL | Intra |
| Fukui (44) | 2001 | Methylene blue | 0.1 mL × 4 | Peri |
| Takami (45) | 2002 | Isosulfan blue | 0.1 mL × 3 | Peri |

Legend:
Intra—injected directly into the primary tumor
Peri—injected around the primary tumor
*Source:* Takami et al. (45). Reprinted with permission from Elsevier.

et al. (45), who injected 0.2 to 0.5 mL of 1% isosulfan or patent blue dye directly into (40,43) or around the thyroid tumor (42,45) (see Table 17-2).

Fukui et al. (44) performed sentinel lymph node biopsy using the method described by Kelemen et al. (37), with minor modifications. At the time of surgery, the thyroid gland and the ipsilateral jugular vein were exposed, and then 0.1 mL of 2% methylene blue was injected with a 27-gauge needle into the parenchyma at the 3, 6, 9, and 12 o'clock positions surrounding the primary tumor. Within seconds, the blue dye was observed spreading to the hemilateral thyroid lobe and passing through the lymphatic channels toward the lymph node.

Although vital dye is useful, the technique also has several disadvantages (46):

1. Even if the initial dissection of the thyroid tumor for vital dye injection is done gently, there is the risk of disruption and interruption of the lymphatics.
2. Lymphatics that drain out of the central compartment cannot be followed through the collar incision for thyroidectomy, making it difficult to find sentinel lymph nodes that lie outside the central compartment.
3. Staining of fat and the parathyroid gland with the dye makes it critical that the parathyroid glands be identified prior to injection. Haigh et al. (1) and Dixon et al. (39) reported that blue dye uptake by a parathyroid gland resulted in its removal as a sentinel node. This complication is not surprising, since the parathyroid glands preferentially take up vital dye.
4. Recognizing a node as being blue is not always easy and requires a steep learning curve.

## Lymphoscintigraphy and Gamma Probe

To overcome the drawbacks of the vital dye technique, some authors have proposed using a combination of lymphoscintigraphy and the intraoperative gamma probe instead of the vital dye alone to localize the sentinel lymph node (42,45–50) (Table 17-3).

Lymphoscintigraphy is an excellent technique to visualize the lymphatic pathways and sentinel nodes (47,49,51). It offers significant advantages over the vital dye technique: 1) the injection of the radiopharmaceutical is done preoperatively, therefore avoiding disruption of the lymphatics during the initial dissection; 2) the use of radiolabeled material permits discovery of sentinel lymph nodes that lie outside the central compartment; and 3) there is no false-positive uptake in the parathyroid glands.

The first study of thyroid sentinel node visualization was reported by Matoba and Kikuchi in 1969 and termed "thyroidolymphography" (52). To examine the pattern of lymphatic drainage from the thyroid, these authors first used the percutaneous injection of a small amount of radiological contrast medium (Lipiodol Ultra-Fluid) directly into the normal thyroid gland. Ten minutes after the injection, the lobe on the side of the injection is completely outlined, and its regional lymph nodes can be visualized by x-rays (52).

Lymphoscintigraphy has been used to study the pattern of lymphatic drainage of thyroid nodules through intranodular injection of 15 to 37 MBq $^{99m}$Tc-nanocolloid particles, with a particle size of 20 to 80 nm in a volume of 0.1 to 0.5 mL normal saline (Table 17-3). The intratumoral injection can be performed using an ultrasound-guided 20-gauge needle, which is particularly useful for small thyroid nodules or those located in a difficult area.

Peritumoral injection does not seem reasonable for thyroid tumors, because of the thyroid gland's rich vascularity and the resulting spillage of the radiotracer outside it (46). Stoeckli et al. (46) used the peritumoral injection in 4 of 10 patients, reporting no sentinel lymph node detection by lymphoscintigraphy. Intraoperatively, high levels of radioactivity were found in both the thyroid lobe and the perithyroid muscular tissue, which impeded detection of a sentinel node with the gamma probe. Sahin et al. (47) reported the presence of the radiopharmaceuti-

TABLE 17-3. Review of literature on radioguided sentinel lymph node dissection in thyroid cancer.

| Author, year | Tracer | Volume | Activity | Injection site |
|---|---|---|---|---|
| Gallowitsch 1999 | $^{99m}$Tc-nanocolloid | 0.1 mL | 15 MBq | Intra |
| Sahin 2001 | $^{99m}$Tc-nanocolloid | 0.4 mL | 15 MBq | Intra |
| Stoeckli 2003 | $^{99m}$Tc-nanocolloid | 0.2 mL | 20 MBq | Peri/Intra |
| Rettenbacher 2000 | $^{99m}$Tc-nanocolloid | 0.5 mL | 37 MBq | Intra |
| Catarci 2001 | $^{99m}$Tc-colloid albumin | 0.1 mL | 22 MBq | Intra |
| Nakano 2004 | $^{99m}$Tc-tin colloid | 0.2 mL × 2 | | Peri |

Legend:
Intra—injected directly into the primary tumor
Peri—injected around the primary tumor
*Source:* Takami et al. (45). Reprinted with permission from Elsevier.

cal in the systemic circulation in 2 of 13 patients, possibly as a result of incorrect peritumoral injection.

Immediately following the intratumoral injection, lymphatic drainage is monitored for up to 10 minutes by dynamic images (1 frame per 15 sec, 64 × 64 matrix) acquired with a low-energy general-purpose collimator in the anterior projection (47). Sahin et al. (47) used a longer dynamic study, acquiring images (1 frame per 60 sec, 128 × 128 matrix) during the first hour.

Lymphoscintigraphy generally outlines the expected lymphatic drainage pattern of the thyroid, according to well-accepted anatomic descriptions, and also may allow sentinel lymph node detection, usually within 30 minutes.

After the dynamic study, additional 5-minute static images are obtained in the anterior, lateral, and oblique views (256 × 256 matrix) for up to 1 to 3 hours from the radiopharmaceutical injection or until the radiotracer accumulates in the sentinel node (47). These late static images permit clear identification of the sentinel nodes, even if the submandibular lymph nodes could not be clearly distinguished from the primary lesion on the planar images.

To localize lymph nodes, images with markers positioned at the chin and sternal notch can be obtained after the last scan, and use of a double tracer technique can improve the correlation of lymphatic drainage to cervical compartments (53).

Using a double-head gamma camera, additional transmission scans with a cobalt-57 sheet source on the opposite detector for better topographic orientation can be acquired (49). After a sentinel lymph node is detected, its location is marked on the patient's skin surface with a water-resistant dye, for the surgeon.

## Gamma Probe

Between 2 hours (46,50) and 24 hours (49) after lymphoscintigraphy, the patient is taken to the operating room where a standard low-collar incision is made for a total or near-total thyroidectomy. Following the thyroidectomy, a handheld gamma probe is inserted through the cervical incision to search the central compartment to verify the presence and location of "hot spots" suggestive of sentinel lymph nodes. Once the central compartment has been examined, the lateral compartments of the neck must be scanned bilaterally with the gamma probe through the intact skin (46).

To search for hot nodes, the probe photopeak must be adjusted appropriately (49,50), and a collimator should be used (49). Even 24 hours following radiotracer injection, the count rate is adequate to view laterocervical nodes with a satisfactorily high lesion-to-background ratio (49).

A lesion-to-background ratio of 2 : 1 or greater can be assumed to be significant for sentinel lymph node identification (50); any node immediately adjacent to the one identified as the sentinel node and not showing a signifi-

cantly lower radioactivity must be considered equivalent to the sentinel node (50). After identification, sentinel lymph nodes are selectively excised, and the activity of the lymphatic bed is monitored to demonstrate a drop of radioactivity counts to background level after node excision (46,49).

It is important to note that the thyroid gland (i.e., the site of the radiocolloid injection) must be excised prior to the sentinel node being removed when a radiotracer sentinel lymph node biopsy technique is performed. In this regard, the shine-through effect is especially problematic in the central neck compartment, where the lymph nodes are located in close proximity to the thyroid (8).

After removal of any sentinel lymph nodes, the specimen must be sent to the pathologist for a detailed histopathologic analysis, and the description of occult metastases can be done according to the technique used by Hermanek and colleagues (54).

## Combination Technique

Catarci et al. (50) used the combination of a vital dye, lymphoscintigraphy, and gamma probe on 6 patients with preoperative cytological evidence of papillary thyroid carcinoma at fine-needle aspiration biopsy. Thyroid nodules were larger than 15 mm at ultrasound study, and there was no clinical or sonographic evidence of lymph node enlargement in the neck.

Ultrasound-guided intratumoral injection of 0.1 mL of $^{99m}$Tc-labelled colloidal albumin (particle size 3 to 80 nm, activity between 11 to 37 MBq) was performed 2 hours before surgery. Immediately after the injection, dynamic scintigraphy followed by serial static scans were performed until sentinel lymph nodes became visible. Two hours later, during surgery, 0.2 to 0.4 mL (0.1 mL per cm of tumoral diameter) of patent blue V (2.5%) was injected directly into the tumor, identified without dissecting any structure (thyroid gland, muscles, vessels, etc.) to preserve all the lymphatic drainage. According to the presumed location at lymphoscintigraphy, sentinel lymph node identification was obtained by the flow and accumulation of the dye; a handheld gamma probe detection was used to verify the presence and location of sentinel nodes and to look for any residual radioactivity at the end of the procedure. No residual activity of the tracer was recorded, thus confirming complete removal of the sentinel lymph node.

Considering all 3 methods, 1 to 2 sentinel lymph nodes were correctly identified in all cases. Preoperative lymphoscintigraphy, intraoperative vital dye, and intraoperative handheld gamma probe revealed the presence and location of the sentinel lymph node in 66%, 83% and 83% of the cases, respectively. These results indicate that in this pilot study the 3 techniques complemented each other. Mean operative time necessary to perform the injection of vital dye and locate the sentinel lymph node was 14.7 minutes (range, 8–19 min). To date, this is the only study on the combination of preoperative lymphoscintigraphy, intraoperative vital dye, and intraoperative handheld gamma probe for sentinel lymph node dissection in DTC.

## Overall Performance

In 1998 at the John Wayne Cancer Institute, Kelemen et al. (37) reported a feasibility study on 17 patients with thyroid nodules ranging from 1.0 to 3.0 cm, in which the final pathological review demonstrated 12 malignant tumors (11 papillary and 1 follicular carcinoma) and 5 benign lesions. Intraoperative lymphatic mapping located at least 1 sentinel lymph node in all but 2 patients, both of whom appeared to have blue lymphatic channels coursing beneath the clavicles. With the exception of these 2 patients, sentinel lymph node dissection was performed in the remaining 15 patients, removing 1 to 5 lymph nodes (median: 2). All the excised sentinel nodes were paratracheal, and 2 patients had additional jugular sentinel lymph nodes that stained blue. In the 12 sentinel lymph node specimens from patients with malignant thyroid nodules, analysis of frozen sections and then permanent sections revealed metastasis in 5 (42%). Central lymph node dissection was performed in 3 patients who had metastasis of the sentinel node diagnosed by frozen section, and in 2 of these the sentinel node was the only positive node.

Haigh et al. (1) updated the John Wayne Cancer Institute experience, performing sentinel lymph node dissection in an ongoing trial on 38 patients with thyroid nodules suspicious for malignancy. They reported a successful detection rate of 87%, finding sentinel lymph nodes in 33 patients, with 5 failed procedures due to fat or a parathyroid gland misidentified as a sentinel node, lymphatic channels coursing retrosternally, or failing dye migration from a nodule. Thyroid carcinomas were identified in 17 out of 38 thyroid nodules; of these 17 malignant lesions, there was 1 failed sentinel lymph node dissection. In the remaining 16 cases, metastases were identified in at least 1 sentinel node in 9 patients (56%). In both of the John Wayne Cancer Institute studies, not all patients had neck dissections after sentinel lymph node dissection, and therefore the false-negative rate is unknown.

Dixon et al. (39) performed sentinel lymph node dissection on 40 clinically N0 patients with thyroid nodules, and identified sentinel nodes in 10 of 12 patients (83%) with papillary thyroid cancer. In 8 of these 10 (80%), the sentinel lymph node status accurately predicted the disease status of the neck. However, among 40 patients studied at the University of Calgary (39), almost 30% had lymphatic channels tracking through the central compartment into the anterior mediastinum or the lateral compartment, and in 13% the sentinel lymph node skipped the central compartment. This phenomenon of initial skipped nodal spread lying outside the central compartment had been demonstrated by Noguchi et al. (32), who found that 7% of nodal metastasis appeared only in the lateral compartment.

Pelizzo et al. (41) identified the sentinel lymph node in 22 of 29 patients (76%) with preoperative cytological diagnoses of papillary thyroid cancer. The location of the sentinel lymph node was in the central compartment in 19 patients (86%), and in the lateral compartment in 3 patients (14%). When identified, the sentinel node accurately predicted the disease status of the neck in all patients, and no false-negative results were reported.

Arch-Ferrer and colleagues (43) studied 22 patients, and a sentinel lymph node was found in 20 patients. Using hematoxylin and eosin staining, metastases were identified in 12 of 20 (60%) sentinel lymph nodes. Eleven patients with a positive sentinel node had additional lymph node metastases, of which 9 were located in the central compartment, 1 in the jugular compartment, and 1 in both. These authors demonstrated that immunostaining the sentinel lymph node with anti-low-molecular-weight cytokeratin antibodies improved the detection of micrometastatic disease.

Johnson et al. (38) carried out sentinel lymph node dissection with isosulfan blue dye on 3 Hürthle cell tumors—1 malignant and 2 benign. Sentinel lymph node as well as central node dissection revealed no lymphatic spread in the patient with Hürthle cell carcinoma.

Four studies have reported on Japanese experience with these techniques (40,42,44,45). First, Fukui and colleagues (44) performed sentinel lymph node biopsy using a dye technique (methylene blue) on 22 patients with papillary carcinoma who underwent subtotal thyroidectomy and modified radical neck dissection of the central compartment and the jugular area. Sentinel nodes were identified in 21 of 22 patients (95.5%), with the number of nodes ranging from 1 to 5 (mean: 1.5). The sentinel nodes were located in the central compartment area in 16 of 21 patients (76.2%), and in the ipsilateral jugular area in 5 patients. The sentinel lymph nodes accurately predicted the disease status of the neck in 19 of 21 patients (90.5%). Two of 21 patients (9.5%) had negative sentinel lymph nodes, but they eventually showed positive nonsentinel nodes.

Takami et al. used the isosulfan blue dye technique to identify sentinel lymph nodes in 48 patients (94.1%) of 51 patients (45). The sentinel lymph nodes were found in the central compartment in 45 of the 48 patients, and within the lateral compartments in 6 patients (3 patients had sentinel nodes in both). In 26 of the 48 patients (54.2%) sentinel nodes were positive for metastases, while 22 patients had negative nodes. There was concordance between the sentinel node status and the final results in the regional lymph nodes in 44 of the 48 patients (91.7%). The sensitivity, specificity, positive predictive value, negative predictive value, and accuracy were 86.7%, 100%, 100%, 81.8%, and 91.7%, respectively (45).

Tsugawa et al. (40) examined the feasibility of sentinel lymph node biopsy for thyroid cancer using patent blue dye in 38 patients with papillary thyroid carcinoma. Sentinel lymph node biopsy removed 1 to 3 lymph nodes (median: 2 nodes). Histologic nodal metastasis was observed in 16 of 27 cases (71%), and the positive rate of cancer metastases in the sentinel node was 58%, which was significantly higher than the 11% value in nonsentinel lymph nodes. Sensitivity was 84%, specificity 100%, and diagnostic accuracy 89%.

In a study by Nakano et al. (42), 32 patients were examined using intraoperative injection around the tumor of 1% isosulfan blue dye, and 23 patients by 1-day preoperative $^{99m}$Tc-colloid injection. In the first method, the sentinel lymph node was identified in 30 (94%) of the 32 patients. Lymph node mapping for detection of sentinel nodes was performed after thyroidectomy, and central and modified lateral neck lymph node dissections. All dissected nodes were then examined postoperatively by hematoxylin and eosin staining to determine whether metastasis was present. This method identified sentinel lymph nodes in 30 (94%) of the 32 patients. Lymph node metastases were found in 14 patients, and some sentinel nodes had papillary cancer metastasis in 13 patients. There was only 1 false-negative case. The sensitivity and accuracy of sentinel lymph node biopsy was 93% and 97%. With the radiotracer method, detection rate, sensitivity, and accuracy of sentinel lymph node biopsy were 96% (22/23), 90% (9/10) and 95% (21/22), respectively.

In the Chow and colleagues (55) series examining 15 consecutive papillary thyroid cancer patients undergoing sentinel lymph node dissection, sentinel nodes were traced in 10 patients, and most were located in the central compartment. The overall accuracy of the sentinel lymph node in predicting nodal status was 90%. The sensitivity, specificity, positive predictive value, and negative predictive value were 88%, 100%, 100%, and 67%, respectively.

In the study reported by Stoeckli et al. involving 10 patients with uninodular thyroid disease and clinically

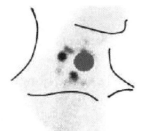 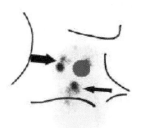

RAO 5 min p.i.                          RAO 18 h p.i.

FIGURE 17-3. Right anterior-oblique (RAO) lymphoscintigraphic images obtained 5 minutes (left) and 18 hours (right) postinjection (P.I.), showing 2 sentinel lymph nodes in the medial jugular region (thick arrow) and 1 sentinel node in the lower jugular region (thin arrow). Injection site is covered with a lead sheet. (Rettenbacher et al. [48], by permission.)

negative lymph node status (46), the overall detection of sentinel lymph nodes was 50% with lymphoscintigraphy and 100% with the gamma probe. The sentinel lymph node was located in the ipsilateral central compartment (level VI) in 50% of the cases, and in the ipsilateral lateral compartment in the remaining 50% (level IV and II). Since a patient experienced a temporary lesion of the recurrent laryngeal nerve during sentinel lymph node dissection, the authors concluded that a search for sentinel nodes in the lower central compartment enhances the risk of injury to this nerve.

Rettenbacher and colleagues (48) identified sentinel lymph nodes (1 to 4 per patient) in 7 of 9 patients, including all 4 patients with papillary thyroid cancer (see Figure 17-3). In 1 patient, no sentinel lymph node was visible with lymphoscintigraphy, but at surgery 3 sentinel lymph nodes were clearly identified using the gamma probe after removal of the primary tumor. There were no false-negative findings.

Table 17-4 summarizes the sensitivity, specificity, and diagnostic accuracy for sentinel lymph node dissection in thyroid cancer reported in the literature (39–45, 48).

TABLE 17-4. Literature data on diagnostic accuracy for sentinel lymph node dissection in thyroid cancer.

| Author, year, reference | Identification (%) | Sensitivity (%) | Specificity (%) | Accuracy (%) |
|---|---|---|---|---|
| Dixon 2000 (39) | 83 (10/12) | 75 | 100 | 80 |
| Tsugawa 2000 (40) | 71 (27/38) | 84 | 100 | 89 |
| Pelizzo 2001 (41) | 76 (22/29) | 100 | 100 | 100 |
| Nakano 2001 (42) | 92 (23/25) | 91 | 100 | 92 |
| Arch-Ferrer 2001 (43) | 91 (20/22) | 71–85 (a) | 100–100 (a) | 75–100 (a) |
| Fukui 2001 (44) | 96 (21/22) | 78 | 100 | 90 |
| Rettenbacher 2000 (48) | 71 (5/7) | 100 | 100 | 100 |
| Nakano 2004 (42) | 100 (11/11) | 80 | 100 | 91 |

Legend:
(a)—Immunohistochemistry with anti-cytocheratin-7 antibody
*Source:* Takami et al. (45). Reprinted with permission from Elsevier.

# The Advantages and Limitations of Sentinel Lymph Node Dissection in Thyroid Carcinoma

Clinical, sonographic, and intraoperative findings have a low predictive value for metastatic nodal involvement in patients with differentiated thyroid cancer. Surgical exploration and palpation are also poor in predicting the nodal spread of disease (39), because lymph node metastases may not be palpable when they are soft or small, or when they are located in the central compartment of the neck or behind the vessels. Occult nodal disease was found in 23% to 69% of patients with apparently negative nodes (8), and 17% of 159 unselected patients with node dissection showed occult disease in the presence of normal macroscopic nodal appearance (32).

In principle, sentinel lymph node dissection offers several advantages:

1. It permits selection of patients who would benefit from compartment-oriented nodal dissection, reducing unnecessary surgery and possible morbidity.
2. It identifies patients with metastatic disease, providing a rationale for the use of high dose postoperative sodium [131]I-iodide treatment to destroy nodal occult micrometastases.
3. It identifies lymph node metastases outside the central compartment, thus allowing a more selective approach and the extension of routine central node dissection to nodes other than the central neck.

However, significant limitations to sentinel lymph node dissection have been reported, including the uncertain prognostic significance of metastatic nodal involvement (which would make this technique unnecessary) and possible low sensitivity in the detection of micrometastasis (7).

## Conclusions

In thyroid carcinoma, sentinel lymph node dissection can be performed successfully and the sentinel nodes easily identified and removed with minimal morbidity using the vital dye technique or especially a combination of lymphoscintigraphy and the intraoperative use of a hand-held gamma probe.

In the untreated neck, lymph node drainage of the thyroid follows a sufficiently predictable pattern, so that the concept of selective treatment and sentinel lymph node dissection has a legitimate rationale. However, unlike with breast cancer and melanoma, the role for sentinel node dissection in the surgical management of patients with DTC has yet to be determined, because the impact of lymph node metastases on prognosis

remains debatable. It is also unlikely that the identification of micrometastatic disease will change care management, since the majority of surgeons only remove clinically involved nodes at surgery.

Further studies on larger sample groups are necessary to ascertain the accuracy of this technique, particularly to assess the actual risk of false-negative results, which are mainly related to the complicated lymphatic streams from the thyroid.

It is likely that sentinel lymph node biopsy will never achieve clinical relevance as a standard treatment for all patients with papillary thyroid cancer. However, it may play a role in specific subgroups of high-risk patients, such as those with nondifferentiated thyroid cancers, Hürthle-cell carcinoma, or medullary thyroid cancers that do not take up sodium [131]I-iodide.

## References

1. Haigh PI, Giuliano AE. Sentinel lymph node dissection for thyroid malignancy. *Recent Results Cancer Res.* 2000; 157:201–205.
2. Gipponi M, Solari N, Di Somma FC, Bertoglio S, Cafiero F. New fields of application of the sentinel lymph node biopsy in the pathologic staging of solid neoplasms: review of literature and surgical perspectives. *J Surg Oncol.* 2004;85:171–179.
3. Lim RB, Wong JH. Sentinel lymphadenectomy in gynaecologic and solid malignancies other than melanoma and breast cancer. *Surg Clin N Am.* 2000;80:1787–1798.
4. Koops HS, Doting MHE, de Vries J, et al. Sentinel node biopsy as a surgical staging method for solid cancers. *Radiother Oncol.* 1999;51:1–7.
5. Shaha AP. Management of the neck in thyroid cancer. *Otorhinolaryngol Clin N Am.* 1998;31:823–831.
6. Delbridge L. Sentinel lymph node biopsy for thyroid cancer: why bother? *Surg Clin N Am.* 2004;74:2.
7. Pasieka JL. Sentinel lymph node biopsy in the management of thyroid disease. *Br J Surg.* 2001;88:321–322.
8. Wiseman SM, Hicks WL Jr, Chu QD, Rigual NR. Sentinel lymph node biopsy in staging of differentiated thyroid cancer: a critical review. *Surg Oncol.* 2002;11:137–142.
9. Gregoire V, Levendag P, Ang KK, et al. CT-based delineation of lymph node levels and related CTVs in the node-negative neck: DAHANCA, EORTC, GORTEC, NCIC, RTOG consensus guidelines. *Radiother Oncol.* 2000;56:135–150.
10. Som PM, Curtin HD, Mancuso AA. An imaging-based classification for the cervical nodes designed as an adjunct to recent clinically based nodal classifications. *Arch Otolaryngol Head Neck Surg.* 1999;125:388–396.
11. Robbins KT, Medina JE, Wolfe GT, Levine PA, Sessions RB, Pruet CW. Standardizing neck dissection terminology. Official report of the academy's committee for head and neck surgery and oncology. *Arch Otolaryngol Head Neck Surg.* 1991;117:601–605.

12. Robbins KT. Classification of neck dissection. Current concepts and future considerations. *Otorhinolaryngol Clin N Am*. 1998;31:639–655.

13. Gregoire V, Coche E, Cosnard G, Hamoir M, Reychler H. Selection and delineation of lymph node target in head and neck conformal radiotherapy. Proposal for standardizing terminology and procedure based on the surgical experience. *Radiother Oncol*. 2000;56:135–150.

14. Robbins KT, Atkinson JLD, Byers RM, Cohen JI, Lavertu P, Pellitteri P. The use and misuse of neck dissection for head and neck cancer. *J Am Coll Surg*. 2001;193:91–102.

15. Guidelines for the management of thyroid cancer in adults. British Thyroid Association, Royal College of Physicians. London: 2002.

16. Sclumberger M, Pacini F. *Thyroid tumors*. Paris: Nucleon; 2003.

17. Shaha AR, Shah JP, Loree TR. Patterns of nodal and distant metastasis based on histologic varieties in differentiated carcinoma of the thyroid. *Am J Surg*. 1996;172:692–694.

18. Mirallie E, Visset J, Sagan C, Hamy A, Le Bodic MF, Paineau J. Localization of cervical node metastasis of papillary thyroid carcinoma. *World J Surg*. 1999;23:970–974.

19. Ozaki O, Hirai K, Maruyama S, Sageshima M, Mori T. Experimental and clinical studies on the thyroid chromolymphography. Part II: clinical study. *Jpn J Surg*. 1982;83:53–59.

20. Frankenthaler RA, Sellin RV, Canqir A, Goepfert H. Lymph node metastasis from papillary-follicular thyroid carcinoma in young patients. *Am J Surg*. 1990;160:341–343.

21. Noguchi M, Kumaki T, Taniya T, et al. Bilateral cervical lymph node metastases in well-differentiated thyroid cancer. *Arch Surg*. 1990;125:804–806.

22. Machens A, Hinze R, Thomusch O, Dralle H. Pattern of nodal metastasis for primary and reoperative thyroid cancer. *World J Surg*. 2002;26:22–27.

23. Sugenoya A, Asanuma K, Shingu K, et al. Clinical evaluation of upper mediastinal dissection for differentiated thyroid carcinoma. *Surgery*. 1993;113:541–544.

24. Noguchi M, Kinami S, Kinoshita K, et al. Risk of bilateral cervical lymph node metastases in papillary thyroid cancer. *J Surg Oncol*. 1993;52:155–159.

25. Ohshima A, Yamashita H, Noguchi S, et al. Indications for bilateral modified radical neck dissection in patients with papillary carcinoma of the thyroid. *Arch Surg*. 2000;135:1194–1199.

26. Noguchi S, Yamashita H, Murakami N, Nakayama I, Toda M, Kawamoto H. Small carcinomas of the thyroid: a long-term follow-up of 867 patients. *Arch Surg*. 1996;131:187–191.

27. Gimm O, Dralle H. Surgical strategies in papillary thyroid carcinoma. *Curr Top Pathol*. 1997;91:51–64.

28. Mazzaferri EL. Thyroid cancer in thyroglossal duct remnants: a diagnostic and therapeutic dilemma. *Thyroid*. 2004;14:335–336.

29. Yamashita H, Noguchi S, Murakami N, Kawamoto H, Watanabe S. Extracapsular invasion of lymph node metastasis is an indicator of distant metastasis and poor prognosis in patients with thyroid papillary carcinoma. *Cancer*. 1997;80:2268–2272.

30. American Joint Committee on Cancer. Thyroid. In: *AJCC Cancer Staging Handbook*. 6th edition. New York: Springer; 2002:89–98.

31. Collins SL. Etiopathogenesis of thyroid cancer. In: *Thyroid Disease: Endocrinology, Surgery, Nuclear Medicine and Radiotherapy*. Falk S, ed. New York: Lippincott Williams & Wilkins, 1990.

32. Noguchi S, Noguchi A, Murakami N. Papillary carcinoma of the thyroid I. Developing patterns of metastasis. II. Value of prophylactic lymph node excision. *Cancer*. 1970;26:1053–1060.

33. Hamming JF, van de Velde CJH, Goslings BM, et al. Preoperative diagnosis and treatment of metastases to the regional lymph nodes in papillary carcinoma of the thyroid gland. *Surg Gynecol Obstet*. 1989;169:107.

34. McHenry CR, Rosen IB, Walfish PG. Prospective management of nodal metastases in differentiated thyroid cancer. *Am J Surg*. 1991;162:353.

35. Coburn MC, Wanebo HJ. Prognostic factors and management considerations in patients with cervical metastases of thyroid cancer. *Am J Surg*. 1992;164:671.

36. Scheumann GFW, Gimm O, Wegener G, Hundeshagen H, Dralle H. Prognostic significance and surgical management of locoregional lymph node metastases in papillary thyroid cancer. *World J Surg*. 1994;18:5591–5994.

37. Kelemen PR, Van Herle AJ, Giuliano AE. Sentinel lymphadenectomy in thyroid malignant neoplasms. *Arch Surg*. 1998;133:288–292.

38. Johnson LW, Sehon J, Benjamin D. Potential utility of sentinel node biopsy in the original surgical assessment of Hürthle cell tumors of the thyroid: 23-year institutional review of Hurthle cell neoplasms. *J Surg Oncol*. 1999;70:100–102.

39. Dixon E, McKinnon JG, Pasieka JL. Feasibility of sentinel lymph node biopsy and lymphatic mapping in nodular thyroid neoplasms. *World J Surg*. 2000;24:1396–1401.

40. Tsugawa K, Ohnishi I, Nakamura M, et al. Intraoperative lymphatic mapping and sentinel lymph node biopsy in patients with papillary carcinoma of the thyroid gland. *Biomed Pharmacother*. 2002;56:100s–103s.

41. Pelizzo MR, Merante Boschin I, Toniato A, et al. The sentinel node procedure with patent blue V dye in the surgical treatment of papillary thyroid carcinoma. *Acta Otolaryngol*. 2001;121:421–424.

42. Nakano S, Uenosono Y, Ehi K, et al. Lymph nodes mapping for detection of sentinel nodes in patients with papillary thyroid cancer. *Gan To Kagaku Ryoho*. 2004;31:801–804.

43. Arch-Ferrer J, Velazquez D, Fajardo R, Gamboa-Dominguez A, Herrera MF. Accuracy of sentinel lymph node in papillary thyroid carcinoma. *Surgery*. 2001;130:907–913.

44. Fukui Y, Yamakawa T, Taniki T, Numoto S, Miki H, Monden Y. Sentinel lymph node biopsy in patients with papillary thyroid carcinoma. *Cancer*. 2001;92:2868–2874.

45. Takami H, Sdasaki K, Ikeda Y, Tajima G, Kameyama K. Sentinel lymph node biopsy in patients with thyroid carcinoma. *Biomed Pharmacother*. 2002;56:83s–87s.

46. Stoeckli SJ, Pfaltz M, Steinert H, Schmid S. Sentinel lymph node biopsy in thyroid tumors: a pilot study. *Eur Arch Otorhinolaryngol.* 2003;260:364–368.

47. Sahin M, Yapici O, Dervisoglu A, et al. Evaluation of lymphatic drainage of cold thyroid nodules with intratumoral injection of Tc-99m nanocolloid. *Clin Nucl Med.* 2001;26:602–605.

48. Rettenbacher L, Sungler P, Gmeiner D, Kassman H, Galvan G. Detecting the sentinel lymph node in patients with differentiated thyroid carcinoma. *Eur J Nucl Med.* 2000;27:1399–1401.

49. Gallowitsch HJ, Mikosch P, Kresnik E, Starlinger M, Lind P. Lymphoscintigraphy and gamma probe-guided surgery in papillary thyroid carcinoma. The sentinel lymph node concept in thyroid carcinoma. *Clin Nucl Med.* 1999;24: 744–746.

50. Catarci M, Zaraca F, Angeloni R, et al. Preoperative lymphoscintigraphy and sentinel lymph node biopsy in papillary thyroid cancer. A pilot study. *J Surg Oncol.* 2001;77:21–24.

51. Balkissoon J, Rasgon BM, Schweitzer L. Lymphatic mapping for staging of head and neck cancer. *Semin Oncol.* 2004;31:382–393.

52. Matoba N, Kikuchi T. Thyroidolymphography: a new technique for visualization of the thyroid and cervical lymph nodes. *Radiology.* 1969;92:339–342.

53. Klutmann S, Bohuslavizki KH, Brenner W, et al. Lymphoscintigraphy in tumors of the head and neck using double tracer technique. *J Nucl Med.* 1999;40:776–782.

54. Hermanek P, Hutter RVP, Sobin LH, Wittekind C. Classification of isolated tumor cells and micrometastasis. *Cancer.* 1999;86:2668–2673.

55. Chow T-L, Lim B-H, Kwok P-YS. Sentinel lymph node dissection in papillary thyroid carcinoma. *Surg Clin N Am.* 2004;74:10–12.

# 18
# Histopathology of Sentinel Lymph Nodes

Giuseppe Viale, Giovanni Mazzarol, and Eugenio Maiorano

To effectively stage patients with clinically node-negative malignancies with minimal morbidity, the sentinel lymph node biopsy must rely on an accurate histopathologic examination of the sentinel nodes (1–7). Intuitively, the rate of identification of metastatic tumors depends on the accuracy and extent of the histopathologic evaluation, i.e., the number of sections scrutinized. The lack of universally adopted protocols for the examination of sentinel lymph nodes has led to broad variation in the procedures currently used in different institutions and in the guidelines or recommendations issued by scientific organizations at the both local and international levels. Unfortunately, this has led to poor reproducibility of data from investigations on different series of patients whose sentinel lymph nodes were evaluated according to different protocols. As a result, despite almost a decade of investigations in sentinel lymph node biopsy and several thousands patients enrolled in clinical studies, a number of questions remain unanswered.

Among these issues, the most important is whether histopathologic examination of sentinel lymph nodes should aim at detecting even minimal lymph node involvement (isolated tumor cells and micrometastases), using all the available technological resources—from traditional serial sectioning, with or without immunohistochemical detection of specific tumor cell markers, to more sophisticated assays, such as reverse-transcription polymerase chain reactions [RT-PCR]). This question can be addressed properly only by following a precise assessment of the clinical implications of minimal lymph node involvement, with regard to both the risk of additional metastases to nonsentinel nodes of the same basin and to the prognostic value of isolated tumor cells and micrometastases for patients' survival (8). Due to the lack of standardization of the histopathologic examination, the clinical implications of minimal sentinel lymph node involvement are still debated, with some studies documenting an important risk of additional involvement of higher-echelon lymph nodes and an unfavorable

clinical outcome, at variance with the results of others (9–16).

Because of this uncertainty of the clinical implications of minimal sentinel lymph node involvement, individual institutions have devised their own protocols for sentinel node examination according to the available resources and cost/benefit analysis, without feeling compelled to adhere to standards of care. A recent survey of the protocols used in Europe for the histopathologic examination of axillary sentinel lymph nodes of breast carcinoma patients unveiled remarkable differences among the 240 laboratories that responded to the questionnaire, with 123 somewhat different histologic protocols reported. Almost 12% of the responding laboratories examined only 1 level per sentinel lymph node, whereas the others performed a multilevel assessment ranging from evaluation of 2 to 5 levels to more than 100 levels separated by 40 µm cutting intervals. Patient outcomes, however, can be optimized only by standardization of the sentinel lymph node biopsy procedure, with particular reference to histopathologic scrutiny (17).

## Sentinel Lymph Node Examination in Different Malignancies

The sentinel lymph node biopsy is a widely accepted procedure to accurately stage patients with clinically node-negative cutaneous melanomas and breast carcinomas, sparing unnecessary lymph node dissection in case of a negative sentinel lymph node biopsy and allowing the choice of the most appropriate adjuvant intervention (18,19). The application of the same procedure for tumors of different organs, including the vulva, colon, and stomach, is promising but has not reached yet unanimous consensus and is still under investigation (20–22).

The first histopathologic approaches to sentinel lymph node examination did not differ from the routine assess-

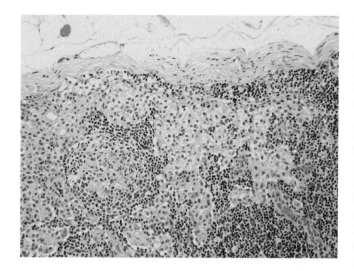

FIGURE 18-1. Subcapsular metastasis from breast carcinoma composed of a large cluster of cohesive tumor cells, circumscribing a residual lymphoid follicle. Hematoxylin and eosin stain on formalin-fixed, paraffin-embedded tissue section, 100×.

ment of regional lymph node status, based on the histologic evaluation of a single or very few sections cut from frozen lymph nodes (in the case of intraoperative diagnosis) or paraffin-embedded tissues (see Figure 18-1). As expected, however, the high false-negative rate of this traditional diagnostic approach was soon highlighted by reports on the higher accuracy of more extensive histopathologic examination of sentinel nodes. Indeed, retrospective studies on sentinel lymph node biopsy of melanoma patients reported a 12% increase in the detection rate of metastases with the examination of further sections, and similar results were obtained in breast cancer patients, in whom a false-negative rate of 17% was documented following the intraoperative examination of only 1 to 3 frozen sections (23,24).

These data prompted a large series of studies to assess the benefit of a more extensive histopathologic examination of sentinel nodes. The aim was to increase the positive and negative predictive value of the sentinel node biopsy by using more demanding histopathologic protocols, based on subserial sectioning of the entire sentinel lymph nodes and use of ancillary immunohistochemical staining techniques, which had to be cost-effective and could not exceed the laboratory workload capacity. Cost-benefit analyses of extensive examination of sentinel nodes vary according to several parameters, including the number of patients evaluated, the amount of the reimbursement, and the availability of dedicated personnel and instrumentation. As a result, several different protocols have been adopted in different institutions, according to their own logistic assets. As a rule, the rate of detection of metastases is dependent on the number

of sections examined from the entire lymph node, so that the prevalence of sentinel node involvement in a given series of patients depends on the adopted histopathologic protocol. To ensure optimization of patient care in different institutions, however, a standardized protocol should be adopted (25–28).

We have devised a demanding protocol for sentinel lymph node examination of breast carcinoma patients that requires histopathologic scrutiny of the entire sentinel lymph node by serial sectioning at very thin cutting intervals. According to this protocol, which is suitable for both frozen and paraffin-embedded lymph nodes, the sentinel node is bisected along the longest axis or cut into 2 to 3 mm slices, if thicker than 5 mm (thinner lymph nodes may be processed uncut). In handling the lymph node, special attention is paid to preserve intact the nodal capsule and the peripheral sinuses, where many metastatic foci may be first seen. Serial sections are then cut at 50 to 100 μm intervals, until examination of the lymph node is completed. Formerly, spare sections for immunohistochemistry were cut at each level, but now immunohistochemical reactions are performed on destained sections, whenever deemed necessary to confirm the metastatic nature of morphologically atypical cells (approximately 5% of the cases) (see Figure 18-2).

The need for complete examination of the sentinel node derives from the observation that while larger (macro-) metastases measuring 2 mm or more usually are detected in the first sections cut from the middle areas of the nodes, smaller (micro-) metastases measuring less than 2 mm are more randomly distributed throughout the node and cannot be detected by examination of sections from the central portions (see Figure

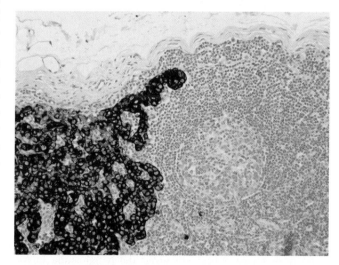

FIGURE 18-2. Immunohistochemical staining for cytokeratins highlights the metastatic epithelial component, leaving unstained resident lymphoid cells. Immunohistochemistry anticytokeratin AE1/AE3, 100×.

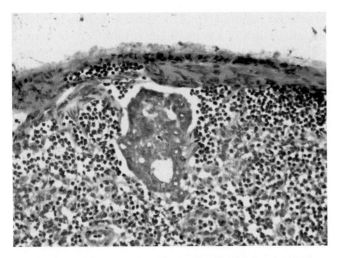

FIGURE 18-3. A single metastatic gland (micrometastasis) from breast carcinoma located just underneath the nodal marginal sinus. Hematoxylin and eosin stain on cryostatic section, 200×.

18-3). Cutting serial sections at 50 to 100 μm intervals aims to identify even minimal lymph node involvement (isolated tumor cells and micrometastases), which could escape detection when only sectioning the node at larger cutting intervals (29,30) (see Figure 18-4).

Such a labor-intensive protocol could not be followed by many other institutions, especially as the clinical implications of minimal sentinel lymph node involvement are still being debated. Thus, it is not surprising that recommendations for sentinel lymph node examination issued by nationwide or international organizations

suggest more affordable protocols (17,31), which emphasize the need for complete examination of the node but allow cutting intervals ranging from 0.5 mm (German Consensus, Committee of the German Society of Senology, 2003) to 1 mm (European Working Group, European Union). The rationale for defining these minimal requirements is to ensure detection of macrometastases only, and not to search for minimal lymph node involvement by isolated tumor cells or micrometastases. Accordingly, use of ancillary diagnostic techniques, such as immunohistochemistry or molecular biology assays, is not recommended. Similar conclusions were reached by the panelists of the Consensus Conference on Sentinel Lymph Node Biopsy in Carcinoma of the Breast held in Philadelphia in 2001 (32). Whether these recommendations will be maintained or changed depends mainly on future progress in unveiling the clinical implications of minimal lymph node involvement (see the following discussion).

The detection of metastatic melanoma in sentinel lymph nodes is more complex, because the morphologic features of melanoma cells are much more variable than breast cancer cells and may mimic normal resident cells, such as lymphocytes and histiocytes. In addition, metastatic melanoma cells often are devoid of melanin pigment, which would be a useful marker to facilitate identification of tumor cells. Accordingly, although detection of larger metastatic deposits in the sentinel nodes is fairly easy on purely morphologic grounds (see Figure 18-5), smaller metastases may be missed if immunohistochemical assays to identify specific cell markers are not performed.

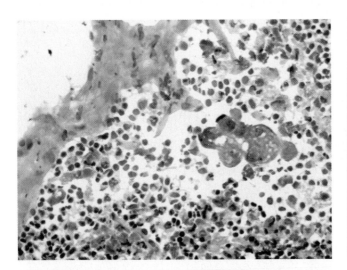

FIGURE 18-4. Rare metastatic epithelial cells (isolated tumor cells) from breast cancer colonized the lymph node in the proximity of the marginal sinus. The tumor cells display cytoplasmic vacuolization, large hyperchromatic nuclei, and prominent nucleoli. Hematoxylin and eosin stain on cryostatic section, 400×.

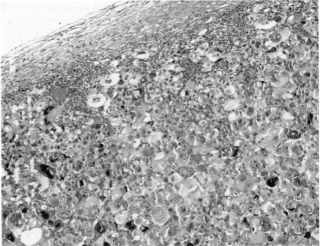

FIGURE 18-5. Nodular metastasis from melanoma. The tumor cells are large and pleomorphic, with distinct cytoplasmic borders, but are less cohesive than true epithelial metastatic cells. Scattered melanoma cells also show intra-cytoplasmic granules of melanin. Hematoxylin and eosin stain on formalin-fixed, paraffin-embedded tissue section, 100×.

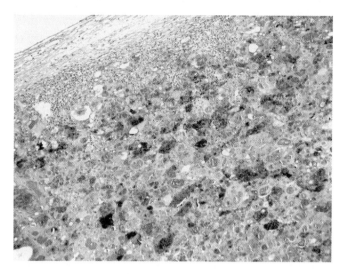

FIGURE 18-6. Nodular metastasis from melanoma. The neoplastic cells display nucleo-cytoplasmic immunostaining for S-100 protein. Immunohistochemistry anti S-100 protein, 100×.

The current protocols for sentinel lymph node examination in melanoma patients invariably include step sectioning of the node and immunohistochemical staining for 1 or more melanoma markers. This combined approach results in a 12% increase in the detection rate of metastases (23). A protocol based on evaluation of at least 10 sections cut from both faces of bisected sentinel lymph nodes, stained with hematoxylin and eosin (H&E), and with immunoreactions for S-100 protein, HMB-45 (see Figures 18-6 and 18-7), and MelanA/Mart-1 antigens has been recommended by the Augsburg Consensus on Techniques of Lymphatic Mapping, Sentinel Lymphadenectomy and Completion Lymphadenectomy in Cutaneous Malignancies, held in Augsburg in 1999 (33). The intraoperative examination of frozen sections has been discouraged, to avoid a high rate of false-negative results due to the unreliability of the morphologic identification of metastatic cells after freezing and to minimize the loss of diagnostic tissue during trimming.

As anticipated, immunohistochemistry plays an important ancillary role in the identification of metastatic melanoma, except for the cases with obvious and large metastases. The value of immunohistochemistry lies not only in its capability of highlighting tumor cells that would escape morphologic recognition, but also in facilitating the distinction between metastatic cells and normal resident nodal cells or benign nodal inclusions. A multimarker approach, with the immunohistochemical detection of S-100 protein, HMB-45, and Mart-1/MelanA antigens ensures maximal specificity and sensitivity. The S-100 protein is detectable in almost 100% of melanoma cells, but it is also expressed by normal resident cells of the lymph nodes. HMB-45 antigen is more specific for melanoma cells, but may not be detectable in up

to 20% of the cases. Mart-1/MelanA antigen is invariable expressed both by nodal nevus and melanoma metastases.

As for metastatic breast carcinoma, the question regarding the extent of histopathologic examination of the sentinel lymph node in melanoma patients remains to be addressed. According to the Augsburg Consensus and to protocols used at the John Wayne Cancer Institute in Santa Monica, analysis should focus on the central portions of the bisected sentinel nodes, examining at least 10 step sections from both moieties. Sections 1, 3, 5, and 10 should be routinely stained with H&E, sections 2 and 4 immunostained for S-100 protein and HMB-45 antigen, respectively, sections 6 and 7 used for negative controls, and sections 8 and 9 spared for further analysis (e.g., Mart-1/MelanA antigen) if necessary.

According to an alternative procedure of the Augsburg Consensus, the sentinel node should be cut along its major axis in 1-mm-thick slices, and 3 sections per slice should be evaluated by both H&E and immunohistochemistry for S-100 protein and HMB-45 antigen. Sections for additional molecular biology studies could also be cut (33).

Cook et al. (6), on behalf of EORTC Melanoma Study Group, proposed a more extensive histopathologic analysis of sentinel nodes in cutaneous melanoma patients, combining immunohistochemistry with an increasing number of cutting levels. Initially, they adopted a protocol similar to the Augsburg Consensus recommendations. Later, they included the examination of 2 additional step sections cut at 50 μm intervals, which lead to an increase in the overall detection rate of metastases from 17.8% to 25% of the cases. When 3 additional sections,

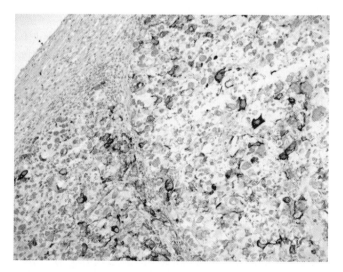

FIGURE 18-7. Nodular metastasis from melanoma. The neoplastic cells display cytoplasmic immunoreactivity for HMB-45 antigen. Immunohistochemistry anti-HMB-45, 100×.

cut at 50 μm intervals, were eventually added to the protocol, the detection rate of metastases rose to 34%.

Somewhat similarly, Spanknebel et al. (7) proposed an enhanced pathologic analysis of the sentinel lymph nodes. Each lymph node was cut at 50 μm intervals for 20 levels, and 3 consecutive sections from each level were stained with H&E and immunostained for S-100 protein and HMB-45 antigen. The enhanced pathologic analysis resulted in the conversion from node-negative to node-positive disease in 14 of 49 patients (28%), with a reported overall detection rate of sentinel lymph node metastases of up to 61% of the cases.

## Diagnostic Accuracy

The assessment of sentinel lymph node status may be affected by both false-negative and false-positive histopathologic results. A false-negative sentinel node biopsy is almost invariably due to a less than optimal scrutiny of the lymph node, either because the number of evaluated sections is not high enough to be truly representative of node status, or because metastases escaped recognition by the pathologist. The issue of a variable detection rate of metastases according to the more or less extensive examination of the sentinel lymph nodes has been dealt with in the preceding paragraphs. It is quite uncommon for an experienced pathologist to overlook lymph node metastases. There are instances, however, where small and/or morphologically unusual metastases from breast carcinoma may be misinterpreted as non-neoplastic resident cells, most likely epithelioid histiocytes of granulomatous lymphadenitis or vessels with high endothelial lining, especially when examining frozen tissue sections. To avoid misdiagnoses, use of ancillary immunohistochemical techniques for specific markers of the epithelial lineage (i.e., cytokeratins) may be extremely useful. These techniques may also be applied to intraoperative frozen section diagnosis, taking advantage of commercially available reagents that allow the reaction to be completed in less than 20 minutes (24,34).

Metastatic melanoma may also be misdiagnosed as benign nevus, if melanoma cells do not show obvious morphological atypia or mitotic activity (see Figure 18-8). Immunohistochemistry may be useful in these instances as well, although it is not as effective as with metastatic breast carcinoma. The HMB-45 antigen is more diffusely and intensely expressed by melanoma cells than by nevus cells, whereas p16 has been reported as a marker of benign nevus cells (35).

Less attention has been paid to the risk of false-positive identification of sentinel lymph node metastases, although this would imply unwarranted lymph node dissection and improper adjuvant treatments. Carter et al. (36) first warned of the possible occurrence

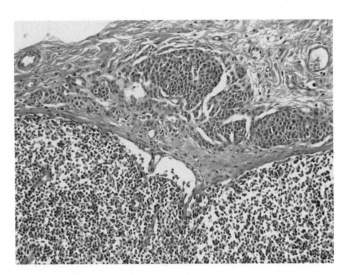

FIGURE 18-8. Occasionally, the perinodal tissues may contain clusters of epithelioid cells, resembling metastatic epithelial cells. This case represents a juxta-capsular nevus and is composed by tightly packed cells, with moderate amounts of nonpigmented cytoplasm and bland-looking nuclei with inconspicuous or absent nucleoli. At variance with true metastatic deposits, which occur more frequently within the lymph node capsule or in the underlying marginal sinus, nevus cells tend to occupy the outer aspect of the lymph node capsule. Hematoxylin and eosin stain on formalin-fixed, paraffin-embedded tissue section, 100×.

of passive transport to the axillary lymph node of normal (and neoplastic) breast tissue following diagnostic needle procedures on the breast. Chiu et al. (37) emphasized inaccurate immunohistochemical procedures as a potential source of false-positive sentinel lymph node biopsy. Also, the immunoreactivity for low-molecular weight cytokeratins of fibroblastic reticulum cells invariably present in normal lymph nodes (38,39) may be responsible for a false identification of metastatic cells. A more subtle cause of false-positive identification of breast metastases is the possible occurrence of benign-appearing breast tissue in the lymph node capsule and/or parenchyma.

The occurrence of ectopic nonneoplastic tissue within lymph nodes is a well-recognized phenomenon, especially for thyroid or salivary structures within latero-cervical lymph nodes or nevus cells in lymph nodes from different basins. Mammary glands are the ectopic structures most frequently detected within axillary lymph nodes (7,18) and, at variance with most of the aforementioned examples that occur intraparenchymally, these are commonly seen in capsular or subcapsular locations or in the perinodal fat tissue. Occasionally, the ectopic tissue has been interpreted as metastatic, leading to overstaging and, eventually, overtreatment of patients (40,41).

We first reported the occurrence of benign epithelial inclusions of ectopic breast tissue in axillary sentinel lymph nodes of 7 breast carcinoma patients with remarkably different morphologic features (42). These benign epithelial inclusions may undergo proliferative changes similar to those encountered in fibrocystic disease (such as florid duct hyperplasia and sclerosing adenosis), making the differential diagnosis with true metastases difficult. Again, use of appropriate immunohistochemical reactions for specific markers (e.g., p63, smooth-muscle myosin, calponin) of the myoepithelial cell component that are invariably present in benign inclusions and absent in metastatic breast carcinoma is instrumental in reaching a correct diagnosis; the examining pathologist should be fully aware of the possible occurrence of such benign inclusions.

False-positive identification of metastatic melanoma may also result from a misinterpretation of the results of the immunohistochemical reactions, which are routinely performed for the assessment of sentinel node status. S-100 protein is the most sensitive marker for melanoma cells, but a substantial background staining is seen almost invariably, and metastatic cells must be differentiated from immigrated Langerhans cells, interdigitating dendritic reticulum cells, nevus cells, and nerve sheath cells, which all share immunoreactivity for S-100 protein. Capsular and trabecular nevi are encountered in 10% to 35% of draining lymph nodes from patients with cutaneous melanoma (43,44). In addition, HMB-45 immunoreactivity may be seen in nodal trabecular calcifications, which are frequently present in the iliac and groin basins (45).

Inaccurate diagnoses of sentinel lymph node biopsies may occur as well in different clinical settings. Hyperplastic mesothelial cell inclusions may be encountered in abdominal lymph nodes scrutinized for metastatic adenocarcinoma of the colon. Mesothelial cells are cytokeratin-immunoreactive and may also show CEA immunoreactivity, which could be incorrectly interpreted as markers of metastatic adenocarcinoma. To avoid misdiagnoses, we could take advantage of calretinin immunoreactivity, which is a marker of mesothelial cells but is almost invariably lacking in adenocarcinoma cells (46,47).

## Predicting the Status of Nonsentinel Lymph Nodes

Extensive examination of sentinel lymph nodes has significantly increased the detection rate of minimal lymph node involvement, and the question has arisen as to whether micrometastases or isolated tumor cells only in the sentinel lymph node predict a risk for additional nonsentinel node metastases that is high enough to justify completion lymph node dissection for these patients. Previous studies had suggested that breast carcinoma

patients with minimal sentinel node involvement could indeed be spared axillary surgery, because of an alleged negligible risk of additional metastases; however, we and other authors have documented a 20% to 24% risk of involvement of further echelon lymph nodes in patients with micrometastatic sentinel nodes (28,48).

More recently, we evaluated a large series of patients with positive sentinel lymph node biopsies followed by completion axillary dissection. Of the 116 patients with isolated tumor cells only in the sentinel node, 17 (14.7%) had further axillary involvement, as did 68 (21.4%) of the 318 patients with sentinel lymph node micrometastases (0.2–2 mm in size) (49). The prevalence of additional metastases was not significantly different between these 2 groups of patients (P = 0.15), whereas patients with macrometastatic disease in the sentinel nodes showed a significantly higher proportion of nonsentinel lymph node metastases, which were detected in 399 of the 794 (50.3%) cases (P < 0.0001). However, when the patients with sentinel node micrometastases were further stratified according to the size of the micrometastases (up to 1 mm vs 1–2 mm), those with larger micrometastases showed a significantly higher prevalence of additional metastases (30.2% versus 17.0%; P = 0.01), thus confirming previous data (13,16). To summarize, patients with a positive sentinel lymph node biopsy can be stratified in 3 groups at significantly different risk for involvement of nonsentinel lymph nodes. Patients with isolated tumor cells or small (up to 1 mm) micrometastases in the sentinel lymph node have the lowest risk of additional metastases (16.2%), which increases to 30.2% and 50.3% for patients with 1 to 2 mm micrometastases or larger metastases, respectively.

In each subgroup of patients with sentinel node metastases, additional metastases to nonsentinel nodes were mostly of the macrometastatic type, i.e., larger than 2 mm (49). Therefore, completion axillary dissection in all patients with positive axillary sentinel lymph node biopsy may be clinically meaningful, because in the vast majority of these patients—including those with isolated tumor cells only or micrometastases in the sentinel lymph nodes—nonsentinel node metastases are larger than 2 mm.

To ascertain whether the identification of minimal sentinel lymph node involvement (with the associated risk of additional nonsentinel lymph node metastases) is informative enough per se to plan an effective adjuvant treatment without the need for further axillary surgery, a randomized clinical trial has been launched by the International Breast Cancer Study Group (IBCSG trial 23-01), whereby patients with micrometastatic disease or isolated tumor cells only in the sentinel node are randomized to further surgery or follow-up. The primary endpoint of the trial is disease-free survival.

In melanoma patients, Starz et al. (50) proposed the so-called S classification as a surrogate of the volumetric determination of the tumor burden in the sentinel lymph node to predict the risk of additional metastases in the remaining nodes of the basin. Originally, it was based on 2 parameters: the number of sentinel lymph node slices in which metastases were detected, and the maximum depth of invasion, measured as the maximum distance in millimeters between intranodal tumor cells and the inner margin of the sentinel lymph node capsule (the S parameter). Subsequent efforts to simplify the method documented that the maximum depth (S) was the most powerful predictive parameter, which is applicable in all laboratories, irrespective of the protocol used for sentinel lymph node examination. The only prerequisite is an adequate number of sections to allow identification of the maximal distance of the metastasis from the inner margin of the sentinel lymph node capsule.

According to this simplified classification method, patients with subcapsular involvement (S-I category) have a 12% risk of additional metastases to nonsentinel lymph nodes, which increases to 13% for S-II patients (those bearing sentinel lymph node metastases with a maximum distance >0.3 mm and <1 mm from the capsule) and to 55% for S-III patients, whose sentinel lymph nodes harbor more distant metastases from the inner margin of the capsule (51,52).

Using a combined assessment of the area of the sentinel lymph node metastases and of the density and distribution of interdigitating dendritic cells, Cochran et al. reported a statistically significant difference in predicting additional metastases to the nodal basin. According to this assessment, 65.4% of patients with high tumor burden in sentinel lymph nodes had additional metastases. Patients with low tumor burden could be further subdivided and were more likely to have additional metastases if a reduced number and density of interdigitating dendritic cells were detected in the sentinel lymph node (45,53).

Dewar et al. (54) described a simpler method, based on the microanatomic location of metastatic melanoma within the sentinel node. Metastatic disease was classified as subcapsular if confined within the subcapsular sinus, parenchymal if located within the paracortical area, combined if both subcapsular and parenchymal, and multifocal or extensive if larger than 5 mm. Patients with subcapsular metastases only did not show any additional metastases to nonsentinel lymph nodes.

# The Role of Molecular Pathology Assays

The increasing adoption of sentinel lymph node biopsy for staging patients with minimal morbidity has raised the question of how best to evaluate the sentinel lymph node, to minimize the risk of false-negative results. Owing also to the lack of standardized and widely accepted protocols for extensive histopathologic examination of the sentinel node, the relative merits of alternative assays based on the identification of tumor-specific mRNA markers over traditional histologic or immunohistochemical methods have been extensively exploited. Initially, qualitative reverse transcription-polymerase chain reaction (RT-PCR) experiments documented that several mRNA markers, either alone or in multimarker assays, were indeed suitable for high-sensitivity detection of metastatic breast cancer or melanoma in sentinel or nonsentinel lymph nodes (55–58).

The specificity of the assays, however, was less than satisfactory, with a high prevalence of positive assays in histologically unaffected lymph nodes, and also in lymph nodes obtained from patients without malignancies (55). Because a possible cause of false-positive identification of lymph node metastases by RT-PCR assays might be the illegitimate expression of low levels of target mRNAs by nonneoplastic cells, real-time quantitative RT-PCR (qRT-PCR) assays have been developed to correctly identify lymph node metastases according to a threshold level of mRNA expression (59–63). Very recently, dedicated kits and instruments for "rapid" qRT-PCR assays have become commercially available for the intraoperative detection of sentinel node metastases from breast carcinoma.

A critical reappraisal of the investigations dealing with the identification of breast carcinoma mRNA markers in axillary sentinel and nonsentinel nodes, however, challenges the possible application of qRT-PCR assays in clinical practice. Indeed, in the studies with the largest series of patients evaluated, the overall concordance between qRT-PCR assays for individual or multiple mRNA markers and morphologic or immunohistochemical findings ranges from 73.2% (62) to 95.7% (63). Discrepancies include both false-negative qRT-PCR results, with histologically detected metastases escaping identification by the assays, and positive assays in lymph nodes not harboring any morphologically identifiable metastasis.

Besides the choice of the molecular assay (qualitative vs quantitative RT-PCR), a likely cause for discrepancies between morphological and molecular findings is the sampling procedure, with part (or half) of the lymph node being subjected to molecular biology assays and another part to morphologic and immunohistochemical examination. As a consequence, the smallest tumor deposits (micrometastases and ITC) may remain confined exclusively to the sample undergoing 1 assay, thus escaping detection by the other.

To minimize the effects of sampling on the final results, we have combined RT-PCR assays with our procedure whereby axillary sentinel lymph nodes of patients with breast carcinoma are snap-frozen and examined completely by serial sectioning at 50 μm intervals. While the frozen sections are examined histologically (including immunohistochemical testing), the interval tissue is subjected to RT-PCR assays. Applying this procedure, we have examined 146 axillary sentinel lymph nodes from 123 patients for the detection of 5 different mRNA tumor markers (cytokeratin 19, CEA, mammaglobin 1, MUC-1, and maspin) by qualitative RT-PCR assays (56). When analyzed individually, the general concordance with the histopathologic findings ranged from 78.8% to 83.6%, with none of the different markers attaining sensitivity higher than 77.8%. Mammaglobin (MGB1) was the mRNA marker most closely correlated with the histopathologic findings, with sensitivity of 77.8% and specificity of 86.1%. We have more recently evaluated the effectiveness of a real-time qRT-PCR assay for MGB1 mRNA in the detection of lymph node metastases in a retrospective series of 81 axillary sentinel nodes from 72 patients for which the results of the previous qualitative assays were known, and validated the results in a prospective series of 61 sentinel nodes from 61 newly diagnosed breast carcinoma patients (69).

In our experimental conditions, qRT-PCR assays were indeed more accurate than conventional RT-PCR in assessing the status of axillary sentinel nodes: 4 of the 6 false-negative cases in conventional RT-PCR assays turned positive in qRT-PCR experiments, whereas 2 of the 5 false-positive cases in conventional RT-PCR assays turned negative in qRT-PCR experiments. Accordingly, qRT-PCR assays were superior to qualitative RT-PCR in terms both of specificity and sensitivity.

The results were compared with the histopathologic findings obtained by an extensive examination of the same nodes, specifically designed to minimize the possible effects of the sampling procedures on the correlation between morphologic and molecular data. The overall concordance with histopathologic findings was 93.8% and 93.4% in the retrospective and validation series, respectively—well in line with previous findings from qRT-PCR assays of individual or multiple tumor markers, indicating a concordance ranging from 73.2% (62) to 95.7% (63). The overall sensitivity of the assay in the 2 combined series was 88.5% and specificity was 94.8%, with a PPV of 79.3% and NPV of 97.3%. The false-negative rate of the assay (3 of 26 histologically positive sentinel lymph nodes, or 11.6%) and the rate of positive detection of MGB1 mRNA (6 of 116, or 5.2%) in lymph nodes not harboring any histologically identifiable metastasis, however, call into question its use in clinical practice as an alternative to histopathologic examination. In the previously mentioned study, we compared the qRT-PCR findings with an extensive histopathologic evaluation of the sentinel node, which makes it unlikely that the molecular assay actually identifies true metastases missed at morphologic scrutiny. Whether the molecular assay may be a valuable and cost-effective tool for identification of breast cancer metastases in axillary sentinel lymph nodes that are not subjected to extensive histopathologic examinations remains to be determined.

Follow-up studies in melanoma patients, however, documented that the assessment of sentinel lymph node status by RT-PCR assays for multiple markers (MAGE-1, tyrosinase, and MelanA/Mart-1) was correlated with prognosis, with RT-PCR-positive patients showing a significantly worse prognosis. Large multicentric, randomized trials are needed to confirm these early reports (64–68).

## Conclusions

This chapter reviewed the role of histopathology in assessing the status of the sentinel lymph node, with the assumption that the detection of even minimal lymph node involvement may be clinically relevant, both for immediate surgical intervention on further echelon lymph nodes, and for prognostic/predictive evaluations.

The mere occurrence of tumor cells in the regional lymph nodes, however, may not be an invariable predictor of clinical progression of the disease. The results of randomized trials (26,70) have shown that the observed number of breast carcinoma patients with clinically overt axillary progression of the disease is much lower than expected based on either the false-negative rate of the sentinel node biopsy or the known prevalence of metastasis to axillary lymph nodes. This suggests that metastatic cells may not progress to clinical disease in all patients, and that only some of these cells have the capability of sustaining tumor progression, consistent with the hypothesis that cancer growth and progression (and hence the clinical outcome of the disease) are dependent on the activation of tumorigenic stem/progenitor breast cancer cells (71,72).

The stem/progenitor cell theory of carcinogenesis and tumor progression conflicts with the traditional stochastic approach, by which all tumor cells in a given patient share the same potential for progression. According to the stochastic approach, prognosis is dictated by the actual amount of invasive or metastatic tumor cells, and therapeutic interventions are intended to minimize their number. This leads pathologists to painstakingly evaluate tumor burden and count tumor cells, using all possible ancillary techniques to identify even individual tumor cells. This attitude may not be truly rewarding. Indeed, the progenitor/stem cell theory predicts that only some (and possibly a minor percentage of) tumor cells are actually responsible for tumor progression and clinical outcome, and that efforts should be made to target these cells with specific interventions. Thus, what is now needed is to unveil specific markers of tumorigenic cells that would allow their identification and quantitation in clinical specimens, and to re-evaluate the prognosis by alternative means.

## References

1. Veronesi U, Paganelli G, Viale G, et al. Sentinel lymph node biopsy and axillary dissection in breast cancer: results in a large series. *J Natl Cancer Inst.* 1999;91:368–373.
2. Kim T, Giuliano AE, Lyman GH. Lymphatic mapping and sentinel lymph node biopsy in early-stage breast carcinoma: a metaanalysis *Cancer.* 2006;106:4–16.
3. Cote RJ, Peterson HF, Chaiwun B, et al. Role of immunohistochemical detection of lymph-node metastases in management of breast cancer. *Lancet.* 1999;354:896–900.
4. Cochran AJ, Wen DR, Huang RR, et al. Prediction of metastatic melanoma in nonsentinel nodes and clinical outcome based on the primary melanoma and the sentinel node. *Mod Pathol.* 2004;17:747–755.
5. Cochran AJ. The pathologist's role in sentinel lymph node evaluation. *Semin Nucl Med.* 2000;30:11–17.
6. Cook MG, Green MA, Anderson B, et al. The development of optimal pathological assessment of sentinel lymph nodes for melanoma. *J Pathol.* 2003;200:314–319.
7. Spanknebel K, Coit DG, Bieligk SC, et al. Characterization of micrometastatic disease in melanoma sentinel lymph nodes by enhanced pathology: recommendations for standardizing pathologic analysis. *Am J Surg Pathol.* 2005;29:305–317.
8. Hermanek P, Hutter RV, Sobin LH, et al. Classification of isolated tumor cells and micrometastasis. *Cancer.* 1999;86: 2668–2673.
9. Rahusen FD, Torrenga H, van Diest PJ, et al. Predictive factors for metastatic involvement of nonsentinel nodes in patients with breast cancer. *Arch Surg.* 2001;136:1059–1063.
10. den Bakker MA, van Weeszenberg A, de Kanter AY, et al. Non-sentinel lymph node involvement in patients with breast cancer and sentinel node micrometastasis: too early to abandon axillary clearance. *J Clin Pathol.* 2002;55: 932–935.
11. Sachdev U, Murphy K, Derzie A, et al. Predictors of nonsentinel lymph node metastasis in breast cancer patients. *Am J Surg.* 2002;183:213–217.
12. Nos C, Harding-MacKean C, Freneaux P, et al. Prediction of tumor involvement in remaining axillary lymph nodes when the sentinel node in a woman with breast cancer contains metastases. *Br J Surg.* 2003;90:1354–1360.
13. de Widt-Levert LM, Tjan-Heijnen VCG, Bult P, et al. Stage migration in breast cancer: surgical decisions concerning isolated tumor cells and micro-metastases in the sentinel lymph node. *Eur J Surg Oncol.* 2003;29:216–220.
14. Liang WC, Sickle-Santanello BJ, Nims TA. Is a completion axillary dissection indicated for micrometastases in the sentinel lymph node? *Am J Surg.* 2001;182:365–368.
15. Guenther JM, Hansen NM, DiFronzo LA, et al. Axillary dissection is not required for all patients with breast cancer and positive sentinel nodes. *Arch Surg.* 2003;138:52–56.
16. Reynolds C, Mick R, Donohue JH, et al. Sentinel lymph node biopsy with metastasis: can axillary dissection be avoided in some patients with breast cancer? *J Clin Oncol.* 1999;17:1720–1726.
17. Cserni G, Amendoeira I, Apostolikas N, et al. Discrepancies in current practice of pathological evaluation of sentinel lymph nodes in breast cancer. Results of a questionnaire-based survey by the European Working Group for Breast Screening Pathology. *J Clin Pathol.* 2004;57:695–701.
18. Roberts AA, Cochran AJ. Pathologic analysis of sentinel lymph nodes in melanoma patients: current and future trends. *J Surg Oncol.* 2004;85:152–161.
19. Veronesi U, Galimberti V, Mariani L, et al. Sentinel node biopsy in breast cancer: early results in 953 patients with negative sentinel node biopsy and no axillary dissection. *Eur J Cancer.* 2005;41:231–237.
20. Hakam A, Nasir A, Raghuwanshi R, et al. Value of multilevel sectioning for improved detection of micrometastases in sentinel lymph nodes in invasive squamous cell carcinoma of the vulva. *Anticancer Res.* 2004;24:1281–1286.
21. Bertagnolli M, Miedema B, Redston M, et al. Sentinel node staging of resectable colon cancer: results of a multicenter study. *Ann Surg.* 2004;240:624–628.
22. Kitagawa Y, Fujii H, Kumai K, et al. Recent advances in sentinel node navigation for gastric cancer: a paradigm shift of surgical management. *J Surg Oncol.* 2005;90:147–151.
23. Cochran AJ. Surgical pathology remains pivotal in the evaluation of 'sentinel' lymph nodes. *Am J Surg Pathol.* 1999;23:1169–1172.
24. Veronesi U, Paganelli G, Galimberti V, et al. Sentinel-node biopsy to avoid axillary dissection in breast cancer with clinically negative lymph nodes. *Lancet.* 1997;349: 1864–1867.
25. Viale G, Maiorano E, Mazzarol G, et al. Histologic detection and clinical implications of micrometastases in axillary sentinel lymph nodes for patients with breast carcinoma. *Cancer.* 2001;92:1378–1384.
26. Veronesi U, Paganelli G, Viale G, et al. A randomized comparison of sentinel-node biopsy with routine axillary dissection in breast cancer. *N Engl J Med.* 2003;349:546–553.
27. Cochran AJ, Morton DL, Stern S, et al. Sentinel lymph nodes show profound down-regulation of antigen-presenting cells of the paracortex: implications for tumor biology and treatment. *Mod Pathol.* 2001;14:604–608.
28. Wong SL, Edwards MJ, Chao C, et al. Predicting the status of the nonsentinel axillary nodes: a multicenter study. *Arch Surg.* 2001;136:563–568.
29. Viale G, Bosari S, Mazzarol G, et al. Intraoperative examination of axillary sentinel lymph nodes in breast carcinoma patients. *Cancer.* 1999;85:2433–2438.
30. Veronesi U, Zurida S, Mazzarol G, et al. Extensive frozen section examination of axillary sentinel nodes to deter-

mine selective axillary dissection. *World J Surg.* 2001;25: 806–808.

31. Kuehn T, Bembenek A, Decker T, et al. Consensus Committee of the German Society of Senology. A concept for the clinical implementation of sentinel lymph node biopsy in patients with breast carcinoma with special regard to quality assurance. *Cancer.* 2005;103:451–461.

32. Schwartz GF, Giuliano AE, Veronesi U, et al. Proceedings of the consensus conference on the role of sentinel lymph node biopsy in carcinoma of the breast, April 19–22, 2001, Philadelphia, Pennsylvania. *Cancer.* 2002;94:2542–2551.

33. Cochran AJ, Balda BR, Starz H, et al. The Augsburg Consensus. Techniques of lymphatic mapping, sentinel lymphadenectomy, and completion lymphadenectomy in cutaneous malignancies. *Cancer.* 2000;89:236–241.

34. Chilosi M, Lestani M, Pedron S, et al. A rapid immunostaining method for frozen sections. *Biotech Histochem.* 1994;69:235–239.

35. Mihic-Probst D, Saremaslani P, Komminoth P, Heitz PU. Immunostaining for the tumor suppressor gene p16 product is a useful marker to differentiate melanoma metastasis from lymph-node nevus. *Virchows Arch.* 2003;443:745–751.

36. Carter BA, Jensen RA, Simpson JF, et al. Benign transport of breast epithelium into axillary lymph nodes after biopsy. *Am J Clin Pathol.* 2000;113:259–265.

37. Chiu A, Hoda SA, Yao DX, et al. A potential source of false-positive sentinel nodes. Immunostain misadventure. *Arch Pathol Lab Med.* 2001;125:1497–1499.

38. Doglioni C, Dell'Orto P, Zanetti G, et al. Cytokeratin-immunoreactive cells of human lymph nodes and spleen in normal and pathological conditions. An immunocytochemical study. *Virchows Arch A Pathol Anat.* 1990;416:479–490.

39. Franke WW, Moll R. Cytoskeletal components of lymphoid organs. I. Synthesis of cytokeratins 8 and 18 and desmin in subpopulations of extrafollicular reticulum cells of human lymph nodes, tonsils and spleen. *Differentiation.* 1987;36:145–163.

40. Fisher CJ, Hill S, Millis RR. Benign lymph node inclusions mimicking metastatic carcinoma. *J Clin Pathol.* 1994;47:245–247.

41. Holdsworth PJ, Hopkinson JM, Leveson SH. Benign axillary epithelial lymph node inclusions—a histological pitfall. *Histopathology.* 1988;13:226–228.

42. Maiorano E, Mazzarol GM, Pruneri G, et al. Ectopic breast tissue as a possible cause of false-positive axillary sentinel lymph node biopsies. *Am J Surg Pathol.* 2003;27:513–518.

43. Carson KF, Wen DR, Li PX, et al. Nodal nevi and cutaneous melanomas. *Am J Surg Pathol.* 1996;20:834–840.

44. Ridolfi RL, Rosen PP, Thaler H. Nevus cell aggregates associated with lymph nodes: estimated frequency and clinical significance. *Cancer.* 1977;39:164–171.

45. Cochran AJ, Roberts A, Wen DR, et al. Optimized assessment of sentinel lymph nodes for metastatic melanoma: implications for regional surgery and overall treatment planning. *Ann Surg Oncol.* 2004;11:156S–161S.

46. Huntrakoon M. Benign glandular inclusions in the abdominal lymph nodes of a man. *Hum Pathol.* 1985;16:644–646.

47. Doglioni C, Tos AP, Laurino L, et al. Calretinin: a novel immunocytochemical marker for mesothelioma. *Am J Surg Pathol.* 1996;20:1037–1046.

48. Turner RR, Chu KU, Qi K, et al. Pathologic features associated with nonsentinel lymph node metastases in patients with metastatic breast carcinoma in a sentinel lymph node. *Cancer.* 2000;89:574–581.

49. Viale G, Maiorano E, Pruneri G et al. Predicting the risk for additional axillary metastases in patients with breast carcinoma and positive sentinel lymph node biopsy. *Ann Surg.* 2005;241:319–325.

50. Starz H, Siedlecki K, Balda BR. Sentinel lymphadenectomy and s-classification: a successful strategy for better prediction and improvement of outcome of melanoma. *Ann Surg Oncol.* 2004;11:162S–168S.

51. Starz H, Balda BR, Kramer KU, et al. A micromorphometry-based concept for routine classification of sentinel lymph node metastases and its clinical relevance for patients with melanoma. *Cancer.* 2001;91:2110–2121.

52. Starz H. Pathology of the sentinel lymph node in melanoma. *Semin Oncol.* 2004;31:357–362.

53. Lana AM, Wen DR, Cochran AJ. The morphology, immunophenotype, and distribution of paracortical dendritic leucocytes in lymph nodes regional to cutaneous melanoma. *Melanoma Res.* 2001;11:401–410.

54. Dewar DJ, Newell B, Green MA, et al. The microanatomic location of metastatic melanoma in sentinel lymph nodes predicts nonsentinel lymph node involvement. *J Clin Oncol.* 2004;22:3345–3349.

55. Bostick PJ, Chatterjee S, Chi DD, et al. Limitations of specific reverse-transcriptase polymerase chain reaction markers in the detection of metastases in the lymph nodes and blood of breast cancer patients. *J Clin Oncol.* 1998;16:2632–2640.

56. Manzotti M, Dell'Orto P, Maisonneuve P, et al. Reverse transcription-polymerase chain reaction assay for multiple mRNA markers in the detection of breast cancer metastases in sentinel lymph nodes. *Int J Cancer.* 2001;95:307–312.

57. Branagan G, Hughes D, Jeffrey M, et al. Detection of micrometastases in lymph nodes from patients with breast cancer. *Br J Surg.* 2002;89:86–89.

58. Ouellette RJ, Richard D, Maicas E. RT-PCR for mammaglobin genes, MGB1 and MGB2, identifies breast cancer micrometastases in sentinel lymph nodes. *Am J Clin Pathol.* 2004;121:637–643.

59. Mitas M, Mikhitarian K, Walters C, et al. Quantitative real-time RT-PCR detection of breast cancer micrometastasis using a multigene marker panel. *Int J Cancer.* 2001;93:162–171.

60. Inokuchi M, Ninomyia I, Tsugawa K, et al. Quantitative evaluation of metastases in axillary lymph nodes of breast cancer. *Br J Cancer.* 2003;89:1750–1756.

61. Schroder CP, Ruiters MHJ, De Jong S, et al. Detection of micrometastatic breast cancer by means of real-time quantitative RT-PCR and immunostaining in perioperative

blood samples and sentinel nodes. *Int J Cancer.* 2003;106: 611–618.

62. Gillanders WE, Mickitarian K, Hebert R, et al. Molecular detection of micrometastatic breast cancer in histopathology-negative axillary lymph nodes correlates with traditional predictors of prognosis. An interim analysis of a prospective multi-institutional cohort study. *Ann Surg.* 2004;239:828–840.

63. Weigelt B, Verduijn AJ, Bosma AJ, et al. Detection of metastases in sentinel lymph nodes of breast cancer patients by multiple mRNA markers. *Br J Cancer.* 2004;90: 1531–1537.

64. Voit C, Kron M, Rademaker J, et al. Molecular staging in stage II and III melanoma patients and its effect on long-term survival. *J Clin Oncol.* 2005;23:1218–1227.

65. Ulrich J, Bonnekoh B, Bockelmann R, et al. Prognostic significance of detecting micrometastases by tyrosinase RT/PCR in sentinel lymph node biopsies: lessons from 322 consecutive melanoma patients. *Eur J Cancer.* 2004;40: 2812–2819.

66. Gradilone A, Ribuffo D, Silvestri I, et al. Detection of melanoma cells in sentinel lymph nodes by reverse transcriptase-polymerase chain reaction: prognostic significance. *Ann Surg Oncol.* 2004;11:983–987.

67. Kammula US, Ghossein R, Bhattacharya S, et al. Serial follow-up and the prognostic significance of reverse transcriptase-polymerase chain reaction—staged sentinel lymph nodes from melanoma patients. *J Clin Oncol.* 2004;22:3989–3996.

68. Takeuchi H, Morton DL, Kuo C, et al. Prognostic significance of molecular upstaging of paraffin-embedded sentinel lymph nodes in melanoma patients. *J Clin Oncol.* 2004;22:2671–2680.

69. Dell'Orto P, Biasi OM, Del Curto B, Zurrida S, Galimberti V, Viale G. Assessing the status of axillary sentinel lymph nodes of breast carcinoma patients by a real-time quantitative RT-PCR assay for mammaglobin 1 mRNA. *Breast Cancer Res Treat.* 2006;98:185–190.

70. Zurrida S, Orecchia R, Galimberti V, et al. Axillary radiotherapy instead of axillary dissection: a randomized trial. Italian Oncological Senology Group. *Ann Surg Oncol.* 2002;9:156–160.

71. Al-Hajj M, Wicha MS, Benito-Hernandez A, et al. Prospective identification of tumorigenic breast cancer cells. *Proc Natl Acad Sci USA.* 2003;100:3983–3988.

72. Dontu G, Abdallah WM, Foley JM, et al. In vitro propagation and transcriptional profiling of human mammary stem/progenitor cells. *Genes Dev.* 2003;17:1253–1270.

# 19
# Frozen Section and Imprint Cytology in Sentinel Lymph Node Biopsy for Breast Cancer

Santo V. Nicosia and Charles E. Cox

Recent trends toward conservative surgery for breast cancer and increasing detection of smaller invasive malignancies have shifted the traditional surgical approach from mastectomy to lumpectomy, and from complete axillary lymph node dissection to sentinel lymph node biopsy to avoid extensive procedures in clinically node-negative women (1,2). Debate continues over radioisotope physical characteristics and the type of dyes, as well as the optimal time of injection and the role of axillary dissection in locoregional disease control (1,3). However, sentinel lymph node biopsy is successful in 92% to 98% of breast cancer patients and is increasingly being used for staging and prognostication, although low-volume micrometastatic disease may be present in up to 15% of nonsentinel nodes when sentinel lymph node biopsy is negative (4,5). Controversy also exists concerning the extent of tissue sampling and the modality of pathological assessment for the most sensitive and accurate detection of metastatic disease (1,6). Although the diagnostic armamentarium of the pathologist is rapidly expanding due to recent advances in molecular techniques, in most laboratories intraoperative assessment of sentinel lymph node histology is routinely done by either frozen section or imprint cytology, with rare and selective use of cytokeratin immunohistochemistry in diagnostically equivocal cases (7–10).

While frozen section is a time-honored technique used at most institutions, lymph node imprint cytology is still limited to those centers with the interest, expertise, and reliance in diagnostic cytopathology (11–16). Nevertheless, imprint cytology has been used for the rapid assessment of axillary node metastases in breast cancer at least since 1984 (17). Building on a longstanding experience with imprint cytology in the intraoperative analysis of lumpectomy margins (18), our group at the Moffitt Cancer Center began applying this technique to the diagnosis of sentinel lymph nodes in 1994 (12). At other institutions, its use was motivated by the need for rapid analysis without loss of nodal tissue and frozen section-related

artifacts. As sentinel lymph node biopsy becomes a standard procedure in the management of breast cancer, it is imperative to better understand the relative diagnostic power of these 2 intraoperative techniques, especially in view of the heterogeneity of some published results. This chapter analyzes the general approach to pathological evaluation of sentinel lymph nodes, and compares the results of 46 published studies with the aim of providing pathologists with a rationale for the adoption of a diagnostic protocol and breast surgeons with a platform to discuss diagnostic expectations with their patients.

## Handling Sentinel Lymph Nodes

An average of 2 sentinel lymph nodes per axilla is removed during a sentinel lymph node biopsy, compared with an approximate average of 15 nodes obtained from a complete axillary lymph node dissection (19,20). A mathematical model suggests that more than 90% of metastases would be detected if a maximum of 6 nodes equal or greater than 6 mm in size were removed from level I–II axillary chains (21). Sentinel lymph nodes should be sent to the pathology grossing room promptly, and preferably wrapped in nonabsorbent, saline-moistened wrappings such as Telfa pads (Kendall Healthcare products, Mansfield, MA). Upon receipt, experienced pathologists or their trained assistants should promptly record the size and morphology of individual nodes(s), as gross evaluation alone can recognize approximately 20% of nodal metastases (22). In 1974, Wilkinson and Hause demonstrated that by obtaining 1-center and 2-quarter sections, the probability of identifying a 0.5 mm metastasis in a node measuring 2 mm is approximately 100% (23) (Figure 19-1A, see Color Plate). Assuming zero observer error, a computer simulation study indicates that a standard 4 μm histologic section has a 64% probability of detecting a 2 mm metastasis in a bivalved node, and that fine slicing the node during

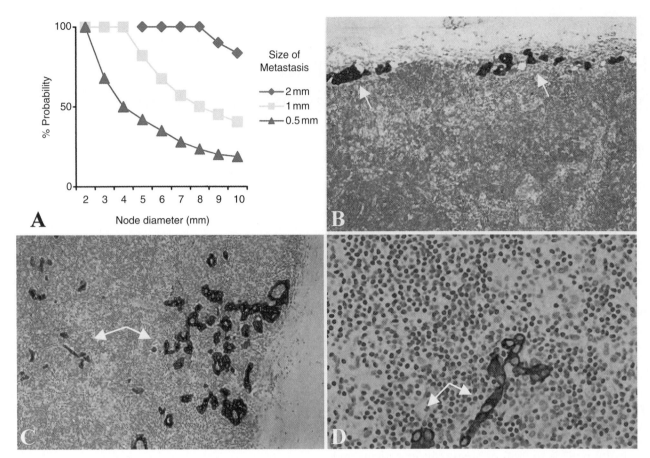

FIGURE 19-1. (A–B) Distribution patterns of metastases in sentinel lymph nodes of patients with breast cancer. Metastases are highlighted by their cytokeratin immunoreactivity. Tumor cells are present in peripheral sinus (A, arrows), the outer cortex (B, arrows), and medulla (C, arrows). The probability of sampling such metastases as a function of their size is illustrated in (A). (B–D). Avidin-biotin complex immunoperoxidase staining. (Original magnification: (B), ×40; (C), ×100; (D), ×200). (A, Wilkinson and Hause, Cancer, Vol. 33, No. 5, 1974, 1269–74 [23]. Copyright 1974 American Cancer Society. This material is reproduced with permission of Wiley-Liss, Inc., a subsidiary of John Wiley & Sons, Inc.) (See Color Plate.)

grossing further improves detection (24). Assuming spherical shapes, a geometrical model also suggests that sections taken 1 mm apart identify almost all macrometastases, while step sectioning at 200 to 250 μm can adequately identify micrometastases (25). These findings provide a rationale for the College of American Pathologists' recommendation that each sentinel lymph node be sectioned along its longitudinal axis in approximately 2 mm-thick sections, and that each sectional surface be carefully evaluated to identify focal lesions (7). However, this approach is not uniformly followed, as representative sentinel node sections may be single (22, 26,27) or multiple and exhaustive of the entire node (28,29).

Although it is recommended that 3 levels be taken from each embedded nodal section, there is wide institutional diversity in the number of final sections, as nodes may only be bivalved and interval levels may not be obtained or taken at 40 to 150 μm (28,30–32). For example, for a 1-cm sentinel lymph node, the number of hematoxylin and eosin (H&E)–stained levels may vary between 2 (1 bivalved node), 15 (3 levels for each of 5 sections, if guidelines are followed) and 250, if levels are obtained at 40 μm intervals. Thus, the final number of H&E sections would differ significantly; a high number would be associated with significant time-management and cost issues but would provide potentially more useful clinical information, as intensive sectioning may discover close to 25% of occult metastases (33).

Figure 19-2 illustrates a sampling protocol that takes into consideration the physical characteristics of individual nodes (34). Sections are submitted for histopathological evaluation, and cytological imprints are obtained from each exposed surface. An awareness of the distribution pattern of metastases is essential for optimal cytological sampling. To this end, gentle but deliberate flattening of cut nodal surfaces by the imprinting glass slide must be applied to obtain representative cellular elements from the peripheral sinus. Following intra-

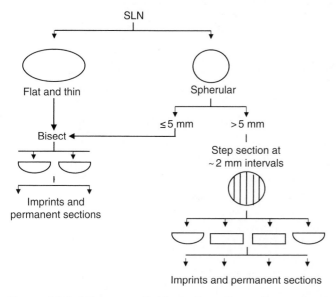

FIGURE 19-2. Diagrammatic illustration of sampling protocol for sentinel lymph nodes in breast cancer.

operative diagnosis, nodal sections are fixed in 10% neutral buffered formalin, embedded in paraffin, and then further sectioned at 4 to 5 μm thickness for final interpretation by H&E or cytokeratin immunostaining. Usually multiple sections from a single node can be embedded in a single cassette.

## Pathologic Evaluation of the Sentinel Lymph Node

Metastases may be localized to the peripheral sinus, in the cortex, or less frequently in the more central compartment of sentinel lymph nodes (Figure 19-1B–D, see Color Plate). Tumor cells may present in aggregates of 0.2 to 2 mm in size (so-called micrometastases, or pathological tumor stage pN1a) or larger than 2 mm in size and visible (so-called macrometastases, or pN1b), or as isolated tumor cells. Surgical pathologists, especially those with oncologic training, are well aware of these characteristics and may recur to cytokeratin immunostaining whenever equivocal cell groups or isolated tumor cells are suspected. Experience in diagnostic cytopathology and progressive learning, as well as good cytopreparation, are necessary for optimal interpretation of sentinel lymph node imprints (35,36). Cells are visualized by a rapid stain of the Romanowski family, including May Grunwald-Giemsa and Diff-Quik, after air-drying, or by rapid Papanicolaou or H&E staining after fixation in ethanol; the first 2 stains are favored by cytopathologists, and the last 2 are preferred by surgical pathologists. Although recommended by some investigators (37,38),

scraping of cut sentinel lymph node surfaces may yield thick cellular areas, and such artifacts may lead to erroneous interpretation (39). An experienced cytopathologist usually scans a cytological imprint under a 4× or a 10× objective if there is a previous history of ductal or lobular carcinoma, respectively; higher magnification is necessary with the latter malignancy because its cells are only slightly larger than the more numerous surrounding lymphocytes (usually >50,000/slide). The average time taken for cytologically evaluating sentinel nodes at our institution is 5 to 6 minutes per node.

It is important to be familiar with the cytology of normal nodal constituents, including lymphocytes at various developmental stages, germinal center cells and immunoblasts, histiocytes, microvascular endothelial cells, dendritic cells, fibroblasts, and mast cells (Figure 19-3A–C, see Color Plate). Mammary cancer metastases occur in cytological imprints in a variety of patterns, such as cohesive cell groups, syncytial groups, acinar or tubular fragments, and single cells (Figure 19-4A–D, see Color Plate). The first 3 patterns usually do not pose a diagnostic challenge, unless associated with low-grade carcinomas; however, the last can escape the scanning eyes of the pathologist or be mistaken for bystander lymphocytes or histiocytes (Figure 19-5C; see Color Plate). In addition, the diffuse single cell pattern may rarely be mistaken for a chronically inflamed or chronically reactive node, when the tumor cells are small in size and imprints are scanned quickly at low power. This pitfall can be avoided through attention to occasional lymphoid follicles and by routinely alternating from low- to high-power microscopic evaluation. The diagnostic challenge presented by lobular carcinoma cells, especially when rare, can be aptly managed through the application of rapid intraoperative immunocytokeratin 40. This procedure can be performed in 16 to 20 minutes and strikingly visualizes the metastatic tumor cells in larger numbers than anticipated on cytomorphological grounds (Figure 19-5A–D, see Color Plate). Benign epithelial and nevus inclusions may also occasionally pose some diagnostic difficulty and be a source of false-positive results (41,42), in the former also due to their morphological phenotype and cytokeratin immunoreactivity. Another potential but as yet unreported problem in imprint cytology is the phenomenon of benign epithelial transport secondary to pre-sentinel lymph node biopsy breast massage (43). The presence of mechanically dislodged epithelial cells in >0.2 mm cell clusters may confound pathological interpretation. Additional false-positive results (usually less than 1%) may be obtained with overlapping histiocytes from areas of sinus histiocytosis (44,45) (Figure 19-6A–B, see Color Plate), immunocytokeratin-positive debris within histiocytes (46) (Figure 19-6C, see Color Plate), germinal center cells (16), and dendritic cells (34,36,47).

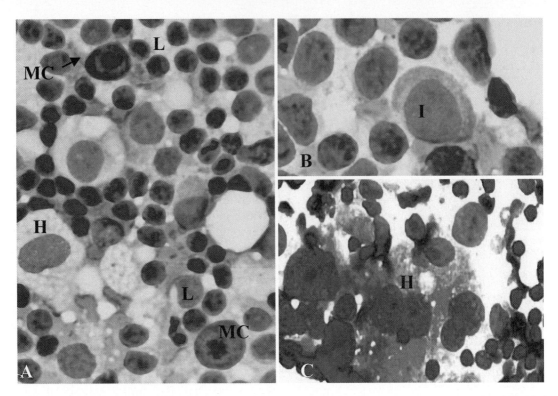

FIGURE 19-3. Normal cytology of sentinel lymph node constituents. Note lymphocytes of different size (L), histiocytes (H), immunoblasts (I), and mast cells (MC). Diff-Quik stain. (A–C, original magnification ×400). (See Color Plate.)

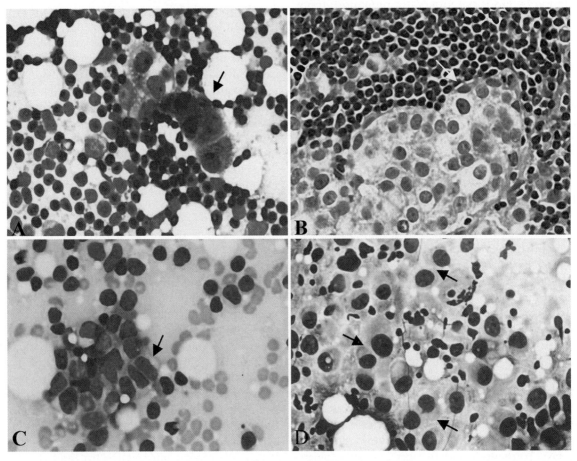

FIGURE 19-4. Cytological patterns of breast cancer metastases. Note cohesive group (A, arrow) and corresponding morphology in permanent section (B), rare (C, arrow) and diffuse (D, arrows) single cell pattern. A, C, and D. Diff-Quik stain (original magnification ×400). B. Hematoxylin and eosin stain (original magnification ×200). (See Color Plate.)

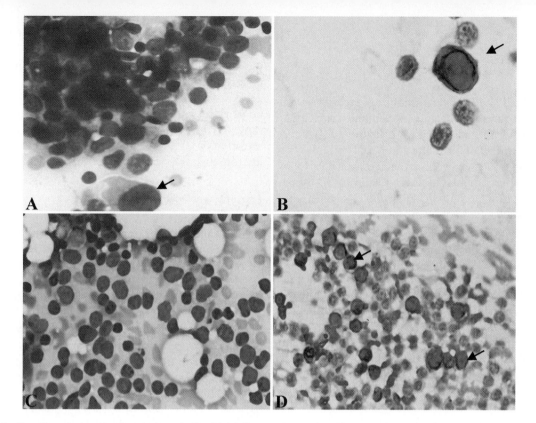

FIGURE 19-5. Cytokeratin expression in cytological imprints from sentinel lymph nodes with an occasional but cytologically evident metastatic tumor cell in a patient with ductal carcinoma (A, arrow), or with frequent but inconspicuous tumor cells in a patient with lobular carcinoma (C, arrow). Note sensitive visualization of tumor cells after application of rapid intraoperative immunocytokeratin staining (B and D, arrows). A and C. Diff-Quik stain. B and D. Avidin-biotin-complex immunoperoxidase. (All original magnifications are ×400.) (See Color Plate.)

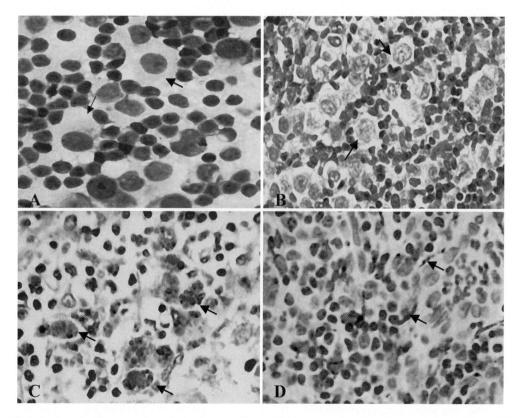

FIGURE 19-6. Histiocytes (A–C, arrows) and dendritic cells (D, arrows) in sentinel lymph nodes. These cells may rarely be a source of diagnostic dilemma due to their overall epithelial-like morphology, especially when in aggregates, or to nonspecific immunoreactivity for cytokeratin (C and D). A. Diff-Quik stain. B. hematoxylin and eosin stain. C–D. Avidin-biotin-complex immunoperoxidase. (All original magnifications are ×400.) (See Color Plate.)

## Literature Data

To analyze the diagnostic performance of frozen section and imprint cytology, 46 peer-reviewed manuscripts identified through a PubMed search were examined. In addition, to collect information on the number of patients with sentinel lymph nodes, as well as the average number of sentinel nodes per patient, data were retrieved from each series on the following statistical parameters: sensitivity, specificity, overall accuracy, positive and negative predictive value, positive and negative likelihood ratios (odds of positive or negative sentinel lymph node independent of disease prevalence, most indicative when ratios have larger numbers or are closest to zero, respectively), and prevalence of disease. Parameters not directly reported were calculated using each series' raw data. Statistical formulas were applied to derive means and standard deviations (available at Tools for Science, www.physics.csbsju.edu/stats/). Whenever data was available, the sensitivity of imprint cytology and frozen section for detecting macrometastases and micrometastases was also recorded.

## Frozen Section

Twenty-two reports on the application of frozen section in the intraoperative evaluation of sentinel lymph nodes in breast cancer were reviewed, spanning from 1993 to 2004 (11,15,16,30,32,45–48,49–61). In total, 4,481 patients and 8,410 lymph nodes were evaluated, for an average of 1.8 nodes per patient (see Table 19-1). Approximately one-third of the nodes harbored metastases (disease prevalence). Statistical data were expressed on a per patient basis, except for 2 studies where this information could not be verified (15,16). The overall average values for sensitivity, specificity, and accuracy of frozen section

were 71.2%, 99.8%, and 90.8%, respectively. Overall positive predictive values were 99.2%, and negative predictive values were 88.1%. The overall negative likelihood ratio was 0.28, and the positive likelihood ratios ranged from 0.62 to infinity (see Table 19-1). The overall sensitivities of frozen section for macrometastases and micrometastases were respectively 90.3% and 21.7%.

## Imprint Cytology

In the application of imprint cytology to the intraoperative diagnosis of sentinel lymph nodes in breast cancer, 29 reports spanning from 1996 to 2003 were reviewed (11–16,22,26,27,35,36,39,49,58,60–76). A total of 6,703 patients and 13,660 lymph nodes were evaluated, for an average of 1.97 nodes per patient (see Table 19-1). Almost one-third of the nodes harbored metastases. Statistical data were expressed on a per patient basis, except for 5 studies where this information could not be verified (15,26,39,61,73). The overall average values for sensitivity, specificity, and accuracy of imprint cytology were 64.18%, 99.44%, and 87.95% respectively. Overall positive predictive values were 98.28%, and negative predictive values 85.16%. The overall negative likelihood ratio was 0.38, and overall positive likelihood ratios ranged from 0.26 to infinity (see Table 19-1). The overall sensitivities of imprint cytology for macrometastases and micrometastases were respectively 80.8% and 18.2%.

## Combined Frozen Section and Imprint Cytology

Three studies from 1999 to 2002 on the diagnostic utility of combined frozen section and imprint cytology were also reviewed (16,44,77). In total, 777 patients and 1,446

TABLE 19-1. Intraoperative pathological analysis of sentinel lymph nodes in breast cancer patients from 46 published series.

| Pathological method | Total number of cases | Total number of SLNs | SLN/Case | Sensitivity % | Specificity % | Accuracy % | PPV % | NPV % | PLR | NLR | Prevalence of metastases§ |
|---|---|---|---|---|---|---|---|---|---|---|---|
| Frozen Section* | 4,481 | 8,410 | 1.80 ± 0.42 | 71.2 ± 14.5 | 99.4 ± 0.44 | 90.8 ± 7.71 | 99.2 ± 2.35 | 88.1 ± 9.90 | 61-infinity | 0.28 ± 0.15 | 32.7 ± 11.2 |
| Imprint Cytology** | 6,703 | 13,660 | 1.97 ± 0.48 | 64.2 ± 20 | 99.4 ± 0.87 | 87.9 ± 7.79 | 98.3 ± 2.83 | 85.2 ± 10.1 | 21-infinity | 0.38 ± 0.19 | 33.3 ± 13.0 |
| Frozen Section + Imprint Cytology*** | 777 | 1,446 | 1.95 ± 0.52 | 81.1 ± 6.62 | 99.4 ± 0.56 | 94.2 ± 1.59 | 98.1 ± 1.93 | 92.8 ± 2.67 | 82-infinity | 0.19 ± 0.06 | 40.33 ± 15. |

*References 11, 15–16, 29–30, 32, 45, 47–61
**References 11–16, 22, 26, 35–36, 39, 48, 57, 59–60, 62–67, 69–75
***References 9, 16, 44
§Reported distribution of micrometastases ranges from 36.2 ± 13.8 (frozen section studies) to 44.8 ± 7.15 (imprint cytology studies) and 40.33 ± 15. (studies on combined frozen section and imprint cytology)

lymph nodes were evaluated, for an average of 1.95 nodes per patient (Table 19-1). Approximately 29% of the nodes disclosed metastatic disease. Statistical data were expressed on a per patient basis. The overall average values for sensitivity, specificity, and accuracy of combined imprint cytology and frozen section were respectively 81.08%, 99.63%, and 94.16%. Overall positive predictive values and negative predictive values were respectively 98.15% and 92.84%. The overall negative likelihood ratio was 0.19, and positive likelihood ratios ranged from 0.82 to infinity (Table 19-1). Sensitivities of combined techniques for macrometastases and micrometastases were reported in 2 of the 3 studies, and ranged from 93.68% to 98%, and from 28% to 60.46%.

## Comparative Analysis of Frozen Section and Imprint Cytology

Sentinel lymph node biopsy has increasingly been used in the management of breast cancer since it was introduced by Krag in 1993 (77) and popularized by other clinical investigators (78,79). Validation studies indicate that sentinel lymph node biopsy accurately and reliably detects axillary metastases in the vast majority of patients and node-positive cases, with most failures secondary to undetected micrometastases (50). Debate continues regarding the role of immediate evaluation of sentinel nodes, and which intraoperative diagnostic modality—frozen section or imprint cytology—is best to identify metastatic disease. Although much literature exists on the use of these 2 techniques, the results are not always readily comparable due to differences in several factors, including: patient population and case selection, node-positive and early-stage disease, the prevalence of micrometastatic disease (range: 38–58%), the frequency of metastatic lobular carcinoma, the number of sentinel nodes and nodal sections evaluated, the type of reagents used, intra- and interobserver variability, diagnostic learning curves, and the effect of time constraints placed on the pathology team (12,27,30,35,36,50,51,58,63,66–69,76). Even with such limitations, a comparison of all series through their reported and extrapolated data offers a useful perspective on the diagnostic utility of frozen section and imprint cytology.

As indicated in Table 19-1, there are no significant differences between the overall diagnostic performance of imprint cytology and frozen section in all parameters evaluated. Sensitivity and negative likelihood ratio estimates show a slight but not significant advantage for frozen section. Both study sets exhibit a similar general prevalence of disease, although more micrometastases are described (when reported) in imprint cytology than in the frozen section series (45% vs. 36%). A lower sen-

TABLE 19-2. Sensitivity of intraoperative pathologic analysis of sentinel lymph nodes in breast cancer patients by size of metastasis.

| Pathologic method | Macrometastases (>2 mm) | Micrometastases (0.2–2 mm) |
|---|---|---|
| Frozen Section* | 90 ± 6.66 | 21.7 ± 5.69 |
| Imprint Cytology** | 80.8 ± 5.62 | 18.2 ± 8.97 |

*References 49–50, 57
**References 12–13, 35–36, 57, 62, 66–67

sitivity of imprint cytology may be secondary to the selection of cytological stains (11,72).

The sensitivity of both techniques usually increases with tumor size, tumor phenotype, and grade, as well as with size of the sentinel lymph node and metastases (12,15,44,45,50,51,53,63,68,69,76,77). Detection of nodal metastases gradually increases, from an average of 17% for T1a (range: 4–40%), 39% for T1b (range: 30–87%), 43% for T1c (range: 28–100%), and 45% for T2 (range: 40–96%), to 80% for T3 lesions (range: 63–100%). Identification of metastases occurs more readily in sentinel lymph nodes larger than 2 cm (77), in ductal rather than in lobular carcinomas and low-grade tumors (12,45,69,75), and in higher grade tumors, as indicated by a sensitivity of 16% with grade 1 versus 45% with grade 2 to 3 tumors (52). In those few series where reported, frozen section is better than imprint cytology for identifying metastases larger than 2 mm (90% versus 81%), but both are imprecise in recognizing metastases smaller than 2 mm (22% versus 18%) (12,30,31,35,36,50,58,63,66–69,76) (see Table 19-2). However, the combined use of frozen section and imprint cytology is associated with improved detection of micrometastases, as indicated by a sensitivity of 44% (95% sensitivity for macrometastases) (16,44,77).

Published data rarely disclose the sensitivity of imprint cytology and frozen section based on a similar number of imprints and sections. Extrapolating from literature where such information is provided, frozen section appears to be more sensitive than imprint cytology (68% versus 53%) when only 1 sample is obtained, but both techniques perform equally when multiple samples are procured (Table 19-3). With multiple sampling, sensitivity of imprint cytology and frozen section rises to 83% and 85%, respectively (Table 19-3). This advantage is

TABLE 19-3. Sensitivity of intraoperative pathologic analysis in breast cancer patients by number of nodal sections or imprints.

| Pathologic method | Single | Multiple |
|---|---|---|
| Frozen Section* | 68.4 ± 14.6 | 84.6 ± 7.60 |
| Imprint Cytology** | 53.2 ± 14.4 | 83.4 ± 14.2 |

*References 11, 15, 29–30, 32, 42, 47, 49, 50–51, 53–55, 57, 59, 60
**References 11–16, 22, 26, 48, 35–36, 39, 57, 59–60, 62, 64–67, 69, 70–75

best illustrated by an overall sensitivity of more than 93% with the use of exhaustive frozen sections (28,29).

## Discussion

This review does not find a definitive advantage for either frozen section or imprint cytology as intraoperative diagnostic adjuncts. As their performance is quite similar, some authors have suggested the combined use of the 2 techniques, or of combining 1 of them with immunocytokeratin (40,67,77). With the exception of 2 studies that suggest individual superiority (60,61), most reports make a case for joint use of imprint cytology and frozen section when comparing their performance in detail (15,16,58,72). The identification of cells immunoreactive for cytokeratin 19 or other breast-associated low-molecular weight keratins upstages 7% to 13% of patients including, unexpectedly, those with in-situ lesions (11,63,80–82), and may extend the capability of conventional pathological evaluation in further predicting axillary nonsentinel node involvement (77,81). However, adequate sampling of sentinel nodes may provide an equally or more satisfactory solution, as indicated by the European Institute of Oncology (Milan, Italy) (20). Although controlled studies comparing this approach for both frozen section and imprint cytology are not available, results with multiple numbers of sections or imprints (Table 19-3) anticipate equivalent performance. Therefore, the choice of diagnostic modality should be based on criteria that include technical advantages and quality assurance, the adequacy of the remaining tissue for adjunctive diagnostic or prognostic studies, turnaround time, cost, and patient satisfaction. Frozen section usually has a lower rate of indeterminate results (76), but it is associated with longer turnaround times, consumption of a significant amount of tissue (up to 50%), additive radioactive contamination of microtomes (83), and freeze-thaw artifacts (54,68,74,76). When applied, serial sectioning may require at least 60 minutes per case, although during this time primary breast surgery would usually take place (20,75). By comparison, imprint cytology has a shorter turnaround (since there is no need for freezing or sectioning), is easy to perform on multiple slides, and does not cause tissue loss or freezing artifacts (68,73,74,76). However, it requires experience in cytopathology that is usually available only in centers with active cytology services, it may yield fewer cells than frozen section, and it has a higher rate of indeterminate results, with 1% to 2% atypical or suspicious diagnoses in a reported series (47,51,54,77). These 2 diagnostic categories should be used sparingly or avoided, as positive results will have untoward clinical implications and clear medicolegal ramifications.

Despite a recent study suggesting no apparent impact on quality of life (31) and the assertion that 70% overall sensitivity may be too low to justify routine intraoperative diagnosis (6,62), frozen section or imprint cytology have sufficient sensitivity to serve not only as screening tools, but also as final diagnostic staging tests by offering the surgeon the opportunity to complete axillary dissection during the same operative setting in at least two-thirds of patients (51). Thus, significant reoperative rates and the associated costs—which exceed the expense of intraoperative diagnosis by 20 to 30 times per case—are avoided (15,50,54,63,84). High levels of diagnostic accuracy must be maintained to ensure acceptance of the intraoperative approach and to avoid the cost of additional sections needed to detect unidentified metastases, as well as to prevent unnecessary axillary dissection.

## Conclusions

Despite its limitations in identifying micrometastases, intraoperative diagnosis eliminates the obligatory delay of several days from sentinel lymph node biopsy to definitive surgery that is encountered with the conventional approach (23). The need for a second surgical procedure is also reduced in a large proportion of patients, resulting in a reoperative rate of 20% to 30%, with approximately 50% of these procedures being performed for cases in which only micrometastases are found (12,19,85). Although micrometastases may have an adverse prognostic effect, their true clinical significance is controversial and hopefully will be resolved by the prospective American College of Surgeons Oncology Group Z0010 and National Surgical Adjuvant Breast Project B32 trials (51). Recent data from the European Institute of Oncology (Milan, Italy) indicate that micrometastatic disease in a single axillary node may be compatible with an excellent prognosis (85). As sentinel node biopsy becomes a common procedure in the management of breast cancer care, it must be standardized. While not addressing the surgical and nuclear medicine aspects of sentinel lymph node biopsy, this review identifies variability in routine and ancillary techniques used in the pathological handling and evaluation of sentinel nodes. These include variations in: (1) the number of sentinel lymph nodes examined, from less than 2 to more than 10 (20,44,54); (2) the number of sections, from less than 2 to more than 30 in a 1-cm node (11,54,68,86,87); (3) the number of interval levels/block, from 2 to 10 μm to 250 to 500 μm steps (88); (4) the number of imprints, from less than 2 to more than 5; (5) the frequency of use and length of intraoperative immunocytokeratin protocols, from 5 to more then 60 minutes (44,67,81,89); (6) the evaluation of sentinel nodes in patients with in-situ lesions; and (7) aliquoting of tissue for molecular assessment (88). At our institution, imprint cytology is preferred over frozen section for its faster turnaround time and the rarity of artifactual results, and we are striving to implement a standard approach using multilevel imprints among 5 cytopathologists (see Figure 19-1; see Color Plate 19-1). As immunocytokeratin and other newer diagnostic adjuncts are increasingly proposed for the evaluation of sentinel nodes (77,88–90), consensus on standardization and related quality control issues become imperative. In the end, however, there is no substitute for good pathological techniques, including careful nodal grossing and sampling, experienced microscopic observation, and inquisitive discussion with astute surgeons who know the importance of sharing their clinical knowledge with team pathologists.

*Acknowledgments.* The authors express their profound appreciation to Dr. Ni Ni K. Ku for contributing illustrations and to Laura White for expert assistance with literature search and inhouse clinical data. Sincere thanks are also due to all the surgeons, pathologists, and grossing room personnel responsible for the procurement and interpretation of more than 7000 sentinel lymph nodes at the Moffitt Cancer Center.

# References

1. Noguchi M. Sentinel lymph node biopsy as an alternative to routine axillary lymph node dissection in breast cancer patients. *J Surg Oncol.* 2001;76:144–156.

2. Mariani G, Moresco L, Viale G, et al. Radioguided sentinel lymph node biopsy in breast cancer surgery. *J Nucl Med.* 2001;42:1198–1215.

3. Sanjuan A, Vidal-Sicart S, Zanon G, et al. Clinical axillary recurrence after sentinel node biopsy in breast cancer: a follow-up study of 220 patients. *Eur J Nucl Med Mol Imaging.* 2005;32:932–936.

4. Viale G, Zurrida S, Maiorano E, et al. Predicting the status of axillary sentinel lymph nodes in 4351 patients with invasive breast carcinoma treated in a single institution. *Cancer.* 2005;103:492–500.

5. Duncan M, Cech A, Wechter D, et al. Criteria for establishing the adequacy of sentinel lymphadenectomy. *Am J Surg.* 2004;187:639–642.

6. Rampaul RS, Miremadi A, Pinder SE, et al. Pathologic validation and significance of micrometastasis in sentinel nodes in primary breast cancer. *J Nucl Med.* 2001;3:113–116.

7. Schwartz GF, Giuliano A, Veronesi U. Proceedings of the consensus conference on the role of sentinel lymph node biopsy in carcinoma of the breast. *Hum Pathol.* 2002;33:579–589.

8. Timar J, Csuka O, Orosz Z, et al. Molecular pathology of tumor metastasis. *Pathol Oncol Res.* 2002;8:204–219.

9. Turner RR. Histopathologic assessment of the sentinel lymph node in breast cancer. *Ann Surg Oncol.* 2001;8(suppl 9):56S–59S.

10. VanDiest P, Torrenga H, Meijer S, et al. Pathologic analysis of sentinel lymph nodes. *Semin Surg Oncol.* 2001;20:238–245.

11. Aihara T, Munakata S, Morino H, et al. Comparison of frozen section and touch imprint cytology for evaluation of sentinel lymph node metastases in breast cancer. *Ann Surg Oncol.* 2004;11:747–750.

12. Cox C, Centeno B, Dickson D, et al. Accuracy of intraoperative imprint cytology for sentinel lymph node evaluation in the treatment of breast carcinoma. *Cancer Cytopath.* 2005;105:13–20.

13. Creager AJ, Geisinger KR, Shiver SA, et al. Intraoperative evaluation of sentinel lymph nodes for metastatic breast carcinoma by imprint cytology. *Mod Pathol.* 2002;15:1140–1147.

14. Deo S, Samaiya A, Jain P, et al. Sentinel lymph node biopsy assessment using intraoperative imprint cytology in breast cancer patients: results of a validation study. *Asian J Surg.* 2004;27:294–298.

15. Henry-Tillman R, Korourian S. Rubio IT, et al. Intraoperative touch preparation for sentinel lymph node biopsy: a 4-year experience. *Ann Surg Oncol.* 2002;9:333–339.

16. Nagashima T, Suzuki M, Yagata H, et al. Intraoperative cytologic diagnosis of sentinel node metastases in breast cancer. *Acta Cytol.* 2003;47:1028–1032.

17. Quill DS, Lehay AL, Lawler RG, et al. Lymph node imprint cytology for the rapid assessment of axillary node metastases in breast cancer. *Br J Surg.* 1984;71:454–455.

18. Weinberg E, Cox C, Dupont E, et al. Local recurrence in lumpectomy patients after imprint cytology margin evaluation. *Am J Surg.* 2004;188:349–354.

19. Viale G, Maiorano E. Pruneri G, et al. Predicting the risk for additional axillary metastases in patients with breast carcinoma and positive sentinel lymph node biopsy. *Ann Surg.* 2005;241:319–325.

20. Viale G, Maiorano E, Mazzarol G, et al. Histologic detection and clinical implications of micrometastases in axillary sentinel lymph nodes for patients with breast carcinoma. *Cancer.* 2001;15:1378–1384.

21. Suzuma T, Sakurai T, Yoshimura G, et al. A mathematic model of axillary lymph node involvement in patients with breast cancer. *Breast Cancer.* 2001;8:206–212.

22. Kane JM 3rd, Edge SB, Winston JS, et al. Intraoperative pathologic evaluation of a breast cancer sentinel lymph node biopsy as a determinant for synchronous axillary lymph node dissection. *Ann Surg Oncol.* 2000;8:361–367.

23. Wilkinson EJ, Hause L. Probability in lymph node sectioning. *Cancer.* 1974;33:1269–1274.

24. Farshid G, Pradhan M, Kollias J, et al. Computer simulations of lymph node metastasis for optimizing the pathologic examination of sentinel lymph nodes in patients with breast carcinoma. *Cancer.* 2000;89:2527–2537.

25. Cserni G, Gregori D, Merletti F, et al. Meta-analysis of non-sentinel node metastases associated with micrometastatic sentinel nodes in breast cancer. *Br J Surg.* 2004;91:1245–1242.

26. Litz CE, Beitsch PD, Roberts CA, et al. Intraoperative cytologic diagnosis of breast sentinel lymph nodes in the routine, nonacademic setting: a highly specific test with limited sensitivity. *Breast J.* 2004;10:383–387.

27. Mullenix PS, Carter PL, Martin MJ, et al. Predictive value of intraoperative touch preparation analysis of sentinel

lymph nodes for axillary metastasis in breast cancer. *Am J Surg*. 2003;185:420–424.

28. Veronesi U, Zurrida S, Mazzarol G, et al. Extensive frozen section examination of axillary sentinel nodes to determine selective axillary dissection. *World J Surg*. 2001;23: 806–808.

29. Viale G, Bosari S, Mazzarol G, et al. Intraoperative examination of axillary sentinel lymph nodes in breast carcinoma patients. *Cancer*. 1999;85:2433–2438.

30. Grabau DA, Rank F, Friis E. Intraoperative frozen section examination of axillary sentinel lymph nodes in breast cancer. *APMIS*. 2005;113:7–12.

31. Chao C, Abell T, Martin RC, et al. Intraoperative frozen section of sentinel nodes: a formal decision analysis. *Am Surg*. 2004;70:215–220.

32. Nahrig J, Richter T, Kowolik J, et al. Comparison of different histopathological methods for the examination of sentinel lymph nodes in breast cancer. *Anticancer Res*. 2000;20:2209–2212.

33. Jannink I, Fan M, Nagy S, et al. Serial sectioning of sentinel nodes in patients with breast cancer: a pilot study. *Ann Surg Oncol*. 1998;5:310–314.

34. Ku MM. Pathologic assessment of sentinel lymph nodes in breast cancer. *Surg Oncol Clin N Am*. 1999;35:14–18.

35. Llatjos M, Castella E, Fraile M, et al. Intraoperative assessment of sentinel lymph nodes in patients with breast carcinoma. *Cancer Cytopathol*. 2002;96:150–156.

36. Pogacnik A, Klopcic U, Grazio-Frkovic S, et al. The reliability and accuracy of intraoperative imprint cytology of sentinel lymph nodes in breast cancer. *Cytopathology*. 2005;16:71–76.

37. Renshaw AA, Gould EW. Concentrated smear techniques for examining sentinel lymph nodes of the breast at the time of frozen section. *Am J Clin Pathol*. 2004;122:944–946.

38. Silverberg SG. Intraoperative assessment of sentinel nodes in breast cancer. *Histopathology*. 2000;36:185–186.

39. Rubio IT, Korourian S, Cowan C, et al. Use of touch preps for intraoperative diagnosis of sentinel lymph node metastases in breast cancer. *Ann Surg Oncol*. 1998;5:689–694.

40. Weinberg ES, Dickson D, White L, et al. Cytokeratin staining for intraoperative evaluation of sentinel lymph nodes in patients with invasive lobular carcinoma. *Am J Surg*. 2004;188:419–422.

41. Chao C. The use of frozen section and immunohistochemistry for sentinel lymph node biopsy in breast cancer. *Am Surg*. 2004;70:414–419.

42. Fisher CJ, Hill S, Lillis RR. Benign lymph node inclusions mimicking metastatic carcinoma. *J Clin Pathol*. 1994;47: 245–247.

43. Diaz NM, Cox CE, Ebert M, et al. Benign mechanical transport of breast epithelial cells to sentinel lymph nodes. *Am J Surg Pathol*. 2004;28:1641–1645.

44. Leidenius M, Krogerus LA, Toivonen T, et al. The feasibility of intraoperative diagnosis of sentinel lymph node metastases in breast cancer. *J Surg Oncol*. 2003;84:68–73.

45. Tanis PJ, Boom RP, Koops HS, et al. Frozen section investigation of the sentinel node in malignant melanoma and breast cancer. *Ann Surg Oncol*. 2001;8:222–226.

46. Rao RS, Taylor J, Palmer J, et al. Breast cancer pseudometastasis in a sentinel lymph node with cytokeratin positive debris. *Breast J*. 2005;11:134–137.

47. Wada N, Imoto S, Hasebe T, et al. Evaluation of intraoperative frozen section diagnosis of sentinel lymph nodes in breast cancer. *Jpn J Clin Oncol*. 2004;34:113–117.

48. Zuo W, Wang Y, Li M. Clinical significance of sentinel lymph node biopsy for breast cancer. *Zhonghua Zhong Liu Za Zhi*. 2001;23:247–250.

49. Weiser M, Montgomery LL, Susnik B, et al. Is routine intraoperative frozen-section examination of sentinel lymph nodes in breast cancer worthwhile? *Ann Surg Oncol*. 2000;7:651–655.

50. Chao C, Wong SL, Ackermann D, et al. Utility of intraoperative frozen section analysis of sentinel lymph nodes in breast cancer. *Am J Surg*. 2002;182:609–615.

51. Cao Y, Paner G, Rajan PB. Sentinel node status and tumor characteristics. A study of 234 invasive breast carcinomas. *Arch Pathol Lab Med*. 2005;129:82–84.

52. Gulec SA, Su J, O'Leary JP, et al. Clinical utility of frozen section in sentinel node biopsy in breast cancer. *Am Surg*. 2001;67:529–532.

53. Mitchell, ML. Frozen section diagnosis for axillary sentinel lymph nodes: the first 6 years. *Mod Pathol*. 2005;18: 58–61.

54. Khalifa K, Pereira B, Thomas VA, et al. The accuracy of intraoperative frozen section analysis of the sentinel lymph nodes during breast cancer surgery. *Int J Fertil Womens Med*. 2004;49:208–211.

55. Flett MM, Going JJ, Stanton PD, et al. Sentinel lymph node localization in patients with breast cancer. *Br J Surg*. 1998;85:991–993.

56. Rahusen FD, Pijpers R, van Diest PJ, et al. The implementation of the sentinel lymph node biopsy as a routine procedure for patients with breast cancer. *Surgery*. 2000;128: 6–12.

57. Menes TS, Tartter PI, Mizrachi H, et al. Touch preparation or frozen section for intraoperative detection of sentinel lymph node metastases from breast cancer. *Ann Surg Oncol*. 2003;10:1166–1170.

58. Yang JH, Nam SJ, Lee TS, et al. Comparison of intraoperative frozen section analysis of sentinel node with preoperative positron emission tomography in the diagnosis of axillary lymph node status in breast cancer patients. *Jpn J Clin Oncol*. 2001;31:1–6.

59. Motomura K, Inaji H, Komoike Y, et al. Intraoperative sentinel lymph node examination by imprint cytology and frozen sectioning during breast surgery. *Br J Surg*. 2000; 87:597–601.

60. VanDiest PJ, Torrenga H, Borgstein PJ, et al. Reliability of intraoperative frozen section and imprint cytological investigation of sentinel lymph nodes in breast cancer. *Histopathology*. 1999;35:14–18.

61. Dixon JM, Mamman U, Thomas J. Accuracy of intraoperative frozen section analysis of axillary nodes. Edinburgh Breast Unit team. *Br J Surg*. 1999;86:392–395.

62. Zgajnar J, Frkovic-Grazio S, Besic N, et al. Low sensitivity of the touch imprint cytology of the sentinel lymph node in breast cancer patients—results of a large series. *J Surg Oncol*. 2004;85:82–86.

63. Cserni G. The potential value of intraoperative imprint cytology of axillary sentinel lymph nodes in breast cancer patients. *Am Surg.* 2001;67:86–91.

64. Karamlou T, Johnson NM, Chan B, et al. Accuracy of intraoperative touch imprint cytologic analysis of sentinel lymph nodes in breast cancer. *Am J Surg.* 2003;185:425–428.

65. Dabbs DJ, Fung M, Johnson R. Intraoperative cytologic examination of breast sentinel lymph nodes: test utility and patient impact. *Breast J.* 2004;10:190–194.

66. Creager AJ, Geisinger KR, Perrier ND, et al. Intraoperative imprint cytologic evaluation of sentinel lymph nodes for lobular carcinoma of the breast. *Ann Surg.* 2004;239: 61–66.

67. Shiver SA, Creager AJ, Geisinger K, et al. Intraoperative analysis of sentinel lymph nodes by imprint cytology for cancer of the breast. *Am J Surg.* 2002;184:424–427.

68. Creager AJ, Geisinger KR. Intraoperative evaluation of sentinel lymph nodes for breast carcinoma: current methodologies. *Adv Anat Path.* 2001;9:233–243.

69. Sauer T, Engh V. Holck AM, et al. Imprint cytology of sentinel lymph nodes in breast cancer. Experience with rapid, intraoperative diagnosis and primary screening by cytotechnologists. *Acta Cytol.* 2003;47:768–773.

70. Ratanawichitrasin A, Biscotti CV, Levy L, et al. Touch imprint cytological analysis of sentinel lymph nodes for detecting axillary metastases in patients with breast cancer. *Br J Surg.* 1999;86:1346–1349.

71. Aihara T, Munakata S, Morino H, et al. Touch imprint cytology and immunohistochemistry for the assessment of sentinel lymph nodes in patients with breast cancer. *Eur J Surg Oncol.* 2003;23:845–848.

72. Baitchev G, Gortchev G, Todorova A. Intraoperative sentinel lymph node examination by imprint cytology during breast surgery. *Curr Med Res Opin.* 2002;18:195–197.

73. Lee A, Krishnamurthy S, Sahin A, et al. Intraoperative touch imprint of sentinel lymph nodes in breast carcinoma patients. *Cancer Cytopathol.* 2002;96:225–231.

74. Mullenix PS, Carter PL, Martin MJ, et al. Predictive value of intraoperative touch preparation analysis of sentinel lymph nodes for axillary metastases in breast cancer. *Am J Surg.* 2003;185:420–424.

75. Barranger E, Antoine M, Grahek D, et al. Intraoperative imprint cytology of sentinel nodes in breast cancer. *J Surg Oncol.* 2004;86:128–133.

76. Turner RR, Hansen NM, Stern SL, et al. Intraoperative examination of the sentinel lymph node for breast carcinoma staging. *Am J Clin Pathol.* 1999;112:627–634.

77. Krag DN, Weaver DL, Alex JC, et al. Surgical resection and radiolocalization of the sentinel lymph node in breast cancer using a gamma probe. *Surg Oncol.* 1993;2:325–339.

78. Albertini JJ, Lyman GH, Cox C, et al. Lymphatic mapping and sentinel node biopsy in the patient with breast cancer. *JAMA.* 1997;12:1818–1822.

79. Liu LH, Siziopikou KP, Gabram S, et al. Evaluation of axillary sentinel lymph node biopsy by immuno-histochemistry and multilevel sectioning in patients with breast carcinoma. *Arch Pathol Lab Med.* 2000;124:1670–1673.

80. Teng S, Dupont E, McCann, C, et al. Do cytokeratin-positive-only sentinel lymph nodes warrant complete axillary lymph node dissection in patients with invasive breast cancer? *Am Surg.* 2000;66:574–578.

81. Gray RJ, Pockaj BA, Conley CR. Sentinel lymph node metastases detected by immunohistochemistry only do not mandate complete axillary lymph node dissection in breast cancer. *Ann Surg Oncol.* 2004;11:1056–1060.

82. Fortunato L, Amini M, Darina M, et al. Intraoperative examination of sentinel nodes in breast cancer: is the glass half full or half empty? *Ann Surg Oncol.* 2004;11:1005–1010.

83. Zurrida S, Mazzarol G, Galimberti V, et al. The problem of the accuracy of intraoperative examination of axillary sentinel nodes in breast cancer. *Ann Surg Oncol.* 2001;8: 817–820.

84. Fitzgibbons PL, LiVolsi VA. Recommendations for handling of radioactive specimens obtained by sentinel lymph-adenectomy. *Am J Surg Path.* 2000;24:1549–1551.

85. Veronesi U, Galimberti V, Mariani L, et al. Sentinel node biopsy in breast cancer: early results in 953 patients with negative sentinel node biopsy and no axillary dissection. *Eur J Cancer.* 2005;41:231–237.

86. Krogerus LA, Leidenius MH, Toivonen TS, et al. Towards reasonable workload in diagnosis of sentinel lymph nodes: comparison of 2 frozen section methods. *Histopathology.* 2004;44:29–34.

87. Cserni G, Amendoeira I, Apostolikas N, et al. Discrepancies in current practice of pathological evaluation of sentinel lymph nodes in breast cancer. Results of a questionnaire based survey by the European Working Group for Breast Screening Pathology. *J Clin Pathol.* 2004;57: 695–701.

88. Richter T, Nahrig J, Komminoth P, et al. Protocol for ultrarapid immunostaining of frozen sections. *J Clin Pathol.* 1999;52:461–463.

89. Ishida M, Kitamura K, Kinoshita J, et al. Detection of micrometastasis in the sentinel lymph nodes in breast cancer. *Surgery.* 2002;131(1suppl):S211–S216.

90. Schroder CP, Ruiters MH, de Jong S, et al. Detection of micrometastatic breast cancer by means of real-time quantitative RT-PCR and immunostaining in perioperative blood samples and sentinel nodes. *Int J Cancer.* 2003;106: 611–618.

# 20
# Molecular Assessment of Sentinel Lymph Nodes

Farin Amersi, Armando E. Giuliano, and Dave S.B. Hoon

Breast cancer will be diagnosed in an estimated 214,640 Americans and cause an estimated 41,430 deaths in 2006 (1). Management of this disease has evolved from the concept of total mastectomy, originally described by Halstead et al. to breast-conserving lumpectomy for early-stage disease. To define a treatment plan for patients with early-stage disease, it is important to determine whether there are metastases in the axillary nodes (2). Imaging modalities such as ultrasound, magnetic resonance imaging (MRI), and position emission tomography (PET) have facilitated detection of distant metastases, but are not reliable in assessing the axillary nodes.

The histopathologic status of axillary lymph nodes is the most significant predictor of overall survival and recurrence, and is used to identify patients who would benefit from adjuvant systemic therapy (3–5). Since a complete axillary lymph node dissection is associated with significant short- and long-term morbidity, it is important to identify node-negative patients who are unlikely to derive therapeutic benefit from this procedure (6–8).

Lymphatic mapping and the technique of the sentinel lymph node biopsy was initially developed by Cabanas et al. in patients with penile cancer (9), and further refined by Morton et al. in patients with melanoma (see further below). The sentinel lymph node is defined as the first lymph node to preferentially receive lymphatic drainage from the primary tumor, and is the first site of lymphatic spread. The sentinel node is localized by a subdermal or peritumoral injection with radiolabeled colloid or vital blue or both together, and its status is highly predictive of that of the remaining lymph nodes in the basin. In 1994, Giuliano et al. applied the technique of lymphatic mapping to breast cancer (10). Sentinel node examination reliably predicts the pathologic status of the regional lymph node basin while reducing functional morbidity, and is more cost-effective than an axillary lymph node dissection (11–13).

Prior to the development of the sentinel lymph node procedure, to pathologically stage the axilla pathologists examined multiple sections from paraffin-embedded lymph nodes obtained from an axillary lymph node dissection. This process of examining multiple sections from lymph nodes to detect micrometastatic disease is time-consuming, arduous, and costly. Furthermore, finding occult metastases in multiple sections can be challenging, and although special techniques such as immunohistochemistry have been used, frequently patients can be understaged (14,15). Immunohistochemistry is also observer dependent and can have low sensitivity, as this analysis entails the use of monoclonal antibodies that are specific for epithelial cells and not breast cancer. Most commonly, cytokeratins (CK) are used as a target for epithelial carcinomas, and can be expressed in normal epithelial cells as intermediate filaments. Anticytokeratin antibodies and cytokeratin antibody cocktails have been used in immunohistochemistry diagnosis, but have been associated with false-positive results. Standard histopathologic techniques in conjunction with immunohistochemistry have limited sensitivity in detecting occult disease; thus, techniques need to be developed that allow clinicians to predict which patients are at risk of developing regional or distant metastases.

## Molecular Assessment for Detecting Tumor Metastases in Sentinel Lymph Nodes

Multiple RNA and DNA markers are currently available to identify patients with occult disease and predict their response to therapy (Tables 20-1 and 20-2). Molecular markers include tumor suppressor genes, oncogenes, tumor-associated antigens, transcription factors, and cellular mediators of apoptosis.

Recently, reverse transcriptase-polymerase chain reaction (RT-PCR) techniques have been developed to detect cancer cells in tissue, lymph nodes, bone marrow, and

TABLE 20-1. RNA molecular markers in breast cancer.

| Markers | Descriptions/Functions |
|---|---|
| Melanoma Antigen Gene A (MAGE-A3) | Encodes for a highly immunogenic protein |
| Muc-1 | Glycosylated membrane glycoprotein expressed by tissues and differentiation marker in development of tissue |
| c-MET | Oncogene that encodes for hepatocyte growth receptor; signal transduction factor |
| ß1 → 4 N-acetylgalactosaminyl transferase (ß1-4-GalNAc-T) | Key enzyme in the biosynthetic pathway of the oncofetal glycolipids GM2/GD2 expressed on cancer cell surfaces |
| ß-Human chorionic gonadotropin (ß-hCG) | Pathophysiologic role unknown |
| Carcinoembryonic antigen (CEA) | Indicates the presence of epithelial cells |
| Mammaglobin 1 and 2 (mam1, mam2) | 93 amino acid proteins, only expressed in breast tissue |
| Prolactin inducible protein (PIP) | Glycoprotein capable of suppressing T-cell apoptosis |
| Cytokeratin (CK-19) | Filament protein marker of epithelial cancers |

blood. In patients with histopathologically negative sentinel lymph nodes by hematoxylin and eosin (H&E) and immunohistochemistry staining, using the RT-PCR technique to identify tumor marker mRNA expression has resulted in the upstaging of a significant number of those with early-stage disease (16–18).

At the John Wayne Cancer Institute in Santa Monica, our group has developed multiple DNA and RNA molecular markers for detecting early disease and predicting disease progression and response to treatment. Tumor marker mRNA expression can be discerned in primary and metastatic tumors, but not in normal lymph nodes or blood. These assays require specific cut-off levels to define the background for individual markers. With the quantitative real-time RT-PCR (qRT), 1 to 5 cancer cells can be detected in $10 \times 10^6$ normal cells (19). Making these assays reliable for clinical use requires meticulous attention to sample preparation, including the steps of nucleic acid extraction and RT and PCR reactions, as well as to sample collection, processing, and storing. With suboptimal conditions, discrepant results can occur. In addition to the technical limitations, there is a biologic heterogeneity of tumor marker expression by tumor cells, even within an individual lesion. Since the expression levels of specific tumor markers may vary with tumor progression, multimarker RT-PCR assays are more inclusive than single marker RT-PCR for detecting occult tumor cells in patients with various cancers (20–22).

## RT-PCR Detection Systems

The John Wayne Cancer Institute laboratory has been developing molecular detection systems to identify occult tumor cells in sentinel lymph nodes obtained from patients with melanoma, colorectal cancer, and breast cancer. Using RT-PCR techniques on frozen tissue sections from these sentinel nodes, we have shown that these techniques are more sensitive than standard H&E staining and immunohistochemistry, and a significant number of patients can be upstaged (23,24). To standardize the results from RT-PCR cDNA examinations, we have developed a multimarker RT-PCR electrochemiluminescence (ECL) assay that is a highly sensitive, solution-phase system for the detection of cDNA product.

TABLE 20-2. DNA molecular markers in breast cancer.

| Markers | Description/Function |
|---|---|
| RAR-ß2, retinoid acid receptor ß2 | Mediates growth inhibition and induction of apoptosis |
| RASSF-1A, ras association domain family protein 1A | Membrane bound GTP/GDP binding protein; protein synthesis and regulation of cell survival, proliferation, and differentiation |
| Rho-GTPases | Maintain normal epithelial polarity; regulate mobility and formation of cell junctions |
| P16 (INK 4a) | Tumor suppressor gene; regulates cell cycle |
| APC | Tumor suppressor gene on chromosome 5q 21; important in Wnt signaling pathway |
| CRBP-I, cellular retinal binding protein-I gene | Regulates retinol and retinoic acid metabolism; important in cellular differentiation growth arrest |
| P14 ARF | Tumor suppressor gene; regulator of cell cycle |
| TWIST | Transcription factor; regulates expression of N-cadherin; important for tumor cell mobility and migration |
| CDH1 | Human E-cadherin gene; maintains architecture in epithelial tissue; important for cellular differentiation |

This semi-quantitative ECL assay isolates specific target PCR cDNA product, and its specificity is increased by hybridization with a probe labeled with the specific cDNA product (25). Amplification of tumor-specific mRNA sequences to specific genes results in increased sensitivity in detecting biomarker expression in tumors, even at lower copy numbers. This probe-based assay allows more sensitive comparative analysis of multiple samples and provides the ability to quantify specific marker copy numbers, unlike ethidium bromide gel and Southern blot cDNA detection systems, which are more subjective and can only detect the presence or absence of a specific marker. In addition, this system enhances detection compared to the gel-based systems by using multiple mRNA markers, since tumor heterogeneity may exist between different patients, as well as expression of different tumor cell clones between the primary tumor and metastases.

## Quantitative Real-Time RT-PCR

Conventional RT-PCR techniques are semi-quantitative and their use in the clinical arena has been fraught with difficulty, as it is hard to ascertain baseline expression of a gene seen in normal tissue with increased expression of that same gene in a tumor specimen. Quantitative real-time RT-PCR (qRT) more efficiently quantitates the number of mRNA copies and can be used to compare differences in gene expression in normal tissue and over-expression in tumor specimens. Our laboratory, as well as other groups, has shown that accurate and reproducible multimarker analysis can be performed, and can be correlated with clinical outcomes as well as prognosis (26–28).

Quantitative real-time RT-PCR requires viable amounts of mRNA based on housekeeping genes such as glyceraldehyde-3-phosphate dehydrogenase (GAPDH), porphobilinogen deaminase (PBGD), and β2-microglobulin (29,30). The integrity of the RNA extracted from tumor specimens is important for establishing the assay's validity. Our approach is to assess the quantity of specific housekeeping gene amplification. In assessment of mRNA copy numbers, we have relied on probe-based assays using primers that detect 1 2-intron region, and a probe that is specific to the open-reading frame cDNA. This is important for detecting a gene that can interfere with results. All primers and probes need to be established initially by gel-based systems to have visualization of the products being amplified. In qRT expression of mRNA copies, we have used ratios of mRNA and housekeeping genes for better normalization. In this approach, mRNA copies are determined by cycle threshold in real-time analysis and a standard curve of mRNA copy numbers is created, which then allows accurate quantification of mRNA copy numbers of the gene of interest in a specimen (31). There is no established method for developing the appropriate standardized curves based on the housekeeping gene, which is a significant factor in the way results are reported. In addition, when performing qRT, appropriate positive and negative controls need to be used to validate the findings of the assay. These controls include different categories of reagent and specimen controls, which are key in evaluating the results.

## Tissue Sampling and Evaluation of Frozen Tissue Sections

Our institute developed a technique for evaluating intraoperative histologic analysis of frozen tissue sections of sentinel lymph nodes (32,33). The presence of tumor cells in the sentinel nodes, identified on frozen sections by immunohistochemistry, would result in a completion lymph node dissection during the operation. Based on this experience, we developed a highly sensitive technique for molecular analysis by RT-PCR on the frozen sections of sentinel nodes from patients with melanoma, breast cancer, and colorectal cancer (34–36).

Bostick et al. assessed the sensitivity and specificity of a multimarker panel, using carcinoembryonic antigen (CEA), cytokeratin 19 and 20 (CK-19 and CK-20), gastrointestinal tumor-associated antigen 733.2 (GA 733.2), and mucin-1 (muc-1) mRNA markers to detect micrometastases in the frozen sections of sentinel nodes from 22 patients with American Joint Committee on Cancer (AJCC) stages I to IIIA breast cancer (37). CEA, a well-studied tumor marker, has been shown to be elevated during tumor progression and metastatic disease (38). CK-19 and CK-20 are intermediate filament proteins expressed by both normal and malignant mammary cells (39). The muc-1 gene is a mucin gene that is aberrantly glycosylated in breast, ovarian, and lung cancers (40). GA 733.2 is a glycoprotein whose cell surface antigen may have clinical utility in immunotherapy for patients with breast cancer (41). The results were compared to standard H&E staining and immunohistochemistry, which demonstrated that when using a multimarker assay, at least 1 marker was positive in 92% of histologically negative sentinel nodes and in 90% of histologically positive ones. This showed that multimarker mRNA RT-PCR can improve the overall sensitivity of detecting occult metastases.

Hoon and colleagues identified β-hCG mRNA expression as a marker for metastatic breast cancer in frozen sections from lymph nodes obtained from 18 AJCC stage I-III breast cancer patients undergoing elective axillary lymph node dissections (42) (they had previously demonstrated the utility of β-hCG as a molecular marker for melanoma [43]). Ten axillary lymph nodes were shown to be involved with metastatic breast cancer using standard H&E technique. Eleven of 18 lymph nodes examined (61%) expressed β-hCG; in addition, β-hCG mRNA expression was not demonstrated in any of the lymph nodes obtained that were not involved with metastases. Furthermore, 2 of 8 sentinel nodes (25%) that were negative by H&E expressed β-hCG mRNA. This study established the potential clinical utility of this marker in RT-PCR assays to detect occult metastatic breast cancer in lymph nodes. The initial approach in the above studies was RT-PCR with Southern blot analysis, but this was converted to a semi-quantitative electrochemiluminescence assay. More recently, the assay has been converted to qRT. β-hCG has been shown to be a good marker for carcinomas and occult tumor cell detection, but its association with breast cancer development and progression remains undetermined. It is believed to be an oncofetal protein that may provide carcinomas an advantage in survival. The complexity of the protein is that it has multiple family members, of which several are pseudogenes.

## Molecular Analysis of Paraffin-Embedded Tissues

As experience was gained in the histopathologic evaluation of sentinel lymph nodes, it became evident that the analysis was more reliable when using paraffin-embedded archival tissues. In sentinel nodes, tumor cells are usually found peripherally in the subcapsular sinus. A whole cross-section would have to be prepared to make an accurate diagnosis. To prepare these cross-sections, however, valuable tissue for confirming a pathologic diagnosis may be lost. In addition, the quality of RNA extracted from frozen sections is inferior to that of paraffin-embedded archival tissue, as frozen tissues undergo nucleic acid degradation if not processed and stored under optimal conditions. In contrast, paraffin-embedded archival tissue specimens do not require special processing protocols or specific storage conditions, and have been found resistant to nucleic acid degradation. Intraoperative frozen section analyses are cumbersome and problematic for accurate diagnosis, and frozen section preparation varies considerably among institutes in the United States and worldwide, leading to problems in comparing histopathology results from different institutions. This same problem is inherent in molecular analysis of frozen section of sentinel lymph nodes.

In 2003, Kuo et al. demonstrated the utility of a multimarker RT-PCR assay in paraffin-embedded archival tissue of 77 sentinel lymph nodes from patients with melanoma metastases (44). The mRNA expression of 4 melanoma-associated antigen markers—tyrosinase (Tyr), melanoma antigen recognized by T cells-1 (MART-1), and tyrosinase-related protein 1 and 2 (TRP-1, TRP-2)—was determined with RT-PCR and the ECL detection assay, using the IGEN Origen Analyzer (IGEN, Bethesda, MD). Tyrosinase is an enzyme that plays an important role in the early stages of melanogenesis. MART-1 is a melanoma-associated antigen recognized by tumor-infiltrating lymphocytes that are HLA-A2-restricted. TRP-1 and -2 are glycoproteins found on the melanosomal membranes that are recognized by T-cells. This study correlated its findings with the patients' clinical and pathological characteristics, including disease recurrence and overall survival, and had long-term follow-up. Of 40 patients with negative sentinel lymph nodes by H&E and/or immunohistochemistry, 55% demonstrated expression of at least 1 marker, and 25% expressed 2 or more markers. Of the 37 patients with positive sentinel lymph nodes, 95% expressed at least 1 marker, and 86% expressed 2 or more markers. After a median follow-up of 55 months, a significant correlation existed between the expression of markers and melanoma recurrences. Patients with negative sentinel lymph nodes that expressed 2 or more mRNA markers had a significantly decreased disease-free survival. Furthermore, of the patients with tumor-free sentinel lymph nodes who expressed 2 or more markers, 80% developed recurrent disease.

## Techniques and Processing of Sentinel Lymph Nodes for Molecular Studies

In evaluating a sentinel lymph node for histopathology, immunohistochemistry, or for molecular analysis for RT-PCR, an important aspect is correct processing of the specimen after the sentinel node has been fixed briefly in 10% formalin. Since most tumor cells are found along the midplane of the sentinel lymph node, the node is bisected through its length, and representative sections of the whole cross-section are then made and submitted for immunohistochemistry. The remaining node is placed into formalin-fixed cassettes for 48 hours, paraffin embedded, and then serially sectioned into 4 μm sections for H&E, immunohistochemistry, and RT-PCR or DNA studies (Figure 20–1).

Lymph nodes metastases have been divided into those that measure >2 mm or <2 mm. The prognostic significance of the presence of micrometastases (<2 mm) in a lymph node remains a topic of debate; however, micrometastatic diseases are currently part of the TNM classification for breast cancer.

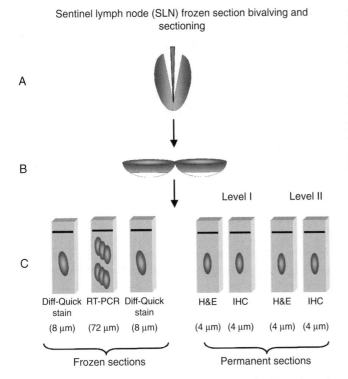

Sentinel lymph node (SLN) frozen section bivalving and sectioning

A

B

Level I    Level II

C

Diff-Quick stain | RT-PCR | Diff-Quick stain | H&E | IHC | H&E | IHC
(8 μm) | (72 μm) | (8 μm) | (4 μm) | (4 μm) | (4 μm) | (4 μm)

Frozen sections          Permanent sections

FIGURE 20-1. Technique of processing the sentinel lymph node for histopathology and molecular studies. (A) Bisect the sentinel lymph node. (B) Section the lymph node. (C) Serial sections for immunohistochemistry, hematoxylin and eosin staining, reverse transcription-polymerase chain reaction studies, and frozen sections.

## Single and Multimarker RT-PCR

Messenger RNA markers are being explored as a potential tool for detecting axillary micrometastases and improving staging in breast cancer patients. Several investigators (40,45,52) have used a single tumor marker to detect occult tumor cells in the sentinel lymph node (Table 20-3).

In 2001, Wascher and colleagues evaluated 121 sentinel nodes obtained from breast cancer patients, where the nodes were examined both by H&E and immunohistochemistry (45). RT-PCR and Southern blot were performed using MAGE-A3, a gene that is commonly expressed in tumors of epithelial origin and which has the capability of inducing cytotoxic T lymphocytes. Fifteen of the 33 positive sentinel lymph nodes expressed MAGE-A3. Of the 88 negative sentinel nodes, 40% were positive for MAGE-A3 expression. In this study, 15 sentinel lymph nodes were upstaged by immunohistochemistry, and 47% of these nodes were positive for MAGE-A3. This study did not correlate expression of MAGE-A3 with recurrence or overall survival.

The expression of a specific tumor-associated mRNA marker has not been shown to have a direct correlation with standard histopathologic techniques. Most single-marker studies lack sensitivity and specificity because of tumor heterogeneity within a population of tumor cells derived from primary tumor or metastases.

However, multiple specific tumor markers improve assay sensitivity and specifically address the issue of tumor heterogeneity among patients, as well as variations in mRNA expression in tumor specimens (46–48). The rationale for multiple markers is that breast tumors consist of a heterogeneous collection of tumor cells, and not all tumor cells express the same level of an individual gene. In addition, the predominant cell type in the tumor or a metastatic focus may not express the specific marker being studied. A tumor may also change genetically in response to adjuvant treatment, further obviating the need for a panel of markers. Studies that have demonstrated significant multimarker expression of tumor-specific mRNA markers in breast cancers are shown in Table 20-4 (37,40,48,50,51,53). Breast cancer is a mixture of many types of histopathology, which makes it difficult to diagnose accurately at early stages where minimal disease is present.

Taback et al. used a study panel of 4 mRNA tumor markers—β-hCG, c-MET, GalNAC-T, and MAGE-A3—that have been studied individually and shown to be expressed in breast cancer (49). Blood from 65 AJCC stage I-IV breast cancer patients and 25 breast tumor specimens were assessed for the 4 mRNA markers. Of

TABLE 20-3. Single mRNA molecular marker studies in sentinel lymph nodes.

| Author, year, reference | Patients | AJCC Stage | Markers | (%) + Patients |
|---|---|---|---|---|
| Mori (1995) (38) | 13 | I–III | CEA | 66% |
| Schoenfeld (1996) (39) | 125 | I–III | CK-19 | 20% |
| Noguchi (1996) (40) | 15 | I–III | Muc-1 | 30% |
| Hoon (1996) (42) | 18 | I–IV | β-hCG | 61% |
| Masuda (2000) (78) | 129 | I–III | CEA | 31% |
| Wascher (2001) (45) | 77 | I–III | MAGE-A3 | 53% |
| Mitas (2002) (52) | 22 | I–IV | PSE | 82% |
| Sakaguchi (2003) (79) | 108 | I–II | CK-19 | 68% |

TABLE 20-4. Multimarker RT-PCR studies in sentinel lymph nodes.

| Author, year, references | Patients | AJCC Stage | Markers | (%) + Patients |
|---|---|---|---|---|
| Noguchi (1996) (40) | 23 | I–III | CK-19, muc-1 | 28% |
| Lockett (1998) (48) | 61 | I–III | CK-19, c-myc, PIP | 40% |
| Bostick (1998) (34) | 57 | I–IIIa | ß1->4, GalNAc-T, c-MET, p97 | 63% |
| Bostick (1998) (37) | 22 | I–IIIa | CEA, CK-19, CK-20, GA 733.2 | 90% |
| Manzotti (2001) (80) | 123 | I–III | maspin, CK-19, CEA, muc-1, mam-1 | 53% |
| Mitas (2001) (51) | 68 | I–IV | mam, mamB, PIP, CEA, CK-19, VEGF, Erbß2, muc-1, c-myc, P97, vim, Ki67 | 79% |
| Zehentner (2002) (53) | 50 | I–III | GABAπ, B305D, B726P | 100% |
| Gillanders (2004) (50) | 489 | I–IIb | CK-19, CEA, muc-1, mam, PIP, PSE | 87% |

the blood samples studied, 69% expressed at least 1 tumor marker, with 20% of the patients expressing 2 or more; GalNAc-T was the more frequently expressed mRNA marker. In addition, 96% of the breast tumors expressed at least 1 marker, and 84% expressed 2. Multimarker combinations were used to determine if correlations existed with known clinical and histopathological factors. Both MAGE-A3 and c-MET mRNA correlated with increasing tumor size and disease stage. The use of c-MET and MAGE-A3 in combination with either ß-hCG or GalNAc-T correlated with advanced stage and increasing tumor size.

Gillanders and colleagues assessed 7 genes in a multimarker panel using qRT analysis of CK-19, CEA, muc-l, mam, mam-B, PIP, and PSE (50). This multi-institutional prospective cohort study included 489 patients with stage I-IIB breast cancer and correlated molecular analysis with clinical outcomes. The 7 genes were selected based on previous studies showing expression of these genes in metastatic breast cancer and not in control lymph nodes (48,51,52). Of the patients enrolled, 145 (30%) had 1 or more positive sentinel lymph nodes, and 344 (70%) had negative sentinel lymph nodes. Of the total, 126 (87%) patients with H&E/immunohistochemistry-positive sentinel nodes expressed a marker, of which mam was the most commonly expressed (114 patients, 90.5%). Using a 2-gene marker panel, mam and CEA were expressed in 123 of the 126 (97%) node-positive patients. Of the 344 node-negative patients, 112 (33%) expressed 1 or more markers, of which mam and CEA were again the most commonly expressed. Analyses correlated marker positivity with known clinical parameters associated with poor outcomes. In the node-negative patients, marker positivity correlated with increasing tumor size, histologic grade, and HER2/neu gene status. The authors hypothesize that marker positivity in node-negative patients will be associated with a higher rate of recurrence at 5 years. This analysis has yet to be completed, but these observations provide evidence that

multimarker studies can be correlated with standard histopathologic techniques, and the findings can help predict patient outcomes.

A multimarker panel consisting of the mam gene, GABAπ, B305D, and B726P was used by Zehentner et al. in a study of 27 tumors and 50 positive sentinel lymph nodes in patients with breast cancer (53). γ-aminobutyrate type A receptor π-subunit GABAπ, B305D, and B726P have been shown to be potential therapeutic targets in breast cancer. Using multigene real-time PCR analysis, all 27 tumor samples expressed all 4 genes when used in a multimarker panel, as compared to 17 of the total specimens with expression of mam in a single marker analysis. Furthermore, all 50 positive lymph nodes showed positive expression signals for all 4 genes, whereas there was no significant expression of these genes in control nodes obtained from patients without cancer.

Mitas et al. assessed 12 genes associated with cancer using a multimarker panel to detect metastatic disease in sentinel lymph nodes obtained from patients with breast cancer (51). RT-PCR was performed to determine the expression levels of mam, PIP, mamB, CEA, CK-19, VEGF, erbB2, muc-1, c-myc, p97, vim, and Ki67 in 17 histopathologically positive nodes and 51 negative nodes. The most diagnostic markers in detecting metastatic disease were mam (99.6%), PIP (93.3%), CK-19 (91.0%), mamB (87.9%), muc-1 (81.5%), and CEA (79.4.0%).

In breast cancer, sentinel lymph node upstaging remains controversial. The major problems have been the reliability of the markers, prognostic significance, specificity/sensitivity issues, standardization, and relevance. With the availability of effective adjuvant treatment for high-risk AJCC stage I, II, and III cancer patients, it is difficult to determine the significance of molecular upstaging over H&E and immunohistochemistry. To date, there is no agreement that immunohistochemistry upstaging of H&E-negative sentinel lymph node carries a greater risk of disease recurrence, so it is no wonder that questions remain over whether molecular upstaging can improve prognosis or be used for patient adjuvant treatment stratification. One critical issue is the development of molecular markers that are predictors of disease outcome, as opposed to just detection of occult tumor cells, and considerable work is still needed in developing breast cancer RT-PCR markers. As debate continues over the relevance of immunohistochemistry in accurately staging minimal disease occurrence in tumor-draining lymph nodes, no doubt molecular staging will also be highly controversial. One major stumbling block is that most laboratories reporting molecular staging of lymph nodes in breast cancer focus on the same markers we have known for the last 10 years, and have not implemented new, more informative ones.

## DNA Molecular Markers

DNA molecular markers are unique in that they are tumor-specific and limited to a single codon. Our laboratory and others have shown circulating tumor DNA in the serum and plasma of patients with various cancers, including breast, melanoma, and gastrointestinal (54–57). Table 20-5 lists most of the DNA tumor markers that have been used to detect occult metastases in sentinel lymph nodes (54,67,69,77); it includes tumor-associated mutations, hypermethylation of CpG islands of promoter regions of tumor suppression genes, loss of heterozygosity of microsatellites, deletions, and amplification. Multiple genetic alterations result in uncontrollable proliferation of epithelial cells, invasion of surrounding tissues, and the ability of cells to escape apoptosis. DNA analysis for mutations, loss of heterozygosity, or hypermethylation has advantages compared to mRNA-based assays, in that DNA is more stable than RNA, and therefore assays are easier to perform technically. In addition, mRNA expression may be variable, due to RNA degradation that can occur during surgical resection and fixa-

tion, making it difficult to quantify objectively in standard RT-PCR assays.

Many studies have demonstrated allelic imbalances, in particular loss of heterozygosity in solid malignancies (58–60). Recent studies have shown that detection of loss of heterozygosity markers at specific chromosome loci correlated with poor outcome in patients with breast cancer (61–63). In addition, loss of heterozygosity and microsatellite instability have been reported to be early events in the growth of the breast tumor and occur with increasing frequency in metastatic disease. Loss of heterozygosity of circulating microsatellite markers—which are highly repetitive, polymorphic sequences of base pairs that occur on chromosomes 3p 25.1, 8p 22, 13q 12, 17p 13.3, and 22q 12—have been associated with breast cancer and correlated with worse prognosis (64–66).

Schwarzenbach et al. performed an analysis of circulating DNA in blood samples collected from 8 patients with primary breast cancer and 26 patients with metastatic disease who had been undergoing chemotherapy (67). Four different microsatellite markers were used—D10S215, D16S421, D17S250, and D17S855, located on chromosomes 10q, 16q, and 17q. Three of the 8 patients (38%) with primary breast cancer and 12 of 26 patients with metastatic disease showed loss of heterozygosity. Of the total patients, 13 (38%) demonstrated loss of heterozygosity in at least 1 of the chromosomal regions, whereas only 2 patients had loss of heterozygosity in 2 or 3 of the regions analyzed. This pattern may identify patients who would benefit from additional therapy.

Taback and colleagues employed a panel of 8 microsatellite markers that had been shown to demonstrate frequent loss of heterozygosity in breast cancer—TP53, D17S5855, D17S849, D16S421, D14S62, D14S51, D10S197, and D8S321, which are located on chromosomes 8, 10, 14, 16, and 17 (68). Blood samples were collected from 30 stage I and 26 stage II patients with breast cancer who underwent breast conservation with lumpectomy and sentinel lymph node biopsy, and from 30 healthy female donors. Of the 56 patients with breast cancer, 12 (21%)

TABLE 20-5. DNA molecular studies of breast cancer patients.

| Author, year, reference | Patients | AJCC Stage | Markers | (%) + Patients |
| --- | --- | --- | --- | --- |
| Gonzalez (1999) (81) | 127 | I–IV | RAD51, RAD52, RAD54, BRCA1, BRCA2 | 32% |
| Silva (1999) (61) | 62 | I–III | D17S85, D17S654, D16S421, TH2, D10S197, D9S161 | 90% |
| Nagahata (2002) (82) | 504 | I–III | 11q23–24, 13q12, 17p13.3, 22q13 | 57% |
| Fackler (2003) (83) | 21 | I–III | RASSF-1A, RAR-ß2, HIN-1, Cyclin D2, TWIST | 89% |
| Taback (2003) (84) | 56 | I–II | D17S489, D14S51, D10S197, D8S321, D4S62, D17S855, D16S421, TP53 | 21% |
| Schwarzenbach (2004) (67) | 34 | I–IV | 10q22–23, 16q22–23, 17q11–12, 17q21 | 34% |
| Shinozaki (2005) (69) | 151 | I–IV | RASSF-1A, APC, TWIST, CDH1, GSTP1, RAR-ß2 | 90% |
| Umetani (2005) (77) | 60 | I–IIIa | ID4 | 67% |

demonstrated loss of heterozygosity of at least 1 micro-satellite marker, with none detected in the remaining patients studied. Stage II patients demonstrated an increase in the presence of circulating microsatellites for loss of heterozygosity when compared to stage I patients (27% vs 17%). Of the 30 controls, none demonstrated loss of heterozygosity for any of the markers assessed. Furthermore, of the 12 patients demonstrating loss of heterozygosity, an analysis was performed to correlate with known histopathologic factors associated with worse outcomes: size, grade, lymphovascular invasion, Bloom-Richardson score, ploidy, DNA index, S phase fraction, MIB-1, HER-2 and p53 protein expression. Ten of the 12 patients had tumors that demonstrated abnormal ploidy, increased DNA index, and MIB-1 overexpression. Loss of heterozygosity analysis of breast cancer tumors can be highly informative and used to predict outcomes, but unfortunately cannot be used to detect occult disease.

# Hypermethylation of CpG Islands of Gene Promoter Regions

Hypermethylation of CpG islands of gene promoter region has become a major focus of current research in molecular oncology. Promoter region CpG islands of specific tumor suppressor genes, where a methylated cytosine 5 is found adjacent to guanine, can contribute to transcriptional silencing resulting in neoplastic development as well as tumor progression. A number of studies have demonstrated the presence of methylated DNA in both the plasma and serum of cancer patients with various malignancies, and not in normal control patients. Hypermethylation of the promoter region of CpG islands has been shown to play a role in the development of breast cancer and tumor progression, and is being used as a predictive marker of disease outcome, as well as response to adjuvant therapy.

Most studies in the literature are descriptive and do not show any correlation with known clinical risk factors. Shinozaki et al. recently reported on promoter hyper-methylation of 6 tumor-related genes that play a role in the progression of early-stage breast cancer: RASSF-1A, APC, TWIST, CDH1, GSTP1, and RAR-β2 (69). Ras-association domain family-1, isoform A gene (RASSF-1A) has been shown to be transcriptionally silenced and frequently hypermethylated in many cancers. It inhibits tumor growth and plays an important role in apoptosis, stabilization of microtubules, and cell-cycle regulation (70). Adenomatous polyposis coli (APC) tumor suppressor gene promotes β-catenin degradation, which is important in the Wnt signal transduction pathway, and has been shown to play a role in carcinogenesis (71). TWIST is a transcription factor that contains a helix-

TABLE 20-6. Methylation status of primary breast tumors and paired sentinel lymph nodes.

| Methylated gene | Primary tumor | Sentinel node |
|---|---|---|
| CDH1 | 53% | 90% |
| RASSF-1A | 81% | 59% |
| RAR-β2 | 24% | 48% |
| APC | 49% | 34% |
| TWIST | 48% | 28% |
| GSTP1 | 21% | 24% |

Source: Data from Shinonzaki M. et al. (69).

loop-helix DNA binding domain and has been shown to regulate the expression of N-cadherin, which is important in tumor cell motility and migration (72). CDH1 is the human E-cadherin gene, which is a key molecule for cellular adhesion and plays a role in cellular differentiation and maintaining architecture in epithelial tissue (73). Glutathione-S-transferase π gene-1 (GSTP-1) protects cells from damage mediated by oxidative stress (74). Retinoic acid receptor-β2 (RAR-β2) is a tumor suppressor gene, and has a part in inhibition of tumor cell growth and apoptosis (75).

DNA extraction and methylation-specific PCR was performed on paraffin-embedded archival tissues from primary tumors of 151 patients who underwent sentinel node biopsy, as well as sentinel lymph nodes from 29 of these patients with nodal metastases. Of the 151 primary tumors, 147 demonstrated promoter region hypermethylation of at least 1 of the 6 genes studied. The frequency of CpG hypermethylation of the 6 genes in the primary tumor and the matched sentinel nodes is shown in Table 20-6. Normal breast tissue specimens from 10 patients showed no evidence of promoter hypermethylation of any of the 6 genes studied. The gene hypermethylation status of each of the 147 hypermethylated tumor specimens was assessed with known prognostic factors to determine if there was any predictive correlation. GSTP1 and RAR-β2 were associated with lymph node metastases and HER-2 receptor positive tumors. Both were also frequently seen in primary tumors that had micrometastases to the sentinel lymph nodes (56% of patients). CDH1 hypermethylation was associated with tumors that were estrogen receptor-negative and with lymphovascular invasion. This study correlating hypermethylation profiling in breast cancer and association with metastases to the lymph nodes may have potential utility in predicting regional metastasis and recurrences in patients with positive sentinel nodes, and thus could help clinicians decide which patients would benefit from a completion axillary lymph node dissection or adjuvant therapy.

The inhibitors of DNA binding (ID) family proteins are members of the helix-loop-helix protein family and have a part in angiogenesis. ID4 gene is involved in growth and cellular differentiation of tumor cells, and in inhibition of DNA binding of transcription factors that contain a basic helix-loop-helix motif, and has been reported to play a role in the progression of advanced-stage breast cancer (76). Umetani et al. assessed the role of ID4 hypermethylation using methylation-specific PCR in primary tumors as well as regional nodes of patients with T1 breast cancers (77). ID4 hypermethylation was observed in 16 of 24 (67%) node-positive breast cancers, 7 of 36 (19%) node-negative tumors, and 2 of 11 (8%) normal control tissue specimens. Hypermethylation of ID4 was significantly higher in tumors from node-positive patients when compared to normal tissue.

Univariate analysis for lymph node metastasis was performed using known clinicopathological risk factors and ID4 methylation status. These studies confirmed that ID4 hypermethylation was a significant risk factor for nodal metastases (odds ratio 8.29, $p < 0.0005$). In addition, lymphovascular invasion and HER2/neu status also correlated with lymph node metastasis (odds ratio 3.62, 3.67, and $p < 0.067$, $p < 0.097$, respectively). On multivariate analysis, only ID4 methylation status significantly correlated with lymph node metastases. Real-time RT-PCR was performed to determine if ID4 mRNA levels would decrease by hypermethylation. Significantly lower mRNA levels of ID4 were seen in hypermethylated than in unmethylated tumors.

## Conclusion

Over the last two decades, we have seen an evolution in the management of breast cancer with surgical procedures becoming increasingly less invasive, improvements in diagnostic imaging, and new adjuvant regimens. The application of molecular technology in the diagnosis of cancer, monitoring a patient's response to therapy, and disease surveillance needs to be established. The risk of recurrence in breast cancer patients is considerable enough to recommend adjuvant therapy for many women, and developing new molecular staging is key to helping identify which patients are at high risk and would benefit from systemic therapy

The potential of both RNA and DNA markers as surrogate markers of disease and disease progression is slowly being realized. However, the markers presently being studied are not ideal, as they lack sensitivity and specificity, and this causes many to be eliminated as a useful tool in the clinical arena. Most single markers are not unique to a specific disease, due to tumor heterogeneity of most cancers. In addition, they are not optimal, in that most detect disease after it has occurred and progressed to advanced stages, resulting in poor outcomes. Markers that can detect cancer at an early stage

of development, or even prior to the onset of disease, need to be identified. A panel of biomarkers may be a better approach as a screening assay for early detection.

Newer molecular techniques to detect cancer-specific alteration in DNA, RNA, and proteins are being developed, including DNA- and RNA-based microarrays. cDNA microarray-based studies correlating tumor characteristics to disease outcome are being performed. Relating gene expression patterns of a specific subset of tumors to specific clinical characteristics, such as resistance to chemotherapy and metastatic potential, is an important issue. These new techniques may uncover biomarkers that have the sensitivity and specificity to be useful in early detection of disease, as well as the ability to differentiate cancer cells from non-cancer cells.

The molecular detection assays using paraffin-embedded archival tissues of sentinel lymph nodes offer a promising future in staging lymph nodes and will improve management of patient care. Molecular detection assays—be it for the primary tumor, metastases, lymph nodes, blood, or bone marrow—will be an invaluable tool for clinicians to individualize treatment protocols for patients. The future of molecular staging of tumors or tumor-draining lymph nodes holds promise, if prospective multicenter trials demonstrate the clinical utility of these markers.

## References

1. Jemal A. Siegel R, Ward E, et al. Cancer statistics. *CA Cancer J Clin*. 2006;56:106–130.
2. Beenken SW, Urist MM, Zhang Y, et al. Axillary lymph node status, but not tumor size predicts locoregional recurrence and overall survival after mastectomy for breast cancer. *Ann Surg*. 2003;237:732–738.
3. Kurtz JM, Kinkel K. Breast conservation in the 21st century. *Eur J Cancer*. 2000;36:1919–1924.
4. Huston TL, Simmons RM. Locally recurrent breast cancer after conservation therapy. *Am J Surg*. 2005;189:229–235.
5. Fortin A, Larochelle M, Laverdiere J, et al. Local failure is responsible for the decrease in survival for patients with breast cancer treated with conservative surgery and postoperative radiotherapy. *J Clin Oncol*. 1999;17:101–109.
6. Schijven MP, Vingerhoets AJ, Rutten HJ, et al. Comparison of morbidity between axillary lymph node dissection and sentinel node biopsy. *Eur J Surg Oncol*. 2003;29:341–350.
7. Swenson KK, Nissen MJ, Ceronsky C, et al. Comparison of side effects between sentinel lymph node and axillary lymph node dissection for breast cancer. *Ann Surg Oncol*. 2002;9:745–753.
8. Burak WE, Hollenbeck ST, Zervos EE, et al. Sentinel lymph node biopsy results in less postoperative morbidity compared with axillary lymph node dissection for breast cancer. *Am J Surg*. 2002;183:23–27.

9. Cabanas RM. An approach to the treatment of penile carcinoma. *Cancer.* 1977;39:456–466.

10. Giuliano AE, Kirgan DM, Guenther JM, Morton DL. Lymphatic mapping and sentinel lymphadenectomy for breast cancer. *Ann Surg.* 1994;220:391–398.

11. Veronesi U, Paganelli G, Viale G, et al. A randomized comparison of sentinel node biopsy with routine axillary dissection in breast cancer. *N Engl J Med.* 2003;349:546–553.

12. McMasters KM, Tuttle TM, Carlson DJ, et al. Sentinel lymph node biopsy for breast cancer: a suitable alternative to routine axillary dissection in multi-institutional practice when optimal technique is used. *J Clin Oncol.* 2000; 18(13):2560–2566.

13. Krag D, Weaver D, Ashikaga T, et al. The sentinel node in breast cancer: a multicenter validation study. *N Engl J Med.* 1998;339:941–946.

14. Gershenwald JE, Colome MI, Lee JE, et al. Patterns of recurrence following a negative sentinel lymph biopsy in 243 patients with stage I or II melanoma. *J Clin Oncol.* 1998;16:2253–2260.

15. Turner RR, Giuliano AE, Hoon DS, et al. Pathologic examination of sentinel lymph node for breast carcinoma. *World J Surg.* 2001;25:798–805.

16. Kammula US, Ghossein R, Bhattacharya S, Coit DG. Serial follow-up and the prognostic significance of reverse transcriptase-polymerase chain reaction-staged sentinel lymph nodes from melanoma patients. *J Clin Oncol.* 2004;22:3989–3996.

17. Palmieri G, Ascierto PA, Cossu A, et al. Detection of occult melanoma cells in paraffin embedded histologically negative sentinel lymph nodes using a reverse transcriptase polymerase chain reaction assay. *J Clin Oncol.* 2001;19:1437–1443.

18. Shivers SC, Wang X, Li W, et al. Molecular staging of malignant melanoma: correlation with clinical outcome. *JAMA.* 1998;280:1410–1415.

19. Hoon DS, Wang Y, Dale PS, et al. Detection of occult melanoma cells in blood with multiple marker polymerase chain reaction assay. *J Clin Oncol.* 1995;13(8):2109–2116.

20. Miyashiro I, Kuo C, Huynh K, et al. Molecular strategy for detecting metastatic cancers with use of multiple tumor-specific MAGE-A genes. *Clinical Chem.* 2001;47: 505–512.

21. Slade MJ, Smith BM, Sinnett HD, Cross NC, Coombes RC. Quantitative polymerase chain reaction for the detection of micrometastases in patients with breast cancer. *J Clin Oncol.* 1999;17:870–879. [Erratum: *J Clin Oncol.* 1999;17:1330].

22. Sarantou T, Chi DD, Garrison DA, et al. Melanoma associated antigens as messenger RNA detection markers for melanoma. *Cancer Res.* 1997;57:1371–1376.

23. Palmieri G, Strazzullo M, Ascierto PA, et al. Polymerase chain reaction-based detection of circulating melanoma cells as an effective marker of tumor progression: Melanoma Cooperative Group. *J Clin Oncol.* 1999;17:304–311.

24. Yamaguchi K, Takagi Y, Aoki S, Futamara M, Saji S. Significant detection of circulating cancer cells in the blood by reverse transcriptase-polymerase chain reaction during colorectal cancer resection. *Ann Surg.* 2000;232:58–65.

25. O'Connell CD, Juhasz A, Kuo C, et al. Detection of tyrosinase mRNA in melanoma by reverse transcription-PCR and electrochemiluminescence. *Clin Chem.* 1998;44:1161–1169.

26. Ioachim E, Kamina S, Athanassiadou S, et al. The prognostic significance of epidermal growth factor receptor (EGFR), C-erbß-2, Ki-67 and PCNA expression in breast cancer. *Anticancer Res.* 1996;16:3141–3147.

27. Manzotti M, Dell'Orto P, Maisonneuve P, et al. Reverse transcription-polymerase chain reaction assay for multiple mRNA markers in the detection of breast cancer metastases in sentinel lymph nodes. *Int J Cancer.* 2001;95:307–312.

28. Sakaguchi M, Virmani A, Dudak MW, et al. Clinical relevance of reverse transcriptase-polymerase chain reaction for the detection of axillary lymph node metastases in breast cancer. *Ann Surg Oncol.* 2003;10:117–125.

29. Takeuchi H, Kuo C, Morton DL, et al. Expression of differentiation melanoma-associated antigen gene is associated with favorable disease outcome in advanced-stage melanomas. *Cancer Res.* 2003;15:441–448.

30. Bilchik A, Miyashiro M, Kelley M, et al. Molecular detection of metastatic pancreatic carcinoma cells using a multimarker reverse transcriptase-polymerase chain reaction assay. *Cancer.* 2000;88:1037–1044.

31. Takeuchi H, Morton DL, Kuo C, et al. Prognostic significance of molecular upstaging of paraffin-embedded sentinel lymph nodes in melanoma patients. *J Clin Oncol.* 2004;22:2671–2680.

32. Morton DL, Wen DR, Wong JH, et al. Technical details of intraoperative lymphatic mapping for early stage melanoma. *Arch Surg.* 1992;127:392–399.

33. Cochran AJ, Wen DR, Morton DL. Occult tumor cells in the lymph nodes of patients with pathological stage I malignant melanoma. An immunohistological study. *Am J Surg Pathol.* 1988;12:612–618.

34. Bostick PJ, Huynh KT, Sarantou T, et al. Detection of metastases in sentinel lymph nodes of breast cancer patients by multiple-marker RT-PCR. *Int J Cancer.* 1998; 79:645–651.

35. Sarantou T, Chi DD, Garrison DA, et al. Melanoma-associated antigens as messenger RNA detection markers for melanoma. *Cancer Res.* 1997;57:1371–1376.

36. Bilchik AJ, Nora DT, Saha S, et al. The use of molecular profiling of early colorectal cancer to predict micrometastases. *Arch Surg.* 2002;137:1377–1383.

37. Bostick PJ, Chatterjee S, Chi D, et al. Limitations of specific reverse-transcriptase polymerase chain reaction markers in the detection of metastases in the lymph nodes and blood of breast cancer patients. *J Clin Oncol.* 1998;16: 2632–2640.

38. Mori M, Mimori K, Inoue H, et al. Detection of cancer micrometastases in lymph nodes by reverse-transcriptase-polymerase chain reaction. *Cancer Res.* 1995;55:3417–3420.

39. Schoenfeld A, Luqmani Y, Sinnett HD, Shousha S, Coombes RC. Keratin 19 mRNA measurement to detect micrometastases in lymph nodes in breast cancer patients. *Br J Cancer.* 1996;74:1639–1642.

40. Noguchi S, Aihara T, Motomura K, et al. Detection of breast cancer micrometastases in axillary lymph nodes by means of reverse transcriptase polymerase chain reaction. Comparison between MUC1 mRNA and keratin 19 mRNA amplification. *Am J Pathol.* 1996;148:649–656.

41. Linnenbach AJ, Wojcierowski J, Wu SA, et al. Sequence investigation of the major gastrointestinal tumor-associated antigen gene family GA733. *Proc Natl Acad Sci USA.* 1989;86:27–31.

42. Hoon DS, Sarantou T, Doi F, et al. Detection of metastatic breast cancer by beta-hCG polymerase chain reaction. *Int J Cancer.* 1996;69:369–374.

43. Doi F, Chi DD, Charuworn BB, et al. Detection of beta-human chorionic gonadotropin mRNA as a marker for cutaneous malignant melanoma. *Int J Cancer.* 1996;65: 454–459.

44. Kuo CT, Hoon DS, Takeuchi H, et al. Prediction of disease outcome in melanoma patients by molecular analysis of paraffin-embedded sentinel lymph nodes. *J Clin Oncol.* 2003;21:3566–3572.

45. Wascher RA, Bostick PJ, Huynh KT, et al. Detection of MAGE-A3 in breast cancer patients' sentinel lymph nodes. *Br J Cancer.* 2001;85:1340–1346.

46. Hoon DS, Bostick PJ, Kuo C, et al. Molecular markers in blood as surrogate prognostic indicators of melanoma recurrence. *Cancer Res.* 2000;60:2253–2257.

47. Baker MK, Mikhitarian K, Osta W, et al. Molecular detection of breast cancer cells in the peripheral blood of advanced-stage breast cancer patients using multi-marker real-time reverse transcription-polymerase chain reaction and a novel porous barrier density gradient centrifugation technology. *Clin Cancer Res.* 2003;9:4865–4871.

48. Lockett MA, Baron PL, O'Brien PH. Detection of occult breast cancer micrometastases in axillary lymph nodes using a multimarker reverse transcriptase-polymerase chain reaction panel. *J Am Coll Surg.* 1998;187:9–16.

49. Taback B, Chan AD, Kuo CT, et al. Detection of occult metastatic breast cancer cells in blood by a multimolecular marker assay: correlation with clinical stage of disease. *Cancer Res.* 2001;61:8845–8850.

50. Gillanders WE, Mikhitarian K, Hebert R, et al. Molecular detection of micrometastatic breast cancer in histopathology-negative axillary lymph nodes correlates with traditional predictors of prognosis: an interim analysis of a prospective multi-institutional cohort study. *Ann Surg.* 2004;239:828–837.

51. Mitas M, Mikhitarian K, Walters C, et al. Quantitative real-time RT-PCR detection of breast cancer micrometastasis using a multigene marker panel. *Int J Cancer.* 2001;93:162–171.

52. Mitas M, Mikhitarian K, Hoover L, et al. Prostate-specific ets (PSE) factor: a novel marker for detection of metastatic breast cancer in axillary lymph nodes. *Br J Cancer.* 2002;86:899–904.

53. Zehentner BK, Dillon DC, Jiang Y, et al. Application of a multigene reverse transcription-PCR assay for detection of mammaglobin and complementary transcribed genes in breast cancer lymph nodes. *Clin Chem.* 2002;48:1225–1231.

54. Silva JM, Dominguez G, Garcia JM, et al. Presence of tumor DNA in plasma of breast cancer patients: clinicopathological correlations. *Cancer Res.* 1999;59:3251–3256.

55. Taback B, O'Day SJ, Hoon DS. Quantification of circulating DNA in the plasma and serum of cancer patients. *Ann N Y Acad Sci.* 2004;1022:17–24.

56. Shapiro B, Chakrabarty M, Cohn EM, et al. Determination of circulating DNA levels in patients with benign or malignant gastrointestinal diseases. *Cancer.* 1983;51:2116–2129.

57. Anker P, Mulcahy H, Chen XQ, Stroun M. Detection of circulating tumor DNA in the blood (plasma/serum) of cancer patients. *Cancer Metastasis Rev.* 1999;18:65–73.

58. Taback B, Fujiwara Y, Wang H, et al. Prognostic significance of circulating microsatellite markers in the plasma of melanoma patients. *Cancer Res.* 2001;61:5723–5726.

59. Hibi K, Robinson CR, Booker S, et al. Molecular detection of genetic alterations in the serum of colorectal cancer patients. *Cancer Res.* 1998;5:1405–1407.

60. Nawroz H, Koch W, Anker P, Stroun M, Sidransky D. Microsatellite alterations in serum DNA of head and neck cancer patients. *Nat Med.* 1996;2:1035–1037.

61. Silva JM, Garica JM, Gonzalez R, et al. Abnormal frequencies of alleles in polymorphic markers of the 17q21 region is associated with breast cancer. *Cancer Lett.* 1999;138:209–215.

62. Hampl M, Hampl JA, Reiss G, et al. Loss of heterozygosity accumulation in primary breast carcinomas and additionally in corresponding distant metastases is associated with poor outcome. *Clin Cancer Res.* 1999;5:1417–1425.

63. Driouch K, Dorion-Bonnet F, Briffod M, et al. Loss of heterozygosity on chromosome arm 16q in breast cancer metastases. *Genes Chromosomes Cancer.* 1997;19:185–191.

64. Emi M, Yoshimoto M, Sato T, et al. Allelic loss at 1p34, 13q12, 17p13.3 and 17q21.1 correlate with poor post-operative prognosis in breast cancer. *Genes Chromosomes Cancer.* 1999;26:134–141.

65. Hirano A, Emi M, Tsuneizumi M, et al. Allelic losses of loci at 3p25.1, 8p22, 13q12, 17p13.3 and 22q13 correlate with post-operative recurrences in breast cancer. *Clin Cancer Res.* 2001;7:876–882.

66. Takita K, Sato T, Miyagi M, et al. Correlation of loss of alleles on the short arms of chromosomes 11 and 17 with metastasis of primary breast cancer to lymph nodes. *Cancer Res.* 1992;52:3914–3917.

67. Schwarzenbach H, Muller V, Stahmann N, Pantel K. Detection and characterization of circulating microsatellite-DNA in blood of patients with breast cancer. *Ann N Y Acad Sci.* 2004;1022:25–32.

68. Taback B, Giuliano AE, Hansen NM, Hoon DS. Microsatellite alterations detected in the serum of early stage breast cancer patients. *Ann N Y Acad Sci.* 2001;945:22–30.

69. Shinozaki M, Hoon DS, Giuliano AE, et al. Distinct hypermethylation profile of primary breast cancer is associated with sentinel lymph node metastasis. *Clin Cancer Res.* 2005;11:2156–2162.

70. Agathanggelou A, Cooper WN, Latif F. Role of the Ras-association domain family 1 tumor suppressor gene in human cancers. *Cancer Res.* 2005;65:3497–3508.

71. Schlosshauer PW, Brown SA, Eisinger K, et al. APC truncation and increased beta-catenin levels in a human breast cancer cell line. *Carcinogenesis.* 2000;21:1453–1456.

72. Martin TA, Goyal A, Watkins G, Jiang WG. Expression of the transcription factors snail, slug, twist and their clinical significance in human breast cancer. *Ann Surg Oncol.* 2005;12:488–496.

73. Koizume S, Tachibana K, Sekiya T, Hirohashi S, Shiraishi M. Heterogeneity in the modification and involvement of chromatin components of the CpG island of the silenced human CDH1 gene in cancer cells. *Nucleic Acids Res.* 2002;30:4770–4780.

74. Zhong S, Tang MW, Yeo W, et al. Silencing of GSTP1 gene by CpG island DNA hypermethylation in HBV-associated hepatocellular carcinomas. *Clin Cancer Res.* 2002;8:1087–1092.

75. Houle B, Rochette-Egly C, Bradley WE. Tumor-suppressive effect of the retinoic acid receptor beta in human epidermoid lung cancer cells. *Proc Natl Acad Sci USA.* 1993;90:985–989.

76. Desprez PY, Sumida T, Coppe JP. Helix-loop-helix proteins in mammary gland development and breast cancer. *J Mammary Gland Biol Neoplasia.* 2003;8:225–239.

77. Umetani N, Mori T, Koynagi K, et al. Aberrant hypermethylation of ID4 gene promoter region increases risk of lymph node metastasis in T1 breast cancer. *Oncogene.* 2005;24:4721–4727.

78. Masuda N, Tamaki Y, Sakita I, et al. Clinical significance of micrometastases in axillary lymph nodes assessed by reverse transcription-polymerase chain reaction in breast cancer patients. *Clin Cancer Res.* 2000;6:4176–4185.

79. Sakaguchi M, Virmani A, Dudak MW, et al. Clinical relevance of reverse transcriptase-polymerase chain reaction for the detection of axillary lymph node metastases in breast cancer. *Ann Surg Oncol.* 2003;10:117–125.

80. Manzotti M, Dell'Orto P, Maisonneuve P, et al. Reverse transcription-polymerase chain reaction assay for multiple mRNA markers in the detection of breast cancer metastases in sentinel lymph nodes. *Int J Cancer.* 2001;95:307–312.

81. Gonzalez R, Silva JM, Dominguez G, et al. Detection of loss of heterozygosity at RAD51, RAD52, RAD54 and BRCA1 and BRCA2 loci in breast cancer: pathological correlations. *Br J Cancer.* 1999;81:503–509.

82. Nagahata T, Hirano A, Utada Y, et al. Correlation of allelic losses and clinicopathological factors in 504 primary breast cancers. *Breast Cancer.* 2002;9:208–215.

83. Fackler MJ, McVeigh M, Evron E, et al. DNA methylation of RASSF1A, HIN-1, RAR-beta, Cyclin D2 and Twist in in situ and invasive lobular breast carcinoma. *Int J Cancer.* 2003;107:970–975.

84. Taback B, Giuliano AE, Hansen NM, et al. Detection of tumor-specific genetic alterations in bone marrow from early-stage breast cancer patients. *Cancer Res.* 2003;63:1884–1887.

# Part III
## Occult Lesion Localization

# 21
# Where It All Began: The Heritage of Radioimmunoguided Surgery

Fausto Badellino, Mario Roselli, Marzio Perri, Fiorella Guadagni, and Giuliano Mariani

*Nowadays some monoclonal antibodies are available that, as magic bullets, are able to reach malignant cells growing in the body and, if carrying appropriate antineoplastic agents, can provide their destruction while sparing normal healthy tissues.*

—Renato Dulbecco, Nobel Laureate for
Physiology and Medicine, 1975

In the mid-1970s, crucial advances in immunology led to widespread fascination with the development of radiolabeled antibodies for immunoscintigraphy of primary or secondary tumors. The availability of these radiolabeled tumor-seeking agents constituted the first step toward radioimmunoguided surgery, as pioneered by Martin et al. (1,2) in patients with colorectal cancer. This chapter provides an overview of the evolution of the radioimmunoguided surgery system, explains its main technical aspects, and outlines its clinical applications.

Intraoperative detection of cancer by means of tumor-specific radiolabeled antibodies evolved from seminal experiments in the early 1970s, which demonstrated the ability of radiolabeled immunoglobulin G against carcinoembryonic antigen (CEA) to localize human GW-39 tumors implanted in hamsters (3,4). After Kohler and Milstein described a method of preparing large numbers of specific monoclonal antibodies (MABs) in 1975 (5), the technique was optimized and, in the beginning of the 1980s, the B72.3 MAB was generated by using membrane-enriched extracts of human metastatic mammary carcinoma lesions (6). The reactivity of this MAB with formalin-fixed, paraffin-embedded tissue sections of human colon adenocarcinomas and adenomas was especially promising (7). The tumor-associated glycoprotein recognized by the B72.3 MAB (TAG-72) is a member of the mucin family.

Shortly thereafter, some research groups began exploring the diagnostic potential of radioimmunodetection, a new technique that combined the administration of radiolabeled antibodies with external imaging to identify clinically occult tumors (8,9). Other groups examined the potential of intraoperative radioactivity counting to detect the uptake of radiolabeled MABs by malignant cells. These latter experiences led to the development of a dedicated handheld gamma-detecting probe for intraoperative use, which improved the sensitivity of external radioimmunodetection (10,11). The first prototypes were tested in 1983–1984 by Martin's group (1,12) at the Comprehensive Cancer Center of the Ohio State University in Columbus. In a pilot clinical study with radiolabeled MAB B72.3 in patients with recurrent colorectal cancer, intraoperative use of the gamma probe localized the tumor-bound antibody in 82% of the patients and detected a clinically occult tumor in 8 of 31 patients (13).

In the following years, the same investigators employed MAB B72.3 in 66 patients with different malignant tumors (2). The gamma probe identified positive counts in 5 of 6 patients with primary colon cancer (83.3%), in 31 of 39 patients with recurrent colon cancer (79.5%), in 4 of 5 patients with gastric cancer (80%), in 3 of 8 patients with breast cancer (37.5%), and in 4 of 8 patients with ovarian cancer (50%). Overall, radioimmunoguided surgery identified tumor lesions in 47 patients (71.2%), was equivocal-positive in 6 patients (9.1%), and failed to detect an occult tumor in 13 (19.7%). By placing the gamma probe directly over the areas of interest, radioimmunoguided surgery had the advantage of minimizing the influence of the inverse-square law on the counting rate for any given radioactive source. Radioimmunoguided surgery allowed accurate clinical assessment of the surgical area before and after treatment, and identified residual disease in a significant number of cases.

In the early 1990s, the development of second-generation MABs specifically for colon cancer led to further improvements in radioimmunoguided surgery for patients with this malignancy. These MABs were characterized by in-vitro immunological assays (14), and 6 of them (CC11, CC30, CC46, CC49, CC83, and CC92) were chosen for in-vivo tumor targeting in a murine model of human colon carcinoma (LS-174T; xenografts in athymic mice) (15). All 6 of these MABs were distinct from B72.3 and from each other by reciprocal competition radioimmunoassays, and all had a higher affinity than B72.3 by either in-vitro assays or in-vivo binding patterns and pharmacokinetics. In addition, they were superior to B72.3 in terms of both the percentage of injected dose delivered per gram of tumor and the tumor-to-normal tissue ratio (15).

Subsequent pilot clinical studies with CC49 revealed efficient tumor localization in 86% of patients with primary colorectal cancer and 97% of patients with recurrent disease (16). In several cases, intraoperative use of the gamma probe with CC49 led to modification of the planned operative procedure, impacting decision making (17). These encouraging findings indicated that the application of radioimmunoguided surgery in patients with primary or recurrent colorectal cancer might yield clinically relevant information regarding the pattern of disease, thus challenging the adequacy of the traditional procedure alone. In a debate published in *Oncology*, the ability of radioimmunoguided surgery to identify a large fraction of colorectal cancers with clinically occult micrometastases was emphasized (18). Moreover, it was outlined that the cumulative data obtained with use of the B72.3 and CC49 MABs proved that this approach was effective in improving both intraoperative surgical decision making and the ability of the surgeon to perform surgical resection at a quasi-microscopic level. They agreed that, at that time, the most relevant clinical and experimental applications of the radioimmunoguided surgery technology were: 1) to aid in intraoperative staging and assist in surgical decision making in patients with primary and recurrent colorectal cancer, 2) to analyse intraabdominal patterns of spread of colorectal cancer and to assess the natural history of clinically occult micrometastases, 3) to localize lymph nodes that contain micrometastatic tumor and/or show tumor antigen, and 4) for an immunologic analysis of host response to microscopic tumor (18). The authors concluded by noting that "in the last years, since the recent diagnostic and surgical improvement, the outcomes are unchanged. Probably the discovering of micrometastasis in lymph nodes will change the clinical results. However, large prospective randomized trials, further improvement in imaging procedures and new targeting molecules are required."

The problems concerning the antigen-antibody binding for radioimmunoguided surgery in the oncologic setting were extensively discussed during a 1992 conference on radioimmunological diagnosis and therapy for cancer (19). Radioimmunoguided surgery was originally carried out using affinity-purified monospecific polyclonal antibodies. Since then, technical advances have improved the quality of immunoreagents and allowed development of MABs and antibody fragments specific for tumor-associated antigens. In general, the "ideal" antibody for tumor radioimmunodetection purposes should exhibit both high affinity and high avidity for antigens expressed in high density only on tumor cells.

Tumor cell heterogeneity is an important consideration when designing clinical protocols using MABs, either for immunodetection or for immunotherapy. One potential approach to circumvent the limitations of these heterogeneous expressions is to identify compounds able to alter cellular differentiation, which also includes changes in surface antigen expression, i.e., biological response modifiers such as interferons. Preclinical studies using human colon carcinoma (HT-29) xenografts in athymic mice as a targeting model demonstrated that the ability of interferon-gamma to enhance TAG-72 expression substantially augmented the antitumor effects of $^{131}$I-CC49 (20). Additional evidence for the use of a radioimmunoconjugate in combination with a cytokine to improve tumor diagnosis and/or therapy derives from clinical studies showing that systemic interferon alpha-2a administration can upregulate TAG-72 and CEA expression at distal tumor sites (21,22). Other implementations introduced to further improve the effectiveness of radioimmunoguided surgery for detecting tumor cells include application of the avidin-biotin system (injection of a non-radiolabeled, biotinylated antibody followed by administration of radiolabeled avidin) (23–25).

One major problem with the therapeutic use of radiolabeled MABs is that the radiolabeled MAB not bound to the tumor remains in the circulation with a half-life of several days, resulting in potential bone marrow toxicity. Thus, a MAB form that clears the blood pool more rapidly would be advantageous. Another concern with the use of large molecules, such as immunoglobulins, as therapeutic agents is their inability to penetrate large tumor masses; a smaller MAB form would be expected to exhibit better penetration. Furthermore, for intraoperative gamma detection the introduction of antibody fragments with shorter biologic half-lives and advances in radiolabeling methods have enabled use of not only halogen radionuclides (such as $^{125}$I, $^{131}$I and $^{123}$I) but also metallic radionuclides (such as $^{111}$In, $^{99m}$Tc, and $^{201}$Tl). In addition, F(ab')$_2$ fragments have been used in radioimmunoguided surgery procedures (26). However, it is often difficult to generate these immunoglobulin forms in a manner that retains their immunoreactivity in vivo. Technologic advances involving the cloning of immunoglobulin genes, the generation of recombinant/chimeric immunoglobulin genes, and their expression in a variety of systems have led to a wide variety of new molecules, including chimeric and humanized antibodies (27), single-chain antigen-binding proteins, and VH-domain and hypervariable-region peptide molecules

(28). The development of these genetically engineered agents allows alterations in immunoglobulin (Ig) domains or glycosylation sites, so that the MAB clears the body faster. Genetic techniques also are being used to insert more efficient binding sites for radionuclide chelate complexes or effector cells; to change immunoglobulin isotypes, e.g., from $IgG_1$ to $IgG_2$; and to alter affinity by modifying the hinge region or the antigen binding region. Antibody fragments with changed or deleted constant regions are less likely to elicit an anti-globulin antibody response (which usually targets the Fc portion). Finally, the development of chimeric MABs and modified constructs should allow repeated administration, making them potentially valuable for radioimmunoimaging follow-up and radioimmunotherapeutic clinical trials.

Since its introduction almost 30 years ago, tumor targeting based on radiolabeled MABs has been tested in nearly 1,400 clinical trials. Most of these trials have focused on patients with colorectal cancer, but radioimmunoguided surgery has also been used for presurgical staging and surgical detection of breast, ovarian, prostatic, and neuroendocrine tumors. Regardless of the type of solid tumor, the success of radioimmunoguided surgery depends on a synergistic combination of the radiopharmaceutical agent, the MAB, the gamma-detecting probe, and the skill of the surgeon. As in other instances where different components of a certain procedure are synergistic, the basic concept of radioimmunoguided surgery is that the whole (global procedure) results in greater performance than the arithmetic sum of its parts does.

Risks related to the injection of anti-TAG antibodies labeled with [125]I or other clinically suitable radionuclides are minimal, and radiation exposure received by personnel in the operating room and the pathology lab is low. The environmental hazard is extremely low or nonexistent (see chapter 5).

In the clinical setting, the guiding principles of radioimmunoguided surgery are the reduction of morbidity and mortality, the amelioration of suffering, and the improvement of quality of life. These principles were the basis of radioimmunoguided surgery clinical research at the Comprehensive Cancer Center of the Ohio State University. The objectives of the first clinical studies were to promote the concept of radioimmunoguided surgery, to clarify pre-enrollment issues (including preoperative evaluation), and to record all intraoperative and pathological data. The investigators were fascinated by the possibility of a new biological staging system, and, in a second phase, locating tumor-reactive cells for adoptive cellular therapy. Over time, radioimmunoguided surgery was extended to growing numbers of patients, and postoperative follow-up was prolonged.

In a study published in 1995, Bertsch et al. (29) reexamined the outcome of radioimmunoguided surgery in 131 patients with recurrent colorectal cancer, who had previously been enrolled in 2 prospective nonrandomized studies. Eighty-six patients had been injected with the B72.3 MAB, and 45 with CC49. Of the 49 patients who underwent resection with curative intent, 55% were alive 2 to 8 years after surgery. By contrast, the overall survival rate was only 2% among patients who underwent palliative surgery. There were no survivors among the 18 patients whose cancers were judged to be resectable based on traditional intraoperative inspection but subsequently found to be unresectable based on radioimmunoguided surgery criteria. These findings confirm the role of radioimmunoguided surgery as a useful intraoperative tool capable of improving the selection of colorectal cancer patients for curative resection.

In January of the same year, Neoprobe Corporation (Dublin, Ohio), manufacturer of the first gamma detector, organized a training and educational program on radioimmunoguided surgery for European investigators. At this meeting in Tel Aviv, Israel, the following issues were discussed: 1) localization of cancer not detected by inspection, palpation, or prior scans; 2) the assessment of surgical margins; 3) the optimal probe design, target agent, and radionuclide; and 4) the processing of radioimmunoguided surgery data. Information pertaining to historical clinical trials on colorectal tumors (pilot studies, and phase I, II, and III studies) was delivered, and a practical guide for investigators was illustrated. The clinical applications and technical characteristics of radioimmunoguided surgery were discussed, with an emphasis on instrumentation, the investigator's responsibility, operative devices, tissue specimen handling, and patient selection. The meeting's underlying theme was radioimmunoguided surgery's ability to aid identification of disease dissemination not identified by traditional staging techniques, with ensuing change in the planned area of resection (30).

Between 1985 and 1995, many patients were enrolled in radioimmunoguided surgery trials. Although a large amount of data and information were collected, some issues remained unsolved. Especially puzzling was the relatively large fraction of lymph nodes that exhibited significant uptake of the radiolabeled MAB, yet had no histologic evidence of metastasis (31). However, use of different MABs and radiotracers (32) helped to define the potential of radioimmunoguided surgery to identify subclinical metastasis. The clinical impact of radioimmunoguided surgery was confirmed by a follow-up study demonstrating significantly improved overall survival after complete surgical removal of all radioimmunoguided surgery-positive tissues in patients with colorectal cancer (33).

The performance of radioimmunoguided surgery can be influenced by immunologic responses, and it may have a certain therapeutic impact by identifying lymph nodes containing tumor-reactive lymphocytes that can be used for adoptive cellular immunotherapy (34). Moreover, immunohistochemical staining of radioimmunoguided surgery-positive lymph nodes with anti-cytokeratin MABs increases the likelihood of identifying occult tumor cells in these nodes (35).

## Current Status and Future Outlook for Radioimmunoguided Surgery

Although the conceptually simple technique of radioimmunoguided surgery has been investigated and refined for almost 30 years, it still has inherent limitations. The poor availability of specific MABs has been overcome only in selected cases, such as colorectal cancer; in the majority of tumors, the efficacy of radioimmunoguided surgery remains uncertain. Other critical issues, such as choice of the radionuclide to label the MAB, are still controversial. Thus, the initial enthusiasm generated by early results with radioimmunoguided surgery has been dampened in the past decade. However, interest in this approach has recently been revived by reports concerning the use of $^{99m}$Tc-peplomycin in lung tumors (36), submucosal injection of radiolabeled anti-CEA MAB in colorectal cancers (37), and pharmacokinetics and clinical evaluation of the $^{125}$I-labeled humanized CC49 MAB (38,39). Moreover, investigations on the targeting of gastric cancer cells by anti-CEA fragments (40) and on its use in a biparatopic form in colon tumors (41) are still in progress.

Experience with the intraoperative gamma probe, originally developed for radioimmunoguided surgery, has paved the way for widespread application of radioguided surgery based on non-antibody tumor-seeking agents and on lymphotropic agents for sentinel lymph node identification (42–44).

Growing knowledge of antigen-antibody relationships and the development of new and superior tumor-targeting agents might constitute the basis for future further advances with radioimmunoguided surgery.

## References

1. Martin EW Jr, Tuttle SE, Rousseau M, et al. Radioimmunoguided surgery: intraoperative use of monoclonal antibody 17–1A in colorectal cancer. *Hybridoma.* 1986;5:S97-S108.
2. Martin EW Jr, Mojzisik CM, Hinkle GH Jr, et al. Radioimmunoguided surgery using monoclonal antibody. *Am J Surg.* 1988;156:386–392.
3. Primus FJ, Wang RH, Goldenberg DM, et al. Localization of human GW-39 tumors in hamsters by radiolabeled heterospecific antibody to carcinoembryonic antigen. *Cancer Res.* 1973;33:2977–2982.
4. Goldenberg DM, Preston DF, Primus FJ, et al. Photoscan localization of GW-39 tumors in hamsters using radiolabeled anticarcinoembryonic antigen immunoglobulin G. *Cancer Res.* 1974;34:1–9.
5. Kohler G, Milstein C. Continuous cultures of fused secreting antibody of redefined specificity. *Nature.* 1975:256;495–497.
6. Colcher D, Hand PH, Nuti M, et al. A spectrum of monoclonal antibodies reactive with human mammary tumor cells. *Proc Natl Acad Sci USA.* 1981;78:3199–3203.
7. Stramignoni D, Bowen R, Atkinson BF, Schlom J. Differential reactivity of monoclonal antibodies with human colon adenocarcinomas and adenomas. *Int J Cancer.* 1983;31:543–552.
8. Moldofsky PJ, Sears HF, Mulhern CB Jr, et al. Detection of metastatic tumor in normal-sized retroperitoneal lymph nodes by monoclonal-antibody imaging. *N Engl J Med.* 1984;311:106–107.
9. Begent RH, Keep PA, Searle F, et al. Radioimmunolocalization and selection for surgery in recurrent colorectal cancer. *Br J Surg.* 1986;73:64–67.
10. Aitken DR, Hinkle GH, Thurston MO, et al. A gamma-detecting probe for radioimmune detection of CEA-producing tumors. Successful experimental use and clinical case report. *Dis Colon Rectum.* 1984;27:279–282.
11. Martin DT, Aitken D, Thurston M, et al. Successful experimental use of a self-contained gamma detecting device. *Curr Surg.* 1984;41:193–194.
12. Martin DT, Hinkle GH, Tuttle S, et al. Intraoperative radioimmunodetection of colorectal tumor with a hand-held radiation detector. *Am J Surg.* 1985;150:672–675.
13. Sickle-Santanello BJ, O'Dwyer PJ, Mojzisik C, et al. Radioimmunoguided surgery using the monoclonal antibody B72.3 in colorectal tumors. *Dis Colon Rectum.* 1987;30:761–764.
14. Molinolo A, Simpson JF, Thor A, et al. Enhanced tumor binding using immunohistochemical analyses by second generation anti-TAG-72 monoclonal antibody against monoclonal antibody B72.3 in human tissue. *Cancer Res.* 1990;50:1291–1298.
15. Colcher D, Minelli MF, Roselli M, Muraro R, Simpson-Milenic D, Schlom J. Radioimmunolocalization of human carcinoma xenografts with B72.3 second generation monoclonal antibodies. *Cancer Res.* 1988;48:4597–4603.
16. Arnold MW, Schneebaum S, Berens A, et al. Intraoperative detection of colorectal cancer with radioimmunoguided surgery and CC49, a second-generation monoclonal antibody. *Ann Surg.* 1992;216:627–632.
17. Arnold MW, Schneebaum S, Berens A, et al. Radioimmunoguided surgery challenges traditional decision making in patients with primary colorectal cancer. *Surgery.* 1992;112:624–629.
18. Kim JA, Triozzi PL, Martin EW Jr. Radioimmunoguided surgery for colorectal cancer. *Oncology (Williston Park, N. Y.).* 1993;7:55–60; discussion 60, 63–64.
19. Goldenberg DM. Introduction to the Fourth Conference on Radioimmunodetection and Radioimmunotherapy of Cancer. *Cancer.* 1994;S73:759–760.

20. Greiner JW, Guadagni F, Roselli M, Ullmann CD, Nieroda C, Schlom J. Improved experimental radioimmunotherapy of colon xenografts by combining [131]I-CC49 and interferon-gamma. *Dis Colon Rectum.* 1994;37:S100–S105.

21. Roselli M, Guadagni F, Buonomo O, et al. Systemic administration of recombinant interferon alfa in carcinoma patients upregulates the expression of the carcinoma-associated antigens tumor-associated glycoprotein-72 and carcinoembryonic antigen. *J Clin Oncol.* 1996;14:2031–2042.

22. Roselli M, Buonomo O, Piazza A, et al. Novel clinical approaches in monoclonal antibody-based management in colorectal cancer patients: radioimmunoguided surgery and antigen augmentation. *Semin Surg Oncol.* 1998;15:254–262.

23. Badellino F. Radioimmunoguided surgery in Italy: 2 years of experience (1996–1998) [foreword]. *Semin Colon Rectal Surg.* 1998;15:203–204.

24. Di Carlo V, De Nardi P, Stella M, et al. Preoperative and intraoperative radioimmunodetection of cancer pretargeted by biotinylated monoclonal antibodies. *Semin Surg Oncol.* 1998;15:235–238.

25. Roselli M, Buonomo O, Piazza A, et al. Novel clinical approaches in monoclonal antibody-based management in colorectal cancer patients: radioimmunoguided surgery and antigen augmentation. *Semin Surg Oncol.* 1998;15:254–262.

26. Roselli M, Guadagni F, Buonomo O, et al. Intraoperative radioimmunolocalization of an anti-CEA MAB F(Ab')$_2$ (FO23C5) in CEA serum-negative colorectal cancer patients. *Anticancer Res.* 1996;16:883–889.

27. Hutzell P, Kashmiri S, Colcher D, et al. Generation and characterization of a recombinant/chimeric B72.3 (human gamma 1). *Cancer Res.* 1991;51:181–189.

28. Colcher D, Bird R, Roselli M, et al. In vivo tumor targeting of a recombinant single-chain antigen-binding protein. *J Natl Cancer Inst.* 1990;82:1191–1197.

29. Bertsch DJ, Burak WE Jr, Young DC, et al. Radioimmunoguided surgery system improves survival for patients with recurrent colorectal cancer. *Surgery.* 1995;118:634–638.

30. Bertsch DJ, Martin EW Jr. Radioimmunoguided surgery (RIGS) challenges the traditional of colorectal cancer surgery. Paper presented at: 48th Annual Cancer Symposium of the Society of Surgical Oncology; March 23–26, 1995; Boston.

31. Arnold MW. The radioimmunoguided diagnosis in surgery for colorectal cancer: introduction. *Semin Colon Rectal Surg.* 1995;6:183–184.

32. Thurston MO, Mojzisik CM. The radioimmunoguided diagnosis in surgery for colorectal cancer: history and development of radioimmunoguided surgery. *Semin Colon Rectal Surg.* 1995;6:185–191.

33. Petty LR, Arnold MW, Martin EW Jr. The radioimmunoguided diagnosis in surgery for colorectal cancer: colon cancer radioimmunoguided surgery technology: diagnosis and prognosis. *Semin Colon Rectal Surg.* 1995;6:198–201.

34. Kim JA. The radioimmunoguided diagnosis in surgery for colorectal cancer: observations on the immunologic basis of the radioimmunoguided surgery system. *Semin Colon Rectal Surg.* 1995;6:202–206.

35. Hitchock CL. The radioimmunoguided diagnosis in surgery for colorectal cancer: radioimmunoguided surgery and the staging of colorectal carcinoma. *Semin Colon Rectal Surg.* 1995;6:207–216.

36. Wang YO, Sun YE, Zhang JM, et al. Clinical practice of Tc[99m]–Peplomycin imaging and radioguided surgery for lung neoplasms. *Ai Zheng.* 2003;22:749–752.

37. Gu J, Zhao J, Li Z, et al. Clinical application of radioimmunoguided surgery in colorectal cancer using [125]I-labeled carcinoembryonic antigen-specific monoclonal antibody submucosally. *Dis Colon Rectum.* 2003;46:1659–1666.

38. Agnese DM, Abdessalam SF, Burak WE Jr, et al. Pilot study using a humanized CC49 monoclonal antibody (HuCC49DeltaCH2) to localize recurrent colorectal carcinoma. *Ann Surg Oncol.* 2004;11:197–202.

39. Xiao J, Horst S, Hinkle G, et al. Pharmacokinetics and clinical evaluation of [125]I-radiolabeled humanized CC49 monoclonal antibody (HuCC49deltaC(H)2) in recurrent and metastatic colorectal cancer patients. *Cancer Biother Radiopharm.* 2005;20:16–26.

40. Kim JC, Hong HK, Roh SA, et al. Efficient targeting of gastric cancer cells using radiolabeled anti-carcinoembryonic antigen-specific T84.66 fragments in experimental radioimmunoguided surgery. *Anticancer Res.* 2004;24:663–670.

41. Kim JC, Hong HK, Roh SA, et al. Preclinical application of radioimmunoguided surgery using anti-carcinoembryonic antigen biparatopic antibody in colon cancer. *Eur Surg Res.* 2005;37:36–44.

42. Krag D, Moffat F. Nuclear medicine and the surgeon. *Lancet.* 1999;354:1019–1022.

43. Buonomo O, Cabassi A, Guadagni F, et al. Radioguided surgery of early breast lesions. *Anticancer Res.* 2001;21:2091–2097.

44. DeNardo SJ. Radioimmunodetection and therapy of breast cancer. *Semin Nucl Med.* 2005;35:143–151.

# 22
# Radioguided Occult Lesion Localization in the Breast

Giovanni Paganelli, Concetta De Cicco, Giovanna Gatti, and Alberto Luini

## General Background

Until recently, noninvasive tumors such as ductal or lobular carcinoma in situ represented a relatively small proportion of diagnosed breast cancers. During the last decade, however, the widespread use of mammography has increased detection of preinvasive cancers; many authors indicate that 15% to 25% of diagnosed breast cancers are intraductal carcinomas, most of which are clinically occult (1–3). Over the next few years, the proportion of nonpalpable lesions is expected to exceed 50% of breast cancers (4–8).

The treatment of occult lesions necessitates close cooperation among the surgeon, the radiologist, and the pathologist, both before and during surgery. The lesion must be carefully located prior to excision, completely removed without unnecessary surgical trauma, and centered in the resected specimen. Intraoperative examination of a frozen section of this specimen may be considered, if definitive treatment can be performed in the same session, or delayed until the histological report is available (5).

## Non-Radionuclide Methods

The technique chosen for preoperative localization of nonpalpable breast lesions (9–17) will depend on the size and other characteristics of the lesion and on the equipment available (9,10,18,19). A breast lesion can be localized by injecting carbon particles or by inserting a hooked wire (Kopans wire, Homer wire, or self-retaining anchor wire) under mammographic or ultrasound guidance (20). Both techniques have shortcomings. Carbon particles in the surgically removed tissue can render histologic evaluation of the specimen problematic. During insertion of a hooked wire, the needle introducing the wire may become displaced (21–23). Attempting to remove and reinsert the wire is unlikely

to be successful and will increase the risk of bleeding and hematoma.

Experience and training are major factors in the successful localization and removal of occult lesions. Accurate placement of the locator is vital. Although the surgeon must follow the path of the wire or the carbon particles, an incision made along this pathway is not necessarily the optimal surgical approach with respect to morbidity or cosmesis. If the wire has been placed correctly, it is possible to "feel" the site of the lesion by pulling slightly on the wire, thus facilitating lesion removal. However, if the wire becomes displaced from its initial position, as often occurs when the breast is fatty, the excised specimen probably will not contain the whole lesion, forcing the surgeon to perform a wider resection. The difficulty of positioning a hooked wire increases with the density of breast tissue, making it more difficult to excise a lesion encircled by adequate margins of normal tissue.

Because the most important problem associated with wire localization is its high incidence of residual disease at the biopsy site (24–26), techniques such as intraoperative ultrasound guidance have been developed to improve the localization and resection of occult breast lesions (27–28). Grey et al. described placement of a radioactive seed in an 18-gauge needle that was then radiographically guided to the lesion; the seed was inserted into the breast parenchyma at the lesion site, the needle was withdrawn, and the seed's position was confirmed with mammography. Up to 5 days later, a handheld gamma probe was used to guide excision of the lesion with the seed. This hybrid technique combines wire localization and radioguided occult lesion localization (29).

Radioguided occult lesion localization was pioneered in 1996 at the European Institute of Oncology in Milan (Italy) for localizing nonpalpable breast lesions. This method marked a natural evolution from earlier studies on radioguided sentinel node biopsy for breast carcinoma. Increasing success and enthusiasm for the sentinel node technique generated great expectations among surgeons of this institute for the potential of nuclear medicine to solve other problems, such as preoperative localization of occult or nonpalpable breast lesions. The first nonpalpable breast lesion was injected under stereotactic guidance in May 1996, using large-size radiolabeled particles (such as those used in lung perfusion scintigraphy) to ensure that the radiotracer would not move from the injection site, and the lesion was removed surgically on the following day. The gamma probe proved just as effective in assisting intraoperative localization and removal here, as in sentinel node biopsy. This was the beginning of the radioguided occult lesion localization technique.

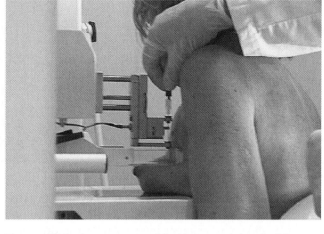

FIGURE 22-1. A mammographic device associated with a stereotactic system to guide the $^{99m}$Tc-MAA injection.

## Technique

### Injection

The original radioguided occult lesion localization technique has been described in detail elsewhere (30). Before surgery, ultrasonography or mammography is used to direct injection of radiolabeled macroaggregates (0.5 µg of human serum albumin, particle size 10–150 µm [Macrotec, GE Healthcare] labeled with 7–10 MBq of $^{99m}$Tc suspended in 0.2 mL of physiological saline) into the center of the lesion. Radiolabeling and quality control are performed according to the manufacturer's instructions.

For microcalcifications, opacities, or other anomalies revealed by mammography and not ultrasonography, a mammographic unit (Senographe DMR, GE Medical Systems) equipped with a computerized stereotactic system is used to guide the injection (Figure 22-1). The x-ray tube is oriented 15° higher and then 15° lower than the reference setting; with the aid of the computerized system, the resulting images are used to calculate the three-dimensional coordinates of the lesion. Craniocaudal projections are used for lesions in the upper quadrants of the breast; external or internal lateral projections are usually acquired for lesions in the outer or inner lower quadrants, respectively.

A 22-gauge spinal needle mounted in the stereotactic frame is introduced into the lesion, so that the position of the needle tip corresponds to the calculated coordinates. A new mammogram is taken to check that the tip is correctly located in the center of the lesion. The mandrel is removed; subsequent injection of the radiotracer is followed immediately by injection of 0.2 mL of radiopaque contrast medium (Iomeron 300, Bracco Imaging, Milan, Italy). The needle is then removed and a standard orthogonal mammogram is obtained to verify correct localization of the contrast medium within the lesion (Figure 22-2). The opaque contrast spot should be superimposed on the lesion; if the distance between the opaque spot and the lesion is more than 2 cm, the needle should be withdrawn and re-inserted for cutaneous mapping or anchor wire.

When the occult lesion is detected ultrasonically, the radiotracer is injected under ultrasonography guidance. The examination is performed with a linear probe at a frequency of 10–13 or 7.5–10 MHz, depending on the breast size. Subsequently, another probe (7.5–10 MHz) is attached to a needle biopsy device. The needle is

FIGURE 22-2. A. Craniocaudal mammogram showing a small radiopaque lesion (arrow). B. The same projection after injection of $^{99m}$Tc-MAA and contrast medium demonstrates the correct position of the tracer.

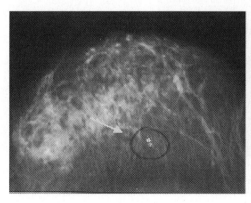
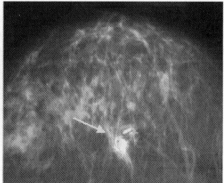

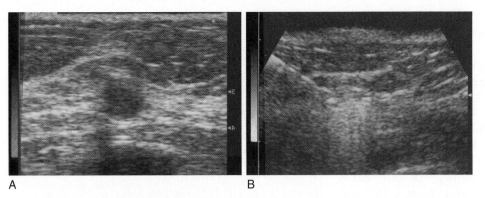

A                                              B

FIGURE 22-3. (A) Radioguided occult lesion localization, guided by ultrasound. A sonogram shows a solid hypoechoic nodule with acoustic shadow (B). Following injection of the radiotracer, the nodule apparently disappears, masked by the liquid injected, which can be identified by the operator as a hyperechoic area.

positioned in the device and manually inserted into the breast; the needle tip is positioned in the center of the lesion, as shown by a change in echogenicity at the lesion site. Radiotracer is then injected, followed by 0.2 mL of saline (Figure 22-3).

If a lesion is visible by both ultrasonography and mammography, the tracer should be injected under ultrasonography control, because of the higher accuracy in centering the lesion. An ink mark placed on the skin over the lesion serves as an initial guide during scintigraphy and surgery.

Audisio et al. (31) have simplified the original radioguided occult lesion localization technique, so that the radiotracer is injected 1 to 4 hours before surgery. This not only decreases the radioactive dose to an amount as small as 1 MBq (corresponding to a radiation burden as low as 0.02 mSv), but also eliminates an overnight stay in the hospital and thereby reduces the cost of the procedure.

## Scintigraphy

Lateral and anterior scintigraphic images are acquired about 10 minutes after radiotracer injection, although the timing varies. The lateral views are obtained while the patient is prone; a polystyrene block holds the breast in position (Figure 22-4). A flexible wire with a $^{57}$Co source is used to outline the breast contour (Figure 22-5). The anterior image is obtained with the patient standing, arms abducted, after placing a $^{57}$Co point source on the nipple as a landmark. Images are acquired for about 5 minutes, collecting 70 Kcounts in a 256 × 256 pixel matrix, with zoom 1.33.

For the first 100 patients entered into the radioguided occult lesion localization protocol, we also acquired a scintigraphic image 5 to 18 hours after radiotracer injection to look for possible migration of the radiotracer. There was no evidence of radioactivity in the breast tissue surrounding the injection site.

The scintigram is evaluated for the absence of areas of contamination. When the hot spot is a small, well-delineated area, the patient can be referred for biopsy (Figure 22-6). If the radiotracer has spread across a large area of breast parenchyma (Figure 22-7), localization should be repeated using a different technique. In case of cutaneous contamination, the scan should be repeated after the skin is cleaned.

Although we strictly adhere to the protocol described above, other groups have questioned the value of systematically acquiring preoperative scintigraphic images. Since the site of injection can be confirmed by imaging

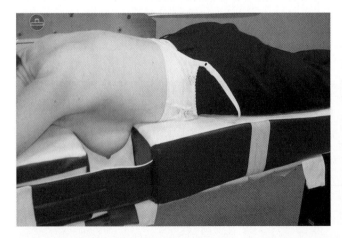

FIGURE 22-4. Scintigraphic lateral scan performed with the patient lying prone over a homemade polystyrene device to hold the breast in position.

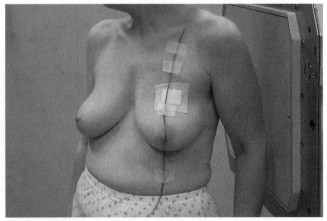

FIGURE 22-5. Scintigraphic lateral scan acquired after positioning a flexible wire $^{57}$Co source to outline the breast contour.

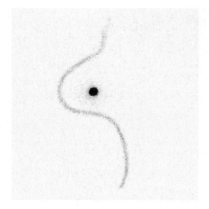

FIGURE 22-6. Scintigraphic lateral scan showing that the injected $^{99m}$Tc-MAA dose is placed in a small, well-delimited area. In this case, the radioguided occult lesion localization procedure is considered correctly performed.

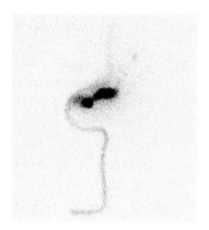

FIGURE 22-7. Scintigraphy with lateral scan, in case of the spread of the radiotracer into the ducts.

the needle tip position under either plain radiographic or ultrasonography control, some authors maintain that scintigraphy is unnecessary (31). The modified technique proposed by Audiso et al. can be useful in any screening unit, without the need for a gamma camera or overnight admission before surgery.

## Surgery

Patients undergo surgical excision of the lesion under general anaesthesia. The incision is guided by the skin mark (Figure 22-8A), by the radioactivity detected with a handheld gamma probe (we employ either

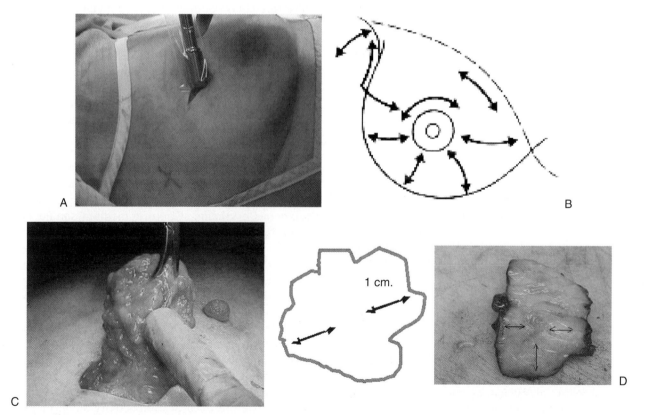

FIGURE 22-8. (A) During surgery, the gamma probe is used to check the position of the hot spot. (B) The surgeon can choose the most appropriate incision, wherever the lesion is located. (C) Another advantage of the method is that the exact site of the radiolabeled lesion can be checked during the operation using the probe. (D) This results in high excision accuracy and centering of the lesion within the specimen, so that it is rarely necessary to radicalize the margins.

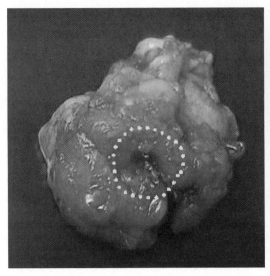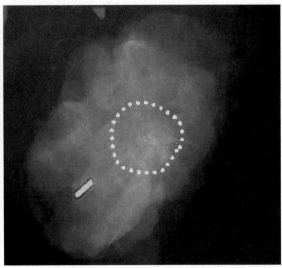

FIGURE 22-9. Specimen x-ray demonstrated the centricity of the lesion in 770 out of 774 (99.5%).

MR 100 [Pol.Hi.Tech, L'Aquila, Italy] or Neo2000 Gamma Detection System [Neoprobe Corp., Dublin, Ohio]), and by cosmetic criteria (Figure 22-8B). The gamma probe is also used to check the position of the hot spot during the excision (Figure 22-8C) and to establish the margins of resection by the points around the hot spot where radioactivity drops abruptly to background levels (1–1.5 counts per second) (Figure 22-8D).

After the lesion is removed, the resection cavity is checked for residual activity. If the level exceeds background, the cavity should be enlarged. In case of microcalcifications, the specimen is tagged with clips on 1 or more margins and x-rayed to verify complete lesion removal and the concentricity of the lesions (Figure 22-9). When the microcalcifications are too close to the margins and/or not centered in the specimen, the cavity should be enlarged. When the resected specimen contains a nonpalpable lesion detected by ultrasonography alone, tissue inked by the pathologist should be cut to verify the presence of the lesion.

## Histopathology

Intraoperative frozen section examination is usually performed only for solid nonpalpable lesions larger than 1 cm; otherwise, permanent hematoxylin and eosin sections are prepared. If an invasive carcinoma is found, the area of resection is expanded to include the breast quadrant. Histological classification follows the World Health Organization classification (32).

## Overall Performance

Our experience is based on 1,778 consecutive procedures performed between January 2001 and December 2004 in women with nonpalpable breast abnormalities. The mean patient age was 54.5 years (range, 25–85 years). Of the 1,778 occult breast lesions, 995 (56%) were clusters of microcalcifications found on mammography; in these cases, the radiotracer was injected under x-ray stereotactic guidance. The remaining 783 lesions (44%) were detected by ultrasonography; thus, the radiotracer was injected under ultrasonography guidance. Radioguided occult lesion localization was generally well tolerated, although needle insertion produced some discomfort. There were no allergic reactions after administration of the radiopharmaceutical, although 1 patient developed a cutaneous erythema. Contrast medium should not be administered to patients with a history of intolerance or allergic reactions to this agent.

Based on the imaging criteria described previously, the procedure was successful in 1,692 of 1,778 lesions (95%). In the remaining 86 cases (5%), the position of the tracer did not coincide with the lesion site (61 cases), or the tracer spread over a large area of the breast parenchyma (25 cases). In these cases, another method of preoperative localization should be used, or the procedure can be repeated a few days later. All 783 procedures performed under ultrasonography guidance were successful. The presence of radioactivity along the needle track (211 cases) did not interfere with correct surgical excision. The hot spot was located by the gamma probe in all 1,717 cases referred to surgery.

In 1,700 of the 1,717 (99%) surgical cases, subsequent x-ray and histopathologic evaluation demonstrated the lesion in the resected specimen. Of the 898 cases (52.8%) of invasive breast cancer, 887 (98.8%) were associated with cancer-free surgical margins; in 11 cases (1.2%), 1 or more margins were extended.

## Final Considerations

Radioguided occult lesion localization is the preferred approach for preoperative localization of nonpalpable breast lesions in our institute. When compared to wire localization, it provides better centering of the lesion within the specimen and reduces the amount of healthy tissue removed (30,33–36). Most importantly, it provides the surgeon with a quick and simple means of locating and removing the lesion in the operating room. The absence of side effects or complications also contributes to its success in our institute and in many others (31,37–41).

However, radioguided occult lesion localization should not be attempted in women with diffuse microcalcifications and multifocal or multicentric lesions. Moreover, the technique requires close collaboration among the radiologist, the nuclear physician, the surgeon, and the pathologist. A team learning curve of 30 procedures is sufficient for correct execution of each step of the procedure.

The best results are obtained when the lesion is localized under ultrasonography guidance; this procedure is simple and fast (5–10 min maximum), with excellent correspondence between location of the hot spot and the lesion's position. The echogenicity changes caused by the presence of both the needle and tracer make it possible to verify that the needle tip is inserted into the lesion and that the tracer is correctly injected.

More problematic and complex is the approach using x-ray stereotaxis. The injection needle is not always inserted to the correct depth. The distance between the injected radiopaque spot and the lesion must always be checked on the standard mammogram taken after injection. Very superficial lesions are difficult to be centered, while another problem is represented by lesions in the central quadrant of the breast, where the probability of injecting the tracer in a galactophore duct is high.

Macroaggregates of albumin do not move from the injection site, and there is no diffusion in the breast tissue around the lesion, provided that the radiotracer has not been introduced into the lymphatic vessels or galactophorous ducts. This allows a large lapse of time prior to surgery, consistent with physical decay of $^{99m}$Tc.

Radioguided occult lesion localization does not require special radioprotection measures. The risk for patients and hospital staff is negligible (42,43). For patients, the mean absorbed dose to the abdomen is 0.45 mGy, which is low compared to doses received from other diagnostic examinations. For surgeons, the mean absorbed dose to the hands after 100 operations is 0.45 mGy and the mean effective dose is 0.09 mSv. Absorbed doses to all hospital personnel involved in the procedure are very low compared to the recommended annual limits established by the International Commission on Radiological Protection (44).

## References

1. Schwartz GF, Feig SA, Patchefsky AS. Significance and staging of nonpalpable carcinomas of the breast. *Surg Gynecol Obstet.* 1988;166:6–10.
2. Franceschi D, Crowe J, Zollinger R, et al. Breast biopsy for calcifications in nonpalpable breast lesions. *Arch Surg.* 1990;125:170–173.
3. Goedde TA, Frykberg ER, Crump JM, et al. The impact of mammography on breast biopsy. *Am Surg.* 1992;58:661–666.
4. Symmonds RE, Roberts JW. Management of nonpalpable breast abnormalities. *Ann Surg.* 1987;205:520–528.
5. Tubiana M, Holland R, Kopans DB, et al. Commission of the European Communities "Europe Against Cancer" Programme. European School of Oncology Advisory Report. Management of nonpalpable and small lesions found in mass breast screening. *Eur J Cancer.* 1994;30:538–547.
6. Schwartz GF, Carter DL, Conant EF, et al. Mammographically detected breast cancer. Nonpalpable is not a synonym for inconsequential. *Cancer.* 1994;73:1660–1665.
7. Brenner RJ. Lesions entirely removed during stereotactic biopsy: preoperative localization on the basis of mammographic landmarks and feasibility of freehand technique— initial experience. *Radiology.* 2000;214:585–590.
8. Liberman L, Kaplan J, Van Zee KJ, et al. Bracketing wires for preoperative breast needle localization. *AJR Am J Roentgenol.* 2001;177:565–572.
9. Frank HA, Hall FM, Steer ML. Preoperative localization of nonpalpable breast lesions demonstrated by mammography. *N Eng J Med.* 1976;295:259–260.
10. Hermann G, Janus G, Lesnick GJ. Percutaneous localization of nonpalpable breast lesions. *Breast.* 1983;9:4–6.
11. Goldberg RP, Hall FM, Simon M. Preoperative localization of nonpalpable breast lesions using a wire marker and perforated mammographic grid. *Radiology.* 1983;146:833–835.
12. Homer MJ. Nonpalpable breast lesion localization using a curved-end retractable wire. *Radiology.* 1985;157:259–260.
13. Silverstein MJ, Gamagami P, Rosser RJ, et al. Hooked-wire-directed breast biopsy and overpenetrated mammography. *Cancer.* 1987;59:715–722.
14. Bellucci MC, Panzarola P. Preoperative localization using a bidimensional mammographic technique of nonpalpable lesions of the breast. *Radiol Med (Torino).* 1990;80:89–92.

15. Mazy S, Galant C, Berliere M, et al. Localization of non-palpable breast lesions with black carbon powder (experience of the Catholic University of Louvain). *J Radiol.* 2001;82:161–164.

16. Allen MJ, Thompson WD, Stuart RC, et al. Management of nonpalpable breast lesions detected mammographically. *Br J Surg.* 1994;81:543–545.

17. Berna-Serna JD, Nieves J, Madrigal M, et al. New system for localization of nonpalpable breast lesions with adhesive marker plate. *Breast.* 2004;13:104–109.

18. Simons N, Lesnick GJ, Lerer WN, et al. Roentgenographic localization of small lesions of the breast by the spot method. *Sur Gynecol Obstet.* 1972;134:572–574.

19. Berger SM, Curcio BM, Gershongohen J, et al. Mammographic localization of unexpected breast cancer. *Am J Roentgenol Radium Ther Nucl Med.* 1996;96:1046–1052.

20. Kopans DB, De Luca S. A modified needle hookwire technique to simplify preoperative localization of occult breast lesions. *Radiology.* 1980;134:781.

21. Bigongiari LR, Fidler W, Skerker LB, et al. Percutaneous needle localization of breast lesions prior to biopsy: analysis of failures. *Clin Radiol.* 1977;28:419–425.

22. Yankaskas BC, Knelson MH, Abernethy ML, et al. Needle localization biopsy of occult lesions of the breast. Experience in 199 cases. *Invest Radiol.* 1988;23:729–733.

23. Tykkä H, Castren-Persons M, Sjöblom SM, et al. Pneumothorax caused by hooked wire localization of an impalpable breast lesion detected by mammography. *Breast.* 1993;2:52–53.

24. Marrujo G, Jolly PC, Hall MH. Nonpalpable breast cancer: needle-localized biopsy for diagnosis and considerations for treatment. *Am J Surg.* 1986;151:599–602.

25. Allen MJ, Thompson WD, Stuart RC, et al. Management of nonpalpable breast lesions detected mammographically. *Br J Surg.* 1994;81:543–545.

26. Vuorela AL, Kettunen S, Punto L. Preoperative hook-wire localization of nonpalpable breast lesions by use of standard and stereotactic technique. *Anticancer Res.* 1993;13:1873–1875.

27. Rahusen FD, Bremers AJ, Fabry HF, van Amerongen AH, Boom RP, Meijer S. Ultrasound-guided lumpectomy of nonpalpable breast cancer versus wire-guided resection: a randomized clinical trial. *Ann Surg Oncol.* 2002;9:994–998.

28. Kaufman CS, Jacobson L, Bachman B, Kaufman LB. Intraoperative ultrasonography guidance is accurate and efficient according to results in 100 breast cancer patients. *Am J Surg.* 2003;186:378–382.

29. Gray RJ, Salud C, Nguyen K, et al. Randomized prospective evaluation of a novel technique for biopsy or lumpectomy of nonpalpable breast lesions: radioactive seed versus wire localization. *Ann Surg Oncol.* 2001;8:711–715.

30. De Cicco C, Pizzamiglio M, Trifiro G, et al. Radioguided occult lesion localization (ROLL) and surgical biopsy in breast cancer. Technical aspects. *Q J Nucl Med.* 2002;46:145–151.

31. Audisio RA, Nadeem R, Harris O, Desmond S, Thind R, Chagla LS. Radioguided occult lesion localization (ROLL) is available in the UK for impalpable breast lesions. *Ann R Coll Surg Engl.* 2005;87:92–95.

32. Tavassoli FA, Devilee P, eds. *Pathology and Genetics of Tumors of the Breast and Female Genital Organs.* Lyon: International Agency for Research on Cancer, 2003.

33. Paganelli G, De Cicco C, Luini A, et al. Radioguided surgery in nonpalpable breast lesions [abstract]. *Eur J Nucl Med.* 1997;24(suppl):893P.

34. Luini A, Zurrida S, Galimberti V, et al. Radioguided surgery of occult breast lesions. *Eur J Cancer.* 1998;34:204–205.

35. Luini A, Zurrida S, Paganelli G, et al. Comparison of radioguided excision with wire localisation of occult breast lesions. *Br J Surg.* 1999;86:522–525.

36. Gennari R, Galimberti V, De Cicco C, et al. Use of Technetium-99m-labeled colloid albumin for preoperative and intraoperative localization of nonpalpable breast lesion. *J Am Coll Surg.* 2000;190:692–699.

37. Feggi L, Basaglia E, Corcione S, et al. An original approach in the diagnosis of early breast cancer: use of the same radiopharmaceutical for both nonpalpable lesions and sentinel node localisation. *Eur J Nucl Med.* 2001;28:1589–1596.

38. Patel A, Pain SJ, Britton P, et al. Radioguided occult lesion localization (ROLL) and sentinel node biopsy for impalpable invasive breast cancer. *Eur J Surg Oncol.* 2004;30:918–923.

39. Rampaul RS, Bagnall M, Burrell H, et al. Randomized clinical trial comparing radioisotope occult lesion localization and wire-guided excision for biopsy of occult breast lesions. *Br J Surg.* 2004;91:1575–1577.

40. Ronka R, Krogerus L, Leppanen E, et al. Radio-guided occult lesion localization in patients undergoing breast-conserving surgery and sentinel node biopsy. *Am J Surg.* 2004;187:491–496.

41. Zgajnar J, Hocevar M, Frkovic-Grazio S, et al. Radioguided occult lesion localization (ROLL) of the nonpalpable breast lesions. *Neoplasma.* 2004;51:385–389.

42. Cremonesi M, Ferrari M, Sacco E, et al. Radiation protection in radioguided surgery of breast cancer. *Nucl Med Commun.* 1999;20:919–924.

43. Rampaul RS, Dudley NJ, Thompson JZ, et al. Radioisotope for occult lesion localisation (ROLL) of the breast does not require extra radiation protection procedures. *Breast.* 2003;12:150–152.

44. ICRP *Publication 60*: Recommendations of the International Commission on Radiological Protection. Annals of the ICRP, Vol. 21/1–3. Elsevier, 1991.

# 23
# Minimally Invasive Radioguided Parathyroidectomy in Primary Hyperparathyroidism

James Norman, Domenico Rubello, Armando E. Giuliano, and Giuliano Mariani

## Epidemiology

Primary hyperparathyroidism is caused by inappropriately high secretion of parathyroid hormone (PTH) by 1 or more enlarged parathyroid glands (1). Diagnosis of primary hyperparathyroidism, especially the asymptomatic form, has dramatically increased worldwide, mainly due to the introduction of automated serum calcium measurement in laboratory screening (2,3). The prevalence of primary hyperparathyroidism in a United States community has increased from about 0.08/1000 to about 0.5/1000, with the proportion of asymptomatic patients rising from 18% to 51% (3). Other United States estimates place the prevalence of primary hyperparathyroidism at 2/1000 women and 0.5/1000 men over age 40 (4). Parallel European estimates in the 1980s indicated an average 10/1000 prevalence in the general population (about 0.3/1000 for men and about 17/1000 for women, with a peak of 33/1000 for women older than 60 years) (5). However, it seems that after such an initial "catch-up effect," this surge in the identification of primary hyperparathyroidism has plateaued or is actually declining, as indicated by the most recent estimates both in the United States (with the annual incidence decreasing in the last decade from 75/100,000 to about 20/100,000) and in Europe (with the present prevalence of 3/1000 in the general population and 21/1000 in women age 55 to 75) (6,7). Although no detailed epidemiological studies have been reported, the incidence of primary hyperparathyroidism seems lower in Asia (8,9).

The last decade has witnessed significant advances both in our understanding of the pathophysiology of primary hyperparathyroidism and in its management. The increased recognition of early, subclinical primary hyperparathyroidism due to the more widespread use of screening tests has led to a new profile of primary hyperparathyroidism, other than the classical clinically overt pattern characterized by recurring nephrolithiasis associated with frank hypercalcemia and low serum phosphate, bone disease, deep weakness, and reduced life expectancy. In the early phases of primary hyperparathyroidism, hypercalcemia is only mild (combined usually with normal or borderline-low serum phosphate) and symptoms are absent or subtle.

Because of such increased recognition of primary hyperparathyroidism, the number of parathyroidectomies performed has increased worldwide. Currently, about one-tenth of all patients with primary hyperparathyroidism undergo surgery in a relatively early phase of the disease.

No other period has witnessed such significant changes in how surgeons manage primary hyperparathyroidism preoperatively and intraoperatively. What once was often a long operation can now be done routinely in less than 20 minutes as a true outpatient procedure, performed with minimal anesthesia. Despite this "lesser" approach, reported cure rates are at their highest (10,11).

The concept of performing a lesser operation to find the offending parathyroid gland has been around for years, but it was not until a number of parathyroid surgeons with the appropriate caseloads undertook prospective studies using physiologic adjuncts in the operating room and documented favorable results that this began to catch on widely. It is the surgeon's ability to operate physiologically, and not just anatomically, that has finally allowed a more directed and confident approach. Subsequently, this has led some centers to minimal use of anesthesia and immediate postoperative discharge—changes that have been embraced enthusiastically by many referring endocrinologists.

## Anatomy and Pathophysiology of Parathyroid Glands

Typically, there are 2 pairs of parathyroid glands in adult humans, with each gland measuring approximately 6 × 4 × 2 mm and weighing about 30 to 50 mg (for a total

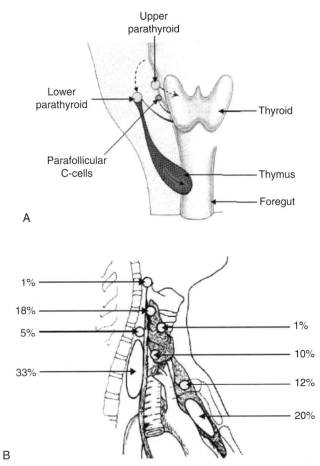

pouch) maintain a close association with the fetal thyroid until descent of both structures to their final locations in the neck, where these parathyroid glands are positioned at the posterolateral surface of the upper poles of the thyroid lobes.

This migration pattern during fetal development explains the variable anatomy that sometimes challenges the surgical approach to the parathyroid glands. While upper glands are most frequently located posterior to the middle and upper third of the thyroid lobe and posterior to the recurrent laryngeal nerves (cranially to the inferior thyroid artery), the location of the inferior parathyroid glands is more variable, posteriorly or laterally to the lower pole of the thyroid lobe (usually within a 20-mm radius) in about 50% of the cases. Other frequent locations of the inferior parathyroid glands include within the thyrothymic ligament, within the thymus in the mediastinum, and the intrathyroidal location (Figure 23-1B).

Ectopic abnormal glands (15% to 20% of the cases) are found in the anterior-superior mediastinum, either within or outside of the thymus, along the esophagus into the posterior-superior mediastinum, or rarely in the mid-lower mediastinum. Other occasional locations include within, or even lateral to, the carotid sheath, while an undescended lower parathyroid gland can be located high in the neck, anterior to the carotid bifurcation. When parathyroid adenomas are located in the mediastinum or high in the neck, in the cervical neurovascular bundle, or even within the thyroid gland (2% to 3% of the cases), the condition is defined as major ectopy. Such a condition can coexist with the presence of 4 parathyroid glands in their normal locations (i.e., the ectopic parathyroid adenoma is frequently an ectopic gland) (12,13).

FIGURE 23-1. (A) Routes of descent of the thymus, parathyroid glands, and ultimopharyngeal body during fetal life. Parathyroid glands originating more cranially in the third pharyngeal pouch migrate closely with the thymus, and are eventually located more caudally to the parathyroid glands originating in the fourth pharyngeal pouch. (B) Location of ectopic parathyroid adenomas, as described by Wang (107) in a series of patients reoperated on because of persistent/recurrent hyperparathyroidism. (Reprinted by permission of the Society of Nuclear Medicine. Mariani G, Gulec SA, Rubello D, et al. Preoperative localization and radioguided parathyroid surgery. J Nucl Med 2003;44:1443–1458. Figures 1 and 2.)

## Calcium Homeostasis and the Parathyroid Hormone

Bone and teeth contain about 95% of all calcium in the body, in the form of calcium phosphate or hydroxyapatite $(Ca_5[PO_4]_3[OH])$, and thus serve as a balancing reservoir for the body fluids, ionized calcium in serum being strictly controlled in the approximate range of 1.15–1.29 mmol/L (or 3.8–4.2 mg/dL).

Thanks to a transmembrane calcium gradient, cells use the calcium ion as an intracellular messenger, carrying information generated by hormones and neurotransmitters. By interacting with a surface receptor on the parathyroid cells (the calcium ion receptor, CaR), the calcium ion has a role both in the secretory balance and in cell proliferation of the parathyroid glands. CaR is also involved in the regulation of calcitonin secretion by parafollicular cells of the thyroid, in the regulation of calcium and water homeostasis by the kidney, in the

parathyroid mass of about 120 to 200 mg). Although more than 4 parathyroid glands (up to 6 to 8 glands) are present in about 1% of individuals, few people have fewer than 4 glands. Embryologically, the parathyroid glands originate as entodermal structures in the third and fourth pharyngeal pouches, inverting their relative position as they migrate during fetal life toward their final location; the glands originally positioned more cranially (in the third pharyngeal pouch) follow the descent of the thymus toward the chest, usually leaving their connection with the thymus as they reach their final location at the posterolateral surface of the lower lobes of the thyroid (see Figure 23-1A). The parathyroids originally positioned more caudally (in the fourth pharyngeal regulation of mineral homeostasis by both the precursors and mature osteoclasts/osteoblasts, and in the regulation of intestinal absorption of calcium. On the other hand, CaR is also expressed in many tissues not known to be directly involved in the regulation of calcium metabolism, such as neurons and keratinocytes, possibly as a calcium sensor regulating hormone secretion, ion channel function, gene expression, cell proliferation, and cell apoptosis.

The main source of calcium in terrestrial vertebrates is dietary. In humans, requirements of dietary calcium intake vary throughout life, beginning with 400 to 600 mg/day in infants, reaching a plateau at about 700 to 800 mg/day in adults, and reaching 1500 mg/day in adults over age 65. However, recommended dietary allowances vary in different countries, depending on different dietary environments (dairy-farming communities versus communities where animal milk is not available, etc.).

Parathyroid hormone (PTH), an 84-amino acid single chain polypeptide with a molecular weight of 9,500 Da, controls the level of ionized calcium in the blood and in extracellular fluid. PTH is synthesized as a larger precursor (115 amino acid), the pre-proparathyroid hormone (pre-pro-PTH). While transiting across the endoplasmic reticulum, the "pre" sequence (a "signal" 25 amino acid peptide) is cleaved and rapidly degraded, thus leaving the pro-PTH peptide of 90 amino acids. Further cleavage of the "pro" sequence (6 amino acids) produces mature PTH, which is concentrated in the secretory vesicles and granules of parathyroid cells. Granules of a distinct subtype also contain cathepsins B and H (2 proteases) in addition to PTH. Because of this co-localization of proteases, a small portion of PTH secreted by the parathyroid cells consists of carboxyterminal PTH fragments that have no clear biologic role in calcium balance. Intracellular fragmentation of PTH probably represents a regulatory inactivating pathway, but its exact role has not yet been fully elucidated.

The major determinant of PTH secretion is the concentration of ionized calcium in the blood; even small reductions in the extracellular calcium concentration cause increased PTH secretion aimed at restoring the calcium levels to normal. PTH has different concomitant effects, primarily in the kidney: 1) increased tubular reabsorption of calcium, 2) increased excretion of phosphorus, and 3) increased transformation of precursors into the active form of vitamin D (which, in turn, stimulates increased absorption of calcium in the gastrointestinal tract). The resulting restoration of normal calcium levels in the extracellular fluid terminates the feedback loop in the parathyroid glands.

It is known that, in the short-term, acute hypocalcemia increases the release of preformed PTH stored in the parathyroid cells (within minutes), while in the longer term (over several hours) there is increased synthesis (and subsequent release) of the hormone, as shown by increased PTH mRNA. Persistent or chronic hypocalcemia increases PTH secretion both by increasing the maximal secretory rate per cell (through enhanced expression of the PTH gene, which in humans is located on chromosome q11) and by stimulating proliferation of the parathyroid cells.

The biological half-life of secreted PTH is 2 to 3 minutes, hormone degradation taking place primarily in the liver (70%) and kidneys (20%), and variations in PTH blood levels are defined mostly by its rate of secretion. PTH receptors on cell surfaces (reacting eventually with less than 1% of secreted hormone) are mainly located in the bone and kidneys, the latter therefore representing both a target organ for triggering responses that increase calcium levels in the blood and an important catabolic site.

## Primary Hyperparathyroidism

In primary hyperparathyroidism, the secretion of PTH is inappropriate with respect to the extracellular calcium concentration. This condition can be caused by either parathyroid adenoma(s) (in 80% to 95% of cases), parathyroid hyperplasia (5% to 20% of cases), or carcinoma (1% of cases or less). Parathyroid cells exhibit both increased proliferative activity, leading to enlarged glands, and decreased sensitivity to the inhibiting effect of increased calcium concentration on PTH secretion (altered set-point). There are some forms of familial hyperparathyroidism, such as multiple endocrine neoplasia (MEN)-1 syndrome (87% to 97%), MEN-2 (5% to 20%), familial hypercalciuric hyper-parathyroidism, the hyperparathyroidism-jaw-tumor syndrome (HPT-JT/HRPT2), and familial isolated hyperparathyroidism.

Molecular biology investigations have shown that sporadic parathyroid tumors are clonal in origin, and there is evidence for oncogene activation and inactivation of tumor suppressor genes.

Because of the characteristic abnormality in primary hyperparathyroidism of the responsiveness of parathyroid cells to the inhibition of PTH secretion normally exerted by calcium, attention has been focused on CaR, both in vivo and in vitro. While the role of this calcium sensor in the development of primary hyperparathyroidism remains unclear, abnormalities in its expression or function as a consequence of some as yet unidentified genetic mutation(s) may contribute to the failure of PTH secretory regulation.

Genetic variations of vitamin D metabolism also have been found to be associated with some primary hyperparathyroidism states. In particular situations, parathyroid cells become less susceptible to inhibition by active vitamin D, and therefore more likely to undergo hyperplastic or adenomatous changes. In addition, irradiation of the neck and upper chest for benign diseases, including [131]I treatment for Graves' disease (but not for malignant disease), has also been found to be a risk factor for the development of primary hyperparathyroidism.

Persistent or recurrent hyperparathyroidism occur in 5% to 10% of all patients who undergo surgery for primary hyperparathyroidism. Persistent hyperparathyroidism is the most common (75%), and is defined as continuing abnormalities of calcium metabolism in the immediate postoperative period. Causes for the immediate failure of surgical treatment include failure in identifying the adenomas, inadequate resection of multiple gland disease unrecognized preoperatively, inexperience of the surgeon, metastatic parathyroid carcinoma, and error on intraoperative frozen section examination. Persistent hyperparathyroidism is particularly frequent in patients with familial hyperparathyroidism, especially the MEN-1 syndrome (usually in less than 25% of the patients, but up to 40% to 60% for less experienced surgeons [13]). Recurrent hyperparathyroidism (i.e., hyperparathyroidism relapsing after more than 6 months of normocalcemia following surgery) is usually linked to continued growth of the remaining parathyroid tissue.

Finally, parathyromatosis—a rare case of recurrent or persistent hyperparathyroidism—is defined as multiple remnants of hyperfunctioning parathyroid tissue scattered throughout the neck or upper mediastinum. This condition is probably due either to inadvertent implantation of parathyroid tissue at the time of parathyroidectomy, or to growth of nests of parathyroid tissue left along the route of descent during embryologic development of the parathyroid glands.

# From Conventional Surgical Approach to Limited Parathyroid Surgery: The Role of Preoperative Localization Imaging

The first successful parathyroidectomy was performed in 1925 with conventional cervicotomy and bilateral neck exploration (14), which has since remained the standard treatment of primary hyperparathyroidism (15). This time-honored approach, based on excision of any grossly enlarged gland with or without biopsy of the remaining glands, yields a 95% success rate with minimal morbidity in the hands of an experienced endocrine surgeon, even with 4-gland hyperplasia (16,17). When more than 1 gland is enlarged, the operative techniques include a resection of at least half of 3 glands (leaving approximately 50 to 100 mg of the most "normal-appearing" gland), excising only those glands that are grossly enlarged at the exploration, and a less common 4-gland parathyroidectomy with subsequent autotransplantation. Success with this approach depends primarily on the

experience and judgment of the surgeon in distinguishing pathologically enlarged from normal glands, although the size of the parathyroid gland does not always correlate well with the secretion of PTH.

In the pre-imaging era, bilateral neck exploration was mandatory, because discrimination between single and multigland disease was based solely on the glands' macroscopic appearance. In general, experienced surgeons believe that by evaluating the size, shape, and color of the parathyroid glands at operation, they can distinguish normal glands from abnormal ones. If 1 gland is enlarged and the others are perfectly normal visually, the diagnosis is "single adenoma," while hyperplasia (multigland disease) should result in enlargement of all 4 glands. However, asymmetric hyperplasia may appear, with 1 or 2 normal size glands confusing the diagnosis, even with biopsy.

The prevalence of hyperplasia varies considerably in different series, and there appears to be a strong influence of clinical (surgical) diagnosis on the pathologist's diagnosis (18). When subtotal parathyroidectomy is performed, final histologic diagnosis is more likely to be hyperplasia. When a focused operation is performed with removal of a single gland, the more likely final histologic diagnosis is adenoma. The importance of mild hyperplasia and the best way of diagnosing this condition are yet to be determined. Parathyroid carcinoma is a rare cause of primary hyperparathyroidism, accounting for less than 1% of all cases.

In the experience of Norman and colleagues from the University of South Florida (19–28)—possibly the largest in the world, with more than 5000 operated patients—the cause of primary hyperparathyroidism is a single adenoma in 95% of cases. In the opinion of these authors, the use of physiologic measures of parathyroid gland activity and the assessment of PTH production (directly or indirectly) in the operating room is responsible for this more accurate accounting of the number of true single adenomas. Historical accounts rely solely on histology and the pathologist's estimation of the percent of fat contained within a gland as the only documentation of a diseased gland. Yet even pathologists cannot agree on what makes a gland hyperplastic on histology. Any surgeon who has interacted with a pathologist during even a handful of parathyroidectomies knows that relying on the pathologist to determine when the patient is cured will surely result in further surgery sooner or later.

Because most patients with sporadic, non-MEN primary hyperparathyroidism have a single tumorous gland, theoretically a full 4-gland exploration was required for only a small subset of the population with this disease. The challenge has always been to establish preoperatively, or even intraoperatively, to which category an individual patient belonged. Did they have a single adenoma, or did they have multigland disease? As mentioned above, since 1925 (14) the accepted standard was for the surgeon to examine all 4 glands through a detailed and meticulous dissection of the neck. For the past several decades, frozen section analysis has supplemented the surgeon's eyes with the microscopic assessment of selected tissues the surgeon deemed important. Usually, the frozen section resulted in the pathologist confirming the presence of parathyroid tissue, but their help in determining cure is limited. This standard operation is, by its nature, one of pure anatomy (gross and microscopic), with the biggest glands being deemed the offending glands and the smaller, normal glands deemed physiologically inactive—and therefore normal.

The principal reason behind the development of limited neck surgery and of minimally invasive radioguided parathyroidectomy is the strong improvement in preoperative localization imaging techniques, especially the parathyroid scintigraphy with $^{99m}$Tc-sestamibi.

## Preoperative Imaging Techniques

### Ultrasonography

Although ultrasound imaging has the advantages of being a noninvasive, low-cost, and non-ionizing procedure, the technique is highly operator-dependent. The accuracy of parathyroid tumor localization by ultrasound imaging varies according to the size and location of the adenoma. In particular, location in the substernal, retrotracheal, and retroesophageal spaces entails poor sensitivity due to acoustic shadowing from overlying bone or air. Parathyroid adenomas are identified by ultrasound with a 60% to 80% sensitivity (29,30), but the range is much wider (30% to 90%) when examining a patient for simply detecting enlarged parathyroid glands (31). Finally, ultrasound imaging sensitivity is reduced to about 40% in patients who have had prior failed surgical exploration (32).

Parathyroid adenomas located behind the thyroid gland or beyond the lower contour of the thyroid are detected by ultrasound imaging with high sensitivity. In contrast, it can be difficult to visualize upper parathyroid glands located medially (close to the larynx and trachea), or located deep in the neck in the para- and retropharyngeal space (31,33–35), or close to the carotid bifurcation (36,37).

Moreover, other structures in the neck, such as muscles, vessels, enlarged lymph nodes, and the esophagus, can mimic parathyroid enlargements (37). Given the non-negligible rate of false-positive ultrasound imaging results, specificity varies widely (40% to 100%) (29–35,38); this variability is probably linked to the fact that this imaging technique is highly operator-dependent.

Combining ultrasound results with those of other imaging procedures (e.g., thyroid scintigraphy) is useful in differentiating enlarged parathyroid glands from thyroid nodule(s) (30,33,38,39). This information is especially important in geographical areas where the prevalence of nodular goiter is high, and can lead to choosing the surgical approach best suited to the individual patients. Minimally invasive radioguided parathyroidectomy is not the best approach when thyroid nodular disease coexists, even in the presence of a single parathyroid adenoma (30,40). The diagnostic value of combined ultrasound imaging and thyroid scintigraphy is limited in the case of intrathyroidal parathyroid adenomas, which usually mimic the pattern of most of the thyroid nodules (hypoechoic, low-uptake areas) (36); in this regard, ultrasound-guided fine-needle aspiration cytology has proven useful to discriminate thyroid nodules from enlarged parathyroids (36). Combined ultrasound imaging and thyroid scintigraphy is of high value in patients with secondary hyperparathyroidism (29,30,34,38,39).

### Computed Tomography and Magnetic Resonance Imaging

Computed tomography (CT) and magnetic resonance (MR) imaging are often employed in the preoperative evaluation of primary hyperparathyroidism patients, especially in those with recurrent or persistent hyperparathyroidism, when the probability of ectopic glands is high. When ectopic adenomas are located in the mediastinum, the high anatomic definition of either CT and/or MR imaging provides useful topographic information for planning the best surgical approach.

While CT is useful for localizing parathyroid adenomas in the retrotracheal, retroesophageal, and mediastinal areas, it performs poorly for other ectopic locations (40–42), and even in discriminating upper from lower parathyroid glands (42–44). The overall sensitivity of CT consistently approaches 80% if the examination is performed with iodinated contrast enhancement (as adenomas and hyperplastic parathyroid glands are hypervascular), especially if performed before any neck surgery. Artifacts caused by metallic clips from previous surgery ("sparkler" effect) lower CT sensitivity to 46% to 58% (36,44,45).

Although MR cannot image normal parathyroid glands (since they are smaller than 5 mm) (46–48), its ability to characterize nodular lesions based on intensity changes in the T1- and T2-weighted images, as well as the possibility of contrast enhancement and three-dimensional reconstruction, makes this technique particularly attractive (41). Enlarged parathyroids display a medium intensity on T1-images (like thyroid tissue or muscle), but have considerably increased intensity on T2- and proton density images (49,50). However, the MR imaging pattern does not discriminate parathyroid adenomas from either simple hyperplasia or carcinoma.

Paired evaluations in the same patients have shown MR sensitivities similar to that of parathyroid scintigraphy—coupled, however, with consistently lower specificities (50–53). Discrepancies reported by different authors likely depend on the different patient populations studied (primary or secondary hyperparathyroidism, before first or second operation, presence or absence of thyroid nodules), and on the different imaging techniques.

Although some authors believe that MR is worth performing when parathyroid scintigraphy is negative or equivocal, or when it suggests an ectopic gland (52–54), others suggest the systematic use of combined MR imaging and parathyroid scintigraphy. Despite the associated high costs, this approach should increase the accuracy and reliability of preoperative identification and localization of parathyroid lesions (49,53).

For a long time, the less-than-optimal sensitivity of both CT and MR imaging has supported the rationale for traditional bilateral neck exploration (see below), in the absence of satisfactory preoperative localization protocols. In 1990, the National Institutes of Health consensus statement on the treatment of primary hyperparathyroidism concluded that preoperative localization in patients without prior neck operation was rarely indicated and not proven to be cost effective, as the surgeon was supposed to localize the glands by direct visualization intraoperatively (55).

This scenario has dramatically changed recently, following the introduction of more effective preoperative localization modalities, especially the parathyroid scintigraphy with $^{99m}$Tc-sestamibi.

## Parathyroid Scintigraphy

### Pre-$^{99m}$Tc-Sestamibi

No radiopharmaceuticals are available that concentrate specifically in the parathyroids, except perhaps in positron emission tomography (PET) for imaging parathyroid carcinoma (56). Scintigraphic exploration of this tissue is complicated by the intrinsic close proximity to—sometimes true "embedding" within—such a metabolically active parenchyma as the thyroid. Early attempts to circumvent this limitation originated the concept of using 2 tracers with different uptake patterns in those 2 tissues, thyroid and parathyroid (57). Although disappointing because of the technical limitations of the imaging equipment available at the time, it is worth mentioning the use of a radiolabeled amino acid ($^{75}$Se-methionine, actively concentrated in both the thyroid

and the parathyroid tissues because of their high metabolic activity), coupled with the simultaneous or sequential administration of a tracer specific for the thyroid tissue, such as $^{131}$I-iodide. After applying some "normalization" factor to the 2 scintigraphic acquisitions, the thyroid-only image (radioiodine) was subtracted from the thyroid + parathyroid image ($^{75}$Se-methionine), thus visualizing residual areas of radioactivity concentration corresponding to abnormal parathyroid glands.

This concept was later refined by Ferlin et al. (58), who opened the avenue to a more efficient modality of parathyroid imaging, so that parathyroid scintigraphy is now almost universally considered the best preoperative localizing method in patients with hyperparathyroidism. This new procedure was also based on dual tracer subtraction, replacing however $^{75}$Se-methionine with $^{201}$Tl-chloride, and $^{131}$I-iodine with $^{99m}$Tc-pertechnetate are both more suitable for gamma-camera imaging. This procedure (dual tracer $^{201}$Tl/$^{99m}$TcO$_4^-$ subtraction technique) proved to be of value for localizing parathyroid adenomas. However, because of its relatively low-energy gamma emission (about 70 to 80 keV) $^{201}$Tl-chloride is not an ideal radionuclide for gamma-camera imaging; furthermore, it entails a non-negligible radiation burden to patients, because of low-energy x-ray emission originated by electron capture. Thus, interest has quickly switched to $^{99m}$Tc-labeled compounds, following the initial reports on the possible use of such compounds for parathyroid scintigraphy, and because the dual isotope $^{201}$Tl/$^{99m}$TcO$_4^-$ procedure failed to demonstrate definite advantages over other imaging modalities, in part due to intrinsic variability and low reproducibility in interpreting the results among different centers (59,60).

## The $^{99m}$Tc-Sestamibi Era

Following the initial experience with $^{99m}$Tc-sestamibi for myocardial perfusion studies, Coakley and colleagues incidentally observed significant uptake and retention of this tracer in the abnormal parathyroids of patients with primary hyperparathyroidism (61). The success of using $^{99m}$Tc-sestamibi for localizing abnormal parathyroid glands (61–65) resulted in parathyroid scintigraphy becoming the standard imaging procedure (66), although with frequent site-to-site modifications of the imaging protocol.

Similarly as it occurs in other tissues, accumulation of $^{99m}$Tc-sestamibi in the parathyroid cells as a function of metabolic activity occurs specifically in the mitochondria. The overall uptake in hyperplastic and/or adenomatous parathyroid glands is linked to blood flow, gland size, and mitochondrial activity (67). $^{99m}$Tc-sestamibi accumulates both in the thyroid and in the parathyroid tissue within a few minutes after intra-

FIGURE 23-2. SPECT/CT images obtained from a patient with primary hyperparathyroidism, about 2 hours after the intravenous administration of $^{99m}$Tc-sestamibi. The lower right panel shows the anterior planar projection of the head and chest, where physiologic uptake in the myocardium and salivary glands is clearly visible; in addition, the parathyroid adenoma is clearly shown as an area of persistent tracer uptake located caudally along the body midline. The upper left, upper right, and lower left panels show the SPECT/CT fusion images, respectively in the transaxial, coronal, and sagittal planes. Both the transaxial and the sagittal sections clearly demonstrate the location of the parathyroid adenoma posteriorly to the trachea, thus providing to the surgeon useful preoperative information for planning the most adequate approach. (See Color Plate.)

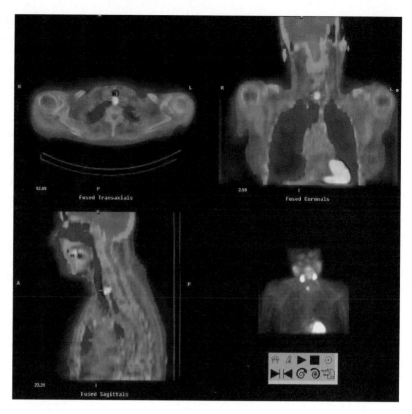

venous administration, but is released much faster from thyroid than from parathyroid tissue, likely due to down-regulation of the P-glycoprotein system (an out-flux carrier molecule for various substrates, including $^{99m}$Tc-sestamibi) in the parathyroid tissue (68–71). Concomitant suppression of thyroidal uptake obviously improves scintigraphic localization of parathyroid lesions with $^{99m}$Tc-sestamibi (72).

It is now generally acknowledged that high-quality scintigraphy with $^{99m}$Tc-sestamibi can accurately localize parathyroid adenomas in 85% to 95% of patients with primary hyperparathyroidism. The addition of single-photon emission computed tomography (SPECT) imaging considerably improves the localization of particular ectopic sites otherwise difficult to explore, such as the retroesophageal space or mediastinum (73–77) (Figure 23-2, see Color Plate). Any imaging protocol based on the use of $^{99m}$Tc-sestamibi intrinsically implies scintigraphic exploration not only of the neck (where parathyroid adenomas are most frequently located, reflecting the normal anatomy of the parathyroid glands), but also of the entire chest to rule out the possible presence of tumors in ectopic locations.

A wealth of information currently supports the use of $^{99m}$Tc-sestamibi scintigraphy as a preoperative localization technique for unilateral neck exploration and minimally invasive radioguided parathyroidectomy

(10,11,19–28,31,40,78–90). Different imaging protocols based on $^{99m}$Tc-sestamibi have developed according to local logistics and experience, as follows:

**Single tracer dual-phase scintigraphy:** This procedure, originally described by Taillefer et al. (91), is based solely on the differential washout rate of $^{99m}$Tc-sestamibi from the thyroid and, respectively, the parathyroid tissue. Scintigraphic acquisitions are recorded 15 minutes, then 2 to 3 hours after the intravenous injection of $^{99m}$Tc-sestamibi (approximately 740 MBq, or 20 mCi). Enlarged parathyroid glands or adenomas appear as areas of increased uptake persisting on late imaging (71) (see example in Figure 23-3). This dual-phase or washout imaging technique is easy to perform and has been shown to be highly sensitive and specific, especially in patients with primary hyperparathyroidism (92).

However, 2 problems may be encountered when systematically employing this procedure. First, solid thyroid nodules can avidly concentrate $^{99m}$Tc-sestamibi, regardless of whether they are benign or malignant, and whether they appear as "hot" or "cold" on the scan (93). Since nodular goiter is frequently associated with hyperparathyroidism in certain geographical areas (in more than 50% of the patients in Italy [94]), this occurrence may produce false-positive results, thus reducing the accuracy of the parathyroid scintigraphy (92,95). In patients with known or suspected concomitant nodular goiter, an

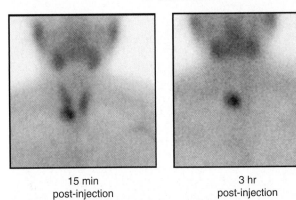

99mTc-Sestamibi

| 15 min | 3 hr |
| post-injection | post-injection |

FIGURE 23-3. Single tracer, dual-phase parathyroid scintigraphy with ⁹⁹ᵐTc-sestamibi. The left panel shows an image obtained 15 minutes postinjection, demonstrating physiologic early uptake in the thyroid gland, with a clear focus of increased uptake at the lower pole of the right thyroid lobe. The right panel shows an image obtained 3 hours postinjection, demonstrating virtually complete washout of ⁹⁹ᵐTc-sestamibi from the thyroid gland, with clear focal retention of radioactivity at the lower pole of the right thyroid lobe, the site of the parathyroid adenoma.

optional late scan with ⁹⁹ᵐTc-pertechnetate or ¹²³I-iodide may contribute to a better interpretation of the first images (92). The second limitation is the occurrence of false-negative results related to the possible (although infrequent) presence of parathyroid adenomas with a rapid ⁹⁹ᵐTc-sestamibi washout, similar to that of thyroid tissue (94,96).

**Dual tracer subtraction scintigraphy:** In this procedure, dual-phase ⁹⁹ᵐTc-sestamibi imaging is combined with administration of a second radiopharmaceutical accumulating solely in the thyroid gland and not in the parathyroid tissue; images are then subtracted to allow detection of focal uptakes specific for abnormal parathyroid tissue. Different protocols have been described, which vary according to the type of thyroid-imaging agent used and the sequence of tracer administration:

1. ¹²³I-iodide/⁹⁹ᵐTc-sestamibi dual-tracer subtraction technique (97)—The thyroid imaging agent ¹²³I (10 MBq) is injected first, followed 2 to 4 hours later by ⁹⁹ᵐTc-sestamibi administration. Imaging is performed at different times or simultaneously (using 2 separate energy windows: 140 keV for ⁹⁹ᵐTc, 159 keV for ¹²³I), and the thyroid image (¹²³I) is subtracted from the combined thyroid-parathyroid image (⁹⁹ᵐTc). Routine application of this procedure is limited by the high cost of ¹²³I (which is, moreover, not always available on a daily basis) and

by the long imaging time required to obtain satisfactory counting statistics in the ¹²³I scanning phase.

2. ⁹⁹ᵐTcO₄⁻/⁹⁹ᵐTc-sestamibi dual-tracer subtraction technique (98)—In this protocol, 185 MBq of ⁹⁹ᵐTc-pertechnetate is injected first, and thyroid imaging is recorded 20 minutes later. The ⁹⁹ᵐTc-sestamibi dose (300 MBq) is injected immediately thereafter without moving the patient, and a 20-minute dynamic acquisition is performed. High sensitivity (89%) and specificity (98%) have been reported with this procedure in patients with primary hyperparathyroidism (98). However, with the radioactive dose ratio as originally described, count rates deriving from ⁹⁹ᵐTc-pertechnetate concentrated in the thyroid tissue are relatively higher than those from ⁹⁹ᵐTc-sestamibi uptake, thus hampering identification of parathyroid adenomas located behind the thyroid contour, especially when planar imaging only is acquired. Geatti et al. (30) modified the technique by reducing the ⁹⁹ᵐTc-pertechnetate dose to 40 MBq, while at the same time increasing the ⁹⁹ᵐTc-sestamibi dose to 400 to 500 MBq. By adopting this modified protocol, 95% sensitivity was achieved in patients with primary hyperparathyroidism, without any false-positive result due to thyroid nodules. A further modification (99,100) aimed at shortening duration of the protocol implies the use of potassium perchlorate (KClO₄⁻) to achieve rapid washout of ⁹⁹ᵐTc-pertechnetate from the thyroid tissue, summarized as follows: 1) 150 MBq of ⁹⁹ᵐTcO₄⁻ is injected intravenously; 2) 20 minutes later, just before positioning the patient under the gamma camera, 400 mg of KClO₄⁻ is administered orally; 3) a 5-minute thyroid scan is acquired; 4) then, without moving the patient, 550 MBq of ⁹⁹ᵐTc-sestamibi is injected intravenously, and a dynamic planar acquisition of 7 5-minute frames covering the neck and the entire mediastinum is obtained. This dynamic sequence is evaluated sequentially, and the most adequate 5-minute frame is selected and used as a static scan for subtraction of the ⁹⁹ᵐTc-pertechnetate scan (after proper normalization), thus searching for possible sites of specific ⁹⁹ᵐTc-sestamibi accumulation; selecting just 1 frame out of the 7 frames recorded dynamically helps in reducing motion artefacts (see Figure 23-4). By applying this protocol (which also included an ultrasound scan of the neck performed in the same imaging session) to a group of 115 patients with primary hyperparathyroidism due to a solitary parathyroid adenoma, Casara et al. achieved 94% sensitivity, and no false-positive results despite concomitant nodular goiter in 29% of the patients (101).

3. ⁹⁹ᵐTc-sestamibi/⁹⁹ᵐTcO₄⁻ dual-tracer subtraction technique—In the case of equivocal discrimination of focal areas of tracer retention pertaining to the thyroid or parathyroid glands, a practicable way for improving interpretation of images acquired during a conventional dual-phase ⁹⁹ᵐTc-sestamibi parathyroid scintigraphy

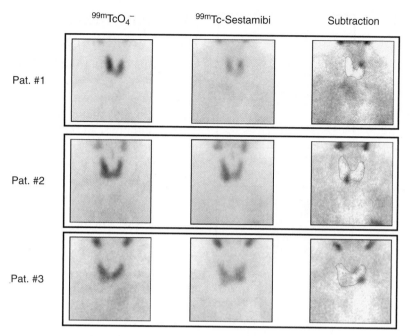

FIGURE 23-4. Parathyroid scintigraphy obtained in 3 different patients according to the dual-tracer protocol ($^{99m}$Tc-pertechnetate and $^{99m}$Tc-sestamibi), with administration of potassium perchlorate at the start of $^{99m}$Tc-pertechnetate imaging. In each row, the left panel shows the $^{99m}$Tc-pertechnetate scan ($^{99m}$TcO$_4^-$), the center panel shows a 5-minute scan recorded within 35 minutes upon $^{99m}$Tc-sestamibi injection (summation scan), and the right panel shows the subtraction scan. Although some indications about the presence of parathyroid adenomas can be derived by the summation scan, the subtraction images clearly delineate the parathyroid adenomas, respectively at the apex of the left lobe of the thyroid (patient 1, upper row), at the base of the right lobe of the thyroid (patient 2, center row), and at the base of the left lobe of the thyroid (patient 3, bottom row). In all these cases, minimally invasive radioguided surgery (performed according to the "low $^{99m}$Tc-sestamibi dose" protocol) confirmed the presence of a parathyroid adenoma at the locations shown by parathyroid scintigraphy.

is to administer the thyroid-imaging agent ($^{99m}$Tc-pertechnetate) after completing acquisition of the late $^{99m}$Tc-sestamibi image (at 2 to 3 hours). At this late time, most of the $^{99m}$Tc-sestamibi has already washed out from the thyroid, which is therefore easily imaged 20 minutes after injecting $^{99m}$TcO$_4^-$; the resulting image combines $^{99m}$Tc-pertechnetate uptake with some residual activity from the earlier $^{99m}$Tc-sestamibi injection, which is subtracted (based on the 2-hour scan) from the combined scan to obtain a "pure" $^{99m}$Tc-pertechnetate image, whose profile is superimposed on the late $^{99m}$Tc-sestamibi scan to resolve the interpretation dilemma (see Figure 23-5).

Experience acquired with the above protocols has demonstrated that different factors affect scintigraphic detection of enlarged parathyroid glands, including size, regional perfusion, functional activity and the corresponding cell cycle phase, and the prevalence of mitochondria-rich oxyphil cells (102,103). Based on a variable combination the above factors, hyperfunctioning parathyroid glands as small as 100 to 150 mg in mass

can be detected, especially when employing SPECT or other technical modalities for improved imaging (101–105).

In particular, the use of a pinhole collimator increases imaging resolution (although prolonging the imaging times), and can reasonably be adopted for a restricted anatomic area such as the neck. A larger area, such as the chest, is better explored with a parallel-hole collimator either in the planar mode or in the SPECT mode, with its added information on the depth of the lesion and topographic correlation with other anatomic structures (see Figure 23-2). Although in principle SPECT offers the advantage of easier discrimination between areas of focal $^{99m}$Tc-sestamibi retention in thyroid nodules and in the parathyroid tissue, in a busy clinical routine this imaging modality is rarely employed for exploring the neck alone. Instead, SPECT is used more frequently when exploring possible sites of ectopic parathyroid glands (primarily the mediastinum), particularly for better guiding the surgeon in preoperative planning. Since detection of parathyroid tumors in ectopic locations is usually not hampered by proximity with the

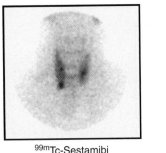

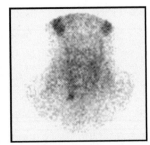

99mTc-Sestamibi
15 min

99mTc-Sestamibi
2.5 hr

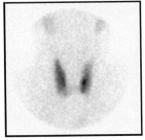

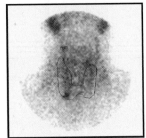

99mTcO₄⁻ with subtraction of
late 99mTc-Sestamibi

Late 99mTc-Sestamibi
with 99mTcO₄⁻ profile

FIGURE 23-5. Dual-phase parathyroid scintigraphy with
99mTc-sestamibi and 99mTc-pertechnetate ($^{99m}TcO_4^-$) in a patient
with primary hyperparathyroidism. The upper left panel shows
the image obtained 15 minutes postinjection of 99mTc-
sestamibi, demonstrating physiologic early uptake in the
thyroid gland, with a clear focus of increased accumulation at
the lower pole of the right thyroid lobe. The upper right panel
shows the late 99mTc-sestamibi scan, with some residual activity
in the thyroid gland and more obvious focal retention at the
lower pole of the right thyroid lobe. The second tracer
($^{99m}TcO_4^-$) is administered after recording the delayed 99mTc-
sestamibi scan. The lower left panel shows the image obtained
by subtracting the delayed scan from the summation scan
recorded after 99mTc-pertechnetate administration: this image
is used to draw the profile of the thyroid gland, which is then
superimposed on the delayed 99mTc-sestamibi scan (lower right
panel) for better anatomic localization of the parathyroid
adenoma (subsequently confirmed by minimally invasive
radioguided surgery).

# Minimally Invasive Radioguided Parathyroid Surgery: Operating Using Physiology in Addition to Anatomy

As described previously, the only reliable and repeatable
preoperative localizing test based upon physiology is the
99mTc-sestamibi scan that was serendipitously discovered
in the late 1980s (61). A test based upon physiology has
a dramatic advantage over other localizing studies, since
essentially all others are based upon anatomy, requiring
the offending gland(s) to be large enough to be detected
by the scan (e.g., ultrasound, CT, MR). 99mTc-sestamibi
scanning works by the systemic intravenous injection of
a 99mTc-labeled lipophilic cationic compound, which is
trapped into mitochondria in every cell of the body wherever adenosine-triphosphate (ATP) is being produced.
Thus, the degree of tracer uptake is related to: 1) the
number of mitochondria contained within each cell, and
2) their activity, i.e., how much ATP is being produced
within mitochondria. As described above, this 99mTc-
labeled compound is in no way specific for parathyroid
glands, but reflects mitochondrial activity and ATP
production. Thus, any localized accumulation of
highly active cells can easily be imaged with a gamma
camera.

In patients with hyperparathyroidism, any parathyroid
gland that is physiologically or supraphysiologically
active and synthesizing hormone will become radioactive after the injection of 99mTc-sestamibi, while those
that are dormant do not. Although normal glands will
take up the radiopharmaceutical similarly, as do all cells
in the body that contain active mitochondria, their small
size combined with a physiological baseline metabolic
activity hampers their scintigraphic visualization and the
possibility of localizing them using a gamma probe in the
operating room. In Norman's opinion, the most important aspect of radioguided parathyroid surgery is not
only the use of a gamma probe to help the surgeon find
the overproducing parathyroid gland, but also the estimation—based on metabolic activity as mirrored by the
uptake of 99mTc-sestamibi—how much hormone any individual parathyroid gland is producing. This indicates
when the patient is cured and the operation can be concluded. In this regard, Norman believes the gamma
probe can distinguish the difference between a normal
parathyroid gland, a hyperplastic parathyroid gland, and
a parathyroid adenoma. In fact, the probe is so accurate
at this determination that frozen sections are necessary
in a minority of Norman's cases (only 2.2% of their last
3000 parathyroid operations). He never uses intraoperative quick PTH assays. Moreover, in their experience the
probe allows the surgeon to know when the operation is
completed and when there is a need to look at other
glands. Norman usually performs 13 parathyroid opera-

thyroid gland, SPECT can easily be performed, with
satisfactory counting statistics, relatively soon after injection of 99mTc-sestamibi (e.g., within 30 to 40 minutes,
immediately after having explored the neck and thorax
with the early planar views). Although only a marginal
improvement in the overall detection rate of parathyroid
adenomas is reported with SPECT (so that the added
cost of its routine use is not always justified), most authors
now favor a wider application of this imaging modality,
especially in patients with recurring hyperparathyroidism
after prior surgery (34,36,67,74,78,103).

tions daily (approximately 1,800 per year), which are completed in an average of 16.6 minutes (skin to skin). In his experience, cure rate for the past 3,500 patients was (99.3%).

## Characteristics of the Gamma Probe for Parathyroid Surgery

In the early 1990s, Norman's group pioneered the use of a gamma probe intraoperatively to locate parathyroid tumors immediately after a $^{99m}$Tc-sestamibi scan (21–24). Others in that group were actively pursuing radioguided surgery and sentinel lymph node biopsy for melanoma and breast cancer. In that center, after much experimentation, it was realized that the probes being developed for sentinel node localization were not optimized for parathyroidectomy. Although the radioactive agent was the same, the associated radiopharmaceutical was unrelated and the means of delivery were dissimilar. Sentinel node localization was accomplished by a subcutaneous injection, whereby the radioactive colloid is transported by lymphatics to the sentinel node. This was in contrast to a systemic intravenous injection for parathyroid localization that causes all tissues in the body to become radioactive to some degree. The optimal probe used for sentinel node localization would be required to locate a radioactive lymph node in a cold background, while that for parathyroid localization was required to find a hot gland in a hot background. An optimal probe was developed in Norman's center and subsequently made widely available. Initially, surgeons performed radioguided parathyroid surgery assuming that the probe used for lymph node mapping could be used for parathyroid surgery as well. However, while these probes will help find large tumors, their use for tumors less than 1 cm is limited. Norman and colleagues are aware of only 1 probe made specifically for parathyroid surgery, and it is produced by U.S. Surgical Corp. (Norwalk, Conn.).

As recently reported by Mariani et al. (106), it is accepted in different centers worldwide that a probe for parathyroid surgery should be characterized by a small diameter (11-mm is ideal), high sensitivity, and high spatial resolution, and should be collimated to avoid "shine-through" effect.

One technical error that may arise is for the surgeon to point the probe into the chest and explore the upper mediastinum, believing that high radioactive counts are due to a large tumor when in fact the high readings are due to the extreme radioactivity of the cardiac ventricles. It is imperative for the surgeon to recognize the interfering radioactivity from other organs trapping $^{99m}$Tc-sestamibi. For this reason and others, the surgeon needs the support of a nuclear medicine physician who is confident with the kinetics and biodistribution of $^{99m}$Tc-sestamibi, thus assuring correct use of the gamma probe intraoperatively.

## The Probe as a Physiologic Tool: Determining Parathyroid Activity Real-Time

All of Norman's early publications regarding the use of a probe to assist with parathyroid surgery were geared toward issues of timing, probe selection, and intraoperative successes (21,22). Norman's minimally invasive radioguided parathyroidectomy protocol is based on a single-day procedure, including the injection of a scintigraphic 20 to 25 mCi dose of $^{99m}$Tc-sestamibi, acquisition of parathyroid scintigraphy with a dual-phase technique, and an operation performed soon thereafter. Ideally, the operation needs to be performed within 3 hours of the injection, with an optimum time of 1 to 2.5 hours postinjection. After the first 100 or so cases, Norman and colleagues noted that the gamma probe did not just tell them where the radioactive parathyroid tumor was located within the neck, it also told them with extremely high accuracy which glands were adenomatous, hyperplastic, or normal based upon the amount of radioactivity they had incorporated (25). The first publication of Norman et al. regarding the use of the probe to determine individual parathyroid gland physiologic activity included 1,336 specimens. The authors have since collected data on more than 15,000 specimens, allowing them to establish rules by which in nearly 98% of their cases intraoperative identification of the hyperfunctioning parathyroid tissue by the gamma probe is not equivocal, and therefore no frozen section examination is required. Based on such experience, they never use intraoperative quick PTH assays, confident that the measurements taken by the probe are more reliable predictors than microscopic anatomical examinations or PTH assays. This information has been lost, however, at least in part, as most surgeons think the probe is used solely to help find the tumor. As stated previously, that is only one aspect of the probe's uses—the surgeon can obtain functional information, other than anatomical, on enlarged parathyroid glands using the probe intraoperatively.

The data obtained with Norman's protocol are presented in Figure 23-6, which shows radioactivity in 14,564 surgical specimens taken during 4000 parathyroid operations. The ex-vivo measures were taken with the tissues removed from the patient and held away from the patient, so that determination of the radioactivity contained in the tissue (expressed as counts per second) was not influenced by the radioactivity emitted by the patient; this measurement cannot be done with the specimen placed on the patient. All measures are expressed as a

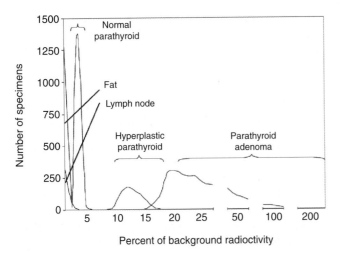

FIGURE 23-6. The 20% rule. Ex-vivo radioactivity of 14,564 specimens removed during 4000 parathyroid operations, expressed as a percentage of background radioactivity. The probe allows normal parathyroid glands, hyperplastic parathyroid glands, and parathyroid adenomas to be differentiated from each other and from other nonparathyroid tissues in the neck. Parathyroid adenomas are the only tissues in the neck to possess 20% or more of background radioactivity. Parathyroid adenomas n = 3889; hyperplastic parathyroids n = 426; normal parathyroids n = 5690; fat n = 3883; thymus n = 399 (not shown); lymph nodes n = 282.

percent of background radioactivity, which was obtained by placing the probe adjacent to the patient's carotid artery aimed at the spine (aiming away from the radioactive submandibular and thyroid glands). Background radioactivity was used as a measure to compensate for the time that had passed from injection, for volume of distribution, and for amount injected. All determinations of tumor and/or background radioactivity were done in patients less than 3.5 hours from the $^{99m}$Tc-sestamibi injection; the surgeon is cautioned that using these measures after 3.5 hours may decrease slightly the specificity of the test. As illustrated in Figure 23-6, certain tissues do not take up radioactivity to such a degree that a surgeon armed with a probe would mistake it as parathyroid tissue and thus waste time performing a frozen section or change the operative approach, thinking a parathyroid gland has been removed. Lymph nodes, fat, muscle, and thymus tissues will not uptake enough radioactivity to possess more than 2% of background radioactivity. If a piece of tissue is removed and the surgeon is not sure if it is a normal parathyroid or a lymph node, he/she simply has to measure its ex-vivo radioactivity. If the surgeon is not sure if the tissue is a piece of fat or a normal parathyroid gland and the probe detects 9 counts per second (given a background of 1000 counts per second), then

this tissue is fat and cannot be parathyroid tissue. These rules hold true for one-half or even one-eighth of a parathyroid gland (as a portion taken as a biopsy, which is how we advise the measures of normal glands to be performed). If there is any question, the surgeon simply measures the radioactivity in a control piece of subcutaneous fat of a similar size removed for this purpose and comparisons are made. This maneuver, which takes several seconds, is 100% accurate in Norman's experience. Thus, in his opinion there should never be a time when a frozen section is required to determine if tissue is parathyroid, a lymph node, or fat. The opposite is true when a parathyroid adenoma is removed. Norman and colleagues established specific guidelines using their protocol for the definitive identification of a parathyroid adenoma without the use of frozen section analysis in their 1999 publication the "Twenty Percent Rule" (25), which they still believe is valid after more than 15,000 specimens. In this series, with 1 exception (discussed below) there are no tissues that can be removed from a patient's neck other than a parathyroid adenoma that will possess 20% or more of that patient's background radioactivity. Therefore, following this protocol and the 20% rule, if tissue is removed and it appears to the trained surgeon to be an adenoma, and it contains 20% or more of background radioactivity, it is a parathyroid adenoma. No frozen section analysis is needed to confirm this, and doing nothing more will provide a cure rate in approximately 97% of all patients with this disease. Documenting at least 1 normal gland in a patient with a single adenoma seen on a preoperative scan will increase the statistical cure rate to more than 99%, as outlined subsequently. As can be seen in Figure 23-6, hyperplastic parathyroid glands will never meet the 20% rule in a patient with sporadic primary hyperparathyroidism. With this approach, Norman and colleagues have not seen a hyperplastic parathyroid gland (parathyroid hyperplasia) meet the 20% rule, therefore in nearly 5000 cases this rule had a 100% accuracy and positive predictive value. When used in patients with sporadic, primary hyperparathyroidism, Norman and colleagues observed only 1 exception to the rule, whereby a surgeon could remove a tumor from a patient's neck that possesses 20% or more of background radioactivity—that being a discrete functioning thyroid adenoma (functioning follicular adenoma). Occasionally, frozen section analysis is used to confirm a parathyroid tumor removed from within the substance of the thyroid gland (an intrathyroid parathyroid adenoma). Furthermore, using Norman's protocol, hyperplastic glands from patients with secondary hyperparathyroidism due to renal insufficiency will often meet the 20% rule (usually 2 or 3 of the glands will meet this criteria). Thus, when operating on patients with secondary or tertiary hyperparathyroidism, the probe will definitively distinguish parathyroid glands from other tissues in the neck and will eliminate the use of frozen section analysis. The surgeon must be aware that these diseases are associated with 4-gland enlargement and hormone overproduction in all 4 of the parathyroid glands. Therefore, finding a single tumor that meets the 20% rule is not an indication for concluding the operation in patients with secondary or tertiary hyperparathyroidism. In Norman's experience, in patients with primary hyperparathyroidism, hyperplastic parathyroid glands will contain between 7% and 18% of background radioactivity. Norman has never seen a case where a hyperplastic gland met the 20% rule in a non-renal failure patient. Thus, Norman concluded that the probe can determine with high accuracy an adenoma from all other parathyroid tissues (100% accuracy, if the 20% rule is met), and can determine with high accuracy a normal parathyroid gland from any other tissues in the neck. There are only 2 areas of overlap, as seen in Figure 23-6: the small hyperplastic gland that can be confused with a normal gland, and a small adenoma that does not meet the 20% rule. About 3.5% of parathyroid adenomas do not meet the 20% rule and will contain between 15% and 19% of background radioactivity. Norman's protocol requires an examination of all 4 parathyroid glands in any patient where removal of a clinically obvious adenoma does not meet the 20% rule. Again, this is the area of overlap between hyperplastic glands and adenomas in Figure 23-1, where the removed tissue contains between 14% and 20% of background radioactivity, which occurs in approximately 3.5% of patients.

# Norman's Minimally Invasive Radioguided Parathyroidectomy Protocol

The following outline is Norman's current protocol for minimally invasive radioguided parathyroidectomy in a patient with sporadic, nonfamilial, non-MEN primary hyperparathyroidism. Following these rules allows for elimination of frozen section analysis in more than 90% of cases, and elimination of intraoperative PTH assays in all cases.

1. The patient undergoes his/her first and only $^{99m}$Tc-sestamibi scan on the morning of the operation.
2. The patient is taken to the operating room within 1.5 to 2 hours of the isotope injection.
3. The side of the neck showing the tumor is explored first (or the side that suggests the tumor, if the scan does not show a definitive tumor).

4. The probe is placed into the field after the strap muscles are lifted off the thyroid gland, in the expected area of the adenoma. Blunt dissection is used exclusively to identify the tumor, with the probe placed into the field as often as necessary.
5. The adenoma is removed, its radioactivity measured, and the percent of background radioactivity calculated.
6. If the patient had a positive $^{99m}$Tc-sestamibi scan (solitary focus of radioactivity distinct from the thyroid) and the tumor meets the 20% rule, the operation is concluded once 1 normal gland can be found. A small piece of the normal gland is removed as a biopsy and it is proven to be a normal parathyroid by measuring its ex-vivo radioactivity (and using a similarly sized piece of fat as a control, if necessary). The thyroid should also be examined during nearly all parathyroid operations. This patient is cured at a statistical rate of 99.8%. No frozen sections are required, and no intraoperative hormone assays are performed.
7. If the preoperative $^{99m}$Tc-sestamibi scan is negative, then the exploration is conducted in a standard fashion and the probe is used to distinguish between normal, hyperplastic, and adenomatous glands. Frozen section analysis is almost always avoided by using the probe to distinguish parathyroid glands from lymph nodes and fat, and to distinguish normal dormant parathyroid glands from overproducing glands. If at any time a parathyroid tumor is found that meets the 20% rule, the operation is concluded provided at least 1 normal gland is located. The only concern is the small chance of a double adenoma. The surgeon's experience and the quality of the preoperative scan will determine whether the third and/or fourth gland should be located. Any parathyroid glands that are located may be biopsied (not removed) and proved to be normal parathyroid glands by comparison to subcutaneous fat, as required by the surgeon's experience.
8. Frozen section analysis should only be necessary in cases that are confusing and/or nonstandard in their presentation—about 3% to 5% for surgeons experienced in the interpretation of the probe data (the area of overlap in Figure 23-6). Intraoperative hormone assays will add nothing to this operation and often will lead to further dissection because of a false-negative reading. At the very least, these measures will delay the operation by 30 minutes. We never use intraoperative PTH assays and strongly discourage their use. Ninety-two percent of the past 220 re-operations that we have performed after another surgeon failed to find the parathyroid gland had originally used intraoperative hormone assays that either did not help or provided significantly incorrect information.

(Note that the techniques and methods described here for performing radioguided parathyroidectomy following Norman's protocol are protected by a United States patent.)

Other authors in Europe have developed a different protocol for minimally invasive radioguided parathyroidectomy. While Norman's protocol is characterized by a single-day scintigraphic imaging and surgery, Rubello and Mariani from the Italian Study Group of Radioguided Surgery and Immunoscintigraphy (GISCRIS) (11,40,83–90) proposed a different-day protocol based on thyroid/parathyroid scintigraphy plus ultrasonography. In the following days (usually within a week), they administer in the operating room a very low (1 mCi) $^{99m}$Tc-sestamibi dose for the purpose of minimally invasive radioguided parathyroidectomy only, without obtaining further scintigraphic imaging the day of the operation. Detailed information on this minimally invasive radioguided parathyroidectomy technique is presented below.

## Rubello and Mariani's Low $^{99m}$Tc-Sestamibi Dose, Minimally Invasive Radioguided Parathyroidectomy Protocol

1. Parathyroid scintigraphy is obtained some days before the operation by dual tracer $^{99m}$TcO$_4^-$/$^{99m}$Tc-sestamibi subtraction technique, using administration of potassium perchlorate to speed $^{99m}$TcO$_4^-$ washout from thyroid tissue, thus obtaining early, good quality $^{99m}$Tc-sestamibi images. They prefer obtaining a $^{99m}$TcO$_4^-$ thyroid scan as well, because of the high prevalence of coexisting thyroid nodules (approximately 30% of cases in their geographic area), which can cause false-positive results with a $^{99m}$Tc-sestamibi scan. In the same session of planar scintigraphy, a high-resolution neck ultrasonogram is obtained and, in cases of discordant scan/ultrasound findings, the imaging workup is completed with a tomographic SPECT head-chest acquisition.

2. The day of the operation, in the operating room blood samples are drawn from the patient from a peripheral vein both before commencing surgery and 10 minutes following parathyroid adenoma removal to measure intraoperative quick PTH levels. Quick PTH is measured because some cases of primary hyperparathyroidism are due to hyperplasia or multiple adenomas, in which Norman's "20% rule" fails. This may be because with this protocol, minimally invasive radioguided parathyroidectomy is performed 10 minutes after $^{99m}$Tc-sestamibi injection, instead of 1.5 to 3 hours later, as in Norman's.

3. The day of surgery, a low (1 mCi) $^{99m}$Tc-sestamibi dose is injected into the patient's forearm vein in the operating room about 10 minutes before the operation;

the injection is followed by a flush of 30 mL of saline to avoid radiotracer stagnation in the veins.

4. Prior to the surgical incision, the patient's neck is scanned with an 11-mm collimated probe to identify the area of maximum count activity in the skin overlying the parathyroid adenoma.

5. A low transverse midline neck incision (approximately 1 cm above the sternal notch) is usually performed to permit easy conversion to bilateral neck exploration, if necessary. High lateral neck access is preferred in some superior adenomas, and in adenomas ectopically located at the carotid bifurcation.

6. A 11-mm collimated probe is repeatedly inserted through the 15-mm skin incision guiding the surgeon to the area of maximum count activity corresponding to the parathyroid adenoma. In some patients with an adenoma located deep in the neck, ligature of the middle thyroid vein and of inferior thyroid artery is required.

7. Radioactivity is measured with the probe on the parathyroid adenoma, thyroid gland, and background.

8. Radioactivity is measured ex vivo on the parathyroid adenoma to evaluate successful removal of parathyroid tissue; frozen section analysis of the surgical specimen is routinely obtained. Although in some centers this is a routine examination for all types of interventions, common experience indicates that this step could be avoided in most patients.

9. Radioactivity is checked on the empty parathyroid bed to evaluate the completeness of the parathyroid tissue resection.

10. Tissue ratios are calculated (parathyroid to background, or P/B; parathyroid to thyroid, or P/T; thyroid to background, or T/B). In particular, in the absence of $^{99m}$Tc-sestamibi-avid thyroid nodules, a P/T ratio higher than 1.5 strongly suggests the presence of a parathyroid adenoma, while typical P/B ratios (excluding the thyroid tissue) range between 2.5 and 4.5. An empty parathyroid bed-to-thyroid ratio approaching 1 is highly indicative of complete removal of abnormal parathyroid tissue; however, this can also be observed when simply hyperplastic parathyroid tissue or even a thyroid nodule is removed, rather than a parathyroid adenoma, so that we prefer to measure intraoperative quick PTH.

11. Finally, assessment of radioactivity in all 4 quadrants before the end of the surgical exploration ensures that all hyperfunctioning glands are removed.

The main advantage of the single-day Norman protocol is that imaging and surgery are obtained in the same session. The main advantages of Rubello and Mariani's protocol are that: 1) using a dual-tracer scintigraphy, they also obtain information about the thyroid gland and identify thyroid nodules that can trap $^{99m}$Tc-sestamibi, potentially giving false-positive results both preoperatively when using the single-tracer $^{99m}$Tc-sestamibi and the dual-phase or wash-out technique, and during minimally invasive radioguided parathyroidectomy; 2) the low $^{99m}$Tc-sestamibi dose injected in the operating room a few minutes before affords minimal radiation exposure to the surgeon and operating room personnel.

The Norman protocol may be preferable in geographic areas with a low prevalence of concomitant thyroid nodules, while Rubello and Mariani's protocol would be preferred in geographic areas with a high prevalence of nodular goiter, such as in central and southern Europe.

## Conclusion

Minimally invasive radioguided parathyroidectomy surgery cures a patient of parathyroid disease in the least invasive and most directed fashion possible. This requires that the surgeon conducts the procedure in such a way that physiology becomes central to the operation, monitoring how much hormone is being produced by any and all removed parathyroid glands. In the experience of some centers, intraoperative radionuclide mapping is the best way that individual parathyroid gland function can be assessed, and this can be done quickly. These rapid assessments allow the surgeon to know when the operation can be concluded and when further dissection is necessary. This quick and simple technique is clearly better for primary hyperparathyroidism patients, is significantly less expensive, and is already leading to a significantly higher percentage of patients with hyperparathyroidism being referred to surgeons by endocrinologists and primary care physicians. Gamma-probe guidance enables the surgeon to perform a rather small skin incision, improved cosmesis being one of the main advantages of this technique, which can also be performed under local anesthesia. The operating time is reduced compared to that for conventional exploration not based on radioguidance, and the patient can be discharged from the hospital earlier.

As with other radioguided surgical procedures (e.g., sentinel lymph node biopsy), the technique requires that the whole team involved (nuclear medicine specialist, surgeon, pathologist, nursing) achieve a satisfactory amount of experience and smooth interaction among team members.

Some recommendations should be followed when considering minimally invasive radioguided parathyroidectomy: 1) the most accurate preoperative scintigraphic modality available should be used, possibly dual-tracer subtraction scintigraphy or dual-phase $^{99m}$Tc-sestamibi SPECT; 2) both in-vivo and ex-vivo gamma probe counting should be obtained to evaluate the success and completeness of the surgery; 3) radiation exposure to

the surgeon and operating room personnel should be minimized by administering the lowest dose of $^{99m}$Tc-sestamibi proved to be effective for performing minimally invasive radioguided parathyroidectomy. Intraoperative quick PTH measurement appears to be strictly related to the minimally invasive radioguided parathyroidectomy protocol used.

The operating surgeon, however, must realize that new techniques and tools are not a substitute for experience, and having a probe in the operating room does not necessarily make an expert out of a surgeon who sees parathyroid patients infrequently. Common sense and a thorough knowledge of parathyroid anatomy are critically important.

## References

1. Bilezikian JP, Silverberg SJ. Clinical spectrum of primary hyperparathyroidism. *Rev Endocr Metab Disord*. 2000;1: 237–245.
2. Sywak MS, Robinson BG, Clifton-Bligh P, et al. Increase in presentations and procedure rates for hyperparathyroidism in Northern Sydney and New South Wales. *Med J Aust*. 2002;177:246–249.
3. Heath H 3rd, Hodgson SF, Kennedy MA. Primary hyperparathyroidism. Incidence, morbidity, and potential economic impact in a community. *N Engl J Med*. 1980;302: 189–193.
4. Clark OH, Siperstein AE. The hypercalcemic syndrome. In: Friesen SR, Thompson NW, eds. *Surgical Endocrinology Clinical Syndromes*. Philadelphia: Lippincott; 1990: 311–339.
5. Palmer M, Jakobsson S, Akerstrom G, Ljunghall S. Prevalence of hypercalcemia in a health survey: a 14-year follow-up study of serum calcium values. *Eur J Clin Invest*. 1988;18:39–46.
6. Melton LJ 3rd. The epidemiology of primary hyperparathyroidism in North America. *J Bone Miner Res*. 2002; 17(suppl 2): N12–N17.
7. Adami S, Marcocci C, Gatti D. Epidemiology of primary hyperparathyroidism in Europe. *J Bone Miner Res*. 2002;17(suppl 2):N18–N23.
8. Cheung PS, Boey JH, Wang CC, Ma JT, Lam KS, Yeung RT. Primary hyperparathyroidism: its clinical pattern and results of surgical treatment in Hong Kong Chinese. *Surgery*. 1988:103:558–562.
9. Bilezikian JP, Meng X, Shi Y, Silverberg SJ. Primary hyperparathyroidism in women: a tale of 2 cities—New York and Beijing. *Int J Fertil Womens Med*. 2000;45: 158–165.
10. Norman J. Minimally invasive parathyroid surgery. Recent trends becoming standard of care yielding smaller, more successful operations at a lower cost. *Otolaryngol Clin North Am*. 2004;37:683–688.
11. Mariani G, Gulec SA, Rubello D, et al. Preoperative localisation and radioguided parathyroid surgery. *J Nucl Med*. 2003;44:1443–1458.

12. Thompson NW, Eckhauser FE, Harness JK. The anatomy of primary hyperparathyroidism. *Surgery*. 1982;92:814–821.

13. Metz D, Jensen R, Allen B, et al. Multiple endocrine neoplasia type 1: clinical features and management. In: Bilezikian J, Levine M, Marcus R, eds. *The Parathyroids*. New York: Raven Press; 1994:591–647.

14. Mandl F. Therapeutischer versuch bei osteitis fibrosa generalisata mittels exstirpation eines epithelkoerpechen tumors. *Wien Klin Wochenschr*. 1925;195:1343–1344.

15. Kaplan EL, Yashiro T, Salti G. Primary hyperparathyroidism in the 1990s. Choice of surgical procedures for this disease. *Ann Surg*. 1992;215:301–317.

16. Rose MD, Wood TF, Van Herle AJ, et al. Long-term management and outcome of parathyroidectomy for sporadic primary multiple gland disease. *Arch Surg*. 2001;136:621–626.

17. Udelsman R. Six hundred fifty-six consecutive explorations for primary hyperparathyroidism. *Ann Surg*. 2002;235:665–672.

18. Lee NC, Norton JA. Multiple gland disease in primary hyperparathyroidism: a function of operative approach? *Arch Surg*. 2002;137:896–900.

19. Norman J. Minimally invasive radioguided parathyroidectomy: an endocrine surgeon's perspective. *J Nucl Med*. 1998;39:15N–24N.

20. Norman J, Jaffray C, Chheda H. The false positive parathyroid sestamibi: a real or perceived problem and a case for radioguided parathyroidectomy. *Ann Surg*. 2000;231:31–37.

21. Norman J, Chheda H. Minimally invasive parathyroidectomy facilitated by intraoperative nuclear mapping. *Surgery*. 1997;122:998–1004.

22. Norman J. The technique of intraoperative nuclear mapping to facilitate minimally invasive parathyroidectomy. *Cancer Control*. 1997;4:500–504.

23. Norman J, Chheda H, Farrell C. Minimally invasive parathyroidectomy for primary hyperparathyroidism: decreasing operative time and potential complications while improving cosmetic results. *Am Surg*. 1998;64:391–396.

24. Costello D, Norman J. Minimally invasive radio-guided parathyroidectomy (MIRP). *Surg Clin North Am*. 1999;8:555–564.

25. Murphy C, Norman J. The 20 percent rule: a simple instantaneous radioactivity measurement defines cure and allows elimination of frozen section and hormone assays during parathyroidectomy. *Surgery*. 1999;126:1023–1029.

26. Denham D, Norman J. Cost effectiveness of preoperative sestamibi scans for primary hyperparathyroidism is dependent solely on surgeon's choice of operative procedure. *J Am Coll Surg*. 1998;186:293–304.

27. Denham DW, Norman J. Cost utility of routine imaging with Tc99m-sestamibi in primary hyperparathyroidism before initial surgery. *Am Surg*. 1999;65:796–797.

28. Gallagher S, Denham D, Murr MM, Norman J. The impact of minimally invasive parathyroidectomy on the way endocrinologists treat primary hyperparathyroidism. *Surgery* 2003;134:910–917.

29. Ammori BJ, Madan M, Gopichandran TD, et al. Ultrasound-guided unilateral neck exploration for sporadic primary hyperparathyroidism: is it worthwhile? *Ann R Coll Surg Engl*. 1998;80:433–437.

30. Geatti O, Shapiro B, Orsolon P, et al. Localization of parathyroid enlargement: experience with technetium 99m methoxyisobutylisonitrile and thallium-201 scintigraphy, ultrasound and computed tomography. *Eur J Nucl Med*. 1994;21:17–23.

31. Casara D, Rubello D, Pelizzo MR, Shapiro B. Role of preoperative imaging with $^{99m}$Tc/MIBI scintigraphy combined with neck ultrasound, and of intraoperative $^{99m}$Tc-sestamibi gamma probe technique in planning unilateral and minimally invasive surgery in primary hyperparathyroidism. *Eur J Nucl Med*. 2001;28:1351–1359.

32. Miller DL, Doppman MD, Shawker MD, et al. Localisation of parathyroid adenomas in patients who have undergone surgery. *Radiology*. 1987;162:133–137.

33. Duh QY, Sancho JJ, Clark OH. Parathyroid localization, clinical review. *Acta Chir Scand*. 1987;153:241–254.

34. Uden P, Aspelin P, Berglund J. Preoperative localization in unilateral parathyroid surgery. A cost-benefit study on ultrasound, computed tomography and scintigraphy. *Acta Chir Scand*. 1990;156:29–35.

35. Gofrit ON, Labensart PD, Pikarsky A, Lackstein D, Gross DJ, Shiloni E. High-resolution ultrasonography: highly sensitive, specific technique for preoperative localization of parathyroid adenoma in the absence of multinodular thyroid disease. *World J Surg*. 1997;21:287–290.

36. Lloyd MNH, Lees WR, Milroy EJG. Preoperative localization in primary hyperparathyroidism. *Clin Radiol*. 1990;41:239–243.

37. Beierwaltes WH. Endocrine imaging: parathyroid, adrenal cortex and medulla, and other endocrine tumors. Part 2. *J Nucl Med*. 1991;32:1627–1639.

38. Tomasella G. Diagnostic imaging in primary hyperparathyroidism. Radiological techniques: US—CT—MR. *Minerva Endocrinol*. 2001;26:3–12.

39. De Feo ML, Colagrande S, Biagini C, et al. Parathyroid glands: combination of $^{99m}$Tc-MIBI scintigraphy and US for demonstration of parathyroid glands and nodules. *Radiology*. 2000;214:393–402.

40. Rubello D, Piotto A, Medi F, et al. Italian Study Group on Radioguided Surgery and Immunoscintigraphy. *Eur J Surg Oncol*. 2005;31:191–196.

41. Udelsman R. Is unilateral neck exploration for parathyroid adenoma appropriate? *Adv Surg*. 2000;34:319–329.

42. Koong HN, Choong LH, Soo KC. The role of preoperative localisation techniques in surgery for hyperparathyroidism. *Ann Acad Med Singapore*. 1998;27:192–195.

43. Mitchell BK, Merrel RC, Kinder BK. Localization studies in patients with hyperpara-thyroidism. *Surg Clin North Am*. 1995;75:483–498.

44. Eisenberg H, Pallotta J, Sacks B, Brickman AS. Parathyroid localisation, three dimensional modelling and percutaneous ablation techniques. *Endocrinol Metab Clin North Am*. 1989;18:659–700.

45. Levin KE, Clark OH. Localisation of parathyroid glands. *Ann Rev Med*. 1988;39:29–40.

46. Stark DD, Moss AA, Gooding GAW, Clark OH. Parathyroid scanning by computed tomography. *Radiology.* 1983;148:297–299.

47. Weber AL, Randolph G, Aksoy FG. The thyroid and parathyroid glands. CT and MR imaging and correlation with pathology and clinical findings. *Radiol Clin North Am.* 2000;38:1105–1129.

48. Kneeland JB, Krubsack AJ, Lawson TL, et al. Enlarged parathyroid glands: high-resolution local coil MR Imaging. *Radiology.* 1987;162:143–146.

49. Stark DD, Clark OH, Moss AA. Magnetic resonance imaging of the thyroid, thymus and parathyroid glands. *Surgery.* 1984;96:1083–1090.

50. Stark DD, Moss AA, Gamsu G, Clark OH, Gooding-GAW, Webb WR. Magnetic resonance imaging of the neck. Part 2: pathologic findings. *Radiology.* 1984;150: 455–461.

51. Lee VS, Spritzer CE, Coleman RE, Wilkinson RH Jr, Coogan AC, Leight GS Jr. The complementary roles of fast spin-echo MR imaging and double-phase $^{99m}$Tc-sestamibi scintigraphy for localization of hyperfunctioning parathyroid glands. *Am J Roentgenol.* 1996;167: 1555–1562.

52. Lee VS, Spritzer CE. MR imaging of abnormal parathyroid glands. *Am J Roentgenol.* 1998;170:1097–1103.

53. Hishibashi M, Nishida H, Hiromatsu Y, Kojima K, Tabuchi E, Hayabuchi N. Comparison of technetium-99m-MIBI, technetium-99m-tetrofosmin, ultrasound, and MRI for localization of abnormal parathyroid glands. *J Nucl Med.* 1988;39:320–324.

54. Fayet P, Hoeffel C, Fulla Y, et al. Technetium-99m-sestamibi, magnetic resonance imaging and venous blood sampling in persistent and recurrent hyperparathyroidism. *Br J Radiol.* 1997;70:459–464.

55. Anonymous. NIH Conference. Diagnosis and management of asymptomatic primary hyperparathyroidism: consensus development conference statement. Consensus Development Conference, NIH. *Ann Intern Med.* 1991;114:593–597.

56. Sundin A, Johansson C, Hellman P, et al. PET and parathyroid L-[carbon-11]methionine accumulation in hyperparathyroidism. *J Nucl Med.* 1996;37:1766–1770.

57. Di Giulio W, Morales J. An evaluation of parathyroid scanning using selenium-75-methionine. *J Nucl Med.* 1966;7:380–384.

58. Ferlin G, Borsato N, Camerani M. New perspectives in localizing enlarged parathyroids by technetium-thallium subtraction scan. *J Nucl Med.* 1983;24:438–441.

59. Samanta A, Wilson B, Iqbal J, Burden AC, Walls J, Cosgriff P. A clinical audit of thallium-technetium subtraction parathyroid scans. *Postgrad Med J.* 1990;66: 441–445.

60. Nicholson DA, Dawson P, Lavender JP. Imaging of the parathyroids. In: Lynn J, Bloom SR, eds. *Surgical Endocrinology.* Oxford: Butterworth-Heinemann; 1993:351–361.

61. Coakley AJ, Kettle AG, Wells CP, O'Doherty MJ, Collins REC. $^{99m}$Tc-sestamibi—a new agent for parathyroid imaging. *Nucl Med Commun.* 1989;10:791–794.

62. O'Doherty MJ, Kettle AG, Wells P, Collins REC, Coakley AJ. Parathyroid imaging with technetium-99m-sestamibi: preoperative localization and tissue uptake studies. *J Nucl Med.* 1992;33:313–319.

63. Taillefer R, Boucher Y, Potvin C, et al. Detection and localization of parathyroid adenomas in patients with hyperparathyroidism using a single radionuclide imaging procedure with technetium-99m-sestamibi (double phase study). *J Nucl Med.* 1992;33:1801–1807.

64. Weber CJ, Vansant J, Alazraki N, et al. Value of technetium 99m sestamibi iodine imaging in reoperative parathyroid surgery. *Surgery.* 1993;114:1011–1018.

65. Casas AT, Burke GJ, Mansberger AR, Wei JP. Impact of technetium-99m sestamibi localization of operative time and success of operations for primary hyperparathyroidism. *Am Surg.* 1994;60:12–17.

66. Feingold DL, Alexander HR, Chen CC, et al. Ultrasound and sestamibi scan as the only preoperative imaging tests in reoperation for parathyroid adenomas. *Surgery.* 2000; 128:1103–1110.

67. Giordano A, Rubello D, Casara D. New trends in parathyroid scintigraphy. *Eur J Nucl Med.* 2001;28:1409–1420.

68. Hetrakul N, Civelek AC, Stag CA, Udelsman R. In vitro accumulation of technetium-99m sestamibi in human parathyroid mitochondria. *Surgery.* 2001;130:1011–1018.

69. Piwnica-Worms D, Chiu ML, Budding M, Kronauge JF, Kramer RA, Croop JM. Functional imaging of multidrug resistant P-glycoprotein with organotechnetium complex. *Cancer Res.* 1993;53:977–984.

70. Mitchell BK, Cornelius EA, Zoghbi S, et al. Mechanism of technetium 99m sestamibi parathyroid imaging and possible role of p-glycoprotein. *Surgery.* 1996;120:1039–1045.

71. Bhatnagar A, Vezza PR, Bryan JA, et al. Technetium-99m-sestamibi parathyroid scintigraphy: effect of P-glycoprotein, histology and tumor size on detectability. *J Nucl Med.* 1998;39:1617–1620.

72. Yamaguchi S, Yachiku S, Hashimoto H, et al. Relation between technetium 99m methoxyisobutylisonitrile accumulation and multidrug resistance protein in the parathyroid glands. *World J Surg.* 2002;26:29–34.

73. Royal RE, Delpassand ES, Shapiro SE, et al. Improving the yield of preoperative parathyroid localization: technetium-99m-sestamibi imaging after thyroid suppression. *Surgery.* 2002;132:968–974.

74. Billotey C, Sarfati E, Aurengo A, et al. Advantages of SPECT in technetium-99m-sestamibi parathyroid scintigraphy. *J Nucl Med.* 1996;37:1773–1778.

75. Carty SE, Worsey MJ, Virji MA, Brown ML, Watson CG. Concise parathyroidectomy: the impact of preoperative SPECT $^{99m}$Tc-sestamibi scanning and intraoperative quick parathormone assay. *Surgery.* 1997;122:1107–1114.

76. Gallowitsch JH, Mikosch P, Kresnik E, et al. Technetium-$^{99m}$-tetrofosmin parathyroid imaging: results with double-phase study and SPECT in primary and secondary hyperparathyroidism. *Invest Radiol.* 1997;32:459–465.

77. Neumann DR, Esselstyn CB Jr, Go RT, Wong CO, Rice TW, Obuchowsky NA. Comparison of double-phase $^{99m}$Tc-sestamibi with $^{123}$I-$^{99m}$Tc-sestamibi subtraction SPECT in hyperparathyroidism. *Am J Roentgenol.* 1997; 169:1671–1674.

78. Francis IS, Loney EL, Buscombe JR, Thakrar DS, Berger L, Hilson AJW. Technetium-99m-sestamibi dual-phase SPECT imaging: concordance with ultrasound. *Nucl Med Commun.* 1999;20:487–488.

79. George EF, Komisar A, Scharf SC, Ferracci A, Blaugrund S. Diagnostic value of the preoperative sestamibi scan in intraoperative localization of parathyroid adenomas: a case study. *Laryngoscope.* 1998;108:627–629.

80. Chen H, Sokoll LJ, Udelsman R. Outpatient minimally invasive parathyroidectomy: a combination of sestamibi-SPECT localization, cervical block anaesthesia, and intraoperative parathyroid hormone assay. *Surgery.* 1999;126:1016–1021.

81. Kumar A, Cozens NJA, Nash JR. Sestamibi scan-directed unilateral neck exploration for primary hyperparathyroidism due to a solitary adenoma. *Eur J Surg Oncol.* 2000;26:785–788.

82. Goldstein R, Blevins L, Delbeke D, Martin W. Effect of minimally invasive radioguided parathyroidectomy on efficacy, length of stay, and costs in the management of primary hyperparathyroidism. *Ann Surg.* 2000;231:732–742.

83. Rubello D, Pelizzo MR, Gross MD, et al. Controversies on minimally invasive procedures for radio-guided surgery of parathyroid tumors. *Minerva Endocrinol.* 2004;29:189–193.

84. Rubello D, Pelizzo MR, Boni G, et al. Radioguided surgery of primary hyperparathyroidism using the low-dose $^{99m}$Tc-sestamibi protocol: multi-institutional experience from the Italian Study Group on Radioguided Surgery and Immunoscintigraphy (GISCRIS). *J Nucl Med.* 2005;46:220–226.

85. Rubello D, Casara D, Giannini S, et al. Minimally invasive radioguided parathyroidectomy: an attractive therapeutic option for elderly patients with primary hyperparathyroidism. *Nucl Med Commun.* 2004;25:901–908.

86. Rubello D, Piotto A, Casara D, Muzzio PC, Shapiro B, Pelizzo MR. Role of gamma probes in performing minimally invasive parathyroidectomy in patients with primary hyperparathyroidism: optimization of preoperative and intraoperative procedures. *Eur J Endocrinol.* 2003;149:7–15.

87. Rubello D, Casara D, Giannini S, et al. Importance of radio-guided minimally invasive parathyroidectomy using hand-held gamma probe and low $^{99m}$Tc-MIBI dose. Technical considerations and long-term clinical results. *Q J Nucl Med.* 2003;47:129–138.

88. Rubello D, Pelizzo MR, Casara D. Nuclear medicine and minimally invasive surgery of parathyroid adenomas: a fair marriage. *Eur J Nucl Med Mol Imaging.* 2003;30: 189–192.

89. Rubello D, Casara D, Pelizzo MR. Optimization of preoperative procedures. *Nucl Med Commun.* 2003;24: 133–140.

90. Rubello D, Giannini S, Martini C, et al. Minimally invasive radioguided parathyroidectomy. *Biomed Pharmacother.* 2006;60:134–138.

91. Taillefer R, Boucher Y, Potvin C, et al. Detection and localization of parathyroid adenomas in patients with hyperparathyroidism using a single radionuclide imaging procedure with technetium-99m-sestamibi (double phase study). *J Nucl Med.* 1992;33:1801–1807.

92. Taillefer R. Technetium-99m-sestamibi parathyroid scintigraphy. In: Freeman L, ed. *Nuclear Medicine Annual 1995.* New York: Raven Press; 1995:51–79.

93. Foldes I, Levay A, Stotz G. Comparative scanning of thyroid nodules with technetium-99m pertechnetate and technetium-99m methoxyisobutylisonitrile. *Eur J Nucl Med.* 1993;20:330–333.

94. dell'Erba L, Bardari S, Borsato N, et al. Retrospective analysis of the association of nodular goiter with primary and secondary hyperparathyroidism. *Eur J Endocrinol.* 2001;145:429–434.

95. Bénard F, Lefebvre B, Beuvon F, Langlois MF, Bisson G. Rapid wash-out of technetium-99m-MIBI from a large parathyroid adenoma. *J Nucl Med.* 1995;36:241–243.

96. Leslie WD, Riese KT, Dupont JO, Teterdy AE. Parathyroid adenomas without sestamibi retention. *Clin Nucl Med.* 1995;20:699–702.

97. Hindié E, Melliere D, Jeanguillaume C, Perlemuter L, Chehade F, Galle P. Parathyroid imaging using simultaneous double-window recording of Technetium-99m-sestamibi and iodine-123. *J Nucl Med.* 1998;39: 1100–1105.

98. Casara D, Rubello D, Saladini G, Piotto A, Toniato A, Pelizzo MR. Procedure di "imaging" nello studio dell'iperparatiroidismo: ruolo della scintigrafia con $^{99m}$Tc-MIBI. In: Rovelli E, Samori G, eds. *L'Iperparatiroidismo Primitivo e Secondario.* Milan: Wichtig Editore; 1992: 133–136.

99. Rubello D, Saladini G, Casara D, et al. Parathyroid imaging with pertechnetate plus perchlorate/MIBI subtraction scintigraphy. A fast and effective technique. *Clin Nucl Med.* 2000;25:527–531.

100. Rubello D, Saladini G, Casara D. The role of scintigraphy with dual tracer and potassium perchlorate ($^{99m}$TcO$_4$ and KClO$_4$/MIBI) in primary hyperparathyroidism. *Minerva Endocrinol.* 2001;26:13–21.

101. Casara D, Rubello D, Cauzzo C, Pelizzo MR. $^{99m}$Tc-MIBI radio-guided minimally invasive parathyroidectomy: experience with patients with normal thyroids and nodular goiters. *Thyroid.* 2002;12:53–61.

102. Carpentier A, Jeannotte S, Verreault J, et al. Preoperative localization of parathyroid lesions in hyperparathyroidism: relationship between technetium-99m-MIBI uptake and oxyphil cell content. *J Nucl Med.* 1998;39:1441–1444.

103. Torregrosa JV, Fernandez-Cruz L, Canaleyo A, et al. $^{99m}$Tc-sestamibi scintigraphy and cell cycle in parathyroid glands of secondary hyperparathyroidism. *World J Surg.* 2000;24:1386–1390.

104. Sfakianakis GN, Irvin GL, Foss J, et al. Efficient parathyroidectomy guided by SPECT-MIBI and hormonal measurements. *J Nucl Med.* 1996;37:798–804.

105. Moka D, Eschner W, Voth E, Dietlein M, Larena-Avellaneda A, Schicha H. Iterative reconstruction: an improvement of technetium-99m-MIBI SPECT for the detection of parathyroid adenoma? *Eur J Nucl Med.* 2000;27:485–489.

106. Mariani G, Vaiano A, Nibale O, Rubello D. Is the "ideal" gamma-probe for intraoperative radioguided surgery conceivable? *J Nucl Med.* 2005;46:388–390.

107. Wang CA, Parathyroid re-exploration. *Ann Surg.* 1977; 186:140–145.

# 24
# Radioguided Surgery of Neuroendocrine Tumors

Richard P. Baum, Sergio Sandrucci, and Stefan Adams

Neuroendocrine tumors constitute a heterogeneous group of neoplasms that have been postulated to originate from a common precursor cell population (1). This kind of tumor can occur sporadically or in a familial context of autosomally inherited syndromes, such as multiple endocrine neoplasms (2,3).

The histopathologic and immunocytochemical examination aims at classifying the tumor according to tissue origin, biochemical behavior, and prognosis (4). In general, most endocrine tumors tend to be relatively slowly growing (well differentiated) and retain many multipotent capacities (5), such as the ability to produce and secrete specific neuroendocrine markers. These include 5-hydroxytryptamine, 5-hydroxytryptophan, glucagon, somatostatin, vasoactive intestinal polypeptide, serotonin, growth hormone, corticotropin melanocyte-stimulating hormone, gastrin, insulin, pancreatic polypeptide, calcitonin, and substance P. Classical symptoms of hormone hyperfunction therefore may be correlated to their precise source (6). Neuroendocrine tumors are named primarily according to the predominant peptide secreted, which can be related to the clinical features. While there is no general marker, some of these products may serve as markers for diagnosis and treatment (7,8).

Somatostatin receptors have been described in many cells of neuroendocrine origin, but mainly in the endocrine glands and in the central nervous system (9,10). Currently, 5 subtypes of somatostatin receptors have been identified, with different tissue distribution (11). Most endocrine tumors (e.g., gastroenteropancreatic tumors, medullary thyroid carcinoma) possess somatostatin receptors that are also expressed in the peritumoral vascular system (12). There are relevant differences in somatostatin receptor expression and profile between different tumor types (13–15). Expression of somatostatin receptors is associated with differentiation and slow proliferation, 2 parameters inversely correlated with the progression of malignancy (16,17). The demonstration of amine uptake mechanisms or a high density of somatostatin receptors on several well-differentiated neuroendocrine tumors as well as their metastases has been used for diagnosis and monitoring by radionuclide techniques (18,19).

Poorly differentiated endocrine tumors (e.g., atypical carcinoids or malignant gastrinomas) with increased mitotic activity often lack somatostatin receptors and show an increased $^{18}$F-2-fluoro-2-deoxy-d-glucose ([$^{18}$F]FDG) uptake. PET imaging using the carbon-11-labeled amine precursors L-dihydroxyphenylalanine and 5-hydroxy-L-tryptophan (5-HTP) is more sensitive to diagnose serotonin-producing tumors than carbon-11-labeled L-DOPA (20–22). Recently, the development of gallium-68-labeled somatostatin analogues such as DOTA-NOC or DOTA-TOC and PET/computed tomograph (CT) have dramatically improved the sensitivity (and specificity) of nuclear medicine diagnosis in neuroendocrine carcinomas (Figures 24-1 and 24-2).

For patients with localized disease, surgery remains the treatment of choice. In patients with metastatic carcinoids presenting with liver and mesenteric metastases, conservative resections of the intestine, mesenteric tumors, and fibrotic areas may considerably improve symptoms and quality of life (23,24). However, it has not been established whether the reduction of tumor mass by surgical intervention improves the outcome (25–27).

Determining the tumor extent (localization and metastases) as well as the primary tumor location is an essential aspect of the management of endocrine tumors, because it is a basic condition for resection. Certain locations, such as the small bowel, can be associated with multicentricity, and care should be taken to ensure adequate resection (28). Intraoperative localization can be accomplished using traditional surgical, radiographic, and endoscopic techniques, including palpation, CT scanning, endoscopic tattooing, and intraoperative ultrasound imaging.

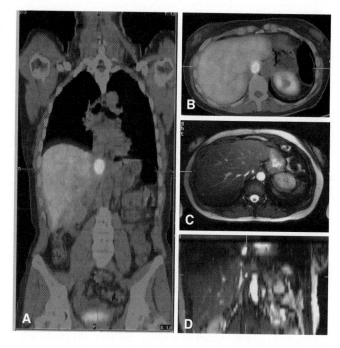

FIGURE 24-1. Positron emission tomography-computed tomography obtained 30 minutes after the intravenous injection of [68]Ga-DOTA-NOC in a patient previously submitted to surgical removal of a pancreatic neuroendocrine tumor. While conventional imaging (including ultrasound, CT, MRI, and [[18]F]FDG-PET) was completely normal, the somatostatin-receptor PET examination revealed a liver metastasis with extremely high expression of somatostatin receptors (SUV = 71). PET/CT image fusion is shown in panels A and B for representative coronal and transaxial sections respectively, while panels C and D show transaxial and coronal fusion sections, respectively, of PET images with the MRI images.

In addition, tumors can be detected using radiolabeled tracers and a gamma-detecting probe (13). Various radiopharmaceuticals are administered prior to surgery. Intraoperatively, the gamma probe can be used to detect the primary tumor, lymph node involvement, or metastatic disease. Postoperatively, scintigraphy can be repeated to detect residual disease.

The intraoperative detection of sentinel lymph nodes of malignant melanoma, sentinel lymph node mapping of breast, vulvar, and penile cancer, the detection of parathyroid adenoma, and the localization of bone tumors have been routinely accepted in surgical practice (29,30). With the preoperative injection of radiolabeled somatostatin analogues, it is possible to identify endocrine tumors intraoperatively and to determine the extent of disease without extensive dissection. Therefore, external scintigraphy combined with intraoperative gamma emission detection might be used to decrease the high rate of unsuccessful surgical explorations. It should be noted that in some series the negative laparotomy rate for patients with pancreatic and ileal endocrine tumors has been reported to be as high as 30% (31,32).

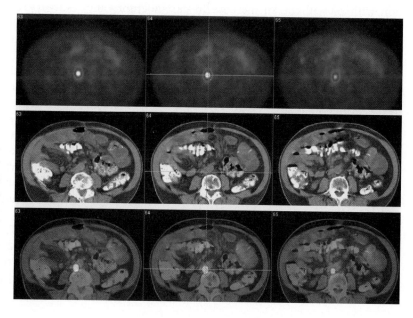

FIGURE 24-2. Positron emission tomography-computed tomography obtained 30 minutes after the injection of [68]Ga-DOTA-NOC in a patient with a pancreatic tumor. Transaxial sections are shown for the PET acquisition (top row), for the CT acquisition (middle row), and for the PET/CT fusion images (bottom row). The somatostatin-receptor PET examination reveals a 5-mm lymph node metastasis that fusion analysis shows to be located in the retro-aorto-caval space.

# Medullary Thyroid Carcinoma and Multiple Endocrine Neoplasia

Medullary thyroid carcinoma is a rare calcitonin-secreting tumor and has its origin in the parafollicular C cells. Medullary thyroid carcinoma occurs in both sporadic (75%) and hereditary forms. Accounting for only 5% to 10% of all thyroid malignancies, it is nevertheless responsible for up to 13.4% of all deaths (33,34). There are 3 distinct hereditary varieties: 1) MEN-IIA syndrome (90% of the cases), characterized by medullary thyroid carcinoma in combination with pheochromocytoma and tumors of the parathyroids; 2) MEN-IIB syndrome, characterized by medullary thyroid carcinoma, pheochromocytoma, ganglioneuromatosis, and a marfanoid habitus; and 3) familial medullary thyroid carcinoma (FMTC), without any other endocrinopathies (35). A germline mutation in the RET protooncogene predisposes individuals to develop MEN-II and FTMC (36). The prognosis of patients with medullary thyroid carcinoma depends on the extent of disease at the time of presentation, the grade of tumor differentiation, and the completeness of surgical resection (36,37). When a thyroid nodule is palpable, cervical lymph node metastases (classified as stage III) are present in at least 50% of patients (36,38). Woolner et al. demonstrated that the 10-year survival rate of patients without lymph node involvement reached 85%; in patients with lymph node metastases, it was significantly reduced to 42% (39). Among the tumor markers described in medullary thyroid carcinoma, calcitonin is the most important in clinical practice (40). Preoperative calcitonin levels correlate with tumor size and are usually above 100 pg/mL in the presence of clinically significant disease (41). Variable loss of calcitonin synthesis and secretion with or without an increase in carcinoembryonic antigen (CEA) may indicate a dedifferentiation and a more aggressive form of medullary thyroid carcinoma (7,42). The initial treatment consists of total thyroidectomy with bilateral cervical lymph node and upper mediastinum dissection (43). Currently, there is no adequate systemic therapy for treating recurrent disease (44), and surgical reoperation or conservative follow-up are the best available options. Complete surgical removal of all tumor tissue may result in normalization of postoperative serum calcitonin levels in only 20% of patients with clinical disease (40). However, stimulated peak plasma calcitonin levels are more useful than basal levels for detecting occult disease after thyroidectomy (35,36). In patients with residual or recurrent disease, further evaluation should be performed by means of high-resolution ultrasonography, with or without fine-needle aspiration; CT and magnetic resonance imaging (MRI) are of limited value in detecting minimal residual disease (45). Selective venous catheterization, with or without pentagastrin stimulation, is recommended for localization of tumor tissue in patients with an elevated serum calcitonin level after initial surgery and clinically occult disease (46).

Preoperative scintigraphy with [131]I-meta-iodobenzylguanidine (MIBG) and [111]In-octreotide has shown a sensitivity of 35% to 50% and 29% to 77%, respectively (19,47–53). One explanation for these divergent results may be that a minority of neuroendocrine tumors—such as medullary thyroid carcinoma and insulinomas—express subtypes of somatostatin receptors characterized by low affinity for [[111]In-DTPA-D-Phe[1]]-pentetreotide (54). Furthermore, endogenous production of somatostatin by part of the tumor in patients with medullary thyroid carcinoma may hamper both the in-vitro and the in-vivo detection of somatostatin receptors (55). The somatostatin analogue [111]In-octreotide has been shown to be more sensitive than MRI scanning in detecting occult medullary thyroid carcinoma recurrence (50), and scintigraphy with this radiopharmaceutical will also visualize chromaffin cell tumors (e.g., pheochromocytomas) in MEN patients (56).

In previously reported data, more than 75% of patients with palpable medullary thyroid carcinoma had associated nodal metastases, which often were not apparent to the surgeon and had no relation to thyroid tumor size. Furthermore, the pattern of lymph node metastatic distribution in neck areas varied between patients, and the number of lymph node metastases is predictive of biological cure after surgery (57,58).

To achieve a good surgical outcome, intraoperative navigation systems (e.g., three-dimensional ultrasound imaging) are useful, because they are more accurate than surgical palpation (59). In 1 of our studies, radioguided surgery using [99m]Tc-Penta-DMSA was able to detect metastases that measured >5 mm in greatest dimension, whereas the palpating finger of the surgeon localized metastases that measured >1 cm in greatest dimension (49). Furthermore, intraoperative scanning was able to localize more tumor-involved lesions (>30%) in patients with recurrent medullary thyroid carcinoma compared with conventional preoperative imaging modalities and surgical findings (Table 24-1).

[99m]Tc-Penta-DMSA uptake has also been confirmed in patients with soft tissue sarcoma, osteosarcoma, prostatic carcinoma, benign and malignant head and neck tumors, and inflammatory lesions (60,61). Therefore, the combined use of different radiopharmaceuticals (e.g., radiolabeled anti-CEA antibodies and somatostatin receptor scintigraphy) has been reported to be more sensitive for tumor localization in patients with recurrent medullary thyroid carcinoma than the use of only 1 tumor-seeking agent (53,62).

TABLE 24-1. Medullary thyroid carcinoma. Comparison of histologically proven lesions detected by preoperative metabolic/receptor imaging, computed tomography, standard surgical exploration, and intraoperative gamma probe localization.

| Method | Sensitivity (%) |
|---|---|
| Computed tomography | 21 (32) |
| [111]In-pentetreotide | 23 (34) |
| [99m]Tc(V)-DMSA | 43 (65) |
| Palpation | 43 (65) |
| Radioguided surgery | 64 (97) |

Legend:
[99m]Tc(V)-DMSA—[99m]Tc (V)-dimercaptosuccinic acid,
[111]In-pentetreotide—[[111]In-DTPA-D-Phe[1]]-pentetreotide
*Source:* Pederzoli et al. (75). Reprinted with permission from Elsevier.

De Groot et al. reported that FDG-PET is superior to conventional nuclear and morphologic imaging, with a lesion-based sensitivity of 96% (63). However, others consider computed tomography superior to FDG-PET in the diagnosis of metastatic medullary thyroid carcinoma (47). Especially in early tumor stages (calcitonin serum levels <20 pg/mL), the morphologic correlation using PET is unsatisfactory. A combination of PET and CT seems to be the most appropriate noninvasive diagnostic approach in patients with medullary thyroid carcinoma (64). MRI exerts equal sensitivity to computed tomography in detecting adrenal tumors, but is superior in detecting extraadrenal tumors (65,66).

Scintigraphy with [123]I-MIBG offers superior specificity, especially for familial and malignant lesions (95–100%), and a sensitivity approximating 90% (67,68). In normal images, [123]I-MIBG shows the medulla as a faint area in dorsal projections, whereas increased uptake is seen in patients with pheochromocytoma. One study has suggested that high tumor-to-background ratios (>5 : 1) can be revealed for intraoperative localization of ectopic tumor sites and small foci [i.e., = 1 cm] (69). Whole-body scanning is limited, however, in part because the dense hepatic and biliary signals intraoperatively overshadow potential sites of pathologic [123]I-MIBG uptake, especially in the subdiaphragmatic/paravertebral region, leading to low tumor-to-background ratios [1.5 : 1] (49). Because pheochromocytomas often express somatostatin receptors, scintigraphy with octreotide can increase sensitivity, particularly in cases of [123]I-MIBG negative lesions (70). The relatively high radioligand accumulation in the kidneys limits the use of [[111]In-DTPA-D-Phe[1]]-pentetreotide for intraoperative detection of tumors in the area of the adrenal gland.

To reduce the renal uptake of [111]In-octreotide, Rolleman et al. suggested the injection of lysine and colchicine. However, liver and blood radioactivity levels were significantly elevated by colchicine, and this can also interfere with intraoperative tumor detection (71).

Positron emission tomography, originally with FDG, [11]C-hydroxyephedrine and 6-[[18]F]-fluorodopamine, and recently with [68]Ga-DOTA-NOC and CT, has been shown to be highly sensitive, and on several occasions better than the established methods, demonstrating almost 100% sensitivity and specificity (72,73).

# Tumors of the Gastroenteropancreatic System

## Pancreatic Endocrine Tumors

Pancreatic endocrine tumors are difficult to localize. The most common functional endocrine pancreatic tumor is insulinoma. These tumors are generally small, and unlike most endocrine tumors, most are benign. As with other pancreatic endocrine tumors, they may occur sporadically or as part of MEN-1. Those arising sporadically are generally solitary lesions, although seemingly sporadic cases with multiple tumors have been reported. These tumors are almost exclusively confined to the pancreas, but they may arise in aberrant pancreatic tissue (74,75).

Gastrinoma is frequently a duodenal tumor. As many as 40% of gastrinomas may occur in the setting of MEN-1. Unlike insulinomas, most sporadic gastrinomas are malignant. They metastasize to regional lymph nodes and the liver, and less commonly to distant sites. Sporadic gastrinomas are usually solitary and vary in size from infra-millimetric to >3 cm in diameter. Most of these tumors are located in the gastrinoma triangle—defined by the confluence of the cystic and common hepatic ducts, the border of the second and third portions of the duodenum, and the neck of the pancreas—but ectopic locations such as the jejunum, stomach, mesentery, spleen, and ovaries have been reported. Surgical exploration is recommended for all sporadic cases of gastrinoma without evidence of hepatic metastasis (76,77).

Endosonography is highly accurate in the localization of gastric and pancreatic neuroendocrine tumors and is cost effective when used early in the preoperative localization strategy (78). Islet cell tumors (e.g., insulinomas) are typically hypervascular, solitary small tumors, with 90% less than 2 cm and 30% measuring 1 cm in diameter (79–81). Successful excision of a benign lesion is associated with normal life expectancy, whereas a 10-year survival of 29% has been described for malignant insulinomas (82,83). Up to 20% of insulinomas are not palpable at the time of surgery, whereas gastrinomas are not found during surgery in up to 40%.

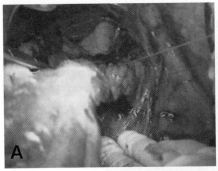
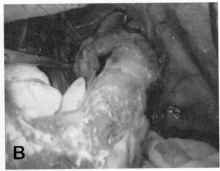
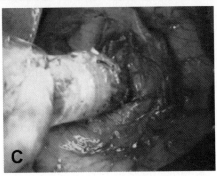

FIGURE 24-3. Intraoperative gamma probe-guided search of a pancreatic gastrinoma of the isthmus aided by a handheld gamma probe (visible inside the sterile plastic sleeve) after injection of the radiolabeled somatostatin analogue [111]In-pentetreotide (Octreo-Scan). Gamma probe counting in the area where intraoperative ultrasound was suspicious for the tumor yielded a 5:1 target-to-background ratio (panel A, where the middle portion of the pancreas is well visible on the right side of the tip of the gamma probe). The target-to-background ratio was 1:1 when counting the pancreatic tail (panel B). After surgical removal of the tumor, repeat gamma probe counting of the tumor bed yielded a 1:1 target-to-background ratio.

Concerning the intraoperative tumor localization rate, Erickson et al. reported that the combination of intraoperative ultrasound and surgical palpation has led to 97% cure rates in patients with benign insulinomas (84). Furthermore, intraoperative ultrasound does not allow accurate detection of small lymph node metastases, because of their normal size. Therefore, the intraoperative use of gamma probes makes it possible to identify recurrent tumor tissue when the normal anatomy was altered or primary tumors in unusual anatomic locations (85) (Figure 24-3). Unfortunately, there is no published experience apart some heterogeneous case reports.

## Gastric Carcinoid Tumors

Gastric carcinoid tumors are relatively rare and are separated into the following 3 categories: type I, associated with chronic atrophic gastritis type A; type II, associated with Zollinger-Ellison syndrome and MEN-I; and type III, sporadic gastric carcinoid tumors (86). Type I and type II tumors are associated with hypergastrinemia, which results in hyperplasia of the enterochromaffin cells in the gastric mucosa. These lesions are generally small (<1 cm in diameter), indolent, and often multifocal (87). Treatment of smaller lesions is usually accomplished with endoscopic resection and close endoscopic surveillance, whereas larger ones sometimes require more extensive resection. Interestingly, antrectomy removes the source of gastrin and may result in tumor regression (88,89). Usually, sporadic (type III) carcinoid tumors are more aggressive; generally, they are greater than 1 cm in diameter at presentation, and are associated with poor outcome because they are often metastatic at the time of presentation. If resection is feasible, a subtotal or radical gastrectomy is usually required (90). In these particular type of gastroenteropancreatic tumors intraoperative detection can be useful only in detecting nodal metastases: multicentricity is not unusual and radioguided techniques do not appear to be useful (91).

## Duodenal Carcinoid Tumors

Duodenal carcinoid tumors are rare and may be classified as either foregut or midgut tumors, depending on the portion of the duodenum from which they are derived (90,92,93). Endoscopic excision can be used for lesions smaller than 1 cm, but transduodenal excision should be employed for lesions between 1 and 2 cm. For larger lesions (>2 cm), pancreaticoduodenectomy or segmental resection should be employed, although all patients with these larger lesions developed recurrent tumors (94). Small endocrine tumors (0.2 to 0.6 cm) in the duodenum have a higher likelihood of not being imaged by intraoperative ultrasound, because of the mixed (gas-liquid-solid) background of the bowel (95). Successful intraoperative radioguided surgery requires tumor-to-background ratios of at least 1.5 to 2 (96,97) (Table 24-2). Measurements with a well-type gamma counter of specimens from intraoperatively detected tumors revealed tumor/normal tissue radioactivity ratios of 2.4–395:1 (96,98).

The high values of specific tracer uptake in tumors relate to factors such as the size of the lesion, its receptor

TABLE 24-2. Gastroenteropancreatic tumors. Intraoperative measurement of tissue radioactivity 24 hours after administration of ($^{111}$In-D-Phe$^1$)-pentetreotide.

| Tissue | Range (cps) | Median (cps) |
|---|---|---|
| Lymph node metastases | 450–1400 | 1100 |
| Primary tumor (ileum) | 400–2200 | 1526 |
| Normal ileum | 50–1100 | 459 |
| Normal liver | 600–1100 | 843 |
| Liver metastases | 1400–2200 | 1857 |
| Lung | 100–300 | 169 |
| Heart/vessels | 300–400 | 351 |
| Kidneys | 1000–4000 | 2753 |
| Spleen | 1500–1950 | 1675 |

Legend:
cps—counts per second
*Source:* Mignon et al. (24), by permission.

specificity, and density. The predominant hepatobiliary excretion of iodine-labeled somatostatin analogues leads to a considerable amount of intestinal activity, reducing the reliability of somatostatin receptor scintigraphy in gastroenteropancreatic tumors. For intraoperative gamma probe counting, the intestinal accumulation of OctreoScan can be overcome by administration of laxatives (96,99,100). Acquisitions at 24 hours post-injection provide better image quality due to improved tumor-to-background ratio; therefore, this is also the optimal time for intraoperative tumor detection (96,101).

## Carcinoid Tumors of the Small Intestine

Carcinoid tumors of the small intestine occur more frequently in the distal ileum and are often multicentric. Most patients present with small bowel obstruction, as malignant carcinoid syndrome is relatively rare, even in patients with metastatic disease. Serum chromogranin A levels are elevated in 80% of these patients (102). Unlike other gastrointestinal carcinoid tumors, size is a less reliable predictor of malignant potential, with a significant metastatic rate identified even with smaller (<2 cm) lesions. Treatment is based on site, size, and metastatic status (20,102). Small (<1 cm) primary tumors without regional lymph node involvement may be removed with segmental intestinal resection (103). For a larger lesion (>1 cm), multicentric disease, or regionally metastatic disease, wide excision of the bowel and mesentery is indicated (23). Lesions of the terminal ileum may require a right hemicolectomy. Five-year survival is approximately 65% in patients with local or regional disease, but this decreases to approximately 35% in patients with metastatic disease.

Small intestinal carcinoids may be multiple: 87% occur within the ileum, and 40% present within 2 feet of the ileocecal valve (104). Primary tumors tend to remain small, and sometimes a metastasis in the liver is the first clinical appearance of a nonfunctioning tumor. In patients with midgut carcinoids, $^{123}$I-MIBG tumor uptake is found with a sensitivity of 40% to 68%, whereas only 37% of foregut carcinoids can be localized (105,106). Somatostatin receptor scintigraphy is currently the investigation of choice for the staging and identification of the primary carcinoid lesion. This functional imaging modality has an 83% diagnostic accuracy and a positive predictive value of 100%, and can also identify lesions not viewed by radiological methods (18,23,107,108). CT and MRI are less sensitive than radionuclide imaging using $^{111}$In-octreotide, because they identify only approximately 50% of the primary tumors (70,107). The combined SPECT-CT device provides both functional and anatomical information; it affected the diagnostic interpretation of somatostatin receptor scintigraphy in 32% of the patients with neuroendocrine tumors and lead to alterations in the therapeutic strategy in 14% of patients (109). Radioguided surgery may be helpful in detecting multicentric disease and to check residual disease to obtain a complete tumor ablation; however, at present no prospective studies are available.

## Carcinoid Tumors of the Appendix

Carcinoid tumors of the appendix often cause partial or complete occlusion of the appendiceal lumen and are most often found after operation for acute appendicitis. In adults, most are asymptomatic until the development of appendicitis, and the tumors are usually smaller than 2 cm (110). Metastatic disease is relatively rare with small lesions; however, with those lesions larger than 2 cm, distant metastatic disease is significantly more common. As with any midgut tumor, hepatic metastasis is a possibility and may result in carcinoid syndrome (110,111). Lymph node metastasis is rare (0.1%) in tumors smaller than 1 cm; therefore, simple appendectomy is the treatment of choice. Carcinoid tumors larger than 2 cm are treated by right hemicolectomy, because lymph node metastases occur in approximately 25% to 50% of patients (111,112).

The treatment of intermediate-sized tumors (1 to 2 cm) is somewhat controversial. The incidence of nodal spread for these tumors is exceedingly low and approaches that of smaller lesions, and many surgeons consider simple appendectomy alone to be adequate, particularly if the tumor is in the mid-appendix or tip (112,113). In contrast, other studies suggest that tumors at the appendiceal base or those with a more aggressive behavior, such as invasion of the mesentery, should be treated with a right hemicolectomy, because this procedure is well tolerated and achieves improved locoregional control

(110,111). Modlin et al. (104) have shown that the 5-year survival is 94% for patients with local disease, 85% for patients with regional invasion, and 34% for patients with distant metastatic disease, respectively. Due to the well-codified surgical procedure, intraoperative radiolocalization does not appear to be useful.

## Colonic and Rectal Carcinoid Tumors

Colonic carcinoid tumors are rare, and are seldom multicentric. They occur more often in the right part of the colon. Patients with colonic carcinoid tumors usually have nonspecific symptoms and present at a later stage than those with small bowel or appendiceal carcinoid tumors (114). Most patients require colonic resection with locoregional lymphadenectomy. Intraoperative gamma probe detection is not of particular interest in this setting.

Rectal carcinoid tumors are usually of hindgut origin and rarely secrete serotonin. Approximately half of the patients with rectal carcinoid tumors present with rectal bleeding, pain, or constipation, whereas the other half are asymptomatic and are diagnosed during screening colonoscopy. Metastatic disease is rare in lesions smaller than 1 cm, but common in those larger than 2 cm (115). Small lesions are managed with local excision or endoscopic resection (116), whereas larger (>2 cm) ones or those that invade the muscularis mucosa are usually treated by a low anterior resection or abdominoperineal resection (117,118).

[$^{123}$I-Tyr$^3$] and $^{111}$In-labeled somatostatin analogues have been successfully used for intraoperative detection of neuroendocrine tumors (96,97,119). Radioguided surgery identified 57% more gastroenteropancreatic tumors when compared to the "palpating finger" of the surgeon (96). Preoperative receptor imaging is particularly efficient for tumors larger than 10 mm, with a detection rate of 92%, in contrast to 38% for gastroenteropancreatic tumors with less than 10 mm in size (99). Use of an intraoperative gamma probe revealed abdominal small endocrine tumor sites accumulating ($^{111}$In-DTPA-D-Phe$^1$)-pentetreotide more efficiently (>90% of all tumors investigated) than somatostatin receptor scintigraphy (68% to 77%), because lesions of more than 5mm in dimension could be identified (96,98). In comparison, $^{111}$In-DTPA-Tyr$^3$-octreotate, a newly synthesized somatostatin analogue, demonstrated higher tumor uptake than $^{111}$In-DTPA-Tyr$^3$-octreotide, whereas kidney uptake was similar (120).

Tracers such as $^{68}$Ga-DOTA-NOC or $^{64}$Cu-TETA-octreotide seem to be of the greatest clinical interest for radioguided surgery, because they exhibit better tumor-to-background ratios than $^{111}$In-octreotide and have demonstrated significantly more lesions in patients with neuroendocrine tumors (121,122).

## References

1. Rindi G, Villanacci V, Ubiali A, et al. Endocrine tumors of the digestive tract and pancreas: histogenesis, diagnosis and molecular basis. *Expert Rev Mol Diagn.* 2001; 1:323–333.
2. Calender A. Molecular genetics of neuroendocrine tumors. *Digestion.* 2000;62(suppl 1):3–18.
3. Calender A, Vercherat C, Gaudray P, et al. Deregulation of genetic pathways in neuroendocrine tumors. *Ann Oncol.* 2001;12(suppl 2):S3–S11.
4. Ahlman H, Wangberg B, Jansson S, et al. Interventional treatment of gastrointestinal neuroendocrine tumors. *Digestion.* 2000;62(suppl 1):59–68.
5. Solcia E, Kloppel G, Sobin LH. Histological typing of endocrine tumors. 2nd ed. Heidelberg: World Health Organization; 2000.
6. Solcia E, Capella C, Fiocca R, et al. The gastropancreatic endocrine system and related tumors. *Gastroenterol Clin North Am.* 1989;4:671–693.
7. Lamberts SW, Hofland LJ, Nobels FR. Neuroendocrine tumor markers. *Front Neuroendocrinol.* 2001;22:309–339.
8. Eriksson B, Oberg K, Stridsberg M. Tumor markers in neuroendocrine tumors. *Digestion.* 2000;62(suppl 1): 33–38.
9. Reubi JC, Maurer R. Autoradiographic mapping of somatostatin receptors in the rat CNS and pituitary. *Neuroscience.* 1985;15:1183–1193.
10. Reubi JC, Laissue J, Waser B, et al. Expression of somatostatin receptors in normal, inflamed and neoplastic human gastrointestinal tissues. *Ann N Y Acad Sci.* 1994; 733:122–137.
11. Yamada Y, Post SR, Wang K, et al. Cloning and functional characterization of a family of human and mouse somatostatin receptors expressed in brain, gastrointestinal tract, and kidney. *Proc Natl Acad Sci USA.* 1992;89: 251–255.
12. Reubi JC, Schaer JC, Laissue J, et al. Somatostatin receptors and their subtypes in human tumors and in peritumoral vessels. *Metabolism.* 1996;458(suppl 1):39–41.
13. Adams S, Baum RP, Hertel A, et al. Intraoperative gamma probe detection of neuroendocrine tumors. *J Nucl Med.* 1998;39:1155.
14. Öhrvall U, Westlin JE, Nilsson S, et al. Intraoperative gamma detection reveals abdominal endocrine tumors more efficiently than somatostatin receptor scintigraphy. *Cancer.* 1997;80:2490–2494.
15. Benjegård SA, Forssell-Aronsson E, Wängberg B, Skånberg J, Nilsson O, Ahlman H. Intraoperative tumour detection using $^{111}$In-DTPA-D-Phe$^1$-octreotide and a scintillation detector. *Eur J Nucl Med.* 2001;28: 1456–1462.
16. Reubi JC, Torhorst J. The relationship between somatostatin, epidermal growth factor and steroid hormone receptors in breast cancer. *Cancer.* 1989;64:1254–1260.
17. Quazzani L, Reubi JC, Volle GE, et al. Evaluation of somatostatin biosynthesis, somatostatin receptors, and tumor growth in murine medullary thyroid carcinoma. *Eur J Endocrinol.* 1994;131:522–530.

18. Krenning EP, Kwekkeboom DJ, Bakker WH, et al. Somatostatin receptor scintigraphy with [$^{111}$In-DTPA-D-Phe$^1$]- and [$^{123}$I-Tyr$^3$]-octreotide: the Rotterdam experience with more than 1000 patients. *Eur J Nucl Med*. 1993:20:716–731.

19. Wiseman GA, Kvols LK. Therapy of neuroendocrine tumors with radiolabeled MIBG and somatostatin analogues. *Semin Nucl Med*. 1995;25:272–278.

20. Adams S, Baum RP, Rink T, et al. Limited value of fluorine-18 fluorodeoxyglucose positron emission tomography for the imaging of neuroendocrine tumors. *Eur J Nucl Med*. 1998;25:79–83.

21. Sundin A, Eriksson B, Bergström M, et al. PET in the diagnosis of neuroendocrine tumors. *Ann N Y Acad Sci*. 2004;1014;246–257.

22. Eriksson B, Bergström M, Sundin A, et al. The role of PET in localization of neuroendocrine tumors and adrenocortical tumors. *Ann N Y Acad Sci*. 2002;970;159–169.

23. Wiedenmann B, Jensen RT, Mignon M, et al. Preoperative diagnosis and surgical management of neuroendocrine gastroenteropancreatic tumors: general recommendations by a consensus workshop. *World J Surg*. 1998 22 309–318.

24. Mignon M. Natural history of neuroendocrine enteropancreatic tumors. *Digestion*. 2000;63:51–58.

25. Gulec SA, Mountcastle TS, Frey D, et al. Cytoreductive surgery in patients with advanced-stage carcinoid tumors. *Am Surg*. 2002;68:667–671.

26. Norton JA, Fraker DL, Alexander HR, et al. Surgery to cure the Zollinger-Ellison syndrome. *N Engl J Med*. 1999;341:635–644.

27. Arnold R. Medical treatment of metastasizing carcinoid tumors. *World J Surg*. 1996;20:203–207.

28. Makridis C, Oberg K, Juhlin C, et al. Surgical treatment of mid-gut carcinoid tumors. *World J Surg*. 1990;14:377–385.

29. Schneebaum S, Even-Sapir E, Meir C, et al. Clinical applications of gamma-detection probes—radioguided surgery. *Eur J Nucl Med*. 1999;26:S26–S35.

30. Colton CL, Hardy JG. Evaluation of a sterilizable radiation probe as an aid to the surgical treatment of osteoid osteoma. *J Bone Joint Surg Am*. 1981;65:1019–1022.

31. Sutton R, Doran HE, Williams EM, et al. Surgery for mid-gut carcinoid. *Endocr Relat Cancer*. 2003;10:469–481.

32. Memon MA, Nelson H. Gastrointestinal carcinoid tumors: current management strategies. *Dis Colon Rectum*. 1997;40:1101–1118.

33. Marsh DJ, Learoyd DL, Robinson BG. Medullary thyroid carcinoma: recent advances and management update. *Thyroid*. 1995;5:407–424.

34. Moley JF. Medullary thyroid cancer. *Surg Clin North Am*. 1995;75:405–420.

35. Raue F. German medullary thyroid carcinoma/multiple endocrine neoplasia registry. German MTC/MEN Study Group. Medullary Thyroid Carcinoma/Multiple Endocrine Neoplasia Type 2. *Langenbecks Arch Surg*. 1998;383:334–336.

36. Kebebew E, Ituarte PH, Siperstein AE, et al. Medullary thyroid carcinoma: clinical characteristics, treatment, prognostic factors, and a comparison of staging systems. *Cancer*. 2000;88:1139–1148.

37. Schröder S, Bocker W, Baisch H, et al. Prognostic factors in medullary thyroid carcinoma. *Cancer*. 1988;62:806–816.

38. Gordon PR, Huvos AG, Strong EW. Medullary carcinoma of the thyroid gland. A clinicopathologic study of 40 cases. *Cancer*. 1973;31:915–924.

39. Woolner LB, Beahrs OH, Black BM, et al. Long-term survival rates. In: Hedinger CHR, ed. *Thyroid Cancer*. Berlin, Heidelberg, New York: Springer; 1969:326–330.

40. Grauer A, Blind E. Tumor markers for medullary thyroid carcinoma. *Rec Results Cancer*. 1992;125:55–89.

41. Cohen R, Campos JM, Salaun C, et al. Preoperative calcitonin levels are predictive of tumor size and postoperative calcitonin normalization in medullary thyroid carcinoma. Groupe d'Etudes des Tumeurs a Calcitonine (GETC). *J Clin Endocrinol Metab*. 2000;85:919–922.

42. Nobels FR, Kwekkeboom DJ, Coopmans W, et al. Chromogranin A as serum marker for neuroendocrine neoplasia: comparison with neuron-specific enolase and the α-subunit of glycoprotein hormones. *J Clin Endocrinol Metab*. 1997;82:2622–2628.

43. Wahl RA, Röher AD. Surgery of C cell carcinoma of the thyroid. *Prog Surg*. 1988;19:100–112.

44. Cohen MS, Moley JF. Surgical treatment of medullary thyroid carcinoma. *J Intern Med*. 2003;253:616–626.

45. Giuffrida D, Gharib H. Current diagnosis and management of medullary thyroid carcinoma. *Ann Oncol*. 1998; 9:695–701.

46. Frank-Raue K, Raue F, Buhr HJ, et al. Localization of occult persisting medullary thyroid carcinoma before microsurgical reoperation: high sensitivity of selective venous catheterization. *Thyroid*. 1992;2:113–117.

47. Gotthardt M, Battmann A, Hoffken H, et al. $^{18}$F-FDG PET, somatostatin receptor scintigraphy, and CT in metastatic medullary thyroid carcinoma: a clinical study and an analysis of the literature. *Nucl Med Commun*. 2004; 25:439–443.

48. Shapiro B, Sisson JC, Shulkin BL, et al. The current status of metaiodobenzylguanidine and related agents for the diagnosis of neuroendocrine tumors. *Q J Nucl Med*. 1995;39:3–8.

49. Adams S, Acker P, Lorenz M, et al. Radioisotope-guided surgery in patients with pheochromocytoma and recurrent medullary thyroid carcinoma. *Cancer*. 2001;92:263–270.

50. Dörr U, Frank-Raue K, Raue F, et al. The potential value of somatostatin receptor scintigraphy in medullary thyroid carcinoma. *Nucl Med Commun*. 1993;14:439–445.

51. Kwekkeboom DJ, Lamberts SWJ, Reubi JC, et al. Tumor localization using $^{111}$In-octreotide scintigraphy. *Eur J Nucl Med*. 1992;19:599.

52. Baudin E, Lumbroso J, Schlumberger M, et al. Comparison of octreotide scintigraphy and conventional imaging in medullary thyroid carcinoma. *J Nucl Med*. 1996;37:912–916.

53. Adams S, Baum RP, Hertel A, et al. Comparison of metabolic and receptor imaging in recurrent medullary thyroid

carcinoma with histopathological findings. *Eur J Nucl Med*. 1998;25:1277–1283.

54. Reubi JC, Krenning E, Lamberts SWJ, et al. In vitro detection of somatostatin receptors in human tumors. *Digestion*. 1993;54:76–83.

55. Kwekkeboom DJ, Reubi JC, Lamberts SW, et al. In vivo somatostatin receptor imaging in medullary thyroid carcinoma. *J Clin Endocrinol Metab*. 1993;76:1413–1417.

56. Rufini V, Salvatori M, Garganese MC, et al. Role of nuclear medicine in the diagnosis and therapy of medullary thyroid carcinoma. *Rays*. 2000;25:273–282.

57. Moley JF, DeBenedetti MK. Patterns of nodal metastases in palpable medullary thyroid carcinoma: recommendations for extent of node dissection. *Ann Surg*. 1999; 229:880–887.

58. Scollo C, Baudin E, Travagli JP, et al. Rationale for central and bilateral lymph node dissection in sporadic and hereditary medullary thyroid cancer. *J Clin Endocrinol Metab*. 2003;88:2070–2075.

59. Inoue T, Tamaki Y, Sato Y, et al. Three-dimensional ultrasound imaging of breast cancer by a real-time intraoperative navigation system. *Breast Cancer*. 2005;12: 122–129.

60. Otha H, Tsuji T, Endo K, et al. SPECT images using $^{99m}$Tc(V)-DMSA in lung metastasis of osteosarcoma. *Ann Nucl Med*. 1989;3:37–40.

61. Ercan MT, Gulaldi NC, Unsal IS, et al. Evaluation of $^{99m}$Tc(V)-DMSA for imaging inflammatory lesions. An experimental study. *Ann Nucl Med*. 1996;10:419–423.

62. Behr TM, Gratz S, Munz DL, et al. Anti-CEA antibodies versus octreotide for the detection of metastatic medullary thyroid cancer: are CEA and somatostatin-receptor-expression prognostic factors? *J Nucl Med*. 1997;38:9P.

63. De Groot JW, Links TP, Jager PL, et al. Impact of $^{18}$F-fluoro-2-deoxy-D-glucose positron emission tomography (FDG-PET) in patients with biochemical evidence of recurrent or residual medullary thyroid cancer. *Ann Surg Oncol*. 2004;11:786.

64. Bockisch A, Brandt-Mainz K, Gorges R, et al. Diagnosis in medullary thyroid cancer with [$^{18}$F]FDG-PET and improvement using a combined PET/CT scanner. *Acta Med Austriaca*. 2003;30:22–25.

65. Goldstein RE, O'Neill Jr JA, Holcomb III GW, et al. Clinical experience over 48 years with pheochromocytoma. *Ann Surg*. 1999;229:755–764.

66. Peppercorn PD, Grossman AB, Reznek RH. Imaging of incidentally discovered adrenal masses. *Clin Endocrinol*. 1998;48:379–388.

67. Hoefnagel CA. Metaiodobenzylguanidine and somatostatin in oncology: role in the management of neural crest tumors. *Eur J Nucl Med*. 1994;21:561–581.

68. Pacak K, Linehan WM, Eisenhofer G, et al. Recent advances in genetics, diagnosis, localization, and treatment of pheochromocytoma. *Ann Intern Med*. 2001; 134:315–329.

69. Ricard M, Tenenbaum F, Schlumberger M, et al. Intraoperative detection of pheochromocytoma with iodine-125 labelled metaiodobenzylguanidine: a feasibility study. *Eur J Nucl Med*. 1993;20:426–430.

70. Kaltsas G, Korbonits M, Heintz E, et al. Comparison of somatostatin analogue and meta-iodobenzylguanidine radionuclides in the diagnosis and localization of advanced neuroendocrine tumors. *J Clin Endocrinol Metab*. 2001;86:895–902.

71. Rolleman E, Krenning EP, van Gameren A, et al. Uptake of $^{111}$In-DTPA-Octreotide in the rat kidney is inhibited by colchicine and not by fructose. *J Nucl Med*. 2004;45: 709–713.

72. Neumann HP, Berger DP, Sigmund G, et al. Pheochromocytomas, multiple endocrine neoplasia type 2, and von Hippel-Lindau disease. *N Engl J Med*. 1993;329: 1531–1538.

73. Pacak K, Goldstein DS, Doppman JL, et al. A "pheo" lurks: novel approaches for locating occult pheochromocytoma. *J Clin Endocrinol Metab*. 2001;86:3641–3646.

74. Proye CAG, Lokey JS. Current concepts in functioning endocrine tumors of the pancreas. *World J Surg*. 2004: 28;1231–1238.

75. Pederzoli P, Falconi M, Bonora A, et al. Cytoreductive surgery in advanced endocrine tumours of the pancreas. *Ital J Gastroenterol Hepatol*. 1999;31:S207–S212.

76. Jensen RT Gastrointestinal endocrine tumors. Gastrinoma. *Baillieres Clin Gastroenterol*. 1996;10:603–643.

77. Viola KV, Sosa JA. Current advances in the diagnosis and treatment of pancreatic endocrine tumors. *Curr Opin Oncol*. 2005;17:24–27.

78. Bansal R, Tiemey W, Carpenter S, et al. EUS should play a primary role in preoperative localization of pancreatic neuroendocrine tumors. *Gastrointest Endosc*. 1999;49: 19–25.

79. Vinik AI, Moattari AR. Treatment of endocrine tumors of the pancreas. *Endocrinol Metab Clin North Am*. 1989;18:483–518.

80. Scott BA, Gatenby RA. Imaging advances in the diagnosis of endocrine neoplasia. *Curr Opin Oncol*. 1998;10: 37–42.

81. Service FJ, McMahon MM, O'Brien PC, et al. Functioning insulinoma: incidence, recurrence, and long-term survival of patients: a 60-year study. *Mayo Clin Proc*. 1991;66:711–719.

82. Grant CS. Gastrointestinal endocrine tumors. Insulinoma. *Baillieres Clin Gastroenterol*. 1996;10:645–671.

83. Service FJ. Classification of hypoglycemic disorders. *Endocrinol Metab Clin North Am*. 1999;28:501–517.

84. Erickson D, Kudva YC, Ebersold MJ, et al. Benign paragangliomas: clinical presentation and treatment outcomes in 236 patients. *J Clin Endocrinol Metab*. 2001;86:5210–5216.

85. Heij HA, Rutgers EJ, de Kraker J, et al. Intraoperative search for neuroblastoma by MIBG and radioguided surgery with the gamma detector. *Med Pediatr Oncol*. 1997;28:171–174.

86. Schindl M, Kaserer K, Niederle B. Treatment of gastric neuroendocrine tumors: the necessity of a type-adapted treatment. *Arch Surg*. 2001;136:49–54.

87. Wolfe MM, Jensen RT. Zollinger-Ellison syndrome. Current concepts in diagnosis and management. *N Engl J Med*. 1987;317:1200–1209.

88. Eckhauser FE, Lloyd RV, Thompson NW, Raper SE, Vinik AI. Antrectomy for multicentric, argyrophil gastric carcinoids: a preliminary report. *Surgery.* 1988;104: 1046–1053.

89. Hirschowitz BI, Griffith J, Pellegrin D, Cummings OW. Rapid regression of enterochromaffin-like cell gastric carcinoids in pernicious anemia after antrectomy. *Gastroenterology.* 1992;102:1409–1418.

90. Akerstrom G. Management of carcinoid tumors of the stomach, duodenum, and pancreas. *World J Surg.* 1996;20:173–182.

91. Norton JA, Alexander HR, Fraker DL, Venzon DJ, Gibril F, Jensen RT. Comparison of surgical results in patients with advanced and limited disease with multiple endocrine neoplasia type 1 and Zollinger-Ellison syndrome. *Ann Surg.* 2001;234:495–506.

92. Modlin IM, Lye KD, Kidd M. A 50-year analysis of 562 gastric carcinoids: small tumor or larger problem? *Am J Gastroenterol.* 2004;99:23–32.

93. Soga J. Endocrinocarcinomas (carcinoids and their variants) of the duodenum. An evaluation of 927 cases. *J Exp Clin Cancer Res.* 2003;22:349–363.

94. Zyromski NJ, Kendrick ML, Nagorney DM, et al. Duodenal carcinoid tumors: how aggressive should we be? *J Gastrointest Surg.* 2001;5:588–593.

95. Norton JA, Cromack DT, Shawher TH, et al. Intraoperative ultrasonographic localization of islet cell tumors. *Ann Surg.* 1988;207:160–168.

96. Adams S, Baum RP, Wenisch HJC, et al. Intraoperative gamma probe detection of neuroendocrine tumors. *J Nucl Med.* 1998;39:1155–1160.

97. Schirner WJ, O'Dorisio TM, Schirner TP, et al. Intraoperative localization of neuroendocrine tumors with $^{125}$I-TYR$^3$-octreotide and a hand-held gamma detecting probe. *Surgery.* 1993;114:745–752.

98. Öhrvall U, Westlin JE, Nilsson S, et al. Intraoperative gamma detection reveals abdominal endocrine tumors more efficiently than somatostatin receptor scintigraphy. *Cancer.* 1997;80:2490–2494.

99. Lebtahi R, Cadiot L, Sarda L, et al. Clinical impact of somatostatin receptor scintigraphy in the management of patients with neuroendocrine gastroenteropancreatic tumors. *J Nucl Med.* 1997;38:853–858.

100. Ind TE, Granowska M, Britton KE, et al. Preoperative radioimmunodetection of ovarian carcinoma using a hand-held gamma detection probe. *Br J Cancer.* 1994;70: 1263–1266.

101. Adams S, Baum RP, Adams M, et al. Untersuchungen zur prä- und intraoperativen Lokalisation von neuroendokrinen Tumoren. *Acta Med Austriaca.* 1997;2:81–86.

102. Burke AP, Thomas RM, Elsayed AM, Sobin LH. Carcinoids of the jejunum and ileum: an immunohistochemical and clinicopathologic study of 167 cases. *Cancer.* 1997;79: 1086–1093.

103. Falconi M, Bettini R, Scarpa A, Capelli P, Pederzoli P. 2001 Surgical strategy in the treatment of gastrointestinal neuroendocrine tumours. *Ann Oncol.* 12(suppl 2):S101–S103.

104. Modlin IM, Lye KD, Kidd M. A 5-decade analysis of 13,715 carcinoid tumors. *Cancer.* 2003;97:934–959.

105. Hanson HW, Feldman JM, Binder RA, et al. Carcinoid tumors: iodine-131 MIBG scintigraphy. *Radiology.* 1989; 17:699–703.

106. Fischer M, Kamanbroo D, Sonderkamp H. Scintigraphic imaging of carcinoid tumors with J-131-metaiodobenzyl-guanidine. *Lancet.* 1984;135:657–662.

107. Ricke J, Klose KJ, Mignon M, et al. Standardization of imaging in neuroendocrine tumors: results of a European Delphi process. *Eur J Radiol.* 2001;37:8–17.

108. Ganim RB, Norton JA. Recent advances in carcinoid pathogenesis, diagnosis, and management. *Surg Oncol.* 2000;9:173–179.

109. Krausz Y, Keidar Z, Kogan I, et al. SPECT/CT hybrid imaging with $^{111}$In-pentetreotide in assessment of neuroendocrine tumors. *Clin Endocrinol.* 2003;59:565–573.

110. Roggo A, Wood WC, Ottinger LW. Carcinoid tumors of the appendix. *Ann Surg.* 1993;217:385–390.

111. Sandor A, Modlin IM. A retrospective analysis of 1570 appendiceal carcinoids. *Am J Gastroenterol.* 1998;93: 422–428.

112. Moertel CG, Weiland LH, Nagorney DM, Dockerty MB. Carcinoid tumor of the appendix: treatment and prognosis. *N Engl J Med.* 1987;317:1699–1701.

113. Butler JA, Houshiar A, Lin F, Wilson SE. Goblet cell carcinoid of the appendix. *Am J Surg.* 1994;168:685–687.

114. Soga J. Carcinoids of the colon and ileocecal region: a statistical evaluation of 363 cases collected from the literature. *J Exp Clin Cancer Res.* 1998;17:139–148.

115. Soga J. Carcinoids of the rectum: an evaluation of 1271 reported cases. *Surg Today.* 1997 27:112–119.

116. Stinner B, Kisker O, Zielke A, Rothmund M. Surgical management for carcinoid tumors of small bowel, appendix, colon, and rectum. *World J Surg.* 1996;20:183–188.

117. Koura AN, Giacco GG, Curley SA, Skibber JM, Feig BW, Ellis LM. Carcinoid tumors of the rectum: effect of size, histopathology, and surgical treatment on metastasis free survival. *Cancer.* 1997 79:1294–1298.

118. Sauven P, Ridge JA, Quan SH, Sigurdson ER. Anorectal carcinoid tumors. Is aggressive surgery warranted? *Ann Surg.* 1990;211:67–71.

119. Woltering EA, Barrie R, O'Dorisio TM, et al. Detection of occult gastrinomas with iodine 125-labeled lanreotide and intraoperative gamma detection. *Surgery.* 1994;116: 1139–1146.

120. Kwekkeboom D, Krenning EP, de Jong M. Peptide receptor imaging and therapy. *J Nucl Med.* 2000;41: 1704–1713.

121. Hofland LJ, Lamberts SW. Somatostatin receptor subtype expression in human tumors. *Ann Oncol.* 2001;12(suppl 2):S31–S36.

122. Anderson CJ, Dehdashti F, Cutler PD, et al. $^{64}$Cu-TETA-octreotide as a PET imaging agent for patients with neuroendocrine tumors. *J Nucl Med.* 2001;42:213–221.

# 25
# Radioguided Surgery of Solitary Pulmonary Nodules

Giuseppe Boni, Franca M.A. Melfi, Gianpiero Manca, Marco Lucchi, Alfredo Mussi, and Giuliano Mariani

## The Clinical Problem

A solitary pulmonary nodule is radiologically defined as an intraparenchymal lung lesion smaller than 3 cm in diameter, not associated with atelectasis or with abnormally enlarged lymph nodes (1). More than 150,000 patients per year in the United States present their physicians with the diagnostic dilemma of a solitary pulmonary nodule, and this number has increased further due to incidental findings of lung nodules discovered on computed tomography (CT) of the chest performed for some unrelated medical reason (2).

Up to 55% of solitary pulmonary nodules are reported to be malignant—either primary lung cancer or pulmonary metastasis of other tumors (3). Poor prognosis of lung cancer is directly associated with its delayed presentation. Signs and symptoms are rarely present until the malignancy has become advanced, and therefore is usually unresectable. Patients with the best prognosis (60% to 75% 5-year survival rate following surgical resection) are those with stage IA disease (T1 N0 M0) (4,5). Unfortunately, approximately half of all lung cancers have already spread to extrapulmonary sites by the time of diagnosis. As a result, the average patient with a newly diagnosed lung cancer has a 5-year survival of only 10% to 15% (6). Therefore, timely and accurate determination of the nature of a solitary pulmonary nodule is essential to provide the patient with malignancy a potential for cancer cure.

The differential diagnosis of a solitary pulmonary nodule includes neoplastic, infectious, inflammatory, vascular, traumatic, and congenital lesions (2). Other benign etiologies for solitary pulmonary nodules are rheumatoid nodules, intrapulmonary lymph nodes, plasma cell granulomas, and sarcoidosis. Although most of these nodules are benign (2,6), primary malignancies are found in approximately 35%, and solitary metastases account for another 23% of solitary pulmonary nodules (3,7–9). Some clinical features, such as older age, history of cigarette smoking, and previous history of cancer all increase the probability that a solitary pulmonary nodule is malignant (10).

Since the solitary pulmonary nodule is by definition a radiographic finding, diagnostic workup is usually based on radiologic findings. However, diagnosing lung cancer based on chest x-ray alone can be quite difficult, with failure rates reported to range from 25% to 90% (11–13).

Spiral CT with intravenous contrast enhancement is the imaging modality of choice, and should be obtained on any newly diagnosed solitary pulmonary nodule, as it provides exact anatomic location as well as some important parameters characterizing the nodule. In case of malignancy, CT has 50% sensitivity and 89% specificity for detecting mediastinal invasion, associated with 14% sensitivity and 99% specificity for identifying invasion of the chest wall (14).

In any patient with a newly discovered solitary pulmonary nodule, a recent history of pneumonia or pulmonary symptoms may warrant simple, noninvasive follow-up of the lesion for 4 to 6 weeks to rule out an infectious etiology. However, persistence of the nodule beyond this time should not further delay thorough diagnostic workup. In a 3-year retrospective study, less than 1% of all solitary pulmonary nodules were found to be infectious (15).

Malignant pulmonary nodules typically exhibit ill-defined, irregular margins and spiculated borders (84% to 90% of spiculated nodules are malignant) (16). Size is an additional useful parameter for defining the likelihood that a lung nodule is malignant: the vast majority of nodules greater than 2 cm in size are malignant, while less than 50% of all nodules smaller than 2 cm are malignant (17). The incidence of malignancy in a lung lesion greater than 3 cm in size is so high that all such lesions should be surgically resected, unless medically contraindicated.

Positron emission tomography (PET) with the glucose analog $^{18}$F-2-fluoro-2-deoxy-d-glucose ($[^{18}F]$FDG) is an excellent mode of tumor imaging (18). Increased [¹⁸F]FDG uptake (with ensuing intracellular retention) is seen in cells with high metabolic rates, which are found in many tumors and areas of moderate to severe inflammation (in addition to tissues with physiologically high glucose consumption, such as the brain cortex). In their meta-analysis of the literature on the diagnostic performance of [¹⁸F]FDG PET in pulmonary nodules and masses (19), Gould et al. found an overall 96.8% sensitivity and 77.8% specificity for detecting malignancy. Conversely, [¹⁸F]FDG PET has 96% sensitivity, 88% specificity, and 94% accuracy for identifying benign nodules. Furthermore, a whole-body [¹⁸F]FDG PET scan has higher diagnostic accuracy than CT for detecting mediastinal lymph node metastases and distant metastases.

Given the 7–8 mm spatial resolution of current PET scanners, some caution should be adopted when imaging solitary pulmonary nodules smaller than 1 cm in size, although even in this group of patients the sensitivity of [¹⁸F]FDG PET has been reported to be as high as 93%, with 77% specificity (20). [¹⁸F]FDG PET can also yield false-negative results for nodules that are carcinoid tumors or bronchoalveolar carcinomas, as these tumors may not have high [¹⁸F]FDG uptake (21). On the other hand, false-positive results can be seen in lung lesions with an infectious or inflammatory etiology, such as tuberculosis, histoplasmosis, or in rheumatoid nodules (19).

The high negative predictive value of [¹⁸F]FDG PET in patients with a solitary pulmonary nodule would support adoption of simple follow-up for any such nodules with a negative scan, especially in low-risk patients. With a 20% pre-test probability of malignancy, the post-test probability of a negative [¹⁸F]FDG PET is extremely low (1%). However, high-risk patients with a pre-test 80% likelihood of malignancy still have a 14% post-test likelihood of malignancy, even with a negative [¹⁸F]FDG PET scan (19).

Percutaneous fine-needle aspiration biopsy has been used for characterizing pulmonary nodules for more than 25 years. CT-guided fine-needle aspiration biopsy has become an important diagnostic tool, particularly for nodules 5 to 15 mm in diameter (22), although its sensitivity and specificity for smaller nodules (ranging from 5 to 10 mm) requires further validation. Furthermore, while sensitivity of fine-needle aspiration biopsy for malignancy is 64% to 100%, it is only 12% to 68% for benign nodules (23,24). Moreover, fine-needle aspiration biopsy is fraught with complications, such as pneumothorax in 25% to 30% of patients (with 5% to 10% of such patients requiring positioning of a chest tube).

Bronchoscopy can be used to perform a diagnostic biopsy in a large central lung mass or in lesions with endobronchial encroachment (with 70% and 90% diagnostic yields, respectively) (25–29). It is also useful in performing fine-needle aspiration biopsy of enlarged mediastinal lymph nodes when staging an already diagnosed non-small cell lung cancer. However, this technique has little to no role for patients with a peripheral solitary pulmonary nodule.

Based on the above considerations, any patient with a newly detected solitary pulmonary nodule not showing benign-looking calcifications should be considered to have a malignancy until proven otherwise. Surgical resection is the ideal approach, as it is both diagnostic and therapeutic. In this regard, thoracoscopic procedures have completely replaced open-chest surgery in the diagnosis of pulmonary, pleural, and mediastinal diseases and in the treatment of benign nodules, especially if located in the peripheral lung regions.

# Video-Assisted Thoracoscopic Surgery and Non-Radionuclide Localization Techniques

Video-assisted thoracoscopic surgery is useful for the diagnosis of peripheral pulmonary nodules eluding diagnosis by other techniques (30,31). It is especially reliable in peripheral solid lesions (within 2 cm of the pleura); nonsolid lesions often produce a normal appearance on surgical inspection and may prove difficult to localize.

Several preoperative methods have been developed to facilitate localization of smaller and deeper pulmonary nodules during video-assisted thoracoscopic surgery, with the purpose of reducing conversion of such a mini-invasive surgical procedure to conventional open-chest surgery. These include CT-guided placement of a percutaneous hookwire (32,33) and placement of a metallic coil (34), or of contrast media under fluoroscopic guidance (35). Although these methods are generally effective, they are not free from complications and limitations. Such possible complications include bleeding (with formation of a hematoma), pneumothorax, and chest pain (36–38). Furthermore, possible displacement of the hookwire is responsible for a certain conversion rate to open surgery.

Alternative preoperative localization techniques include CT-guided intralesional injection of methylene blue (39–41) or of a colored collagen (42). Both procedures provide satisfactory results, with the advantage of fewer complications than the techniques outlined above. However, in some patients the injected dye is not easily detected when performing video-assisted thoracoscopic surgery, either because the lung is anthracotic or because the dye has simply diffused away from the injection site on the pleural surface (especially if surgery is performed more than 3 hours after injection of the dye). This causes conversion of the mini-invasive video-assisted thoracoscopic surgery to a conventional thoracotomic surgical approach (40,43).

Finally, endothoracic ultrasonography has been reported to be useful for localizing peripheral lung lesions to be resected during video-assisted thoracoscopic surgery (44), although its application can be limited by coexistent lung emphysema (45,46).

All the preoperative localization procedures described above have limitations that in several instances make it necessary to convert a mini-invasive video-assisted thoracoscopic surgery procedure to open-chest surgery, thus involving possible higher morbidity, longer hospital stays, and higher overall costs.

## Radioguided Localization of Occult Lung Lesions

In the 1990s, development of a procedure for radioguided occult lesion localization by interstitial injection of $^{99m}$Tc-labeled human albumin macroaggregates in patients with nonpalpable breast tumors (see chapter 22) (47,48) spurred interest in this approach for lesions outside the breast as well. Although few reports have been published on this matter so far (49–52), clinical experience is increasing, so that it is now possible to set some guidelines for performing this procedure. The information provided here is based on our experience with more than 220 procedures performed at the University of Pisa Medical School, Italy, between 1997 and 2005.

### Preoperative Phase

As a general rule in video-assisted thoracoscopic surgery with radioguidance, we selected pulmonary nodules smaller than 2 cm, situated in the lung parenchyma

(>5 mm and <3 cm from the pleural surface), and therefore expected to be neither visible nor palpable with endoscopic instruments during thoracoscopy.

Injection of the radiolabeled particles into the solitary pulmonary nodule can be performed either on the same day of surgery (single-day procedure) or 24 to 36 hours before surgery (2-day procedure). After localizing the pulmonary nodule by means of high-resolution axial CT sections, local anaesthesia of the thoracic wall is performed and a 22-gauge needle of adequate length is introduced into the lesion, or just in contact with it, under CT guidance. Approximately 0.3 to 0.5 mL of a suspension—composed of 0.1 to 0.2 mL of either 5 MBq (single-day procedure) or 10–15 MBq (2-day procedure) $^{99m}$Tc-albumin macroaggregates (>90% of particles in the 10–90 µm size range) and 0.2 to 0.3 mL of non-ionic contrast medium—is injected (see Figure 25-1). A CT scan is repeated after injection to confirm exact placement of the injectate, based on visualization of the contrast medium in the solitary pulmonary nodule or close to it, as well as to exclude possible complications of the procedure (bleeding and/or pneumothorax).

### Operative Phase

Either immediately after intranodular injection (single-day procedure), or the next day (2-day procedure), the patient is transferred to the operating room for video-assisted thoracoscopic surgery. Under general anesthesia with selective orotracheal intubation, and with the patient in a lateral position, pneumothorax is induced on the affected side and a 7-mm trocar is introduced for the videothoracoscope, usually in the sixth or seventh intercostal space along the mid-axillary line. After a first exploration of the pleural space, a second 11.5-mm trocar is placed in the most adequate position according to location of the nodule and anatomy of the pulmonary lobes on thoracoscopic vision. Through this second trocar, an

Back

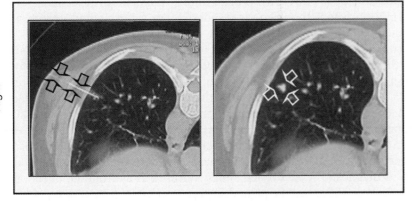

Right

Left

Front

FIGURE 25-1. Selected computed tomographic (CT) images of the preoperative phase of radioguided surgery in a patient with a small solitary nodule at the lower lobe of the right lung (prone position). The left panel shows CT-guided transthoracic insertion of the needle (indicated by open black arrows) in the nodule. The right panel shows correct deposition of the $^{99m}$Tc-albumin macroaggregates (as visualized by co-injected contrast medium, indicated by the open white arrows) at the site of the nodule.

FIGURE 25-2. Intraoperative survey of detectable radioactivity with the thoracoscopic gamma probe during video-assisted thoracoscopic surgery. (A) Identification of the nodule is based on high count rate (actual reading visible in upper right panel). (B) Definition of the correct level for endostapler resection is based on low count rate (background reading visible in upper right panel) below the planned resection margin.

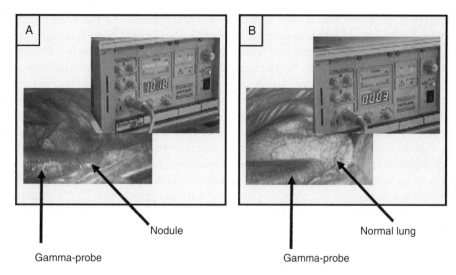

Nodule

Normal lung

Gamma-probe

Gamma-probe

11-mm diameter collimated thoracoscopic gamma probe is introduced (Figure 25-2), measuring first background radioactivity on an area of the lung far from the suspected lesion site. Then pleural surface is systematically scanned to detect the "radioactive focus" with the highest count rate and target/background ratio (Figure 25-3). Once the target area is identified, a third trocar is introduced, choosing a site that allows maximum maneuverability of the endostapler device (Endopath ET45B, Ethicon Endo-Surgery) for wedge resection. Before "firing" the endostapler, careful instrumental palpation of the area identified by gamma-probe counting is performed. In addition, the gamma probe is placed below the stapler to ensure that all radioactivity counts are included within the resection level. Once wedge resec-tion is performed, the nodule is extracted from the pleural cavity into an endoscopic bag through the largest porthole, to avoid possible tumor seeding to the chest wall. Intraoperative frozen-section histology is immediately performed and, if a primary lung cancer is identified, the procedure is completed by a completion thoracotomic lobectomy (if the patient has an adequate pulmonary reserve).

## Institutional Experience

Based on more than 220 consecutive procedures carried out between January 1997 and June 2005 in patients with solitary or multiple small pulmonary nodules, it can be

FIGURE 25-3. $^{99m}$Tc-Depreotide single photon emission computed tomography showing selected transaxial sections (upper panel), sagittal sections (center panel), and coronal sections (lower panel) obtained in a male 45-year-old heavy smoker, in whom computed tomography had revealed a 1-cm solitary pulmonary nodule in the left lung. Images clearly show high uptake of the radiopharmaceutical in the lesion, with a 3.5 maximum target-to-background ratio. Because of the tumor's central location, open-chest surgery was performed, during which the lesion was searched with the aid of an intraoperative gamma probe. This procedure quickly directed the surgeon to the mass to be removed, with a 3.2 target-to-background intraoperative counting ratio.

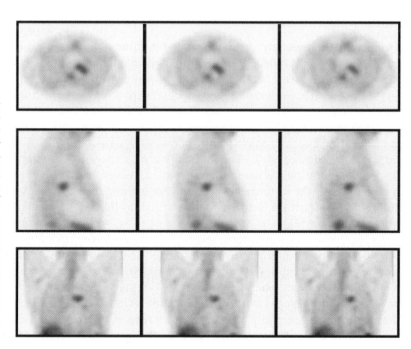

stated that, after a learning phase of 20 procedures (which is necessary to harmonize the team, composed of specialists in radiology, nuclear medicine, and thoracic surgery), video-assisted thoracoscopic surgery with radioguidance can be safely performed in patients with nodules within 3 cm of the visceral pleura surface or near the edge of a pulmonary lobe, to make resection by endostapler possible. In our experience, the mean time for the CT-guided intranodular injection is 17 minutes (range 13–42 min), while it takes only about 3 minutes (range 1–5 min) to localize the nodule with endoscopic gamma-probe scanning, and duration of the entire surgical procedure is about 50 minutes (range 20–100 min) for wedge resection.

The success rate of video-assisted thoracoscopic surgery with radioguidance in our series is 99%; in 2 patients, conversion to minimal thoracotomy was necessary because of some spread of the radiotracer in emphysematous bullae around the lesion. Neither mortality nor morbidity related to the procedure was observed in our series, while partial pneumothorax (a possible complication when performing a transcutaneous procedure) was observed in 6 patients, none of which required pleural drainage.

Although this proportion can obviously change depending on selection and preoperative characterization of the patients (aided, for instance, by [18F]FDG PET, which was not performed systematically in our center), in our experience 51.5% of the nodules were benign, while 34.5% were metastatic tumors and 14% were primary lung cancers.

## Conclusions

Thoracoscopic resection of small peripheral pulmonary nodules is easy and quick when the nodule is in contact with the pleural surface. In this case, it is generally visible on thoracoscopic exploration or palpable with endoscopic instruments. However, when the nodule is either too small or too deep beneath the pleural surface, failure in localization and, as a consequence, conversion to open surgery may be necessary. When relying only on thoracoscopic exploration and endoscopic palpation, this event is more likely if the distance between the nodule and the nearest pleural surface is >5 mm and/or if the nodule is <10 mm in size (53).

To overcome such limitations, several techniques have been developed for preoperative or intraoperative localization of deeper nodules. Percutaneous hookwire placement and methylene blue injection under CT guidance have been widely used, alone or in association. Although these procedures generally yield satisfactory results, they are however fraught with failures (due to displacement of the wire or diffusion of the dye, for example) and/or complications (such as pneumothorax and/or hemothorax). Moreover, when employing such localization techniques, the time elapsed between preoperative placement of the hookwire or blue dye injection and the surgery itself must be kept to a minimum, while intranodular injection of radiolabeled particles for gamma-probe guidance during video-assisted thoracoscopic surgery can be performed up to 24 to 36 hours before surgery.

In our experience, thoracoscopic radioguidance following CT-guided intranodular injection of radiolabeled particles proved to be practicable and efficient for resecting solitary pulmonary nodules during video-assisted thoracoscopic surgery. Only 6 patients developed an asymptomatic pneumothorax (which was, nevertheless, asymptomatic and required no specific treatment), but neither hemothorax nor chest pain have been reported.

The most important advantages of radioguided localization of occult lung lesions as described above can be summarized as follows: 1) exact location of the nodule and its depth from the pleural surface can be defined by CT-guided transthoracic placement of radiolabeled particles that do not move from the site of injection ($^{99m}$Tc-albumin macroaggregates); 2) a safe and sufficient surgical margin can be ensured if the resection line is far enough from the radiolabeled mark; and 3) thoracotomy (even minimal) for palpation to search for location of a nodule can be avoided in virtually all cases.

On the other hand, the possibility remains open to achieve a target-to-background ratio sufficiently high to enable radioguided surgery of solitary pulmonary nodules during video-assisted thoracoscopic surgery to be performed also after systemic administration of a radiopharmaceutical with optimal tumor-localizing properties. This possibility would thus avoid local, transthoracic deposition of nonspecific, large-size radiolabeled particles as described above. [18F]FDG certainly constitutes one such potential radiopharmaceutical, as it has already been explored for occult tumor lesions in other regions of the body (54–56). As this tracer has not been available in our center until recently, we explored the tumor-localizing potential for radioguided surgery of solitary pulmonary nodules of a $^{99m}$Tc-labeled somatostatin analog ($^{99m}$Tc-Deprotide) whose diagnostic performance in patients with a solitary pulmonary nodules has been reported to be almost equivalent to that of [18F]FDG (57–59). In a preliminary study involving 17 patients, we observed high uptake of $^{99m}$Tc-Deprotide in 14 of 17 solitary pulmonary nodules, with target-to-background ratios evaluated on the SPECT images equal to 2.8 ± 1.2. All the patients with a positive scan underwent radioguided surgery (either open chest or video-assisted thoracoscopic surgery) on the next day. Intraoperative radioguidance was successful for localizing the solitary pulmonary nodules in all cases with a positive SPECT except 1, with intraoperative target-to-background gamma probe count ratios equal to $2.3 \pm 0.8$ (see Figure 25-3), therefore closely mirroring the corresponding values evaluated on the SPECT images (60,61).

# References

1. Tuddenham WI. Glossary of terms for thoracic radiology: recommendations of the Nomenclature Committee of the Fleischner Society. *Am J Roentgenol.* 1984;43:509–517.
2. Leef JL 3rd, Klein IS. The solitary pulmonary nodule. *Radiol Clin North Am.* 2002;40:123–143.
3. Mack MJ, Hazelrigg SR, Landreneau RJ, Acuff TE. Thoracoscopy for the diagnosis of the indetermined solitary pulmonary nodule. *Ann Thorac Surg.* 1993;56:825–832.
4. Mountain CF. Revisions in the international system for staging lung cancer. *Chest.* 1997;111:1710–1717.
5. Abeloff MD, Annitage IO, Lichter AS, et al. *Clinical Oncology.* 2nd edition. New York: WB Saunders; 2000: 1398–1464.
6. Yankelvitz DF, Hensche CI. Lung cancer: small solitary pulmonary nodules. *Radiol Clin North Am.* 2000;38:1–9.
7. Greenlee RT, Hill-Harmon MB, Murray T, et al. Cancer statistics, 2001. *CA Cancer J Clin.* 2001;51:15–36.
8. Jemal A, Murray T, Thun LA. Cancer statistics, 2002. *CA Cancer J Clin.* 2002;52:23–47.
9. Swanson SI, Iaklitsch MT, Mentzer SI, et al. Management of the solitary pulmonary nodule: role of thoracoscopy in diagnosis and therapy. *Chest.* 1999;116:523S–524S.
10. Swenson SI, Silverstein MD, Ilstrup DM, et al. The probability of malignancy in solitary pulmonary nodules: application to small radiologically indeterminate nodules. *Arch Intern Med.* 1997;57:849–855.
11. Stitik FP, Tockrnan MS. Radiologic screening in the early detection of lung cancer. *Radiol Clin North Am.* 1978; 16:347–366.
12. Muhm JR, Miller WE, Fontana RS, et al. Lung cancer detected during a screening program using 4-month chest radiographs. *Radiology.* 1983;143:609–615.
13. Heenan RT, Flehinger BJ, Melamed MR, et al. Non-small cell lung cancer: results of the New York screening program. *Radiology.* 1984;151:289–293.
14. White P, Adams H, Crane M, et al. Preoperative staging of carcinoma of the bronchus: can computed tomographic scanning reliably identify stage II tumors. *Thorax.* 1994; 49:951–957.
15. Rolston KV, Rodriguez S, Dholakia N, et al. Pulmonary infections mimicking cancer: a retrospective 3-year review. *Support Care Cancer.* 1997;5:590–593.
16. Zwirewich CV, Vedal S, Miller RR, et al. Solitary pulmonary nodule: high resolution CT and radiologic-pathologic correlation. *Radiology.* 1991;179:469–481.
17. Shure D, Fedullo PF. Transbronchial needle aspiration of peripheral masses. *Am Rev Respir Dis.* 1983;728:1090–1092.
18. Gambhir SS, Czernin J, Schwimmer J, Silverman DH, Coleman RE, Phelps ME. A tabulated summary of the FDG PET literature. *J Nucl Med.* 2001;4(suppl 5):1S–93S.
19. Gould MK, Maclean CC, Kuschner WG, et al. Accuracy of positron emission tomography for diagnosis of pulmonary nodules and mass lesions: a meta-analysis. *JAMA.* 2001;285:914–924.
20. Herder GJ, Golding RP, Hoekstra OS, et al. The performance of $^{18}$F-fluorodeoxyglucose positron emission tomography in small solitary pulmonary nodules. *Eur J Nucl Med Mol Imaging.* 2004;31:1231–1236.
21. Goldsmith SI, Kostakoglu L. Nuclear medicine imaging of lung cancer. *Radiol Clin North Am.* 2000;38:511–524.
22. Yankelevitz DF, Henschke CI, Koizumi JH, et al. CT-guided transthoracic needle biopsy of small solitary pulmonary nodules. *Clin Imaging.* 1997;21:107–110.
23. Sanders C. Transthoracic needle aspiration. *Clin Chest Med.* 1992;13:11–16.
24. Weisbrod GL. Transthoracic needle biopsy. *World J Surg.* 1993;17:705–711.
25. Stringfield JT, Markowitz DJ, Bentz RR, et al. The effect of tumor size and location on diagnosis by fiberoptic bronchoscopy. *Chest.* 1977;72:474–476.
26. Arroliga AC, Matthay RA. The role of bronchoscopy in lung cancer. *Clin Chest Med.* 1993;14:87–98.
27. Torrington KG, Kern JD. The utility of fiberoptic bronchoscopy in the evaluation of solitary pulmonary nodules. *Chest.* 1993;104:1021–1024.
28. American Thoracic Society/European Respiratory Society. Pretreatment evaluation of non-small-cell lung cancer. *Am J Respir Crit Care Med.* 1997;156:320–332.
29. Baaklini WA, Reinoso MA, Gorin AB, et al. Diagnostic yield of fiber-optic bronchoscopy in evaluating solitary pulmonary nodules. *Chest.* 2000;117:1049–1054.
30. Mack MJ, Hazelrigg SR, Landreneau RJ, Acuff TE. Thoracoscopy for the diagnosis of the indetermined solitary pulmonary nodule. *Ann Thorac Surg.* 1993;56: 825–832.
31. Shulkin AN. Management of the indetermined solitary pulmonary nodule: a pneumologist's view. *Ann Thorac Surg.* 1993;56:743–744.
32. Shah RM, Spirn PW, Salazar AM, et al. Localization of peripheral pulmonary nodules for thoracoscopic excision: value of CT-guided wire placement. *AJR Am J Roentgenol.* 1993;161:279–283.
33. Shepard JO, Mathisen DJ, Muse VV, Bhalla M, McLoud TC. Needle localization of peripheral lung nodules for video-assisted thoracoscopic surgery. *Chest.* 1994;105: 1559–1563.
34. Asamura H, Kondo H, Naruke T, et al. Computed tomography-guided coil injection and thoracoscopic pulmonary resection under roentgenographic fluoroscopy. *Ann Thorac Surg.* 1994;58:1542–1544.
35. Moon S, Wang Y, Jo K, et al. Fluoroscopy-aided thoracoscopic resection of pulmonary nodule localized with contrast media. *Ann Thorac Surg.* 1999;68:1815–1820.
36. De Kerviler E, Gossot D, Frija J. Localization techniques for the thoracoscopic resection of pulmonary nodules. *Int Surg.* 1996;81:241–244.
37. Kunazawa S, Ando A, Yasui K, et al. Localization of pulmonary nodules for thoracoscopic resection: experience

with a system using a short hookwire and suture. *AJR Am J Roentgenol.* 1998;170:332–334.

38. Horan TA, Pinheiro PM, Araujo LM, Santiago FF, Rodriguez MR. Massive gas embolism during pulmonary nodule hook wire localization. *Ann Thorac Surg.* 2002;73:1647–1649.

39. Lenglinger FX, Schwarz CD, Artmann W. Localization of pulmonary nodules before thoracoscopic surgery: value of percutaneous staining with methylene blue. *AJR Am J Roentgenol.* 1994;163:297–300.

40. Wicky S, Mayor B, Schnyder P. Methylene blue localizations of pulmonary nodules under CT-guidance: a new procedure used before thoracoscopic resections. *Int Surg.* 1997;82:15–17.

41. Vandoni RE, Cuttat JF, Wicky S, Suter M. CT-guided methylene-blue labelling before thoracoscopic resection of pulmonary nodules. *Eur J Cardio-Thorac Surg* 1998;14:265–270.

42. Nomori H, Horio H. Colored collagen is a long-lasting point marker for small pulmonary nodules in thoracoscopic operation. *Ann Thorac Surg.* 1996;61:1070–1073.

43. Saito H, Minamiya Y, Matsuzaki I, et al. Indication for preoperative localization of small peripheral pulmonary nodules in thoracoscopic surgery. *J Thorac Cardiovasc Surg* 2002;124:1198–1202.

44. Greenfield AL, Steiner RM, Liu JB, et al. Sonographic guidance for the localization of peripheral pulmonary nodules during thoracoscopy. *AJR Am J Roentgenol* 1997;168:1057–1060.

45. Kerviler E, Gossot D, Celerier M, Frija J. Limitations of intraoperative sonography for the localization of pulmonary nodules during thoracoscopy. *AJR Am J Roentgenol.* 1998;170:214–215.

46. Santambrogio R, Montorsi M, Bianchi P, Mantovani A, Ghelma F, Mezzetti M. Intraoperative ultrasound during thoracoscopic procedures for solitary pulmonary nodules. *Ann Thorac Surg.* 1999;68:218–222.

47. Luini A, Zurrida S, Galimberti V, et al. Radioguided surgery of occult breast lesions. *Eur J Cancer.* 1998;34:204–205.

48. Luini A, Zurrida S, Paganelli G, et al. Comparison of radioguided excision with wire localisation of occult breast lesions. *Br J Surg.* 1999;86:522–525.

49. Boni G, Bellina CR, Grosso M, et al. Gamma probe-guided thoracoscopic surgery of small pulmonary nodules. *Tumori.* 2000;86:364–366.

50. Chella A, Lucchi M, Ambrogi MC, et al. A pilot study of the role of Tc-99m radionuclide in localization of pulmonary nodular lesions for thoracoscopic resection. *Eur J Cardio-Thorac Surg.* 2000;18:17–21.

51. Sortini D, Feo CV, Carrella G, et al. Thoracoscopic localization techniques for patients with a single pulmonary nodule and positive oncological anamnesis: a prospective study. *J Laparoendosc Adv Surg Tech A.* 2003;13:371–375.

52. Ambrogi MC, Dini P, Boni G, et al. A strategy for thoracosscopic resection of small pulmonary nodules. *Surg Endosc.* 2005;19:1644–1647.

53. Suzuki K, Nagai K, Yoshida J, et al. Video assisted thoracoscopic surgery for small indeterminate pulmonary nodules: indications for preoperative marking. *Chest.* 1999;115:563–568.

54. Essner R, Hsueh E-C, Haigh P-I, et al. Application of an [18]F-fluorodeoxyglucose-sensitive probe for the intraoperative detection of malignancy. *J Surg Res.* 2001;96:120–126.

55. Zervos EE, Desai DC, De Palatis LR, et al. [18]F-labeled fluorodeoxyglucose positron emission tomography-guided surgery for recurrent colorectal cancer. *J Surg Res.* 2001;97:9–13.

56. Meller B, Sahlmann C, Horstmann O, Gerl J, Bahere M, Meller J. Conventional gamma and high-energy probes for radioguided dissection of metastases in a patient with recurrent thyroid carcinoma with [99m]Tc-MIBI and [18]F-FDG. *Nuklearmedizin.* 2005;44:N23–N25.

57. Blum J, Handmaker H, Lister-James J, Rinne N; the NeoTect Solitary Pulmonary Nodule Study Group. A multicenter trial with a somatostatin analog [99m]Tc Depreotide in the evaluation of solitary pulmonary nodules. *Chest.* 2000;117:1232–1238.

58. Kahn D, Menda Y, Kernstine K, et al. The utility of [99m]Tc-depreotide compared with F-18 Fluorodeoxyglucose positron emission tomography and surgical staging in patients with suspected non-small cell lung cancer. *Chest.* 2004;125:494–501.

59. Halley A, Hugentobler A, Icard P, et al. Efficiency of [18]F-FDG and [99m]Tc-depreotide SPECT in the diagnosis of malignancy of solitary pulmonary nodules. *Eur J Nucl Med Mol Imaging.* 2005;32:1026–1032.

60. Boni G, Melfi FMA, Givigliano F, et al. [99m]Tc-Depreotide in the surgical patients with pulmonary malignancy: correlation between scintigraphic data and intrasurgical findings [Abstract]. *Q J Nucl Med.* 2004;48 (suppl 1):43.

61. Boni G, Bertolaccini P, Melfi FMA, et al. Clinical utility of [99m]Tc-depreotide as diagnostic procedure and intraoperative marker for radioguided surgery in patients with pulmonary malignancy. *Eur J Nucl Med Mol Imaging.* 2005;32(suppl 1):S49–S50.

# 26
# Radioguided Surgery of Occult Lesions in Patients with Thyroid Cancer

Domenico Rubello, Massimo Salvatori, Maria Rosa Pelizzo, Giuseppe Boni, and Giuliano Mariani

In patients with well-differentiated thyroid carcinoma, poorly differentiated thyroid carcinoma, and medullary thyroid carcinoma, surgery is the first and most important modality of treatment (1). The extent of the surgery is debatable, although most clinicians currently recommend total or near-total thyroidectomy for all clinically obvious thyroid tumors (2), to reduce local recurrence rates. This is supported by follow-up studies demonstrating that the completeness of surgical excision is an independent prognostic indicator for survival (3).

In patients with well-differentiated thyroid carcinoma, initial surgery is often followed by radioiodine ($^{131}$I) ablation. Postoperative remnant ablation is performed for 3 reasons: 1) to eradicate microscopic residual tumor foci, 2) to facilitate follow-up by serial evaluations of serum thyroglobulin (Tg) and $^{131}$I whole-body scans, and 3) to perform a highly sensitive $^{131}$I whole-body scan 3 to 7 days after administration of the therapeutic dose to detect metastases (4).

The frequency of lymph node metastasis at initial staging is related to the tumor histologic type, the size of the primary tumor, the extent of lymph node dissection, and the method of histologic analysis (2). In most studies, lymph node involvement is associated with a higher risk of locoregional recurrences and of distant metastases, so that the 2002 TNM classification analyzes its prognostic impact according to the extent of the primary tumor (5).

While the impact of lymph node metastases on the survival of patients with well-differentiated thyroid carcinoma is still controversial, several studies have shown that survival of patients with medullary thyroid carcinoma is correlated with the adequacy of the initial, extensive lymph node dissection of the neck (6). Nevertheless, despite complete initial treatment, 5% to 20% of patients with well-differentiated thyroid carcinoma and nearly 50% of patients with medullary thyroid carcinoma show residual or recurrent disease, which is respon-

sible for a higher incidence of distant metastases and worse survival rates (7).

Surgery is the main modality of treatment for locoregional recurrences. Planning this requires a preoperative work-up for the site(s) and the extent of the metastases. Ultrasonography, computed tomography (CT), and magnetic resonance imaging (MRI) are sensitive, but are often difficult to interpret. Scarring in the thyroid bed from prior thyroidectomy and in the previously dissected areas alters anatomy (8), making the usual landmarks difficult to recognize. Furthermore, despite their relatively high spatial resolution, ultrasonography, CT, and MRI have limited ability in discriminating mass lesions as being viable tumor or scar, in determining whether mildly enlarged lymph nodes represent tumor or a non-malignant process, and in detecting cancer foci less than 1 cm in diameter.

While often capable of distinguishing residual disease from scar tissue, scintigraphic imaging with specific and nonspecific tumor-seeking agents suffers from inadequate sensitivity, primarily because of the limited spatial resolution of the gamma camera. Like single photon imaging, positron emission tomography (PET) with [$^{18}$F]-2-fluoro-2-deoxy-d-glucose ([$^{18}$F]FDG) has been advocated to detect metastasis in lymph nodes. Unfortunately, the entire node usually has to be involved to see the lesion. If there are only a few tumor cells in the node, it is usually not identified on the [$^{18}$F]FDG-PET scan. In addition, in the early phase of well-differentiated thyroid carcinoma, when the tumor cells are iodine avid, the lesions are rarely [$^{18}$F]FDG avid (9).

To overcome these difficulties, several authors have proposed radioguidance with an intraoperative gamma probe following the administration of specific or nonspecific tumor-seeking radiopharmaceuticals to detect and dissect metastatic lymph nodes during operations for locoregional recurrences in patients with thyroid carcinomas.

This chapter discusses the techniques, results, advantages, and limitations of various radioguided surgical

TABLE 26-1. Radiopharmaceuticals for radioguided surgery in thyroid cancer.

| Tumor-seeking radiopharmaceuticals for radioguided surgery in thyroid cancer |
| --- |
| Differentiated thyroid carcinoma |
| [131]I-iodine |
| [123]I-iodide |
| Nonfunctioning thyroid carcinoma |
| [99m]Tc-sestamibi |
| [[18]F]FDG |
| Medullary thyroid carcinoma |
| [111]In-pentetreotide |
| [99m]Tc (V)-DMSA |
| Monoclonal antibodies |

procedures applied in patients with well-differentiated thyroid carcinoma (8,10,11), iodine-negative thyroid cancer (12,13), and medullary thyroid carcinoma (14–19) (Table 26-1).

# Differentiated Thyroid Carcinoma

Total or near-total thyroidectomy followed by [131]I ablation of the thyroid remnants is widely accepted as the most effective modality of treatment for patients with well-differentiated thyroid carcinoma. However, after such combined initial treatment, locoregional recurrences appear in 5% to 20% of patients (about twice the frequency of distant metastases) (4). In general, these recurrences are the result of incomplete initial treatment or of particularly aggressive tumors, and usually appear early during follow-up, although some may be detected later (4).

Lymph node metastases, the most frequent site of the locoregional recurrences, can occur in the thyroid bed, in the soft tissue of the neck, or invading the aerodigestive tract, the strap muscles, recurrent laryngeal nerves, and esophagus (2).

Some patients have a higher risk of developing local and regional recurrences, especially: 1) patients under age 16 or over age 45; 2) those with special histologic subtypes, tumors greater than 3 cm, or tumors extending beyond the thyroid capsule; and 3) those with large, bilateral and multiple lymph nodes metastases at the initial diagnosis (2).

Although a locoregional recurrence may not be an unfavorable independent prognostic factor, the tumor-specific mortality after lymph nodal recurrence is increased in most series, especially in patients over age 45 years (20). The treatment for lymph nodal recurrences includes radioiodine therapy, surgery, and external radiotherapy, depending on the lesion's morpho-functional features and the clinical characteristics of the disease.

The efficacy of the radioiodine therapy is conditioned essentially by size of the lesion, radioiodine uptake and retention, and the absorbed dose by residual or recurrent thyroid tissue. At Memorial Sloan-Kettering Cancer Center, New York, Robbins et al. (21) found that a single dose of radioiodine can abolish subsequent uptake of radioiodine in approximately 65% of patients. However, for macroscopic tumor deposits and for absorbed doses below 3500 cGy, the chances of cure are reduced (22).

The role of adjuvant external beam radiotherapy in lymph nodal recurrences remains controversial, and it is clearly not indicated in patients younger than 45 years with elevated [131]I uptake. However, it can be recommended for patients older than age 45 years with papillary carcinoma and extrathyroidal invasion who fail to demonstrate significant [131]I uptake in the neck (4).

Surgery is the treatment of choice for both iodine avid and non-iodine avid recurrent lymph node metastases >1 cm in diameter, since usually these lesions only have a partial response to [131]I treatment (21).

However, often reoperation is problematic when tumor foci are present in regions of previous surgery or at unusual sites adjacent to vessels or in the mediastinum (8). If possible, neck dissection for locoregional recurrences should be performed in a single session, avoiding subsequent surgical procedures and the consequent higher possibility of surgical complications.

To get around these difficulties, various authors use radioguided surgery with an intraoperative gamma probe following radioiodine administration ([131]I or [123]I) to identify involved nodes at the time of dissection (8,10,11,23,24). Because of the thyroid stimulating hormone (TSH)-dependent iodine uptake (25), a short withdrawal of L-thyroxine therapy or treatment with rhTSH is helpful for preoperative preparation.

## [131]I-Iodide

Since 1988, at the Institut Gustave-Roussy in Villejuif, France, Travagli et al. have designed and advocated a protocol that combines the administration of high doses of [131]I and use of an intraoperative probe to detect and then radically dissect lymph node recurrences in a single session (8). The same protocol with minor modifications was adopted by Lippi et al. (10) and Salvatori et al. (11) for a smaller number of patients with local and regional recurrences of well-differentiated thyroid carcinoma.

Together, the 3 studies evaluated 70 patients; 57 patients had papillary thyroid carcinoma, 2 had minimally invasive follicular cancer, and 6 had widely invasive, poorly differentiated thyroid carcinoma (8,10,11). All patients had total (or near-total) thyroidectomy and often also had dissections of lymph nodes; lymph node metastases were found in about 75% of patients at initial surgery (8,10,11).

The time elapsed from initial surgery to inclusion in the protocol ranged from 5 months to 29 years (mean, 5 years) at the Institut Gustave-Roussy (8), and 14 to 60 months (mean, 28.7 months) in the series of Salvatori et al. (11), respectively.

After initial surgical treatment and before radioguided surgery, all patients from the Institut Gustave-Roussy received a number of [131]I treatments, ranging from 1 to 7, for ablation of thyroid remnants and/or treatment of functioning metastases (8). The main inclusion criterion in the series reported by Salvatori et al. was the presence of persistent or recurrent radioiodine-positive lymph node metastases after at least 2 radioiodine treatments (11). Other criteria were clinical evidence of lymph node metastases, positive neck ultrasound or neck and chest computed tomography (CT) studies, and detectable serum Tg levels (11).

The protocol designed by Travagli et al. (8) takes place over a week, beginning on day 0 when hypothyroid patients receive 3,700 MBq (or 100 mCi, that is, a full therapeutic dose) of [131]I. Hypothyroidism (TSH >30 μIU/mL) is obtained by discontinuing treatment with L-thyroxine (L-T4) and maintaining on triiodothyronine until 2 weeks prior to administration of the radioiodine (Figure 26-1).

On day 4, a highly sensitive presurgery whole-body scan is performed, using a double head gamma camera equipped with a high-energy collimator. The neck spot scan is also performed in each patient, using a rectilinear scanner with a high-energy collimator for precise anatomical localization of each focus of uptake. In spite of its limitations, the rectilinear scanner has the advantage of producing a life-size image of the neck and permitting precise localization of recurrent or residual functioning thyroid disease (Figure 26-2). The whole-body scan provides accurate localization of well-known functional

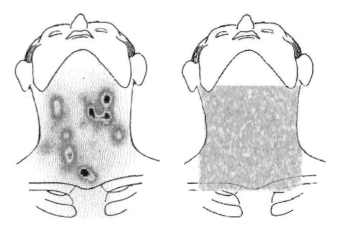

FIGURE 26-2. Preoperative (A) and postoperative (B) scans of the neck (obtained with a rectilinear scanner) in a patient submitted to radioguided surgery after iodine [131]I administration (3.7 GBq) for functioning lymph node metastases. (Salvatori et al. 2003 [11], by permission.)

neoplastic foci and often allows identification of additional tissue that should be removed.

Five days after radioiodine administration and 1 day after scanning, a complete dissection of previously undissected neoplastic areas is performed using an intraoperative handheld gamma detection probe that permits both identification and localization of metastases in unusual sites or embedded in sclerosis. Guided according to the [131]I spot view of the neck obtained during the whole-body scan, the patient's neck is scanned with the probe to localize the cutaneous projection of the radioiodine focal uptake sites. During surgery, the probe is placed in direct contact with any suspect tumor site and also is used to search any other area demonstrating a high lesion-to-background count ratio. Activities in the main vessels (aorta) and in normal soft tissues are used as background values. After nodes are removed, radioactivity is also measured in the lesion bed looking for any residual activity of the tracer to verify the completeness of resection. The protocol is completed after 7 days, when a postoperative neck scan is performed, using the remaining radioactivity to verify the completeness of the surgical resection.

Salvatori et al. only minimally modified this protocol, performing the presurgery whole-body scan 3 days after [131]I administration (instead of 4 days) when the patients were discharged from isolation because the radiation exposure rate was >30 μSv/hr at 1 m (11).

Travagli et al. (8) considered radioguided surgery decisive in 20 of 54 patients, revealing neoplastic foci either inside the postoperative scar (n = 9), at unusual sites behind vessels or in the mediastinum (n = 10), or both (n = 1). The probe facilitated the intraoperative detection

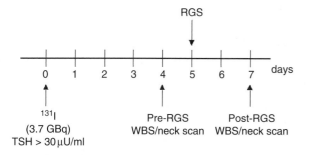

RGS: radioguided surgery with intraoperative gamma probe
WBS: highly sensitive whole body scan

FIGURE 26-1. Design of the protocol for radioguided surgery of lymph node metastases adopted at the Institut Gustave Roussy, Villejuif, France.

of foci of [131]I uptake previously depicted by preoperative whole-body scan in 26 additional patients. The usefulness of the protocol was confirmed by the postoperative whole-body scan, which indicated the completeness of excision in all 46 patients, as [131]I uptake had disappeared. Furthermore, in 22 of the 46 patients, the probe permitted the discovery and excision of 38 metastatic lymph nodes (ranging from 1 to 6 nodes per patient) not seen on the preoperative whole-body scan. These neoplastic nodes were located in the central compartment of the neck (13 patients), the jugulocarotid chain (8 patients), and the internal mammary chain (1 patient) (8).

The radiation doses received by the surgeon's hands and neck during surgery and the contamination of surfaces and surgical tools were measured by thermoluminescent dosimeters and a portable dedicated device, respectively (8). The mean radiation dose received during each surgical procedure was 40 μSv to the left hand, and 13 to 15 μSv to the neck. Therefore, the radiation dose received by the surgeon, and particularly by the surgeon's fingers, in 1 surgical procedure was low and clearly acceptable, equivalent to 3 days of exposure to natural radiation in Western Europe (8).

The apparent complete remission rate observed during the long-term follow-up for the whole series of patients after radioguided surgery was higher (85%) than that reported in previous series in which a traditional surgical procedure or radioiodine treatment alone were performed (40%) (8).

In the study by Lippi et al. (10), the radioactivity detected during radioguided surgery varied considerably among the 6 patients studied and in the same patient among different sites of uptake. Correlation with histology showed that 11 of 13 tissue specimens removed by the surgeon were metastatic. It is worth noting that the 2 samples that proved to be non-neoplastic lymph nodes histologically had the lowest site/background ratio (0.95 and 0.75), while all the metastatic lesions had higher ratios, ranging between 1.4 and 25.8 (10). The post-surgery scan performed 48 hours later showed the disappearance of all areas of [131]I uptake recorded at the presurgery whole-body scan.

In the 10 patients who had radioguided surgery with [131]I by Salvatori et al. (11), the preoperative whole-body scan was positive in all patients, with a total of 33 scintigraphic focal sites of radioiodine uptake (average of 3.3 sites per patient) in the lateral cervical compartments of all patients, in the central compartment of 3 patients, and in the supraclavicular compartments of 2 patients.

The final histologic examination showed the presence of metastases in 78 lymph nodes, with a mean of 7.8 per patient (range 4 to 12); among these, 33 were evident on whole-body scan and gamma probe evaluation, while 41 were identified only by gamma probe and 4 were not seen

either with the whole-body scan or gamma probe evaluation (11).

For most operations, the surgeon found the radioguided surgery procedure decisive (showing tumor foci otherwise undetectable) or favorable (intraoperative detection of tumor foci already shown by preoperative diagnostic methods) in 8 patients, and irrelevant (unimportant contribution to the surgical operation) in 2 patients. Salvatori et al. (11) did not observe a significant lengthening of the normal operative times necessary to perform a radical lymph node dissection, reporting a mean time of 102 minutes (range 60 to 180).

No surgical morbidity was observed, and the dosimetric measurements were confirmed in all cases, with very low levels of exposure to the surgeon's hands (less than 40 μSv) and no radioactive contamination of surfaces or surgical instruments (11).

The published results demonstrate that radioguided surgery with [131]I identifies neoplastic foci with high sensitivity and specificity. The procedure does not lengthen the duration of the operation, and is not associated with significant morbidity (8). The radiation dose received in 1 surgical procedure by the surgeon, and in particular by the surgeon's fingers, is low and clearly acceptable (8,11).

Due to the physical properties of [131]I, the gamma probe shows a suboptimal performance using this radiopharmaceutical. Better performance has been obtained using a gamma probe after injection of [99m]Tc-sestamibi or [123]I (12,13,23,24). Wartofsky observed that it might be preferable to employ [123]I (an isotope that would be associated with less radiation exposure and less potential for stunning) to guide the intraoperative gamma probe (26). In most countries, radioprotection regulations do not permit the use of a large dose of [131]I on an outpatient basis, requiring hospitalization, with the resultant increased costs and patient disadvantages.

Finally, both Travagli et al. (8) and Salvatori et al. (11) reported lymph node metastases that were not revealed by either the whole-body scan or the probe, but were found only at histologic examination of surgical specimens. These false-negative results suggest that a complete node dissection is necessary to remove the greatest number of lymph nodes, irrespective of the counts measured by the gamma probe.

## [123]I-Iodide

Gallowitsh et al. (23) described their findings in a 27-year-old woman who had had a thyroidectomy, [131]I ablation (2,960 MBq), and external beam radiotherapy (50 Gy) in fractionated doses of 2 Gy for invasive papillary thyroid cancer with lymph node metastases in the neck. One year after initial treatment, a reoperation for disease in the neck was performed 4 hours after administration of 74 MBq of iodine [123]I, using a handheld gamma probe designed for the energy peak of [99m]Tc (140 keV, with a 20% window) and a collimator reducing the field of view to 5 mm. Mean count rates were measured over the sternocleidomastoid muscle, the metastasis in-situ and ex-situ, and the tumor bed. The lymph node metastasis was correctly located within the scarred tissue. Complete resection was verified by monitoring the thyroid bed, and histologic examination confirmed the diagnosis of a completely resected nodular metastasis of papillary carcinoma (1.5 × 1.2 × 1.0 cm in diameter).

Gulec et al. (24) performed radioguided surgery after administration of [123]I, using the gamma probe to guide lymph node dissection ("gamma picking") in a 52-year-old man with papillary thyroid cancer scheduled to undergo total thyroidectomy. Eighteen hours before the planned thyroidectomy, the patient was given 37 MBq (1 mCi) of iodine [123]I orally. Operative exploration revealed multiple tumor nodules in both thyroid lobes, but no palpable lymph nodes in the neck. Gamma probe scanning of the thyroid bed and the central and lateral lymph node basins performed after total thyroidectomy revealed 4 distinct foci of increased activity, with counts ten-fold higher than background activity. Histologic examination of the thyroid revealed bilateral, multifocal papillary thyroid cancer, with the largest tumor focus measuring 0.6 cm. Two of 4 hot spots proved to be metastatic tumor in small lymph nodes measuring less than 0.5 cm, while the other 2 showed no nodal tissue (24).

Both studies demonstrate the intraoperative utility of probe-guided surgery with [123]I. Its 13-hour half-life allows optimization of target-to-background ratio with a fairly strong target signal over a period of 12 to 24 hours, permitting flexible operating room scheduling. The gamma energy (159-keV gamma photon) of [123]I is better for use with the probe, and reduces radiation exposure to both the patient and the surgeon.

## Iodine-Negative Thyroid Cancers

Radioiodide ([131]I or [123]I) is the main radiopharmaceutical used in the evaluation and management of suspected recurrent differentiated thyroid cancer. Although radioiodine has high specificity (99% to 100%), only a moderate percentage of recurrences are iodine-avid (50%-60% of papillary and 64%-67% of follicular cancers) (27).

Significant limitations both in diagnostic procedures and radioiodine treatment are present in patients with metastases that have lost the capability of trapping radioiodine (iodine-negative or nonfunctioning metastases). Nonfunctioning metastases can be found at all ages, but their prevalence increases in patients who are elderly or have poorly differentiated or aggressive tumors (4). In these patients, the precise localization of nonfunctioning neck or mediastinal metastases is crucial, because only resection can offer an improvement in the survival rate and the possibility of a complete cure.

Radiologic imaging modalities such as CT and MRI have shown a relatively low sensitivity in detecting locoregional metastases of well-differentiated thyroid carcinoma (28,29). In contrast, high-resolution ultrasonography examination of the neck and some tumor-seeking scintigraphic methods, such as [99m]Tc-sestamibi scan, have proven highly sensitive in revealing cervical and mediastinal well-differentiated thyroid carcinoma recurrences (28–31). These tumor-targeting properties have prompted clinical trials aimed at exploring the potential of radioguided surgery in patients with non-functioning well-differentiated thyroid carcinoma recurrences, as initially proposed by Boz et al. (12). Subsequent reports on a larger scale have confirmed the feasibility and high success rate of radioguided surgery following administration of [99m]Tc-sestamibi in such patients (13,32).

On the other hand, it is now well known that as well-differentiated thyroid carcinoma lesions lose their iodine-trapping capability (thus becoming less amenable to efficient therapy with [131]I), their more aggressive pattern of growth is mirrored by increasing uptake of [[18]F]FDG (9,33–35), the mainstay radiopharmaceutical for clinical positron emission tomography (PET). Similarly as described for other tumors (36–42), this observation has opened an additional route of performing radioguided surgery in patients with nonfunctioning well-differentiated thyroid carcinoma, based on the high tumor-targeting potential of [[18]F]FDG. Although so far this approach has been described in a single case report (43) and in a small series of patients (44), it has good potential, especially for employing dedicated beta-sensitive probes instead of the common gamma probes used with conventional radiopharmaceuticals.

In the case described by Meller et al. (43), radioguided surgery of recurrent metastases from a nonfunctioning oxyphilic follicular thyroid carcinoma was performed both under [99m]Tc-sestamibi guidance (using a conventional intraoperative gamma probe) and, on a separate occasion and using a beta-sensitive prototype to detect high-energy gamma quanta as well as positron emission annihilation quanta, under [[18]F]FDG guidance (220 MBq administered 60 minutes before initiating surgery), following stimulation with exogenous rhTSH. [[18]F]FDG guidance was successful in identifying and localizing for radical excision cervical metastatic lymph nodes, with target-to-background ratios of about 1.5 during in-vivo counting, and about 8 in ex-vivo counting.

In their series of 10 patients undergoing radioguided surgery under [18F]FDG guidance, Kraeber-Bodéré et al. (44) employed a conventional handheld gamma probe (equipped with a bismuth germanite oxide scintillator), initiating surgery 30 minutes after tracer administration (165 to 526 MBq, mean 365 MBq). Exogenous rhTSH stimulation was performed in 6 of the 10 patients, and presurgical localization of the metastatic lesions was achieved by PET/CT fusion images obtained a few days before surgery with a full diagnostic dose of [18F]FDG. Although the gamma probe was helpful in guiding the surgeon to remove metastatic lesions, intraoperative counting did not allow detection of lesions that were not detected in the diagnostic [18F]FDG PET/CT scan. The mean in-vivo target-to-background count ratios evaluated using 2 different sites—the neck and the shoulder—as background were 1.40 (range, 0.76 to 2.59) and 1.73 (range, 1.19 to 2.84), respectively, while the average ex-vivo tumor-to-normal tissue count ratio was 2.4 (range, 1.18 to 7.89). Dose exposure for the surgeon (hands) ranged from 90 to 270 µSv, somewhat higher than the corresponding value reported for radioguided surgery performed after administration of [131]I (8,11).

# Medullary Thyroid Carcinoma

Medullary thyroid cancer has its origin in the parafollicular C cells and represents 5% to 10% of all thyroid malignancies. This neuroendocrine tumor tends to grow slowly and occurs either in a sporadic (80%) or in a familial (20%) form that is associated with other endocrine abnormalities (2).

Many authorities advocate that patients with medullary thyroid carcinoma should be surgically treated in an aggressive fashion with initial total thyroidectomy and standard en-bloc dissection of the central and superior mediastinal lymphatic compartment, regardless of nodal status (45). In addition, selective lymph node dissection might be required if further lymph nodes are thought to be involved (7). The presence of lymph node metastases and the completeness of initial tumor resection are the most important prognostic factors affecting the survival of patients with medullary thyroid carcinoma (46).

For patients with gross or microscopic residual disease, or extensive regional lymph node involvement, adjuvant external beam radiotherapy to the thyroid bed and regional nodal tissue may be used to reduce the local recurrence rate (47). However, local control rate after external beam radiotherapy is as low as 20%; therefore, every attempt should be made to achieve complete resection (47).

During surgery, microscopic and occult disease that cannot be found by inspection and palpation may remain, leading to recurrences and shortened survival for the patient (19). Many radiopharmaceuticals have been employed to visualize recurrent medullary thyroid carcinoma, but none has shown optimal sensitivity for scintigraphic imaging (Table 26-1).

Intraoperative radio-detection of recurrent medullary thyroid carcinoma demonstrated a higher sensitivity than conventional radiological and scintigraphic imaging, and a range of radioguided surgery techniques using different radiopharmaceuticals ([123]I-MIBG, [99m]Tc-V-DMSA [111]In-pentetreotide, [111]In-monoclonal antibodies) has been employed (14–19).

None of these radiopharmaceuticals alone demonstrate sufficient sensitivity. The combined use of different radiopharmaceuticals has been reported to be more sensitive than the use of only 1 tumor-seeking agent (17).

## [111]In-Pentetreotide and [99m]Tc-V-DMSA

Medullary thyroid carcinomas usually express somatostatin receptors (SSTRs), and tumors with a high expression of SSTRs can be localized by [[111]In-DTPA-D-Phe[1]]-pentetreotide ([111]In-pentetreotide) (48). [111]In-pentetreotide has been shown to bind preferentially to SSTR2 and SSTR5 subtypes, with the highest affinity to SSTR2 (41). Medullary thyroid carcinomas visualized by it are usually larger and more aggressive than those that cannot be visualized scintigraphically.

Waddington et al. (49), using radioguided surgery with [111]In-pentetreotide in a 44-year-old male patient, demonstrated the successful localization of recurrent medullary thyroid carcinoma. These lesions showed no uptake with prior [123]I-MIBG and [99m]Tc-V-DMSA scans.

Ahlman (50) and Wangberg et al. (51) reported their experiences in a total of 23 patients with somatostatin receptor-positive neuroendocrine tumors, including 10 patients with residual medullary thyroid carcinomas. All patients had previously undergone total thyroidectomy and had been subjected to 1 to 4 neck dissections for recurrent tumor in lymph nodes. All had elevated calcitonin levels with pentagastrin provocation. As the optimal interval between injection of [111]In-pentetreotide (activity 140 to 300 MBq) and surgery had not yet been established, 5 different time intervals (24, 48, 72, 120, and 168 hours) were explored. The tumor-to-background ratios were not affected by the interval between injection and surgery (24 to 168 hours). Unfortunately, medullary thyroid carcinoma patients often had lymph nodes with microscopic tumor burden and consequently less total [111]In content than the large lymph node metastases of midgut carcinoid tumors, making the smaller lesions difficult to detect in some patients. Subsequent reports by the same group on radioguided surgery using [111]In-pentetreotide in patients with a variety of neuroendocrine tumors (including patients with medullary thyroid carcinoma) have confirmed the feasibility and usefulness of this approach for recurrent/metastatic medullary thyroid carcinoma (52).

In 2001, Adams et al. (19) described 25 patients suspected of having, or at risk of having, recurrent medullary thyroid carcinoma. All patients previously had undergone total thyroidectomy, and 18 had undergone repeated cervical lymph node dissections. These authors used either $^{111}$In-pentetreotide or $^{99m}$Tc-V-DMSA for radioguided surgery, depending on which tumor-seeking agent showed the greatest preoperative tumor uptake. This approach confirmed the high accuracy of radioguided surgery, reporting a lesion-wise 97% sensitivity for radioguided surgery and 65% sensitivity for surgical palpation, while preoperative imaging had sensitivities of 32% for CT, 34% for $^{111}$In-pentetreotide scintigraphy, and 65% for $^{99m}$Tc-V-DMSA scintigraphy. Altogether, among 71 lesions removed on the basis of intraoperative radio-detection, only 3 false-positive results identified as lymphadenitis were reported. Radioguided surgery using $^{99m}$Tc-V-DMSA guidance detected medullary thyroid carcinoma metastases measuring 5 mm or more, whereas the palpation during surgery only localized metastases that measured 1 cm or more (19). Radioguided surgery was able to localize more residual tumoral tissue (>30%) compared to conventional preoperative imaging modality and surgical findings. Using $^{99m}$Tc-V-DMSA, intraoperative lesion-to-background ratios were higher compared with the ratios for $^{111}$In-pentetreotide (median 1200 vs 850 counts per second, respectively) (19).

Benjegard et al. (52) evaluated 5 patients with medullary thyroid carcinoma, 5 patients with papillary thyroid carcinoma, and 5 patients with various other thyroid diseases (Hürthle cell carcinoma, follicular carcinoma, and Hashimoto thyroiditis). Preoperative scintigraphy was performed 1 day after intravenous injection of $^{111}$In-pentetreotide and intraoperative tumor detection 1 to 7 days after injection. The preoperative $^{111}$In-pentetreotide scan showed clear radioactivity uptake in all patients, except for 1 patient who was eventually diagnosed (at histopathologic examination) as bearing a nodular goiter. Altogether, thyroid tumors showed low uptake with preoperative scintigraphy. The intraoperative gamma probe detection yielded correct information in 70% of patients with medullary thyroid carcinoma. The authors concluded that this method has low sensitivity for thyroid cancer (including medullary thyroid carcinoma) and that the better results reported by Adams et al. (19) could be due to the combined use of 2 radiopharmaceuticals at the same time ($^{111}$In-pentetreotide and $^{99m}$Tc-V-DMSA), which seemed to increase the sensitivity significantly as intraoperative radioguidance was based on the agent showing better tumor localization on the preoperative scan.

## Monoclonal Antibodies

Abnormally high serum levels of the carcinoembryonic antigen (CEA) are frequently associated with increased mitotic activity, and this marker has been proposed as a prognostic factor for patients with recurrent medullary thyroid carcinoma (53). In most cases, the surface of the tumor cells expresses high levels of CEA, and labelled monoclonal antibodies or antibody fragments specific for CEA have been used in clinical studies for radioimmunodetection and radioimmunotherapy of recurrent/metastatic medullary thyroid carcinoma (54,55).

De Labriolet-Vaylet et al. performed radioguided surgery in patients with suspected occult metastases from medullary thyroid carcinoma after injection of $^{111}$In-labeled bivalent haptens targeted to cancer cells by means of bispecific monoclonal antibodies (the so-called Affinity Enhancement System) (18). A bispecific antibody was administered to 13 patients with elevated circulating levels of CEA and calcitonin levels at $4 \pm 1$ days before the intravenous injection of $^{111}$In-labeled di-DTPA-TL agent (118–370 MBq). Whole-body scan, planar spot views, and single photon emission computed tomography (SPECT) images were performed at 5 and 24 hours after tracer injection before surgery, being repeated after surgery as well in 3 of the patients. Radioguided surgery was performed $3 \pm 1$ day after tracer injection. The signal was considered positive when the mean radioactivity counts were greater than the normal adjacent tissue counts plus twice the standard deviation of normal tissue counts (i.e., the square root of the counts). Altogether, the results of gamma probe exploration for 208 locations (11 patients) provided 86% accuracy, 75% sensitivity, and 90% specificity. Taking into account only the results concerning lymph nodes greater than 0.5 cm in diameter (n = 45), accuracy was 98%, sensitivity 100%, and specificity 94%. The false-positive signal reported in 13 of 208 locations (6.2%) was attributed to blood vessels or to non-tumor tissue with histiocytosis or fibrous reactions. However, in 3 cases, tissue containing histiocytes-macrophages that stained positive for CEA was detected.

Radioguided surgery allowed detection of small tumors, including those too small to be detected by immunoscintigraphy. The smallest detected metastatic lymph nodes were 0.2 to 0.3 cm in diameter (5 to 15 mg), some only partially infiltrated with tumor cells, and in 6 cases radioguided surgery allowed resection of tumor sites that otherwise would not have been resected. The largest false-negative resected sites were of the same mass as the smallest true-positive lesions, except for 2 samples of 450 and 600 mg of fibroadipose tissue infiltrated with tumor cells and attached to the jugular vein and carotid artery. The authors concluded that Affinity Enhancement System immunoscintigraphy and radioguided surgery allow the resection even of very small, often unanticipated tumors and therefore represent new and powerful tools for the surgical management of patients with recurrent medullary thyroid carcinoma (18).

# References

1. Shaha AP. Management of the neck in thyroid cancer. *Otorhinolaryngol Clin North Am.* 1998;31:823–831.
2. Schlumberger M, Pacini F. *Thyroid Tumors.* Paris: Editions Nucleon; 2003.
3. Hay ID, Bergstrahl EJ, Goellner JR, Ebersold JR, Grant CS. Predicting outcome in papillary thyroid carcinoma: development of a reliable prognostic scoring system in a cohort of 1779 patients treated at one institution during 1940 through 1989. *Surgery.* 1993;114:1050–1058.
4. Mazzaferri EL, Kloos RT. Current approaches to primary therapy for papillary and follicular thyroid cancer. *J Clin Endocrinol Metab.* 2001;86:1447–1463.
5. American Joint Committee on Cancer. Thyroid. In: *AJCC Cancer Staging Handbook.* 6th edition. New York: Springer; 2002:89–98.
6. Kebebew E, Ituarte PHG, Siperstein AE, Duh QY, Clark OH. Medullary thyroid carcinoma. Clinical characteristics, treatment, prognostic factors, and comparison of staging systems. *Cancer.* 2000;88:1139–1148.
7. Tisell LE, Hansson G, Jansson S, Salander H. Reoperation in the treatment of asymptomatic metastasizing medullary thyroid carcinoma. *Surgery.* 1986;99:60–66.
8. Travagli JP, Cailleux AF, Ricard M, et al. Combination of radioiodine ($^{131}$I) and probe-guided surgery for persistent or recurrent thyroid carcinoma. *J Clin Endocrinol Metab.* 1998;83:2675–2860.
9. Wang W, Larson SM, Fazzari M, et al. Prognostic value of [$^{18}$F]fluoro-deoxyglucose positron emission tomographic scanning in patients with thyroid cancer. *J Clin Endocrinol Metab.* 2000;85:1107–1113.
10. Lippi F, Capezzone M, Miccoli P, et al. Use of surgical gamma probe for the detection of lymph node metastases in differentiated thyroid cancer. *Tumori.* 2000;86:367–369.
11. Salvatori M, Rufini V, Reale F, et al. Radio-guided surgery for lymph node recurrences of differentiated thyroid cancer. *World J Surg.* 2003;27:770–775.
12. Boz A, Arici C, Güngör F, et al. Gamma probe-guided resection and scanning with Tc-99m MIBI of a local recurrence of follicular thyroid carcinoma. *Clin Nucl Med.* 2001;26:820–822.
13. Rubello D, Piotto A, Pagetta C, Pelizzo MR, Casara D. $^{99m}$Tc-MIBI radio-guided surgery for recurrent thyroid carcinoma: technical feasibility and procedure, and preliminary clinical results. *Eur J Nucl Med.* 2002;29:1201–1205.
14. Peltier P, Curtet C, Chatal JF, et al. Radioimmunodetection of medullary thyroid cancer using a bispecific anti-CEA/anti-Indium-DTPA antibody and a Indium-111-labeled DTPA dimer. *J Nucl Med.* 1993;34:1267–1273.
15. Adams S, Baum RP, Hertel A, et al. Intraoperative gamma probe detection of neuroendocrine tumors. *J Nucl Med.* 1998;39:1155–1160.
16. Barbet J, Peltier P, Bardet S, et al. Radioimmunodetection of medullary thyroid carcinoma using Indium-111 bivalent hapten and anti-CEA anti-DTPA-Indium bispecific antibody. *J Nucl Med.* 1998;39:1172–1178.
17. Adams S, Baum RP. Intraoperative use of gamma-detecting probes to localize neuroendocrine tumors. *Q J Nucl Med.* 2000;44:59–67.
18. de Labriolet-Vaylet C, Cattan P, Sarfati E, et al. Successful surgical removal of occult metastases of medullary thyroid carcinoma recurrences with the help of immunoscintigraphy and radioimmunoguided surgery. *Clin Cancer Res.* 2000;6:363–371.
19. Adams S, Acker P, Lorenz M, Staib-Sebler E, Hor G. Radioisotope-guided surgery in patients with pheochromocytoma and recurrent medullary thyroid carcinoma. *Cancer.* 2001;92:263–270.
20. Voutilainen PE, Multanen MM, Leppaniemi AK, et al. Prognosis after lymph node recurrence in papillary thyroid carcinoma depends on age. *Thyroid.* 2001;11:953–957.
21. Robbins RJ, Schlumberger MJ. The evolving role of $^{131}$I for the treatment of differentiated thyroid carcinoma. *J Nucl Med.* 2005;46:28S-37S.
22. Maxon HR, Englaro EE, Thomas SR, et al. Radioiodine-131 therapy for well differentiated thyroid cancer. A quantitative radiation dosimetric approach: outcome and validation in 85 patients. *J Nucl Med.* 1992;33:1132–1136.
23. Gallowitsh HJ, Fellinger J, Mikosch P, et al. Gamma probe-guided resection of a lymph node metastasis with I-123 in papillary thyroid carcinoma. *Clin Nucl Med.* 1997;22:591–592.
24. Gulec SA, Eckert M, Woltering EA. Gamma probe-guided node dissection ("gamma picking") in differentiated thyroid carcinoma. *Clin Nucl Med.* 2002;12:859–861.
25. Staub JJ, Althaus BU, Engler H, et al. Spectrum of subclinical and overt hypothyroidism: effect on thyrotropin, prolactin and thyroid reserve, and metabolic impact on peripheral target tissues. *Am J Med.* 1992;92:631–642.
26. Wartofsky L, Sherman SI, Gopal J, et al. Therapeutic controversy. The use of radioactive iodine in patients with papillary and follicular thyroid cancer. *J Clin Endocrinol Metab.* 1998;83:4195–4203.
27. Schluter B, Bohuslavizki KH, Beyer W, Plotkin M, Buchert R, Clausen M. Impact of FDG PET on patients with differentiated thyroid cancer who present with elevated thyroglobulin and negative $^{131}$I scan. *J Nucl Med.* 2001;42:71–76.
28. Elser H, Henze M, Hermann C, Eckert W, Mende U. $^{99m}$Tc-MIBI for recurrent and metastatic differentiated thyroid carcinoma. *Nucklearmedizin.* 1997;37:7–12.
29. Rubello D, Mazzarotto R, Casara D. The role of technetium-99m methoxy-isobutylisonitrile scintigraphy in the planning of therapy and follow-up of patients with differentiated thyroid carcinoma after surgery. *Eur J Nucl Med.* 1999;27:431–440.

30. Yen TC, Lin HD, Lee CH, Chang SL, Yeh SH. The role of technetium-99m sestamibi whole-body scans in diagnosis of metastatic Hürthle cell carcinoma of the thyroid gland after total thyroidectomy: a comparison with iodine-131 and thallium-201. *Eur J Nucl Med.* 1994;21:980–983.

31. Franceschi M, Kusic Z, Franceschi D, Luiniac L, Roncevic S. Thyroglobulin determination, neck ultrasonography and iodine-131 whole body scintigraphy in differentiated thyroid carcinoma. *J Nucl Med.* 1996;37:446–451.

32. Rubello D, Salvatori M, Pelizzo MR, et al. Radio-guided surgery of differentiated thyroid cancer using [131]I or [99m]Tc-Sestamibi. *Nucl Med Commun.* 2006;27:1–4.

33. Wang W, Macapinlac H, Larson SM, et al. [[18]F]-2-Fluoro-2-deoxy-D-glucose positron emission tomography localizes residual thyroid cancer in patients with negative diagnostic [131]I whole-body scans and elevated serum thyroglobulin levels. *J Clin Endocrinol Metab.* 1999;84:2291–2302.

34. Schluter B, Bohuslavizki KH, Beyer W, Plotkin M, Buchert R, Clausen M. Impact of FDG PET on patients with differentiated thyroid cancer who present with elevated thyroglobulin and negative [131]I scan. *J Nucl Med.* 2001;42:71–76.

35. Al-Nahhas A. Dedifferentiated thyroid carcinoma: the imaging role of [18]F-FDG PET and non-iodine radiopharmaceuticals. *Nucl Med Commun.* 2004;25:891–895.

36. Desai DC, Arnold M, Saha S, et al. Correlative whole-body FDG-PET and intraoperative gamma detection of FDG distribution in colorectal cancer. *Clin Positron Imaging.* 2000;3:189–196.

37. Essner R, Hsueh E-C, Haigh P-I, et al. Application of an [18]F-fluorodeoxyglucose-sensitive probe for the intraoperative detection of malignancy. *J Surg Res.* 2001;96:120–126.

38. Zervos EE, Desai DC, De Palatis LR, et al. [18]F-labeled fluorodeoxyglucose positron emission tomography-guided surgery for recurrent colorectal cancer. *J Surg Res.* 2001;97:9–13.

39. Essner R, Daghighian F, Giuliano AE. Advances in FDG PET probes in surgical oncology. *Cancer J.* 2002;8:100–108.

40. Barranger E, Kerrou K, Petegnief Y, David-Montefiore E, Cortez A, Darai E. Laparoscopic resection of occult metastasis using the combination of FDG-positron emission tomography/computed tomography image fusion with intraoperative probe guidance in a woman with recurrent ovarian cancer. *Gynecol Oncol.* 2005;96:241–244.

41. Carrera D, Fernandez A, Estrada J, Martin-Comin J, Gamez C. Detection of occult malignant melanoma by [18]F-FDG PET-CT and gamma probe. *Rev Esp Med Nucl.* 2005;24:410–413.

42. Franc BL, Mari C, Johnson D, Leong SP. The role of a positron- and high-energy gamma photon probe in intra-operative localization of recurrent melanoma. *Clin Nucl Med.* 2005;30:787–791.

43. Meller B, Sahlmann C, Horstmann O, Gerl J, Bahere M, Meller J. Conventional gamma and high-energy probe for radioguided dissection of metastases in a patient with recurrent thyroid carcinoma with [99m]Tc-MIBI and [18]F-FDG. *Nuklearmedizin.* 2005;44:N23-N25.

44. Kraeber-Bodéré F, Cariou B, Curtet C, et al. Feasibility and benefit of fluorine 18-fluoro-2-deoxyglucose-guided surgery in the management of radioiodine-negative differentiated thyroid carcinoma metastases. *Surgery.* 2005;138:1176–1182 (discussion 1182).

45. Robbins KT, Atkinson JLD, Byers RM, Cohen JI, Lavertu P, Pellitteri P. The use and misuse of neck dissection for head and neck cancer. *J Am Coll Surg.* 2001;193:91–102.

46. Gordon PR, Huvos AG, Strong EW. Medullary carcinoma of the thyroid gland. A clinicopathology study of 40 cases. *Cancer.* 1973;31:915–924.

47. Wilson PC, Millar BM, Brierley JD. The management of advanced thyroid cancer. *Clin Oncol.* 2004;16:561–568.

48. Tisell LE, Ahlman H, Wangberg B, et al. Somatostatin receptor scintigraphy in medullary thyroid carcinoma. *Br J Surg.* 1997;84:543–547.

49. Waddington WA, Kettle AG, Heddle RM, Coakley AJ. Intraoperative localization of recurrent medullary carcinoma of the thyroid using indium-111 pentetreotide and a nuclear surgical probe. *Eur J Nucl Med.* 1994;21:363–364.

50. Ahlman H. Radioisotope-guided surgery in patients with neuroendocrine tumors. *Digestion.* 1996;57(suppl 1):88–89.

51. Wangberg B, Forssel-Aronsson E, Tisell LE, Nilsson O, Fjalling M, Ahlman H. Intraoperative detection of somatostatin-receptor positive neuroendocrine tumors using indium-111 labelled DTPA-D-Phe[1]-octreotide. *Br J Cancer.* 1996;73:770–775.

52. Benjegard SA, Forssell-Aronsson E, Wangberg B, Skanberg J, Nilsson O, Ahlman H. Intraoperative tumor detection using [111]In-DTPA-D-Phe[1]-octreotide and a scintillation detector. *Eur J Nucl Med.* 2001;28:1456–1462.

53. Busnardo B, Girelli ME, Simonini N, Nacamulli D, Busetto E. Nonparallel patterns of calcitonin and carcinoembryonic antigen levels in the follow-up of medullary thyroid carcinoma. *Cancer.* 1984;53:278–285.

54. O'Byrne KJ, Hamilton D, Robinson I, Sweeney E, Freyne PJ, Cullen MJ. Imaging of medullary carcinoma of the thyroid using [111]In-labelled anti-CEA monoclonal antibody fragments. *Nucl Med Commun.* 1992;13:142–148.

55. Juweid M, Sharkey R, Behr RM, et al. Radioimmunotherapy of medullary thyroid carcinoma with iodine-131-labeled anti-CEA antibodies. *J Nucl Med.* 1996;37:905–911.

# 27
# Radioguided Bone Lesion Localization

Gianpiero Manca, Giuliano Mariani, and Lary A. Robinson

## Background

Accurate cancer staging is necessary to guide the clinician in selecting the most suitable therapy for each patient in the particular phase of the disease. Staging is especially important when considering surgical treatment, since the presence of metastases may alter the extent of the resection. The presence of bone metastases from a solid tumor classifies the cancer as stage IV (1), which is generally treated with systemic therapy, reserving radiation therapy (either external radiation and/or radiometabolic therapy with bone-seeking agents) as a palliative option for symptomatic lesions.

Although bone scintigraphy (which is widely employed to stage patients with malignant disease) is characterized by high sensitivity, its low specificity causes a relatively high false-positive rate (2–4) for suspected bone metastases, possibly leading to overstaging of some cancer patients. For this reason, suspected osseous metastases should be confirmed with other imaging techniques (5), or preferably with biopsy and histologic confirmation when potential lesions are identified only by scintigraphy.

## Bone Metastases

Although primary bone cancers are rather rare, osseous metastases from other malignancies are frequent, especially in patients over age 45 years. Bone metastases develop in areas with persistent red marrow, and in particular in the axial skeleton, due to the higher local flow of blood (6) than that of fatty (yellow) marrow. A milestone study involving approximately 2000 patients with bone metastases showed that the vertebrae, pelvis and sacrum, femur, ribs, skull, humerus, scapula, and sternum are, in descending frequency, the most common sites of metastatic disease (7). Breast and prostate cancer have the highest frequency of osseous metastases (73% and 68%, respectively), followed by neoplasms of the kidney,

thyroid, lung, esophagus (6%), and gastrointestinal tract (5–11%) (6). When followed over their lifetime, bone metastases occur eventually in 67% of patients with breast cancer, 50% of prostate cancer patients, 25% of lung and kidney cancer patients, and in less than 10% patients with the remaining types of cancer (6).

Patients with metastatic bone disease are often asymptomatic. Frequently, patients with osseous metastases have numerous lesions. As the lesions progress in late-stage disease, bone pain may develop in a few of the metastatic sites. Cancer-induced bone pain consists of "a triad of background pain, spontaneous pain, and movement-induced pain" (8). When bone pain develops, patients frequently have all 3 types of pain.

Histologically, the majority of bone metastases demonstrate both bone destruction and new bone formation. Often, both processes take place, but 1 is dominant. Radiographically, the net amount of residual calcium in the region of the lesion is seen. When bone metastases cause destruction leading to bone lysis, standard radiography may not detect the lesion until at least 50% of the trabecular bone (e.g., in a vertebral body) has been destroyed. Depending on the lesion, bone lesions may appear osteolytic or osteoblastic. An elevated serum alkaline phosphatase level is seen in about one-third of patients with osseous metastases, but this enzyme elevation can also occur in a series of other pathological conditions ranging from hyperparathyroidism to osteomalacia, osteitis deformans, osteogenic sarcoma, rickets, healing fractures, pregnancy, normal growth, and various hepatobiliary diseases (9).

## Bone Scintigraphy

Scintigraphy with $^{99m}$Tc-labeled hydroxy ethylidene diphosphonate (HEDP) or with methylene diphosphonate (medronate, MDP) is the most sensitive indicator of bone metastases, as it shows positive results when the tumor has destroyed as little as 10% of the trabecular bone (6). Therefore, this diagnostic tool is more sensitive than standard x-rays and can show bone metastases very early. Clinical experience and numerous experimental studies have combined to provide an understanding of the mechanisms involved in the uptake of the $^{99m}$Tc-phosphate complexes into the skeleton and the manner in which abnormalities are demonstrated. Although the exact mechanism of tracer accumulation at the site of a osseous metastasis is not completely clear, increased

capillary permeability, increased bone surface area, enhanced formation of new bone, and increased blood flow are the main factors responsible for indirect visualization (as hot spots) of bone metastases on the scan image. Although quite rare, a cold area with diminished uptake of the radiopharmaceutical may be seen at a metastatic lesion, or a doughnut-type pattern of uptake is also possible (Figure 27-1, see Color Plate) (10). Although in principle locally increased blood flow allows

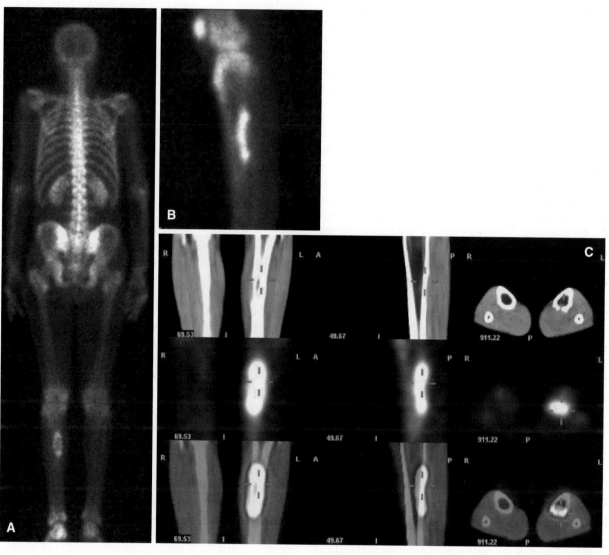

FIGURE 27-1. In a 56-year-old man, an unusual presentation of a single metastatic lesion at the diaphyseal portion of the left tibia from a previously unnoticed breast cancer. The posterior view of the $^{99m}$Tc-labeled methylene diphosphonate whole-body scan (A) shows a quite large area of increased uptake with a doughnut-type pattern (peripheral rim of increased uptake with central area of decreased uptake) that the left lateral spot view (B) demonstrates to be located posteriorly in the diaphyseal portion of the left tibia. There is also alteration in the longitudinal profile of the bone, suggesting possible extension to adjacent soft tissue. A SPECT-CT examination (panel C) better demonstrates the boundaries of the lesion in the 3 standard reconstruction planes (coronal, sagittal, transversal). The CT images (upper row) show important erosion of cortical bone in the posterior aspect of the left tibia and extension of the lesion also to adjacent soft tissue. The fusion images (bottom row) elucidate anatomic correspondence between the structural abnormality and the pattern of abnormal uptake of the bone-seeking radiopharmaceutical. Left, center, and right columns in panel C depict, respectively, the coronal, sagittal, and transverse section planes for the CT (upper row), the SPECT (middle row), and the fusion images (bottom row). (See Color Plate.)

for increased extraction of the tracer, it does not represent the rate-limiting factor, since increased vascularity alone does not account for increased activity in bone lesions.

The extraction process requires movement of tracers from the blood through a series of biological structures and/or compartments including the endothelial cells, extracellular fluid, osteocytes, bone fluid, and finally bone. While the exact mechanism of the extraction process in the bone fluid is unknown, $^{99m}$Tc-labeled phosphates are most likely actively transported into a matrix vesicle as an intact complex. While phosphates are thought to bind to $Ca^{2+}$ ions via one set of oxygen atoms of the phosphate groups, $^{99m}$Tc probably binds to the other set. The complex would then be incorporated within the matrix milieu into the amorphous (noncrystalline) calcium phosphate (ACP) before membrane rupture. As the ACP is formed, the $^{99m}$Tc-labeled phosphates would bind onto the growing crystalline material. An alternative hypothesis postulates that the $^{99m}$Tc-labeled phosphates passively interact with the crystalline hydroxyapatite (HA) material after membrane rupture. These compounds bind primarily to bone mineral, and not to the osteoid component (nor to the actual tumor cells). In addition, $^{99m}$Tc-labeled phosphates preferentially bind to ACP rather than to HA. Although both pathways most likely occur simultaneously, the active nature of transport into vesicles causes more accumulation in ACP.

Despite an exquisitely high sensitivity, bone scintigraphy is not equally specific for the definitive diagnosis of bone metastasis, as many benign bone lesions, including Paget disease, and degenerative changes can cause increased tracer uptake. Therefore, a nonspecific positive bone scintigraphic pattern, especially in the absence of definite abnormal plain bone radiographs (or other more advanced imaging modalities), mandates a biopsy to confirm histologically suspected metastases.

## Bone Identification

Plain radiographs are the initial imaging procedure recommended for patients with bone pain or local swelling. If the plain films are abnormal, computed tomography (CT) or magnetic resonance (MR) imaging of the site might be required for further evaluation of the bone and adjacent tissues. If the lesions appear to be metastatic, bone scintigraphy is indicated to search for additional areas of asymptomatic metastasis. Even for patients with known bone lesions, whole-body bone scintigraphy is useful to identify metastases in weight-bearing bones (such as the femurs), to facilitate early treatment to prevent pathologic fractures.

Histologic confirmation of lesions seen on a bone scan can be obtained with percutaneous needle biopsy. In some cases, open surgical biopsy for histologic evaluation of the lesions is necessary to confirm the etiology. Generally, intraoperative identification of the exact area to biopsy is simple in symptomatic lesions with obvious radiologic evidence of osseous metastasis, especially in those patients who are not muscular or obese. However, performing a bone biopsy in asymptomatic patients with positive bone scintigraphy and a negative standard x-ray can be quite challenging for the surgeon. In these patients, there is a high incidence of false-positive results (reported to range from 47% to 71%) with bone scintigraphy (3,4,11,12). Therefore, performing a biopsy with only the bone scan as a guide can be problematic from a technical point of view, as it is rather difficult to identify the correct site for bone biopsy. On the other hand, using an intraoperative probe can help accurately localize the lesion.

## Techniques for Open Bone Biopsy

### Standard Open Biopsy

From a technical point of view, the ribs are the most accessible bones for biopsy, but exact localization of the lesion can be difficult, especially if the patient is muscular or obese. Furthermore, it may be challenging to correctly define on a bone scan which rib is hot, and to spot the precise location of the lesion along the rib. Therefore, wide excision of grossly normal-appearing tissue of 1 or more ribs is sometimes needed to be sure that the lesion previously observed on the bone scintigraphy is included in the specimen for histologic analysis. Often, it is helpful to specifically mark the lesion while the patient is under the gamma camera. In 1983, Little et al. described a technique they employed to mark preoperatively the target rib to biopsy (13). Following a whole-body bone scan, the potential biopsy sites are identified. When the most accessible site is selected, the patient is again placed on the imaging table with the lesion facing the detector, and a radioactive source is moved slowly over the patient while viewing the persistence screen. When the source is aligned with the lesion seen on the scan, the site of increased uptake is specifically identified. Local anesthesia is administered, and a dose of a colored dye (such as methylene blue) is injected directly into the bone. Immediately following the procedure, the patient is brought to the operating room for open biopsy.

Hybrid imaging equipment, such as single photon emission computed tomography combined with CT (SPECT-CT) is also helpful for guiding the biopsy, especially when the lesion is located close to deeper organs (liver or spleen) in the lower section of the ribcage (Figure 27-2, see Color Plate). Intraoperative frozen

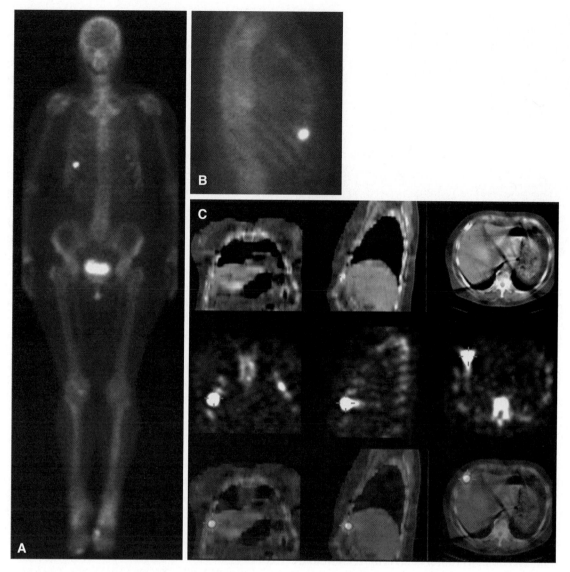

FIGURE 27-2. Markedly increased uptake of $^{99m}$Tc-labeled methylene diphosphonate in the anterior portion of the tenth right rib in a 53-year-old woman, well delineated both in the whole-body scan (A) and in the right lateral spot view of the chest (B). A SPECT-CT examination (C) clearly demonstrates close topographic correlation of the rib lesion with the liver underneath the ribcage, especially in the fusion images (lower section of panel C). Such anatomic relations should be taken into account when planning biopsy of the bone lesion in the rib. Left, center, and right columns in panel C depict, respectively, the coronal, sagittal, and transverse section planes for the CT (upper row), the SPECT (middle row), and fusion images (bottom row). (See Color Plate.)

section histology of bone biopsies is virtually impossible, because decalcification of the specimens is necessary before preparing histologic sections for staining. Therefore, several days must elapse before the surgeon even knows if he has biopsied the correct site. It should be noted that a negative or normal histological report sheds doubt on the accuracy of the biopsy site.

## Gamma Probe Intraoperative Localization

In 1998, Robinson et al. first described the surgical technique of radioguided localization of bone lesions for biopsy (especially for the ribs and sternum) (14). This technique involves preoperative administration of a standard diagnostic dose of a $^{99m}$Tc-labelled bone-imaging agent, with surgery planned for 3 to 4 hours after injection of the tracer. Based on the diagnostic total body bone scan, the region of the lesion is identified. Following anesthesia and preparation of the patient, a small handheld gamma probe in a sterile sleeve on the operative field is used to locate the zone of greatest tracer activity. An incision (about 3 cm) is performed in this area, and, using an intraoperative probe, the site with the highest target-to-background ratio (generally ranging

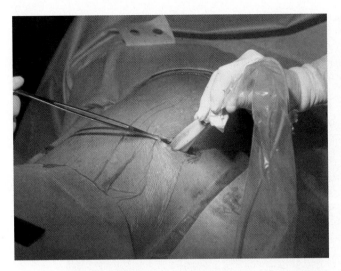

FIGURE 27-3. Intraoperative view of the handheld gamma probe in a sterile sleeve being used by the surgeon to measure counts directly on the left eighth rib laterally. The patient is in the right lateral decubitus position, with the head superiorly to the right in this photograph.

between 2.5 and 10) is identified and resected (Figure 27-3) (15).

This method has been employed in more than 50 patients with cancer who had a positive bone scan with no x-ray-detectable abnormalities (14–16). Only about 30% of these lesions were proven to be bone metastases, with a false-positive rate of bone scintigraphy of approximately 70%. Enchondroma was the most common benign tumor (about 23%) in this clinical experience. This asymptomatic cartilaginous tumor represents more than 13% of all benign osseous tumors and is most commonly located in the small bones of the hands and feet, although it can also affect long thin bones, such as the ribs (17). Besides being generally asymptomatic, enchondroma—especially if small—is also undetectable on standard bone x-ray examination, whereas on the bone scan it appears as a focal area of markedly increased uptake whose diagnostic differential can be problematic in cancer patients. Therefore, a gamma probe-directed biopsy can easily solve this clinical problem.

## Conclusions

The presence of an asymptomatic area of increased uptake on bone scintigraphy in a patient with known or suspected malignancy, but with normal plain bone radiographs, does not necessarily verify the presence of bone metastasis. In this setting, the suspicion of metastatic disease raised by a positive bone scan needs to be confirmed histologically, as the incidence of false-positive bone scan abnormalities is quite high (in the 46% to 71% range).

Locating a bone lesion for open biopsy using only bone scintigraphy as a guide is problematic, while the method of methylene blue tattooing of the target bone (12) is effective but time-consuming and rather cumbersome. As described by Robinson et al. and Thurman et al. the method incorporating an intraoperative handheld gamma probe has been used reliably with excellent results to biopsy rib or sternal lesions suspected as metastases (14–16). Presumably, this technique could also be adapted for radioguided identification of bone abnormalities in the appendicular skeleton. Moreover, this technique could be useful to spot symptomatic and/or radiographically visible osseous lesions in patients whose body structure or the anatomic site of the lesion makes localization difficult. The procedure requires minimal interdepartmental coordination (intravenous injection of a radioisotope 2 to 3 hours before surgery) and is free of serious side effects. Since the handheld gamma probe is commonly found in the operating rooms of most major hospitals (employed for sentinel node biopsies in breast cancer and melanoma), this technique should be readily available to any thoracic surgeon consulted to perform an open rib biopsy. The technique is reliable and offers the advantage of short operative times and easy implementation.

## References

1. Greene FL, Page DL, Fleming ID, et al. *AJCC Cancer Staging Manual*. 6th edition. New York: Springer; 2002.
2. Corcoran RJ, Thrall, JH, Kyle RW, Kaminski RJ, Johnson MC. Solitary abnormalities in bone scans of patients with extraosseous malignancies. *Radiology*. 1976;121:663–667.
3. Harbert JC. The musculoskeletal system. In: Harbert JC, Eckelman WC, Neumann RD, eds. *Nuclear Medicine—Diagnosis and Therapy*. New York: Thieme; 1996:801–863.
4. Van del Wall H, Clarke S. The evaluation of malignancy: metastatic bone disease. In: Ell PJ, Gambhir SS, eds. *Nuclear Medicine in Clinical Diagnosis and Treatment*. 3rd Edition. Edinburgh: Churchill Livingstone; 2004: 641–655.
5. Even-Sapir E. Imaging of malignant bone involvement by morphologic, scintigraphic, and hybrid modalities. *J Nucl Med*. 2005;46:1356–1367.
6. Rogers LF. Secondary malignancies of bone. In: Juhl JH, Crummy AB, eds. *Paul and Juhl's Essentials of Radiologic Imaging*. 6th edition. Philadelphia: JB Lippincott; 1993:164–165.
7. Clain A. Secondary malignant disease of bone. *Br J Cancer*. 1965;19:15–29.
8. Urch C. The pathophysiology of cancer induced bone pain: current understanding. *Palliat Med*. 2004;18:267–274.
9. Henry JB, ed. *Clinical Diagnosis and Management by Laboratory Methods*. 19th edition. Philadelphia: WB Saunders; 1996:277.

10. Wahner HW, Brown ML. Role of bone scanning. In: Sim FH, ed. *Diagnosis and Management of Metastatic Bone Disease*. 1st edition. New York: Raven Press; 1988:5 1–67.

11. Ichinose Y, Hara N, Ohta M, et al. Preoperative examination to detect distant metastasis is not advocated for asymptomatic patients with stages 1 and 2 non-small cell lung cancer. *Chest*. 1989;96:1104–1109.

12. Moores DWO, Line B, Dziuban SW Jr, McKneally MF. Nuclear scan guided rib biopsy. *J Thorac Cardiovasc Surg*. 1990;90:620–621.

13. Little AG, DeMeester TR, Kirchner PT, et al. Guided biopsies of abnormalities on nuclear bone scans: techniques and indications. *J Thorac Cardiovasc Surg*. 1983; 85:396–403.

14. Robinson LA, Preksto D, Muro-Cacho C, Hubbell DS. Intraoperative gamma probe-directed biopsy of asymptomatic suspected bone metastases. *Ann Thorac Surg*. 1998;65:1426–1432.

15. Robinson LA. Radio-guided surgical biopsy for the diagnosis of suspected osseous metastases. *Q J Nucl Med*. 2001;45:38–46.

16. Thurman SA, Robinson LA, Ahmad N, Pow-Sang JM, Lockhart JL, Seigne J. Investigation on the safety and accuracy of intraoperative gamma probe directed biopsy of bone scan detected rib abnormalities in prostatic adenocarcinoma. *J Urol*. 2003;169:1341–1344.

17. Unni KK. Chondroma. In: Unni KK, ed. *Dahlin's Bone Tumors*. 5th edition. Philadelphia: Lippincott-Raven; 1996: 25–45.

# Index

Printed in the United States of America.